# Anxiety, Gut Microbiome, and Nutraceuticals

Healthy gut function is associated with normal central nervous system (CNS) function. Hormones, neurotransmitters, and immunological factors released from the gut are known to send signals to the brain either directly or via autonomic neurons. Recently, studies have emerged focusing on variations in the microbiome and the effect on various CNS disorders, including, but not limited to anxiety, depressive disorders, schizophrenia, and autism. *Anxiety, Gut Microbiome, and Nutraceuticals: Recent Trends and Clinical Evidence* is focused on understanding the role of gut microbiomes on anxiety and how it can be treated using various nutraceuticals. It covers recent trends and clinical evidence in application of nutraceuticals in treating anxiety and related disorders.

**Key Features**

- Explains various factors related to anxiety and anxiety-related disorders including pathophysiological and pharmacological factors
- Discusses the pharmacology behind anxiety and related disorders
- Explores the role of gut microbiota and its relationship with anxiety and related disorders
- Describes different nutraceuticals and classes of nutraceuticals which can be useful to treat anxiety and related disorders

In recent years, there has been an increased interest in nutraceuticals and their applications in treating many diseases and disorders. The market has grown tremendously, and this book focuses on the many clinical studies reporting on the usefulness of nutraceuticals in treating such health conditions.

# Nutraceuticals: Basic Research and Clinical Applications
Series Editor: Yashwant Pathak, PhD

For more information about this series, please visit: https://www.crcpress.com/Nutraceuticals/book-series/CRCNUTBASRES

# Anxiety, Gut Microbiome, and Nutraceuticals

## Recent Trends and Clinical Evidence

Edited by
Yashwant V. Pathak, Sarvadaman Pathak,
and Con Stough

**CRC Press**
Taylor & Francis Group
Boca Raton  London  New York

CRC Press is an imprint of the
Taylor & Francis Group, an **informa** business

First edition published 2024
by CRC Press
6000 Broken Sound Parkway NW, Suite 300, Boca Raton, FL 33487-2742

and by CRC Press
4 Park Square, Milton Park, Abingdon, Oxon, OX14 4RN

*CRC Press is an imprint of Taylor & Francis Group, LLC*

*Library of Congress Cataloging-in-Publication Data*
Names: Pathak, Yashwant V., editor. | Pathak, Sarvadaman, editor. | Stough, Con, editor.
Title: Anxiety, gut microbiome, and nutraceuticals : recent trends and clinical evidence / edited by Yashwant V. Pathak, Sarvadaman Pathak, and Con Stough.
Description: First edition. | Boca Raton, FL : CRC Press, 2024. | Series: Nutraceuticals | Includes bibliographical references and index.
Identifiers: LCCN 2023012749 (print) | LCCN 2023012750 (ebook) | ISBN 9781032367958 (hardback) | ISBN 9781032368009 (paperback) | ISBN 9781003333821 (ebook)
Subjects: LCSH: Anxiety disorders--Diet therapy. | Anxiety--Diet therapy. | Functional foods. | Nutrition--Psychological aspects.
Classification: LCC RC531 .A595 2024 (print) | LCC RC531 (ebook) | DDC 616.85/220654--dc23/eng/20230710
LC record available at https://lccn.loc.gov/2023012749
LC ebook record available at https://lccn.loc.gov/2023012750

ISBN: 9781032367958 (hbk)
ISBN: 9781032368009 (pbk)
ISBN: 9781003333821 (ebk)

DOI: 10.1201/9781003333821

Typeset in Garamond
by Deanta Global Publishing Services, Chennai, India

*Dedicated to all the rishis, sages, shamans, medicine men and women, and people of ancient traditions and cultures who contributed to the development of drugs and nutraceuticals worldwide and kept the science of health alive for the past several millennia.*

# Contents

# Foreword

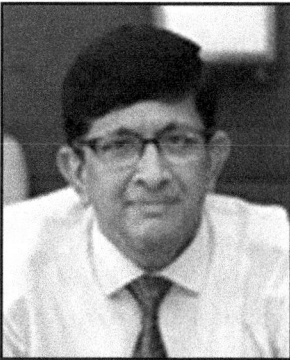

Foreword from the desk of the Vice-Chancellor, Dibrugarh University, Dibrugarh, Assam, India

If you suffer from anxiety, then you are part of the one-fifth of the population who has suffered from anxiety disorders. Recent statistics revealed that anxiety disorders and mental health conditions are almost on the pandemic level around the world.

An anxiety disorder involves excessive, irrational fear and worry beyond what a typical person would experience with everyday stressors.

In the United States adult population, the prevalence of anxiety disorders was 19.1 percent within the past year, meaning that during a 12-month period, 19.1 percent of adults had an anxiety disorder. Lifetime rates are even higher at 31.1 percent, according to the National Institute of Mental Health (NIMH). The NIMH reports that the incidence of anxiety disorders varies by age. Anxiety disorders in adults are seen in 22.3 percent of those aged 18–29 and 22.7 percent of people ages 30–44. The prevalence of anxiety disorders drops to 20.6 percent for individuals ages 45–59. Anxiety in older adults is less common, affecting only 9 percent of people 60 years or older. Anxiety disorders in teens are relatively common. Lifetime prevalence rates of anxiety disorders in adolescents, based on age, are as follows: age 13–14: 31.4 percent, age 15–16: 32.1 percent, and age 17–18: 32.3 percent. Anxiety disorders in women are more common than anxiety disorders in men. In the past year, 23.4 percent of women experienced an anxiety disorder, compared to 14.3 percent of men, according to NIMH (www.therecoveryvillage.com/mental-health/anxiety/anxiety/) disorder statistics.

Some of the common anxiety disorders include generalized anxiety disorders, panic disorders, social anxiety disorders, obsessive-compulsive disorders, phobias, and post-traumatic stress disorders. Most of the Western medicine depends on addictive psychiatric drugs which have demonstrated long-term side effects and people have shown suicidal traits.

Anxiety symptoms are common in mental diseases and a variety of physical disorders, especially in disorders related to stress. More and more basic studies have indicated that gut microbiota can regulate brain function through the gut–brain axis, and dysbiosis of intestinal microbiota is related to anxiety. However, there is no specific evidence to support treatment of anxiety by regulating intestinal microbiota. The trillions of microorganisms located in the gut are called gut microbiota, and they perform important functions in the immune system and metabolism by providing essential inflammatory mediators, nutrients, and vitamins.

More than half of the clinical studies related to gut microbiota and anxiety showed positive results when treating anxiety symptoms by regulation of intestinal microbiota. The BGM (Brain Gut Microbiome) system is made up of neuroendocrine, neural, and immune communication channels which establish a network of bidirectional interactions between the brain, the gut, and its microbiome. Diet not only plays a crucial role in shaping the gut microbiome, but it can modulate structure and function of the brain through these communication channels (Horn, J., Mayer, D.E., Chen, S. et al. "Role of diet and its effects on the gut microbiome in the pathophysiology of mental disorders." *Transl. Psychiatry* **12**, 164 (2022) https://doi.org/10.1038/s41398-022-01922-0).

Several nutraceutical products are available to treat such anxiety disorders such as prebiotics, probiotics, and many herbal preparations. These are found to be very useful to treat anxiety disorders but without any of the side effects of the psychiatric or positronic drugs.

I would like to congratulate the editors of this book, Yashwant V. Pathak PhD, Sarvadaman Pathak, MD, and Con Stough, PhD, who have taken significant effort to bring this volume to market for the consumption of scientists, academicians, and also the common people on the road. This book has 21 chapters contributed by leading scientists working in this area and who also have a passion for promoting nutraceutical and herbal products.

I would like to congratulate the editors and the contributors of the chapters for their excellent work, and I am sure this book contributes a wealth of information to the world of science.

The readers will definitely enjoy reading the book.

With best wishes,

**Prof. Jiten Hazarika**

# Preface

The microbiome is defined as all microorganisms in the human body and their respective genetic material. The microbiota is defined as all microorganisms in a particular location, such as the Gastrointestinal (GI) tract or skin. The microbiota is disturbed due to many reasons including disturbances in nervous systems, use of antibiotics, development of stress, and many other physiological and pharmacological factors.

Healthy gut function is associated with normal central nervous system (CNS) function. Hormones, neurotransmitters, and immunological factors released from the gut are known to send signals to the brain directly or via autonomic neurons.

It was discovered and reported that the impaired stress response in germ-free mice propose the existence of the gut–brain axis. Other studies using germ-free mice not only supported this existence, but also the idea that the gut–brain axis (GBA) extends even beyond these two systems into the endocrine, neural, and immune pathways. Recently, studies have emerged focusing on variations in the microbiome and the effect on various CNS disorders, including, but not limited to, anxiety, depressive disorders, schizophrenia, and autism.

Several reviews on the GBA in the context of anxiety and depressive disorders have been published. Therapeutic interventions to treat dysbiosis, or disturbance in the gut, and mitigate its effects on the GBA are only recently coming to the forefront, as more is known about this unique relationship. The use of probiotics in treatment of anxiety and depression both as standalone therapy and as adjunct to commonly prescribed medications is significantly increasing.

In recent years, there has been an increased interest in nutraceuticals and their applications in treating many diseases and disorders. The market has grown tremendously and there are many clinical studies reporting on the usefulness of nutraceuticals in treating such health conditions.

This book is dedicated to exploring links between anxiety and gut microbiome and how these are interdependent. Applications of nutraceuticals are discussed in detail in many of the book chapters. The relationship between gut microbiome and anxiety is discussed in detail.

The book consists of a total of 21 chapters written by the leading scientists in this field. Chapters 1 to 6 covers nutraceuticals and their applications, various anxiety disorders, symptoms and causes of anxiety, pharmacology of human anxiety, and gut microbiota and mental health.

Chapters 7 to 12 cover stress, depression, diet, and gut microbiota, evidence of applications of nutraceuticals, nutraceuticals as modulators of gut microbiota, and stress disorders and gut microbiota.

Chapters 13 to 21 cover various applications of nutraceuticals in treating anxiety symptoms and their mechanisms. The chapter includes discussion about polyphenolic nutraceuticals and combat of oxidative stress, role of functional foods and nutraceuticals in health, prebiotic and probiotic therapies for anxiety disorders, and several other aspects.

The editors are indebted to all the chapter authors and the lead scientists who have contributed their wisdom to this book in the form of individual chapters. We are sure it will contribute to the wealth of knowledge in this field.

We are extremely thankful to CRC press, Steve Zollo, Ms Laura Piedrahita, and many others, who have been diligently working to make this book faultless. These printing press colleagues are the key players behind the scenes and we wish to express our gratitude to all of them.

Our sincere thanks to our respective families who were witness to the growth of this concept and it finally coming to reality in the form of this book.

If our readers find any faults kindly inform us, we take all responsibility for them and will try to improve in the next edition.

We feel very proud to hand over the hard work of all the authors and editors into the hands of our colleagues and hope they will enjoy the book for sure.

Yashwant V. Pathak

Sarvadaman Pathak

Con Stough

# Editor Biographies

**Sarvadaman Pathak, MD,** went to the University of Houston for undergraduate studies, with a concentration in biochemistry and pre-medicine. Following that he pursued a Doctor of Medicine degree from Avalon University School of Medicine summa cum laude. He was educated partially in Belize, Mexico with all clinical experience in Chicago, Illinois. After graduating from medical school, he focused on research and worked at the University of South Florida. In 2013 he completed a one-year clinical fellowship in Traditional Chinese Medicine, including Chinese herbalism, with a focus on Eastern and Western integrative medicine at the Dalian Medical University in Dalian, Liaoning province in Mainland China. Currently he works for Veterans Affairs and University of South Florida, Internal Medicine, and focuses on cancer research and pediatrics research.

**Yashwant V. Pathak, PhD,** is currently the Associate Dean for Faculty Affairs at the College of Pharmacy, University of South Florida, Tampa. Pathak earned his MS and PhD degrees in pharmaceutical technology from Nagpur University, India, and EMBA and MS degrees in conflict management from Sullivan University, Louisville, Kentucky. With extensive experience in academia and industry, Pathak has over 150 publications, research papers, abstracts, book chapters, and reviews to his credit. He has presented over 180 talks, posters, and lectures worldwide in the field of pharmaceuticals, drug delivery systems, and other related topics. He has received several national and international awards including Fulbright Senior Scholar Fellowship for Indonesia, Endeavour Executive Fellowship from the Australian government, the CNPQ research award from the Brazilian government and also was recognized by USF (University of South Florida) through the Outstanding Faculty Award and Global Engagement Achievement Award.

**Con Stough, PhD,** is Professor of Cognitive Neuroscience and Psychology and Director, Centre for Human Psychopharmacology. He earned his Bachelor of Science (Hons) and his PhD at the University of Adelaide, Australia. Professor Con Stough's research interest lies in understanding human intelligence and cognition. He examines this central question from both psychological and biological perspectives, particularly using pharmacological methods.

A significant part of this research aims towards a better understanding of the cognitive and psychological effects of pharmacologically active substances ranging from illicit drugs to herbal and nutrient medicines. This includes validating new and existing nutritional products that may have a pharmacological profile useful in cognitive enhancement—for example, the bacopa extract CDRI08. More broadly, Professor Stough's research contributes to the development of nutritional products that can improve brain and cognitive function in Australia and overseas. In other research, Professor Stough has been working closely with partner schools from Australia and New Zealand to develop measures of emotional intelligence that can be used as development programs for children of all ages. This school-based research and development coalition is known as Aristotle Emotional Intelligence.

# Contributors

**Abdullah Abdelkawi**
University of South Florida
Tampa, Florida

**Sathya Amarasena**
Memorial University of
    Newfoundland
St John's, Newfoundland and
    Labrador

**Carlos Bellido**
University of South Florida Morsani
    College of Medicine
Tampa, Florida

**Jonathan Charles**
University of South Florida Morsani
    College of Medicine
Tampa, Florida

**Patrick Chan**
University of South Florida Morsani
    College of Medicine
Tampa, Florida

**Aaishwarya B. Deshmukh**
Smt. Kashibai Navale College of
    Pharmacy
Maharashtra, India

**Dan DuBourdieu**
R&D Life Sciences
Menomonie, Wisconsin

**Debopriya Dutta**
Delhi Pharmaceutical Sciences and
    Research University
New Delhi, India

**Emily Evangelista**
University of South Florida Morsani
    College of Medicine
Tampa, Florida

**Erik Feldtmann**
University of South Florida Morsani
    College of Medicine
Tampa, Florida

**Namrata Gautam**
Delhi Pharmaceutical Sciences and
    Research University
New Delhi, India

**Ramesh C. Gupta**
Murray State University
Hopkinsville, Kentucky

**Steven Herd-Bond**
University of South Florida Morsani
    College of Medicine
Tampa, Florida

**Muhamed Hobi**
University of South Florida
Tampa, Florida

**Rena Jiang**
University of South Florida Morsani
    College of Medicine
Tampa, Florida

**Jesna John**
University of South Florida
Tampa, Florida

**Rajiv Lall**
R&D Life Sciences
Menomonie, Wisconsin

**Vivek Patel**
Sun Pharmaceutical Industries Ltd.,
Vadodara, India

**Dhara Patel**
Pioneer Pharmacy Degree College
Vadodara, India

**Jayvadan K. Patel**
Aavis Pharmaceuticals
Hoschton, United States

**Jean-Pierre Perez Martinez**
University of South Florida
Tampa, Florida

**Shyamchand Mayengbam**
Memorial University of
    Newfoundland
St John's, Newfoundland and
    Labrador
University of South Florida
Tampa, Florida

**Philopateer Messeha**
University of South Florida
Tampa, Florida

**Rahul Mhaskar**
University of South Florida Morsani
    College of Medicine
Tampa, Florida

**Monalisa Mishra**
NIT Rourkela
Rourkela, Odisha, India

**Grant Morrison**
University of South Florida Morsani
    College of Medicine
Tampa, Florida

**Jad Mouslle**
University of South Florida
Tampa, Florida

**Nicole Nesto**
University of South Florida Morsani
    College of Medicine
Tampa, Florida

**Ashley Oake**
University of South Florida Morsani
    College of Medicine
Tampa, Florida

and

Lake Erie College of Osteopathic
    Medicine
Bradenton, Florida

**Malcolm Padgett**
University of South Florida
Tampa, Florida

**Rupali Joshi Panse**
Orlando, Florida
University of South Florida
Tampa, Florida

**Komal Parmar**
ROFEL Shri G.M. Bilakhia College
of Pharmacy
Vapi, Gujarat, India

**Jayvadan K. Patel**
Aavis Pharmaceuticals
Hoschton, Georgia

**Sai Patel**
Ganpat University
Mehasana, Gujarat, India

**Sarvadaman Pathak**
Pathak Group Inc.
Lutz, Florida

**Yashwant V. Pathak**
University of South Florida
Tampa, Florida
Adjunct professor, Faculty of
Pharmacy, Airlangga University,
Surabaya, Indonesia

**Addie Pitts**
University of South Florida
Tampa, Florida

**Pier Pointdujour**
University of South Florida Morsani
College of Medicine
Tampa, Florida USA

**Charles Preuss**
University of South Florida Morsani
College of Medicine
Tampa, Florida

**Diban Sabbagh**
University of South Florida
Tampa, Florida

**Shilpi Saxena**
Delhi Pharmaceutical Sciences and
Research University
New Delhi, India

**Sonal Setya**
SGT University
Gurugram, Haryana, India

**Kevin Sneed**
University of South Florida
Tampa, Florida

**Roshni Singh**
Delhi Pharmaceutical Sciences and
Research University
Delhi, India

**Ajay Srivastava**
R&D Life Sciences
Menomonie, Wisconsin

**Sabrina Strelow**
University of South Florida Morsani
College of Medicine
Tampa, Florida

**Jamil Talukder**
R&D Life Sciences
Menomonie, Wisconsin

**Triveni Shelke**
NIT Rourkela
Rourkela, Odisha, India

**Thomas Shen**
University of South Florida Morsani
  College of Medicine
Tampa, Florida

**Sushama Talegaonkar**
Delhi Pharma Sciences and
  Research University
New Delhi, India

**Katherine Tsay**
University of South Florida Morsani
  College of Medicine
Tampa, Florida

**Carrie Wang**
University of South Florida Morsani
  College of Medicine
Tampa, Florida

**Thomas Wotherspoon**
University of South Florida Morsani
  College of Medicine
Tampa, Florida

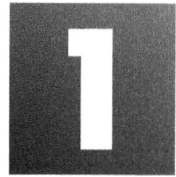

# Nutraceuticals and Their Applications

## Recent Trends and Challenges

Shilpi Saxena, Roshni Singh, Debopriya Dutta, Namrata Gautam, Sonal Setya, and Sushama Talegaonkar

## Contents

DOI: 10.1201/9781003333821-1

## 1.1 Introduction

The word "nutraceutical" is a portmanteau of two words, nutrition and pharmaceutical: "nutra" means *nutrition* and "ceutical" pertains to *therapy for
healing*. This term, in broad, signifies the role of food and related products in
providing several physiological benefits along with protection against acute
as well as chronic diseases, thus, considered as a reliable approach for accomplishing complete wellness [Das et al., 2012]. The idea of nutraceuticals origi-
nated in the year 1989 by *Stephen DeFelice*, the founder and chairman of The
Foundation for Innovation in Medicine (FIM), Cranford, NJ. He explained the
term nutraceutical as "a food or a part of a food, that provides medical or
health benefits including the prevention and treatment of disease" [Nasri et
al., 2014].

"Let food be thy medicine and medicine be thy food," a quote given by the
Greek physician Hippocrates about 2,500 years ago is proving to be the doc-
trine of the current world scenario with nutraceuticals as an alternative option
to combat health ailments to maintain the normal functioning of the body,
thus avoiding complex, expensive, and sometimes unaffordable modern medicine system. Nutraceuticals promise to improve overall health and increase
life expectancy by serving as a potential nutritional and safe face of therapeutics [AlAli et *al.*, 2021].

The routine lifestyle nowadays is such that we are opting for less healthy ways
of living in terms of working and eating. Sitting for hours and working is
proving to have deleterious impacts on our body system. Additionally, regular
consumption of unhealthy and junk food items contribute, leading to several
complications, with deficiency of macro- and micronutrients being one of the
reasons for them. So, nutraceuticals provide a rationale to cover up these deficiencies in easy ways and thus have the following advantages:

• Fulfilment of nutritional deficiencies and combating of various related
  problems
• Perceived by consumers as "food-like" substances
• Promote the use of natural products rather than synthetic consumptions
• Lesser or no side effects when compared to synthetic drugs
• Can be safely consumed for the long term.

Nutraceuticals are derived conjointly from different segments of industries
like food, pharmaceutical, and herbal-based industries [Fig. 1.1] to give us

NUTRACEUTICALS ARE ARISING FROM VARIOUS SEGMENTS LIKE...

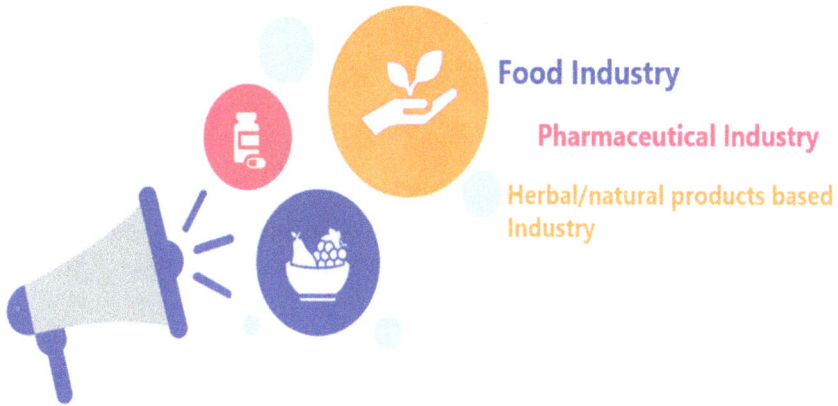

**Figure 1.1** *Arising segments of nutraceuticals in different industries.*

## Nutraceuticals Market Report Scope

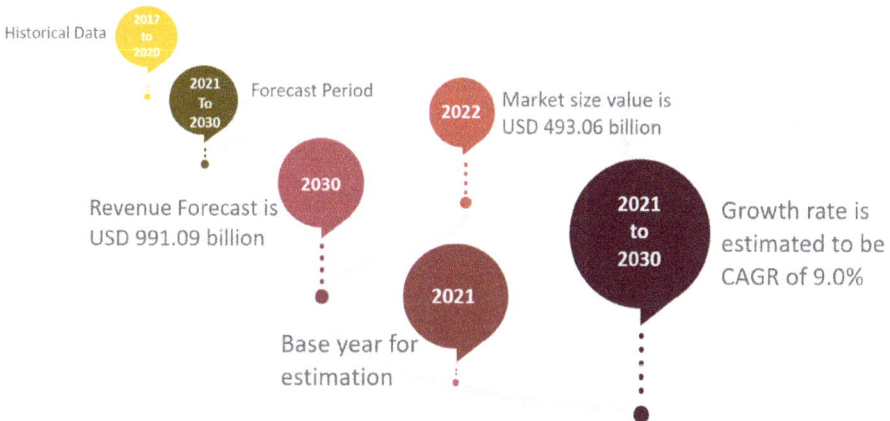

**Figure 1.2** *Nutraceuticals market report and growth rate estimation.*

products of natural origin that showcase therapeutic efficacy assuring several health benefits with no adverse effects.

As metabolic dysfunction is arising among populations across the globe, the need for safer options is prevailing day by day. By having a look into this scenario, a 10-year (2021–2030) forecast has been generated indicating the rate of growth of the nutraceutical market in upcoming years.

The global nutraceutical market was valued at $289.8 billion in the year 2021 and is expected to grow to $438.9 billion by the year 2026, at a compound annual growth rate of 8.7% [BCC Research] [Fig. 1.2]. The ongoing pandemic has further contributed to the rise in the nutraceutical market, due to the possible beneficial effects of these products on the human immune system function [Mordor Intelligence, 2022].

## 1.2 Regulations for Nutraceuticals in India

Nutraceuticals are needed to be regulated in our country due to their rising demands in the market. So, it has become a necessity to maintain the quality and safety of the products to avoid any adverse effects, toxic effects, and misuse of some products, and monitor that their proper dose is being sold by the manufacturer and the seller and consumed by the consumer [Gulati et al., 2021].

In our country, nutraceutical products are regulated by the Food Safety and Standards Authority of India (FSSAI), implemented under the Ministry of Health and Family Welfare, Government of India. This authority furnishes an act that consists of 21 chapters detailing guidelines for the approval of nutraceutical products in the Indian market. Accordingly, the following information is required for any novel food:

1. Chemical composition of engineered food
2. Surface modifications
3. Particle size of constituents
4. Solubility
5. Digestibility
6. Proportion of nanomaterial, if any
7. Specific claims, if any

A 2011 amendment of FSS regulation issued guidelines and regulations for the following segments listed below: [Gulati et al., 2021]

- Registering and licensing of food business
- Packing and labeling
- Standards of food products and additives
- Restrictions on sales
- Prohibited products
- Contaminations
- Toxins
- Adulterants
- Residues
- Sample analysis
- Laboratory techniques

There are six schedules under the food act that list the class of ingredients to be considered for a nutraceutical product. These schedules are stated in Table 1.1 [Gulati et al., 2021].

**Table 1.1** Schedules under the Food Act

| Schedule | Class of Ingredients |
|---|---|
| Schedule I | Minerals & vitamins |
| Schedule II | Essential amino acids & other nutrients |
| Schedule IV | List of botanical ingredients |
| Schedule VI | List of ingredients as nutraceuticals |
| Schedule VII | List of strains for probiotics |
| Schedule VIII | List of prebiotic compounds |

## 1.3 Types of Nutraceuticals

Nutraceuticals can be categorized basically in two ways *traditional* and *nontraditional*. The traditional ones are those obtained in natural ways and include functional foods, dietary fibers, spices, and others (listed in next section) whereas the nontraditional ones are the artificial products that are prepared by adding some bioactive components meant for curing health ailments. This can be stated as described in Figure 1.3 [Das et al., 2012].

### 1.3.1 Dietary Fibers

Dietary fibers, typically plant materials, are also called by the names "bulks" or "roughages" and constitute the undigestible and unabsorbable class of nutraceuticals [AlAli et al., 2021]. These are present in legumes, fruits, vegetables, whole grain cereals, isabgol husk, etc., and provide multiple health benefits from maintaining a healthy weight to treating digestive anomalies [Table 1.2 and 1.3]. These are basically non-starch carbohydrates and include lignin, cellulose, hemicellulose, pectin, dextrin, and many more and can be further classified as *soluble* and *insoluble* dietary fibers:

- **Soluble dietary fibers:** those which can be dissolved in water to obtain a gel-like material and could get fermented in the colon. Examples include fibers like mucilage, pectin, β-glucans, and hemicellulose that are generally present in apples, oats, beans, nuts, citrus fruits, peas, psyllium, barley, carrots, etc.
- **Insoluble dietary fibers:** those which cannot be dissolved in water, form bulk in the intestine, and help in promoting the passage of stool out of the digestive tract. These are unable to get fully fermented in the colon. Examples include lignin, cellulose present in whole wheat flour, wheat bran, and vegetables such as cauliflower, green beans, and potatoes.

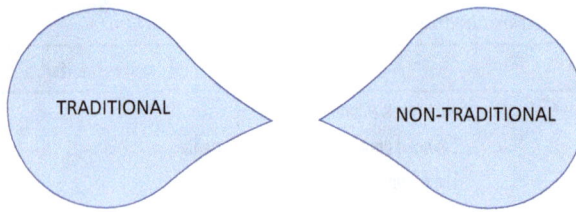

TRADITIONAL

NON-TRADITIONAL

- Dietary fibres
- Probiotics
- Poly-phenols
- Poly-unsaturated fatty acids
- Vitamins
- Prebiotic
- Spices

- Fortified foods
- Recombinants

**Figure 1.3** *Classification of nutraceuticals.*

**Table 1.2** Daily Recommendation of Fiber Intake [Barber et al., 2020]

| Sex | Adults | Aged 51 and Above |
|---|---|---|
| Male | 35–40 grams | 25–30 grams |
| Female | 25–30 grams | 15–20 grams |

**Table 1.3** Some of the Marketed Products in the Form of Dietary Fibers

| Product | Company |
|---|---|
| Crunchy muesli fruit & nut | Lawrence Mills |
| Everyday Fiber | TruNativ |
| Nutralite Fiber | Nutralite |
| Hi Fibre Protein Crackers | Bites of Bliss |

Together, they perform the function of increasing fecal bulk by increasing water retention and promoting the flourishment of beneficial bifidobacteria in the gut [Barber et al., 2020].

The various benefits associated with a high-fiber diet intake are:

1. **Efficient bowel movement:** by absorbing water, these fibers form bulk thus helping to clean the digestive tract and preventing constipation and the risk of developing hemorrhoids.
2. **Lower cholesterol levels:** soluble fibers are found to lower the levels of "bad" cholesterol in the body, thereby maintaining cardiovascular health.

3. **Controlled blood sugar levels:** by reducing the absorption of sugar, fibers regulate the blood sugar levels in diabetics.
4. **Maintenance of a healthy weight:** fibers provide the feeling of fullness in the abdomen, thus restricting unhealthy food intake for longer periods which helps to manage weight efficiently.

## 1.3.2 Probiotics and Prebiotics

### 1.3.2.1 Probiotics

Prebiotics are the live microorganisms like bacteria and yeast that are used in the form of feed supplement to maintain the overall balance in gut microflora and enhance gut functions. These are nontoxic, nonpathogenic, acid-resistant microbes that affect gut nerves and control gut motility. Following are the classes of bacteria that usually serve as probiotics *gram-positive cocci*: *Lactococcus lactis, Streptococcus salivarius, Enterococcus feacium*, etc [Amara & Shibl, 2015].

1. ***Lactobacilli:*** L.casie, L.acidophillus, L.delbrueckii, L.cellobiosus, L.brevis, etc.
2. ***Saccharomyces boulardii:*** a yeast
3. ***Bifidobacteria:*** B.adolescentis, B.infantis, B.bifidun, B.thermophillum, B.longum, etc.

### 1.3.2.2 Pre-biotics

Pre-biotics are generally short-chain polysaccharides that are crucial for promoting healthy growth of *good bacteria* in our lower digestive tract. This results in faster fermentation of food and prevention of constipation and related problems. These remain undigestible in our body and can be found naturally or in added forms in food items known as *fortified foods* (to be discussed later in this chapter) [Davani-Davari et al., 2019]. Prebiotics are obtained naturally from fruits, vegetables, and whole grains like berries, tomatoes, bananas, apples, barley, flaxseeds, garlic, beans, peas, and many more. Structurally they are oligosaccharides having groups like fructose, galactose, raffinose, stachyose, etc., and aid in calcium absorption, relief from irritable bowel syndrome, and enhanced metabolism through gut microflora [Helal et al., 2019] (Fig. 1.4, Table 1.4).

**Table 1.4** Some Prebiotic and Probiotic Products in the Market

| Product | Company |
| --- | --- |
| Nutrifit Probitic Dahi | Mother Dairy |
| Enzyme Miracle | Nusentia |
| Progut 50 Billion CFU | Pure Nutrition |
| Yakult | LcS Probiotics |

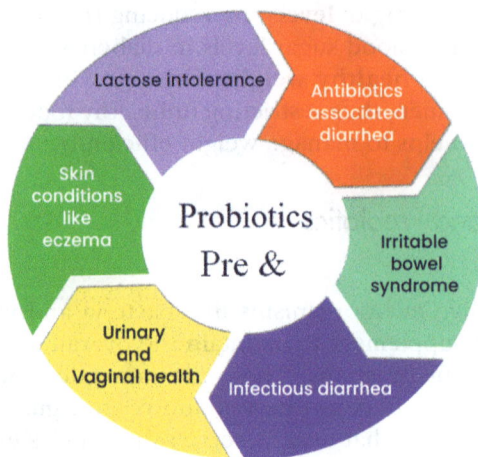

**Figure 1.4** *Various indications of pre and probiotics.*

### 1.3.3 Polyphenols

Polyphenols are secondary metabolites of plants that protect them from reactive oxygen species being formed from photosynthetic stress. This antioxidant property helps to combat many harmful effects of reactive oxygen species in humans as well [Cory et al., 2018] (Fig. 1.5).

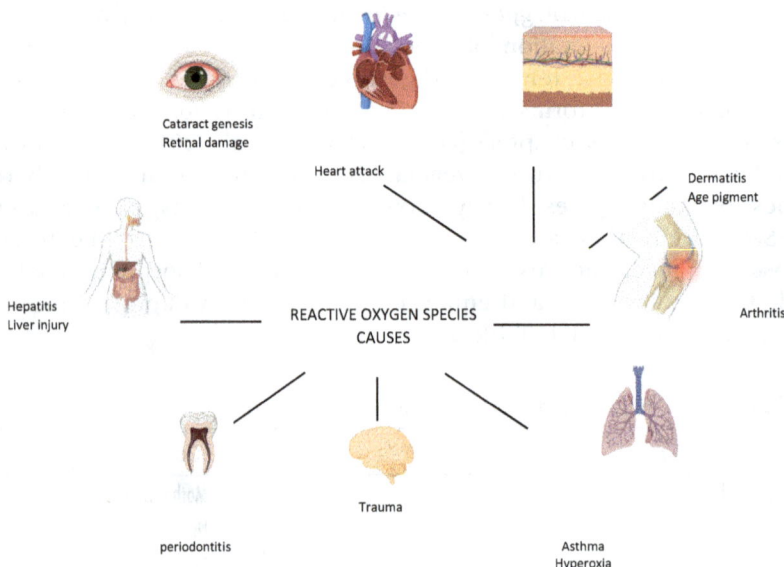

**Figure 1.5** *Antioxidant properties of polyphenols and their effects on several disorders.*

Other than antioxidant properties, these compounds possess anti-inflammatory, cardioprotective, immune-protective, and anti-neurodegenerative properties as well.

Nearly 8,000 polyphenolic compounds have been identified out of which some are immensely important for our body and are present in a variety of food items (see Table 1.5).

There are other daily consumed food items that contain polyphenols in good amounts to exert beneficial health effects.

## 1.3.4 Polyunsaturated Fatty Acids [PUFAs]

PUFAs are the kind of *essential fatty acids* not produced inside our bodies and thus to be taken from outside. These are a salient class of chemical constituents in the form of nutraceuticals as they exert important consequences on a variety of health conditions. The two main types of PUFAs mostly discussed are *omega-3-fatty acids* and *omega-6-fatty acids* [Das et al., 2012; Kapoor et al., 2021].

**Table 1.5** Food and Beverages Having Polyphenolic Contents (Shahidi & Ambigaipalan 2015)

| Food/ Beverage | Polyphenol Present | Physiological Effect | References |
|---|---|---|---|
| Soybean | Genistein and Daidzein | • Controls hormone-dependent breast, prostate, and skin cancer. (Mouse model) | • [Kumar & Goel, 2019] |
| Whole grains like barley, oats, etc. | Lignans and Stillenes | • Antimicrobial, anti-inflammatory, antioxidant | • [Rodriguez-Garcia et al., 2019] |
| Red wine | Reservitol, Catechins, Gallic acid | • Inhibits coronary atherosclerosis<br>• Controls carcinogenesis by inhibiting COX-2 activity<br>• Anti-tumor profile<br>• Anti-tumor profile | • [Das et al., 2012] |
| Tea | Catechins, Quercetins, Myricetins | • Antioxidant and anticancerous profile | • [Das et al., 2012] |
| Hyacinth bean | Kievitone | • Anti-breast cancer | • [Das et al., 2012] |
| Winged bean | Agmatine and Isovitexin | • Antimicrobial | • [Das et al., 2012] |
| Litchi | Flavonoids | • Anti-inflammatory & antioxidant | • [Ullah et al., 2020] |
| Chili pepper | Capsaicinoids | • May relief neuralgia and pain associated with arthritis | • [Saleh et al., 2018] |
| Berries | Ellagic acid | • Anti-inflammatory, anti-oxidant, anti-cancer | [Kang et al., 2016] |

### 1.3.4.1 Omega-3-Fatty Acids

The main subtypes are α-linolenic acid (ALA), eicosapentaenoic acid (EPA), and docosahexaenoic acid (DHA) [Table 1.6].

#### 1.3.4.1.1 α-Linolenic Acid

An essential fatty acid that is present in nuts and seeds generally. It is good for the overall functioning of the body and the nourishment of cells. It also acts as a precursor for the next two fatty acids, i.e, EPA and DHA [Blondeau et al., 2015].

#### 1.3.4.1.2 Eicosapentaenoic Acid

It is commonly obtained from aquatic organisms like fish and algae and is known to exert beneficial effects on blood and cardiovascular functioning. It is a US-FDA-approved drug for lowering the cholesterol levels in the body [Swanson et al., 2012].

*Docosahexaenoic Acid*

It is an essential fatty acid that occurs along with EPA in aquatic foods. It acts well to protect the immune system, cardiovascular system, neuronal functioning, and cognitive functions [Swanson et al., 2012].

**Table 1.6** Subtypes of Omega-3 and Omega-6 Fatty Acids [Cholewski et al., 2018]

| Subtype | Role | Source |
|---|---|---|
| EPA (eicosapentaenoic acid) | • Immunomodulator<br>• Cardioprotective<br>• Neuroprotective | Salmon, seabass, oyster, seaweed and algae, shrimp, sardines |
| DHA (docosahexaenoic acid) | • Immunomodulator<br>• Cardioprotective<br>• Neuroprotective<br>• Improves cognitive functions | Mackerel, shrimp, sardines, salmons, bluefin tuna, herrings |
| ALA (α-linolenic acid) | • Hypoglycaemic<br>• Hypotensive<br>• Anti-atherosclerotic | Soybean, walnuts, canola, flaxseeds, red meat, chia seeds, hemp seeds |
| LA (linoleic acid) | • Cardioprotective<br>• Nourishes brain cells<br>• Nourishes skin cells<br>• Improves reproductive health<br>• Boosts immune functions<br>• Protects bone density | Nuts, vegetable oils, meat, eggs |
| GLA (γ-linolenic acid | • Hypotensive<br>• Anti-allergic<br>• Helps in diabetic neuropathy | Spirulina, primrose, black currant, borage |
| ARA (arachidonic acid) | • Regulates cell membrane fluidity<br>• Regulates important receptor pathways<br>• Important structural component of cell membranes | Chicken, pork, beef, eggs, fish, cheese, cream |

### 1.3.4.2 Omega-6 Fatty Acids

Those mainly discussed are linoleic acid (LA), Υ-linolenic acid (GLA) and arachidonic acid (ARA) [Das et al., 2012; Kapoor et al., 2021] [Table 1.6].

*1.3.4.2.1 Linoleic Acid*   This is found in a variety of vegetable oils in the form of glycerides and plays an important role in conducting regular functioning of the body [Jandacek, 2017; Whelan & Fritsche, 2013].

*1.3.4.2.2 Υ-linolenic Acid*   It is obtained readily from seeds and oils and acts as a precursor for dihomo-Υ-linolenic acid (DGLA) which is further responsible for the production of prostaglandins and thromboxanes in our body that importantly serves as inflammatory markers [Van Hoorn et al., 2008].

*1.3.4.2.3 Arachidonic Acid*   It serves as an important component of phospholipid bilayers in the cells and thus regulates cellular stability and functioning. It is abundantly present in poultry and dairy products [Tallima & Ridi, 2018].

## 1.3.5 Vitamins and Carotenoids

Vitamin C, vitamin E, and carotenoids like β-carotene, lutein, zeaxanthin, etc. altogether comprise this class of nutraceuticals called antioxidants. These are indispensable for the vital functioning of the body since they prevent various degenerative diseases that may arise due to the presence of free radicals in the body. Free radicals are *unstable molecules*. Free radicals are *unstable molecules* that are formed in the body due to internal factors like the breakdown of food to energy or restlessness in the body along with harmful effects of pollution, sunlight, etc. that contribute to the external factors. This results in *oxidative stress* to the body that leads to serious health issues like neuronal disorders such as Parkinson's and Alzheimer's, diseases arising from cellular damage like cancer, and anomalies related to the heart, lungs, skin, joints, eye, etc. [Rutjes et al., 2018].

Vitamins and carotenoids play a crucial role in scavenging these free radicals thus promoting healthy ways of living. These are abundantly present in fruits and vegetables [Tables 1.7 and 1.8].

### 1.3.5.1 Vitamin E

Vitamin E is also known as the beauty vitamin and this group of tocopherols serves the blood, brain, skin, hair, and healthy reproductive system. Food items rich in vitamin E are olive oil, almonds, peanuts, pumpkin, spinach,

**Table 1.7** Recommended Dietary Intake of Vitamin C [Abdullah et al., 2022]

| Age | Male | Female | Pregnancy | Lactation |
|---|---|---|---|---|
| 0–6 months | 40 mg | 40 mg | — | — |
| 7–12 months | 50 mg | 50 mg | — | — |
| 1–3 years | 15 mg | 15 mg | — | — |
| 4– years | 25 mg | 25 mg | — | — |
| 9–13 years | 45 mg | 45 mg | — | — |
| 14–18 years | 75 mg | 65 mg | 80 mg | 115 mg |
| 19+ years | 90 mg | 75 mg | 85 mg | 120 mg |

**Table 1.8** Some of the Marketed Products Containing Vitamins

| Product | Company |
|---|---|
| HK Vitals Vitamin E Capsules | Healthkart |
| Vitamin C Tablets | Pure Nutrition Natural Treasures |
| Daily Immune Support Tablets | Swisse |
| Betatene Natural Mixed Carotenoids Softgels | Swanson |
| Beta-Carotene Capsules | Nimbose Nutrition |

soybean oil, sunflower seeds, and many more. These are known to prevent the peroxidation of PUFA within the biological membranes and quench the singlet oxygen species through the transfer of hydrogen atoms by tocotrienols [Rizvi et al., 2014].

### 1.3.5.2 Vitamin C

Vitamin C, known by another name "ascorbic acid," plays an essential role in promoting a healthy immune system, teeth, skin, blood, and blood vessels, and boosts up collagen synthesis in the body which is crucial for wound healing and skin firmness. It is also well known for its antioxidant property along with the ability to impart better absorption of nonheme iron. Vitamin C is found abundantly in citrus fruits like lemons, oranges, strawberries, grapefruits, kiwis, tomatoes, etc. [Chambial et al., 2013] [Table 1.7].

### 1.3.5.3 Carotenoids

These are the pigments present in plants and photosynthetic bacteria and perform the function of reflecting the bright colors of vegetables and fruits we consume [Johnson, 2002]. These are best known for helping to fight different types of cancer and severe eye disorders caused due to macular degeneration and retinal damage. Rich sources of carotenoids include corn, pumpkin, spinach, avocado, egg yolks, etc. [Black et al., 2020].

## 1.3.6 Fortified foods

Fortified foods are "designer foods" which are prepared by the addition of essential minerals, vitamins, and other micronutrients into normal food products to enhance their nutritional values and the overall benefit they provide to our bodies. The concept of food fortification arose in the USA in the 1940s and is now classified under *nonconventional/nontraditional nutraceuticals* [Helal et al., 2019]. The aim is to cover up nutritional deficiency in children as well as in adults by transforming the usual food products into nutritional inventory in exciting ways without disturbing the normal habits of food intake in the population.

Also, these promise to be safe and provide a high benefit-to-cost ratio. Some examples of fortified foods are given in Figure 1.6 and Table 1.9.

## 1.3.7 Recombinant Nutraceuticals

The substances that are meant for providing nutrition and treating ailments and produced with the help of *genetic modulations* in food items are called "recombinant nutraceuticals." The recombined formulae of food serve as great alternatives to many usual food items that a certain group of people could not afford due to unacceptable nutritional qualities. For example, cow-milk allergy was identified in many infants and adults because of the presence of β-lactoglobulin. Thus, to resolve this problem, Orcajo et al. produced

**Table 1.9** Marketed Products in Fortified Foods

| Products | Company |
|---|---|
| Kellogg's Real Almond Honey Cornflakes | Kellogg's |
| Gritzo Super Milk | Healthkart |
| Immuneiveda Golden Turmeric Milk Mix | Saffola |
| Maggie | Nestlé |

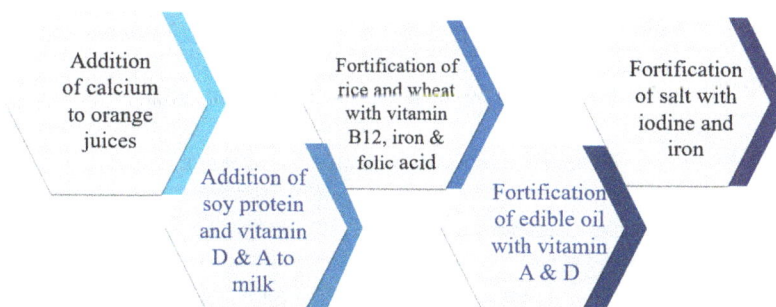

*Figure 1.6* *Examples of fortified foods.*

beta-lactoglobulin-free cow milk using recombinant technology that led to more easily digestible milk. Another example is the production of *gold kiwifruit* which possesses higher levels of ascorbic acid, lutein, carotenoids, and zeaxanthins [AlAli et al., 2021].

## 1.3.8 Spices

Our country India is the largest producer, consumer, and exporter of spices globally because they are responsible for immense flavoring, seasoning, and aromatizing of dishes. Apart from that, they have great potential as a nutraceutical to improve the overall health of individuals [Srinivasan, 2005]. The various constituents present in spices possess qualities that have good physiological impacts on us. Some of these can be stated as follows [Table 1.10] [Shylaja et al., 2007]:

**Table 1.10** Spices with Their Beneficial Effects [Dubey 2017].

| Spices | Biological Source | Physiological Effects |
|---|---|---|
| Asafoetida | Oleo-gum-resin obtained from rhizomes and roots of *Ferula asafoetida* (Family — Umbelliferae) | Carminative, Digestive stimulant |
| Ajowan | Dried ripe fruits of *Trachyspermum ammi* (Family — Umbelliferae) | Carminative, Digestive stimulant |
| Coriander | Dried ripe fruits of *Coriandrum sativum* (Family — Umbelliferae) | Anti-dyspeptic, Digestive stimulant |
| Cumin | Cumin seeds are obtained from the herb *Cuminum cyminum* (Family — Apiaceae) | Antispasmodic, Carminative, Hypoglycaemic, Digestive stimulant |
| Fennel | Dried ripe fruits of *Foeniculum vulgare* (Family — Umbelliferae) | Carminative, Digestive stimulant |
| Fenugreek | Dried seeds of *Trigonella foennum* graecum (Family — Fabaceae) | Antidiabetic, Diuretic, Emmenagogue, Emollient, Hypoglycaemic, Hypotensive |
| Garlic | Ripe bulbs of *Allium sativum* (Family — Liliaceae) | Anti-dyspeptic, Antiflatulent, Antimicrobial, Antimutagenic, Hypoglycaemic, Rubefacient |
| Ginger | Rhizomes of *Zingiber officinale* (Family — Zingiberaceae) | Antitussive, Digestive stimulant, Sialagogue |
| Mint | Fresh or dried leaves of *Mentha piperita* Linn. (Family — Labiatae) | Antispasmodic, Digestive stimulant, Carminative |
| Mustard | Seeds of Brassica nigra or *Brassica juncea* (Family — Cruceferae) | Antidiabetic, Anti-psoriatic, Antimutagenic |
| Onion | Bulb of *Allium cepa* (Family — Amaryllidaceae) | Digestive stimulant, Diuretic, Emmenagogue, Expectorant |
| Pepper | Dried unripe fruits of *Piper nigrum* (Family — Piperaceae) | Antipyretic, dissolves gallstones, Rubefacient |
| Red pepper | Ripe fruits of plant *Capsicum Britannica* | Anti-inflammatory, Antipyretic, Rubefacient |
| Turmeric | Dried rhizomes of Curcuma longa (Family — Zingiberaceae) | Anti-inflammatory, Antimicrobial, Antioxidant, Antimutagenic, Diuretic, Laxative, Jaundice |

## 1.4 Applications of Nutraceuticals in Improving Human Health

Humans have always been curious about their health and improving it in every way possible. People are more leaning towards using medications derived from herbal origin rather than synthetic medicines or any other preparations which have multiple side effects. They want cures and prevention of diseases by using dietary supplements and nutraceutical-based products which can give the same effects without causing as many adverse effects. A major role of nutraceuticals in human health is in the prevention and cure of several diseases [Fig. 1.7 and Table 1.11] [Bergamin et al., 2019; Gupta et al., 2015].

### 1.4.1 Nutraceutical for Allergic Disorders

Berberine which is extracted from Oregon grape, barberry, goldenseal, coptis, and tree turmeric, by activating Activated protein kinase (AMPK), inhibits mast cell degranulation. AMPK suppresses SYK (spleen tyrosine kinase) which plays a major role in promoting mast cell degranulation [McCarty et al., 2021] [Zhang et al., 2020]. Lipoic acid and sulforaphane extracted from broccoli are phase-2 inducers which inhibits mast cell Nicotinamide adenine dinucleotide phosphate (NADPH) oxidase activity. Melatonin promotes phase-2 induction acting on Nrf2 expression and increasing it, also can boost AMPK activity by inducing Sirt1 and inhibiting the NF-kappa β-mediated phase of mast cell activation [McCarty et al., 2021]. Paeoniflorin, extracted from peony flowers, is a bioactive component and is a mast stabilizer. Phycocyanobilin (PCB), found in cyanobacteria, is a light-absorbing chromophore and has an inhibitory effect on NADPH oxidase, which ultimately reduces histamine release and lowers the symptoms of allergic rhinitis. Biotin is also effective in stabilizing mast cells and lowering symptoms of allergy. Supplemental N-acetylcysteine (NAC) and taurine have been found to induce cystathionine γ-lyase (CSE) and cystathionine βsynthase (CBS) [Mc Carty et al., 2021]. Benifuuki tea has been shown to have clinical efficacy in seasonal allergies.

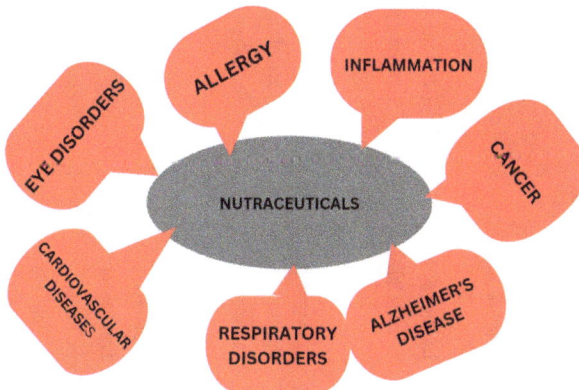

*Figure 1.7* *Applications of nutraceuticals in human health.*

**Table 1.11** Some Marketed Products with Their Active Ingredients, Manufacturers, and Indications

| Sr. No. | Product Name | Ingredients/Active Constituents | Manufacturer | Indication |
|---|---|---|---|---|
| 1. | Gingever | Ginger extract | Omni active | Immune health<br>Gastrointestinal health |
| | Curcuwin ultra | Curcumin | | Bone, joint, and muscle heath<br>Immune health<br>Heart health |
| | Metavive | Salacia extract | | Blood glucose management<br>Weight management |
| | Lutemax skin Glo | Lutein and zeaxanthin | | Skin, hair, and nails health |
| | Lutemax 2020 | Lutein and zeaxanthin | | Eye disorders and vision performance<br>Sleep health<br>Mental health<br>Mood support |
| | Omnixan | Zeaxanthin | | Eye health |
| | Capsimax | Red chili pepper extract | | Weight management<br>Sports nutrition |
| 2. | PeptiStrong<br>PeptiForce<br>PeptiTension | | Nurita's | Muscle health<br>Maintaining glucose level<br>Muscle health |
| 3. | Tru niagen | Nicotinamide riboside chloride | Chromadex | Vital resource of cellular energy and repair |
| 4. | Amifull forte capsules | Vitamins and calcium | Bionova life sciences | Bone health |
| | Elvin-o soft gel | Wheat germ oil<br>Omega-3 fatty acid<br>Vitamin E | | Immune health<br>Anti-inflammatory<br>Antioxidant |
| | Glutagut powder | L-glutamine | | Weight loss |
| 5. | Nutrisyd | | Sydler | Stress and anxiety |

| Sr. No. | Product Name | Ingredients/Active Constituents | Manufacturer | Indication |
|---|---|---|---|---|
| 6. | Megatein smoothie | Algal biomass plus fruits and vegetables protein | Zivo bioscience | Source of protein and vitamin |
| 7. | Zarbees cough syrup | Grade A dark honey<br>Ivy leaves<br>Elderberry | Zarbees | Cough and mucus clearance<br>Immunity booster |
| | Zarbees elderberry immune support gummies | Elderberry extract with burst of vitamins and antioxidants | | Immunity booster |
| | Zarbees sleep with melatonin | Dark honey<br>melatonin | | Promote restful sleep |
| 8. | Coenzyme Q10 liquid bulk | Coenzyme Q10 Liquid oil of USP grade | Agati healthcare pvt ltd. | Heart failure<br>Congestive heart failure (CHF)<br>Chest pain<br>Angina pectoris<br>High blood pressure. |
| | Apro adult powder | Natural cow colostrum with added vitamins and minerals 350 mg | | Diarrhoea, Alzheimer's disease, acne, and anaemia due to Folate deficiency. |
| | Panag Ig capsules | | | Nutrition |
| 9. | Femargin sachet | l-Arginine<br>Docosahexaenoic acid<br>Vitamins | Lactonova nutripharm | Placental blood flow and foetal development |
| | Carnicare | L-carnitine<br>L-tartrate | | Increases heart muscle viability, prevents the risk of arteriosclerosis, and improves cardiac function |

*(Continued)*

**Table 1.11 (Continued)** Some Marketed Products with Their Active Ingredients, Manufacturers, and Indications

| Sr. No. | Product Name | Ingredients/Active Constituents | Manufacturer | Indication |
|---------|-------------|--------------------------------|--------------|------------|
| | Lactomega | Omega-3 fatty acids (Docosahexaenoic acid) EPA (Eicosapentaenoic acid) | | Reduces LDL (Low density lipoprotein) Increases HDL (High density lipoprotein) |
| | Maxvision | Zeaxanthin Luteine Anthrocyanins Lycopene Ginkgo biloba extract Vitamin B₁₂ Citrus bioflavonoids | | Age-related macular degeneration (ADMR) Cataract Dry eye syndrome |
| 10. | Probiotic+ Isabgol husk | Probiotics Isabgol husk | United laboratories ltd | Digestive supplements/appetizer |
| | L- Arginine- 3 G | L-Arginine | | Cardiac health |
| | Bioactive Collagen Peptide Sachet | Collagen+ nettle leaf+ biotin+ green tea+ green apple+ MSM+ Ginkgo biloba+ Vitamins and minerals | | Dermatology |
| | Berberine, Purslane, Gymneva Sylvestre, and Banaba leaf extract Tablets | Berberine+ Purslane+ Gymneva Sylvestre+ banaba leaf extracts+ Vitamins and minerals | | Antidiabetic Orthopaedics |
| 11. | Crunchy muesli — Fruit and Nut | High in fibre and protein 85% fruit and nuts | Lawrence mills | Sources of protein and fibre Gastrointestinal health |
| 12. | Kellogg's Corn flakes | Roasted corn flakes | Kellogg's | Energy rich food Helps in weight loss |

## 1.4.2 Nutraceuticals in Alzheimer's Disease

Several studies show that oxidative stress may be the reason for neurological disorders like AD (Alzheimer's disease). Antioxidants taken as dietary supplements have been found to decrease AD in most patients. Nutraceutical antioxidants such as lutein, curcumin, lycopene, β carotene, and turmerine have beneficial effects on particular disorders by lowering oxidative stress. Several currently written documents show the therapeutic effects of various nutraceutical plants such as *Zizyphus jujube* and *Lavandula officinalis* for the prevention and management of AD and memory loss. Vitamin E and C in combination reduce the risk of AD. Phosphatidyl serine can be used for a significant improvement in dementia and age-related cognitive decline and AD. It has received FDA approval for early-age dementia and memory decline [Das et al., 2012].

Alpha-lipoic acid (ALA) improves blood circulation in the brain and is a powerful antioxidant. Dietary omega-3 fatty acids show a significant effect in improving the functions of the brain. People who eat fish are 60% at less risk than those who rarely eat fish or never eat fish. Flavonoids are present in most fruits, vegetables, and natural drinks (tea, cocoa, and wine). They have antioxidant properties and induce changes in cerebral blood flow. Isoflavones (Soy-Genistein, Daidzein, Glycitin) from soybean improve memory.

Berries, such as blueberry, cranberry, bilberry, elderberry, strawberry, and raspberry seeds, are sources of natural anthocyanin [Calfio et al 2020]. They have neuroprotectant action. B vitamins, Folate, Cobalamin, and Pyridoxin, improve brain functions by repairing damaged cells and preventing AD [Fig. 1.8] [Das et al., 2012].

## 1.4.3 Nutraceuticals in Cardiovascular Diseases

List of nutraceuticals that improves heart health:

- Sterols/stanols
- Polyphenols
- Spirulina
- Resveratrol
- Catechins

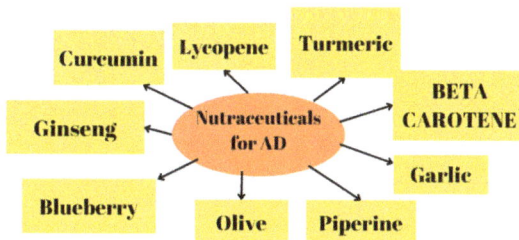

**Figure 1.8** *Some examples of nutraceuticals used in Alzheimer's disease.*

Nutraceuticals like vitamins, antioxidants, minerals, self-restraint from snack fiber, and n-53 polyunsaturated fatty acids (n-3 PUFA) are recommended for the management of Cardiovascular diseases (CVD). Exercise will help to fasten the process. The polyphenols change instinctive assimilation and signaling trusted to lower arterial blockage. Flavonoids present in various fruits and vegetables and in beverages like tea, coffee, etc. are said to prevent cardiovascular diseases [Sosnowska et al., 2017]. Anthocyanins, tetrahydro β carbolines, tannins, stilbenes, serotonin, indoleamine, and melatonin from foodstuffs have health benefits.

Hesperidin is used for the situation of arterial blockage and hemorrhoids. Hesperidin is a flavanone glycoside obtained from citrus fruits (family Rutaceae), various unripe, sweet and sour oranges, Citrus sinensis, Citrus mitis, Citrus aurantium, and Citrus unshiu, lemons, grapefruits, and clementine. The orange and lemon peel has a higher concentration of hesperidin. Flavonoids, mostly present in the pulp of oranges and in constantly used foodstuffs, weakens the risk of heart failure, mostly in elderly people.

Ginger has shown effects on CVD. Ginger has potent anti-inflammatory and antioxidant actions and has a curative effect on hypertension and palpitation [Alissa & Ferns, 2012; Sosnowska et al., 2017].

Buckwheat proteins help in reducing blood cholesterol level and show an effect in reducing hypertension. N-3 fatty acids obtained from fish show an effect on plasma lipids and CVD, such as arrhythmias. Octacosanol from grains and different plants lowers lipids and has fewer side effects [Fig. 1.9] [Donato et al., 2021].

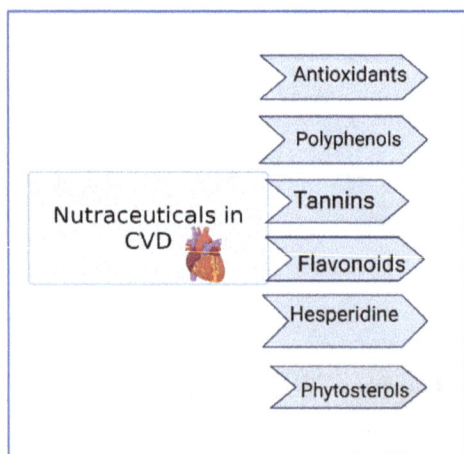

*Figure 1.9* *Nutraceuticals in CVD. Created with BioRender.com.*

## 1.4.4 Nutraceuticals in Cancer

Carotenoids, a group of phytochemicals, are the cause of various colors of food. They have antioxidant activity and thus help in preventing cancer [Das et al., 2012]. Lycopene-held legumes and fruits decrease oxidative stress and damage to DNA and prevent malignancies. They are mostly obtained from a variety of fruits and vegetables like tomatoes, guava, pink grapefruit, papaya, and watermelon.

Ginseng possesses anti-inflammatory properties and hence marks as a key performer in reducing inflammation-induced cancer.

Phytoestrogens inhibit prostate and breast cancers. Soybean appears to offer protection against breast cancer, uterine cancer, pleural cancer, prostate cancer, and colorectal cancer.

β carotene, found in colorful vegetables and fruits like tomatoes, oranges, sweet potatoes, muskmelons, carrots, and those lettuces, oranges, alfalfa, spinach, cantaloupes, broccoli, and winter squash, has anticancer activity [Roudebush et al., 2004].

Garlic containing sulphur compound has been reported as an immunity booster, reduces atherogenesis and platelet cohesion, and prevents cancer.

Broccoli containing sulforaphane (SFN) is a potent phase-2 enzyme inducer. It produces D-gluconolactone, which prevents breast cancer. It is also an antioxidant and stimulus of organic detoxifying enzymes. SFN reduces the risk of prostate cancer. Curcumin has anti-inflammatory, anticarcinogenic and antioxidant activity. It has been stated that it weakens the risk of prostate cancer [Xu et al., 2012].

Saponins are stated to show anti-tumor activities and antimutagenic effects and help to manage cancer.

Ellagic acid found in walnuts, cranberries, strawberries, raspberries, pecans, and pomegranate acts as an anticancer agent [Zhang et al., 2020].

Soluble fiber, pectin found in apples, has proved to prevent cancer metastasis. Phenolic compounds and their derivatives, curcumin, gallic acids, ferulic acid, and caffeic acid carry the anticancer activity [Roudebush et al., 2004]. Broccoli containing sulforaphane is a potent phase-2 enzyme inducer. It produces D gluconolactone, which prevents breast cancer. It is also an antioxidant and stimulus of organic detoxifying enzymes [Zhang et al., 2020].

Curcumin has anti-inflammatory, anticarcinogenic and antioxidant activity [Fig. 1.10].

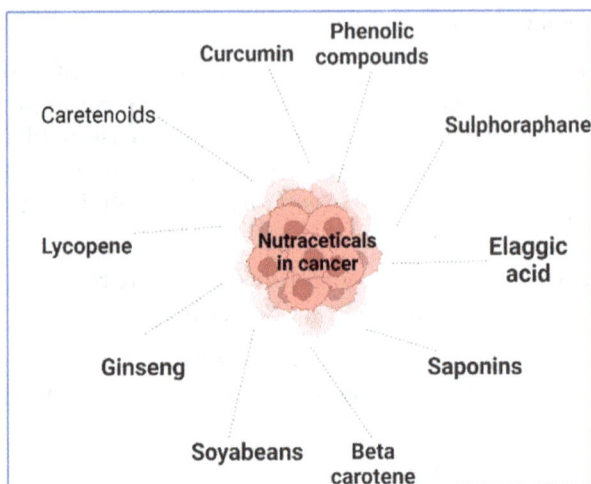

*Figure 1.10* *Nutraceuticals used in cancer treatment. Created with BioRender.com.*

## 1.4.5 Nutraceuticals in Diabetes

Isoflavones, found in soybeans, chickpeas, peanuts, and other fruits and nuts, are phytoestrogens that have fundamental resemblances to human estrogen. Consuming soy isoflavones lowers the rate of type 2 diabetes, myocardial infarction, cancers, and osteoporosis [Das et al., 2012]. Lipoic acid is an antioxidant that is used for the management of diabetic neuropathy. It also appears beneficial when taken as a dietary supplement for the management and prevention of diabetes. Dietary fibers from psyllium have been widely used as dietary supplements, main ingredients in foods, and processed foods to encourage weight loss, for monitoring glucose levels in diabetic patients, and lower lipid levels in hyperlipidemia. Lots of plants such as Teucrium polium, bitter melon, and cinnamon extract have proven their use in the treatment of diabetes [Bertuccioli et al., 2021]. Omega-3 fatty acids have been reported to decrease glucose tolerance in patients with diabetes. Berberine, a compound derived from certain medicinal herbs like Oregon grape, barberry, goldenseal, coptis, and tree turmeric, is currently widely used both for glycemic control in type 2 diabetes and as a hypolipidemic agent. [Hannon et al., 2020]

## 1.4.6 Nutraceuticals in Eye Disorders

Higher concentrations of polyphenolic flavonoids in nutraceuticals, herbaceous extracts, like green tea, *Allium* spp., vitamins C and E, coenzyme Q10, and carotenoids (lycopene and β carotene) retain antioxidant properties and are persuasive in age-associated macular deterioration (AMD) [Mares, J. 2016]. Astaxanthin, a potent antioxidant, is a carotenoid mainly found in the marine world, its main sources are sea bream, salmon, shrimps, and trout. Lutein is a carotenoid, present in several herbs and fruits, such as sweet vegetables, carrots, squash, mangoes, grain, tomatoes, and leafy vegetables. Zeaxanthin is present in egg yolks, corn, green vegetables, peas, broccoli, kiwi, collard greens, spinach, cabbage, lettuce, sprouts, kale, and honeydew. Lutein and zeaxanthin are widely used in supplements for the management of visual disorders [Mares, 2016].

## 1.4.7 Nutraceuticals in the Immune System

Nutraceuticals can be used as immune boosters and they are beneficial for immune functions. Extracts from the cone flowers or herbs of *Echinacea angustifolia*, *Echinacea pillida*, and *Echinacea purpurea* help in boosting immunity [Das et al., 2012]. Phytoestrogens are used mostly for the management of different hormone-associated disorders. Soy isoflavones can also be used as potential alternatives to the artificial estrogen receptor modulator and are presently used for hormonal replacement therapy. Nutraceuticals, morphine, and garlic are suppressors as well as stimulators of the immune system. Probiotics show effects in improving infectious diarrhoea (in infants) and contaminations induced by recurrent clostridium. Functional foods having probiotics (live microorganisms) modulate the functions of dendritic cells, macrophages, and T and B lymphocytes. They also activate toll-like receptors and activate innate immunity. They alter the intestinal microflora to maintain a favorable environment by balancing pathogenic and nonpathogenic bacteria [Basak & Gokhale, 2022].

## 1.4.8 Nutraceuticals in Inflammation

Nutraceuticals, soybean, ginger, glucosamine, chondroitin, and S-adenosylmethionine are effective in managing osteoarthritis. Cat's claw is an effective anti-inflammatory agent. Scientists have ascribed the effectiveness of cat's claw plant and the compounds called oxindole alkaloids are trusted to have anti-inflammatory actions [Das et al., 2012]. Sirtuins are chemical compounds that prevent cyclooxygenase catalyst and can increase the life span of yeast and fruit flies. They possess anti-inflammatory and antifungal properties. [Inan & Inan 2019].

Gentian root containing gentianine is a productive anti-inflammatory power. Bromelain, a proteolytic enzyme obtained from the stinging nettle, turmeric, and pineapple, has anti-inflammatory actions. Examples of fruits, vegetables, herbs, beverages, and spices having antioxidative properties are grapes, blueberries, citrus fruits, strawberries, blackberries, crowberries, tomatoes, broccoli, beans, beetroot, mushrooms, white cabbage, corn, kale, cauliflower, garlic, onions, spinach, cacao beans, rosemary, oregano and thyme, sage, tea, and wine. They can reduce the level of reactive oxygen species and free radicals. They also show an effect in the process of lipid oxidation that inhibits or downregulates the formation of free alkyl radicals and inhibits the chain reactions of free radical. They have intracellular signaling pathway modular effect [Inan & Inan 2019].

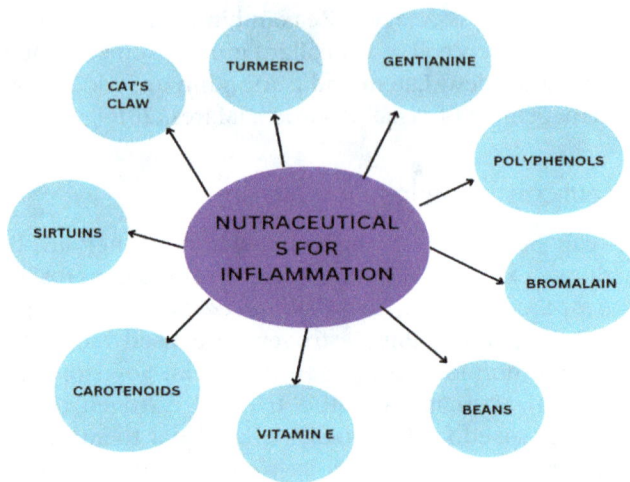

*Figure 1.11* *Nutraceuticals used for inflammation.*

Vitamin E, carotenoids (xanthophylls and carotenes), and polyphenols (fla-vonoids) are both anti-inflammatory and antioxidative in nature, they can be used for the treatment of rheumatoid arthritis, cancer, and other inflammatory and oxidative stress-induced diseases [Fig. 1.11].

## 1.4.9 Nutraceuticals in Obesity

Causes of obesity:

- High fat
- Energy-dense food
- Less physical activity
- More junk food consumption

The prevalence of obesity is increasing globally and that is the reason why nutrition and exercise play a major role in the management of body weight [Das et al., 2012]. Nutraceuticals, capsaicin-conjugated linoleic acid, psyllium fiber, and Momordica charantia have efficacy against obesity. An effective nutraceutical that can increase energy and decrease caloric consumption proves to be a good option for losing weight easily. Herbal stimulants, a hot beverage made from beans, ephedrine, chitosan, and green tea are helpful in weight loss.

Ginseng, both Asian and American, has been studied in various animal mod-els for its role in weight loss and for the improvement of glucose-lipidemic profile [Bertuccioli et al., 2021]. The evidence proposes that β-glucans have an optimistic effect on gut microbiota and improve lipid and glucose levels, offer-ing an outstanding adjunct to less caloric diets.

Psyllium, a water-soluble fiber obtained from the husks of seeds of *Plantago ovate*, is able to form a gelatinous liquid. It is used for reducing appetite and intestinal irregularity. It also interferes with the absorption of carbohydrates, lipids, and bile salt.

## 1.4.10 Nutraceuticals in Parkinson's Disease

Parkinson's disease (PD) is the most common neurodegenerative disorder caused by genetic and environmental factors [Das et al., 2012; Lama et al., 2020]. Nutrients like coenzyme Q10, fish oils, lycopene, and resveratrol show neuroprotective actions by reducing oxidative stress and mitochondrial damage. Phytochemicals such as eppigallocatechin-3 gallate, vincamine, ginsenosides, and vinpocetine protect against the toxic effects of dopamine metabolites. Palmitoylethanolamide, vitamin A, β carotene, coenzyme Q10, crocin, rosmarinic acid, gallic acid, resveratrol, and salidroside reduce endoplasmic reticulum stress (ER stress).

Nutraceuticals targeting neuroinflammation in PD include curcumin, silymarin, glucocalyxin B Asiatic acid, *Mucuna pruriens*, and quercetin. Dietary soy and peanut products have also been reported to have similar effects. Another powerful nutraceutical that has been proven to show actions against PD and other neurotoxicity is Ginko biloba extract [Hang et al., 2016].

## 1.4.11 Nutraceuticals in Respiratory Diseases

The important health and financial problems, nowadays, are asthma, chronic obstructive pulmonary disease (COPD), bronchitis, acute respiratory distress syndrome (ARDS), and lung cancer (LC). The leaves, roots, flowers, and bark of *Adhatoda vasica* (family Acanthaceae) have useful effects on cough, colds, asthma, mucus, bronchial communicable disease, bronchitis, and seasonal infection [Rahman et al., 2022].

Vasicine, an alkaloid, has antioxidant, anti-inflammatory, and bronchodilatory properties. The liquid extract of *Albizia lebbeck* displayed anti-asthmatic and anti-anaphylactic effects in recent studies.

Extract of *Boswellia serrata* (family Burseraceae) is a traditional medicine for the treatment of asthma.

*Kalanchoe integra* (family Crassulaceae) has proved to have various pharmacological actions like anthelmintic, immunosuppressive, wound restorative, hepatoprotective, antagonistic-instigative, antidiabetic, nephroprotective, antioxidant, antimicrobial, anticonvulsant, analgesic and antipyretic effects.

Curcumin studies (both *in vivo* and *in vitro*) showed that it has anti-asthmatic activity. Liquorice root is effective in treating coughs. It contains chalcones, glycyrrhizin and glycyrrhetinic acid, flavonoids, and isoflavonoids. They give symptomatic relief from coughs, colds, asthma, SARS-CoV, and COPD [Allam et al., 2022]

The rhizome of the *Hedychium spicatum* has existed in use since ancient times to treat cough, asthma, and other respiratory diseases, and is clinically used for the management of asthma. *Ocimum sanctum* (family Lamiaceae), usually famous as tulsi, is used for cough, cold, asthma, and bronchitis. *Piper longum* has been reported as a good remedy for respiratory infections and is also helpful in the treatment of tuberculosis. *Tylophora Indica* (family Apocynaceae) is used for the treatment of coughs. The extracts of the leaves of *T. indica* have anti-asthmatic and anti-allergic potential [Chavda et al., 2022]

The rhizome of the plant *Zingiber officinale* (family Zingiberaceae) has been used to treat colds, asthma, and bronchitis. Foods containing zinc, vitamins, garlic, turmeric, ginger, selenium, etc. are immunity boosters and effectively prevent Covid-19. They also help in combating aftereffects of Covid-19. The use of vitamins C, D, and E helps to prevent Covid-19. Lifestyle modifications like healthy eating and taking immunity-boosting supplements help to prevent Covid-19 [Subedi et al., 2021].

*In vitro* studies have proved that zinc inhibits the replication of SARS-CoV by inhibiting the Ribonucleic acid (RNA) synthesizing activity of the replication and transcription complex (RTC) of the virus. Melatonin (N-acetyl-5-methoxytryptamine), having anti-inflammatory, antioxidative, and immunomodulatory properties, may also be advantageous in relieving Covid-19 symptoms. Tetrandrine, extracted from *Stephania tetrandra*, inhibits viral replication by blocking the two-pore channel 2 (TPC2) in host cells. TPC2 channels are used by the virus for egress and replication.

Flavonoids from *Camellia sinensis*, extract of *Dioscoreae rhizoma*, *Taxillus Chinensis*, and *Cibotium barometz* also play a major role in preventing SARS-CoV.

Medicinal plants such as *Scutettaria baicalensis* and *Toona sinensis* have also been reported to inhibit viral replication of SARS-CoV [Subedi et al., 2021].

Honey is a functional food that is supposed to have antibacterial, antiviral, antioxidant, and anti-inflammatory properties [Fig. 1.12].

## 1.5 Recent Trends and Challenges

Nutraceuticals have gained popularity over the past few decades because of their health-promoting role and diverse application in the prevention and treatment of diseases. Recent times have witnessed a massive increase in the number of commercially available nutraceuticals, nutraceutical-based patents, and manuscripts published on nutraceuticals [Tsiaka et al., 2022]. Current trends include the use of nano-scaled materials and nano-delivery systems in the domain of food and health sciences, such as nanoengineered materials

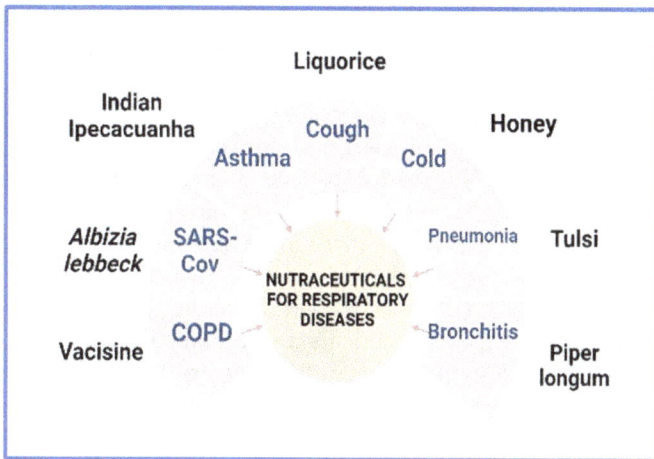

**Figure 1.12** *Nutraceuticals used for the treatment of respiratory disorders. Created with BioRender.com.*

being employed for nanopacking, improvement of the sensory attributes, targeted or slow and controlled delivery of foods, protection of encapsulated bioactive molecules from oxidation or the action of gastrointestinal tract enzymes and thus improved bioefficacy, nano-fortification of functional and fortified products[Aguilar-Pérez et al., 2021; Paolino et al., 2021]. The use of *in silico* methods and computational techniques are still at a nascent stage in the field of nutraceuticals, thereby offering a unique opportunity for further investigation and exploitation [Tsiaka et al., 2022]

Presently the nutraceutical industry faces certain challenges such as the fragmentary nature of regulations, undefined privileges in labeling, and false advertising. A proper system for quality checks for identification of the authentic source of raw materials, purity of compounds, presence of other active compounds, and interactions between supplements and drugs is lacking [Siddiqui & Moghadasian, 2020]. A few nutraceuticals have been reported to be adulterated with hazardous heavy metals toxicants, pesticides, toxic plants, fertilizers, and mycotoxins. Detailed clinical studies including safety profiles for a large number of nutraceutical products are yet to be explored. This would also be useful to validate the possible medicinal or health benefits of these products [Murugan, 2022]. Additionally, consumer education is required to avoid the inappropriate and/or overuse of nutraceuticals that may carry some health risks.

## 1.6 Future Prospects

Nutraceuticals are functional foods or part of them that offer several health aids that may inhibit and cure diseases. There are different types of nutraceuticals, such as dietary fibers, probiotics, polyphenols, polyunsaturated fatty acids, vitamins, prebiotics, fortified foods, recombinants, and spices, which may have important roles in strategizing human health as discussed in this chapter. The cause of the increasing demand for nutraceuticals may be changing lifestyles of people and increased awareness about nutraceuticals. Recent studies have proved that nutraceuticals may be used in the future for maintaining health and combating various diseases like cardiovascular disorders, mental health, allergies, respiratory diseases, Alzheimer's disease, Parkinson's disease, gastrointestinal health, skin health, eye disorders, inflammatory diseases, diabetes, immune health, and cancer, as well as obesity. The number of companies manufacturing nutraceuticals and dietary supplements is increasing rapidly as they may be an important support in the healthcare segment.

## Refernces

Abdullah, M., Jamil, R. T., & Attia, F. N. (2022). Vitamin C (Ascorbic Acid). *Encyclopedia of Toxicology: Third Edition*, 962–963. https://doi.org/10.1016/B978-0-12-386454-3.01250-1

Aguilar-Pérez, K. M., Ruiz-Pulido, G., Medina, D. I., Parra-Saldivar, R., & Iqbal, H. M. (2021). Insight of Nanotechnological Processing for Nano-fortified Functional Foods and Nutraceutical—Opportunities, Challenges, and Future Scope in Food for Better Health. *Critical Reviews in Food Science and Nutrition*, 1–18. DOI: 10.1080/10408398.2021.2004994

AlAli, M., Alqubaisy, M., Aljaafari, M. N., AlAli, A. O., Baqais, L., Molouki, A., Abushelaibi, A., Lai, K.-S., & Lim, S.-H. E. (2021). Nutraceuticals: Transformation of Conventional Foods into Health Promoters/Disease Preventers and Safety Considerations. *Molecules*, 26(9), 2540. https://doi.org/10.3390/molecules26092540

Alissa, E. M., & Ferns, G. A. (2012). Functional Foods and Nutraceuticals in the Primary Prevention of Cardiovascular Diseases. *Journal of Nutrition and Metabolism*, 2012, 569486. https://doi.org/10.1155/2012/569486

Allam, V. S. R. R., Chellappan, D. K., Jha, N. K., Shastri, M. D., Gupta, G., Shukla, S. D., Singh, S. K., Sunkara, K., Chitranshi, N., Gupta, V., Wich, P. R., MacLoughlin, R., Oliver, B. G. G., Wernersson, S., Pejler, G., & Dua, K. (2022). Treatment of Chronic Airway Diseases Using Nutraceuticals: Mechanistic Insight. *Critical Reviews in Food Science and Nutrition*, 62(27), 7576–7590. https://doi.org/10.1080/10408398.2021.1915744

Amara, A. A., & Shibl, A. (2015). Role of Probiotics in Health Improvement, Infection Control and Disease Treatment and Management. *Saudi Pharmaceutical Journal*, 23(2), 107–114. https://doi.org/10.1016/j.jsps.2013.07.001

Barber, T. M., Kabisch, S., Pfeiffer, A. F. H., & Weickert, M. O. (2020). The Health Benefits of Dietary Fibre. *Nutrients*, 12(10), 3209. https://doi.org/10.3390/nu12103209

Basak, S., & Gokhale, J. (2022). Immunity Boosting Nutraceuticals: Current Trends and Challenges. *Journal of Food Biochemistry*, 46(3). https://doi.org/10.1111/jfbc.13902

BCC Research. Nutraceuticals Market Size, Share & Growth Analysis Report. Available Online: https://www.bccresearch.com/ market-research/food-and-beverage/nutraceuticals-global-markets.html (accessed on 13 March 2022).

Bergamin, A., Mantzioris, E., Cross, G., Deo, P., Garg, S., & Hill, A. M. (2019). Nutraceuticals: Reviewing Their Role in Chronic Disease Prevention and Management. *Pharmaceutical Medicine*, 33(4), 291–309. https://doi.org/10.1007/s40290-019-00289-w

Bertuccioli, A., Cardinali, M., Biagi, M., Moricoli, S., Morganti, I., Zonzini, G. B., & Rigillo, G. (2021). Nutraceuticals and Herbal Food Supplements for Weight Loss: Is There a Prebiotic Role in the Mechanism of Action? *Microorganisms*, 9(12). https://doi.org/10.3390/MICROORGANISMS9122427

Black, H. S., Boehm, F., Edge, R., & Truscott, T. G. (2020). The Benefits and Risks of Certain Dietary Carotenoids That Exhibit Both Anti- and Pro-oxidative Mechanisms—A Comprehensive Review. *Antioxidants*, *9*(3), 264. https://doi.org/10.3390/antiox9030264

Blondeau, N., Lipsky, R. H., Bourourou, M., Duncan, M. W., Gorelick, P. B., & Marini, A. M. (2015). Alpha-Linolenic Acid: An Omega-3 Fatty Acid with Neuroprotective Properties—Ready for Use in the Stroke Clinic? *BioMed Research International, 2015*, 1–8. https://doi.org/10.1155/2015/519830

Calfio, C., Gonzalez, A., Singh, S. K., Rojo, L. E., & Maccioni, R. B. (2020). The Emerging Role of Nutraceuticals and Phytochemicals in the Prevention and Treatment of Alzheimer's Disease. *Journal of Alzheimer's Disease: JAD*, *77*(1), 33–51. https://doi.org/10.3233/JAD-200443

Chambial, S., Dwivedi, S., Shukla, K. K., John, P. J., & Sharma, P. (2013). Vitamin C in Disease Prevention and Cure: An Overview. *Indian Journal of Clinical Biochemistry: IJCB, 28*(4), 314–328. https://doi.org/10.1007/s12291-013-0375-3

Chavda, V. P., Patel, A. B., Vihol, D., Vaghasiya, D. D., Ahmed, K. M. S. B., Trivedi, K. U., & Dave, D. J. (2022). Herbal Remedies, Nutraceuticals, and Dietary Supplements for COVID-19 Management: An Update. *Clinical Complementary Medicine and Pharmacology, 2*(1), 100021. https://doi.org/10.1016/j.ccmp.2022.100021

Cholewski, M., Tomczykowa, M., & Tomczyk, M. (2018). A Comprehensive Review of Chemistry, Sources and Bioavailability of Omega-3 Fatty Acids. *Nutrients, 10*(11). https://doi.org/10.3390/NU10111662

Cory, H., Passarelli, S., Szeto, J., Tamez, M., & Mattei, J. (2018). The Role of Polyphenols in Human Health and Food Systems: A Mini-Review. *Frontiers in Nutrition, 5*. https://doi.org/10.3389/fnut.2018.00087

Das, L., Bhaumik, E., Raychaudhuri, U., & Chakraborty, R. (2012). Role of Nutraceuticals in Human Health. *Journal of Food Science and Technology, 49*(2), 173–183. https://doi.org/10.1007/s13197-011-0269-4

Davani-Davari, D., Negahdaripour, M., Karimzadeh, I., Seifan, M., Mohkam, M., Masoumi, S., Berenjian, A., & Ghasemi, Y. (2019). Prebiotics: Definition, Types, Sources, Mechanisms, and Clinical Applications. *Foods, 8*(3), 92. https://doi.org/10.3390/foods8030092

Dubey, S. (2017). Indian Spices and their Medicinal Value. *Indian Journal of Pharmaceutical Education and Research*, *51*(3), S330–S332. https://doi.org/10.5530/IJPER.51.3S.41

Donato, M., Faggin, E., Cinetto, F., Felice, C., Lupo, M. G., Ferri, N., & Rattazzi, M. (2021). The Emerging Role of Nutraceuticals in Cardiovascular Calcification: Evidence from Preclinical and Clinical Studies. *Nutrients, 13*(8), 2603. https://doi.org/10.3390/nu13082603

Gulati, K., Thokchom, S. K., Joshi, J. C., & Ray, A. (2021). Regulatory Guidelines for Nutraceuticals in India: An Overview. *Nutraceuticals: Efficacy, Safety and Toxicity*, 1273–1280. https://doi.org/10.1016/B978-0-12-821038-3.00074-4

Gupta, S., Parvez, N., & Sharma, P. (2015). Nutraceuticals as Functional Foods. *Journal of Nutritional Therapeutics, 4*(2), 64–72. https://doi.org/10.6000/1929-5634.2015.04.02.4

Hang, L., Basil, A. H., & Lim, K. L. (2016). Nutraceuticals in Parkinson's Disease. *NeuroMolecular Medicine, 18*(3), 306. https://doi.org/10.1007/S12017-016-8398-6

Hannon, B. A., Fairfield, W. D., Adams, B., Kyle, T., Crow, M., & Thomas, D. M. (2020). Use and Abuse of Dietary Supplements in Persons with Diabetes. *Nutrition and Diabetes, 10*(1). https://doi.org/10.1038/s41387-020-0117-6

Helal, N. A., Eassa, H. A., Amer, A. M., Eltokhy, M. A., Edafiogho, I., & Nounou, M. I. (2019). Nutraceuticals' Novel Formulations: The Good, the Bad, the Unknown and Patents Involved. *Recent Patents on Drug Delivery and Formulation, 13*(2), 105–156. https://doi.org/10.2174/1872211313666190503112040

Inan, S., & Inan, S. (2019). The Potential Role of Nutraceuticals in Inflammation and Oxidative Stress. *Nutraceuticals - Past, Present and Future*. https://doi.org/10.5772/INTECHOPEN.83797

Jandacek, R. J. (2017). Linoleic Acid: A Nutritional Quandary. *Healthcare, 5*(2), 25. https://doi.org/10.3390/healthcare5020025

Johnson, E. J. (2002). The Role of Carotenoids in Human Health. *Nutrition in Clinical Care: An Official Publication of Tufts University, 5*(2), 56–65. https://doi.org/10.1046/j.1523-5408.2002.00004.x

Kang, I., Buckner, T., Shay, N. F., Gu, L., & Chung, S. (2016). Improvements in Metabolic Health with Consumption of Ellagic Acid and Subsequent Conversion into Urolithins: Evidence and Mechanisms. *Advances in Nutrition, 7*(5), 961–972. https://doi.org/10.3945/an.116.012575

Kapoor, B., Kapoor, D., Gautam, S., Singh, R., & Bhardwaj, S. (2021). Dietary Polyunsaturated Fatty Acids (PUFAs): Uses and Potential Health Benefits. *Current Nutrition Reports, 10*(3), 232–242. https://doi.org/10.1007/s13668-021-00363-3

Kumar, N., & Goel, N. (2019). Phenolic Acids: Natural Versatile Molecules with Promising Therapeutic Applications. *Biotechnology Reports (Amsterdam, Netherlands), 24*, e00370. https://doi.org/10.1016/j.btre.2019.e00370

Lama, A., Pirozzi, C., Avagliano, C., Annunziata, C., Mollica, M. P., Calignano, A., Meli, R., & Mattace Raso, G. (2020). Nutraceuticals: An Integrative Approach to Starve Parkinson's Disease. *Brain, Behavior, & Immunity - Health, 2*, 100037. https://doi.org/10.1016/J.BBIH.2020.100037

Mares, J. (2016). Lutein and Zeaxanthin Isomers in Eye Health and Disease. *Annual Review of Nutrition, 36*, 571–602. https://doi.org/10.1146/annurev-nutr-071715-051110

McCarty, M. F., Lerner, A., Dinicolantonio, J. J., & Benzvi, C. (2021). Nutraceutical Aid for Allergies - Strategies for Down-Regulating Mast Cell Degranulation. *Journal of Asthma and Allergy, 14*, 1257–1266. https://doi.org/10.2147/JAA.S332307

Mordor Intelligence. Global Nutraceuticals Market Size, Share, Trends, Growth. (2022–27). Available Online: https://www. mordorintelligence.com/industry-reports/global-nutraceuticals-market-industry (accessed on 13 March 2022).

Murugan, R. (2022). Nutraceuticals: Pros and Cons. *Chettinad Health City Medical Journal, 11*(1), 41–44.

Nasri, H., Baradaran, A., Shirzad, H., & Rafieian-Kopaei, M. (2014). New Concepts in Nutraceuticals as Alternative for Pharmaceuticals. *International Journal of Preventive Medicine, 5*(12), 1487–1499.

Orcajo, J., Martinez de Marañon, I., & Lavilla, M. (2015). Cow's milk allergen β-lactoglobulin immunoreactivity affected by pulsed light treatment. *Clinical and Translational Allergy, 5*(S3). https://doi.org/10.1186/2045-7022-5-S3-P50

Paolino, D., Mancuso, A., Cristiano, M. C., Froiio, F., Lammari, N., Celia, C., & Fresta, M. (2021). Nanonutraceuticals: The New Frontier of Supplementary Food. *Nanomaterials, 11*(3), 792.

Rahman, M. M., Bibi, S., Rahaman, M. S., Rahman, F., Islam, F., Khan, M. S., Hasan, M. M., Parvez, A., Hossain, M. A., Maeesa, S. K., Islam, M. R., Najda, A., Al-malky, H. S., Mohamed, H. R. H., AlGwaiz, H. I. M., Awaji, A. A., Germoush, M. O., Kensara, O. A., Abdel-Daim, M. M., Saeed, M., & Kamal, M. A. (2022). Natural Therapeutics and Nutraceuticals for Lung Diseases: Traditional Significance, Phytochemistry, and Pharmacology. *Biomedicine and Pharmacotherapy, 150*, 113041. https://doi.org/10.1016/J.BIOPHA.2022.113041

Rizvi, S., Raza, S. T., Ahmed, F., Ahmad, A., Abbas, S., & Mahdi, F. (2014). The Role of Vitamin E in Human Health and Some Diseases. *Sultan Qaboos University Medical Journal, 14*(2), e157–e165.

Rodríguez-García, C., Sánchez-Quesada, C., Toledo, E., Delgado-Rodríguez, M., & Gaforio, J. J. (2019). Naturally Lignan-Rich Foods: A Dietary Tool for Health Promotion? *Molecules (Basel, Switzerland), 24*(5). https://doi.org/10.3390/molecules24050917

Roudebush, P., Davenport, D. J., & Novotny, B. J. (2004). The Use of Nutraceuticals in Cancer Therapy. *The Veterinary Clinics of North America. Small Animal Practice, 34*(1), 249–269. https://doi.org/10.1016/J.CVSM.2003.09.001

Rutjes, A. W., Denton, D. A., di Nisio, M., Chong, L.-Y., Abraham, R. P., Al-Assaf, A. S., Anderson, J. L., Malik, M. A., Vernooij, R. W., Martínez, G., Tabet, N., & McCleery, J. (2018). Vitamin and Mineral Supplementation for Maintaining Cognitive Function in Cognitively Healthy People in Mid and Late Life. *Cochrane Database of Systematic Reviews, 2019*(1). https://doi.org/10.1002/14651858.CD011906.pub2

Saleh, B. K., Omer, A., & Teweldemedhin, B. (2018). Medicinal Uses and Health Benefits of Chili Pepper (Capsicum spp.): A Review. *MOJ Food Processing & Technology, 6*(4). https://doi.org/10.15406/mojfpt.2018.06.00183

Shahidi, F., & Ambigaipalan, P. (2015). Phenolics and Polyphenolics in Foods, Beverages and Spices: Antioxidant Activity and Health Effects – A Review. *Journal of Functional Foods*, 820–897. https://doi.org/10.1016/j.jff.2015.06.018

Shylaja, M. R., & Peter, K. V. (2007). Spices in the Nutraceutical and Health Food Industry. *Acta Horticulturae, 756*, 369–378. https://doi.org/10.17660/ActaHortic.2007.756.39

Siddiqui, R. A., & Moghadasian, M. H. (2020). Nutraceuticals and Nutrition Supplements: Challenges and Opportunities. *Nutrients, 12*(6), 1593.

Sosnowska, B., Penson, P., & Banach, M. (2017). The Role of Nutraceuticals in the Prevention of Cardiovascular Disease. *Cardiovascular Diagnosis and Therapy, 7*(Suppl 1), S21–S31. https://doi.org/10.21037/CDT.2017.03.20

Srinivasan, K. (2005). Role of Spices Beyond Food Flavoring: Nutraceuticals with Multiple Health Effects. *Food Reviews International, 21*(2), 167–188. https://doi.org/10.1081/FRI-200051872

Subedi, L., Tchen, S., Gaire, B. P., Hu, B., & Hu, K. (2021). Adjunctive Nutraceutical Therapies for COVID-19. *International Journal of Molecular Sciences, 22*(4), 1963. https://doi.org/10.3390/ijms22041963

Swanson, D., Block, R., & Mousa, S. A. (2012). Omega-3 Fatty Acids EPA and DHA: Health Benefits throughout Life. *Advances in Nutrition (Bethesda, Md.), 3*(1), 1–7. https://doi.org/10.3945/an.111.000893

Tallima, H., & el Ridi, R. (2018). Arachidonic Acid: Physiological Roles and Potential Health Benefits - A Review. *Journal of Advanced Research, 11*, 33–41. https://doi.org/10.1016/j.jare.2017.11.004

Tsiaka, T., Kritsi, E., Tsiantas, K., Christodoulou, P., Sinanoglou, V. J., & Zoumpoulakis, P. (2022). Design and Development of Novel Nutraceuticals: Current Trends and Methodologies. *Nutraceuticals, 2*(2), 71–90. https://doi.org/10.3390/nutraceuticals2020006

Ullah, A., Munir, S., Badshah, S. L., Khan, N., Ghani, L., Poulson, B. G., Emwas, A.-H., & Jaremko, M. (2020). Important Flavonoids and Their Role as a Therapeutic Agent. *Molecules, 25*(22), 5243. https://doi.org/10.3390/molecules25225243

van Hoorn, R., Kapoor, R., & Kamphuis, J. (2008). A Short Review on Sources and Health Benefits of GLA, *the GOOD Omega-6. Oléagineux, Corps Gras, Lipides, 15*(4), 262–264. https://doi.org/10.1051/ocl.2008.0207

Whelan, J., & Fritsche, K. (2013). Linoleic Acid. *Advances in Nutrition (Bethesda, Md.), 4*(3), 311–312. https://doi.org/10.3945/an.113.003772

Xu, T., Ren, D., Sun, X., & Yang, G. (2012). Dual Roles of Sulforaphane in Cancer Treatment. *Anti-Cancer Agents in Medicinal Chemistry, 12*(9), 1132–1142. https://doi.org/10.2174/187152012803529691

Zhang, C., Sheng, J., Li, G., Zhao, L., Wang, Y., Yang, W., Yao, X., Sun, L., Zhang, Z., & Cui, R. (2020). Effects of Berberine and Its Derivatives on Cancer: A Systems Pharmacology Review. In *Frontiers in Pharmacology* (Vol. 10). Frontiers Media S.A. https://doi.org/10.3389/fphar.2019.01461

Zhang, F. F., Barr, S. I., McNulty, H., Li, D., & Blumberg, J. B. (2020). Health Effects of Vitamin and Mineral Supplements. *BMJ*, m2511. https://doi.org/10.1136/bmj.m2511

# 2

# Anxiety Disorders: Background, Anatomy, and Pathophysiology

Ashley Oake and Yashwant V. Pathak

## Contents

## 2.1 Introduction

Anxiety is defined in the Diagnostic and Statistical Manuel for mental disorders (DSM-5) as the excess worry and apprehension of generalized activities, occurring for the majority of a 6-month period (1). This was first acknowledged as a psychiatric disorder in the 20th century (2). The way individuals experience anxiety is a combination of the emotional component (fear or worry) and the physical symptoms (increased heart rate and sweating) (3). Clinical presentations of anxiety can include headaches, trembling, shortness of breath, perspiration, restlessness, nausea, and palpitations (3). During an acute episode of anxiety, the extreme thoughts of fear and a racing heartbeat with chest tightness may cause a person to feel as if they are having a heart attack (3). Chronic forms of anxiety present with a more negative or blunt affect, with signs of depression (3).

The American Psychiatric Association has reported that anxiety disorders are the most common type of psychiatric disorder across the United States, with one in five adults reporting a history (3). In the DSM-5, anxiety is categorized into twelve different subtypes ranging from generalized anxiety disorder to

DOI: 10.1201/9781003333821-2

specific phobias (3). Each subtype is clearly explained with clinical features, prevalence, epidemiology, comorbidities, and risk factors (3). For social anxiety, the age of onset is 11 years old and over 75% are diagnosed by the age of 20 (3). Certain subsets of anxiety disorders, including separation anxiety, start at a young age and predisposition the individual for panic disorders, while others, like agoraphobia, develop closer to 30 years of age (3). Women commonly develop anxiety with a 3:2 ratio against men, possibly due to the imbalance of hormones, although there is no difference in prevalence across races (3).

An individual's risk for anxiety is influenced by both inheritance of genetic factors and an environmental impact throughout their lifetime (4). Family studies suggest that there is a higher incidence in twins, especially monozygotic, and certain anxiety disorders may be attributed to a higher genetic component (ex. generalized anxiety demonstrates about 30% while phobias may have up to 60%) (4). Peptide and hormone signaling genes are commonly researched for their association with anxiety disorders when dysregulated, single nucleotide polymorphisms being of high prevalence (4). One study found that mutations in the NPSR1, RGS2, and CRHR1 genes were all highly associated with panic disorders, while OXTR, SLC6A4, MAOA, and HTR1A were all links to Social Anxiety Disorder (4).

Social factors that may increase an individual's risk for developing anxiety range from childhood trauma to substance abuse (3). Environmental influences contribute to the theory that anxiety is a learned behavior and may result from an inability to adapt or develop socially (3). Certain personality traits, such as avoiding social situations and expressing shyness, and physical abnormalities including hyperthyroidism and arrhythmias can act as precursors for development of anxiety disorders. (3). Long-term stress caused by traumatic events can alter the chemical balance for controlling emotion, leading to trouble regulating it long term (3). Anxiety may be referred to differently across cultures, like the "wind attacks" in Cambodia and *Ataque de Nervios* in Puerto Rico (3). The symptoms that individuals present with are similar, but the cultural view on causative agents may differ so consulting a cultural specialist is important in the treatment process (3).

Theories regarding the causative agents of anxiety disorders are mainly centered around the dysregulation of neurotransmitters (3). Imaging studies have shown a hyperactivity of the amygdala, which controls fear and aggression, in most subtypes along with an imbalance of norepinephrine, serotonin, dopamine, and GABA (Gamma-aminobutyric acid) (3). Norepinephrine is responsible for the "fight or flight" mode that are body encounters during stressful situations or increased sympathetic activity (3). The hypothalamic-pituitary-adrenal (HPA) axis is thought to be overstimulated and leads to an excess release of cortisol by the adrenals (3). The imbalance of norepinephrine can also encourage the decrease in serotonin and increase of dopamine levels to cause changes in an individual's mood (3).

Although small amounts of anxiety in situations where danger may present is something all individuals experience, it becomes a pathological complication when there is severe distress and dysfunction (3). Diagnoses of anxiety are highly associated with comorbidities such as phobias, depression, alcohol abuse, suicide, and drug use (3). Chronic anxiety can increase the risk of hypertension and arrhythmias which eventually can lead to a myocardial infarction and mortality (3). Anxiety is a precursor for substance abuse as well as a symptom of, as substance-induced anxiety is frequently misdiagnosed by physicians (3). When diagnosing a patient with an anxiety disorder, other medical conditions can present with physical symptoms, such as hyperthyroidism and cardiovascular complications, and need to be ruled out (3). Abnormal physical symptoms during panic-like attacks, including lack of bladder control or ataxia, can indicate that there may be another underlying cause (3).

Treatment for anxiety disorders is initially focused on therapy before prescription of medications and hospitalization (3). Cognitive behavioral therapy has proven very effective for most generalized anxiety, social anxiety, and panic disorder, although some psychologists believe group therapy is better for specific conditions like social anxiety (3). Other approaches include interpersonal psychotherapy, virtual therapy, insight-oriented psychotherapy, and supportive psychotherapy (3). When medications are indicated, the first-line treatment for most subtypes is selective serotonin reuptake inhibitors (SSRIs) (3). There will be a few weeks before these medications start to take full effect, so benzodiazepines are used for short-term therapy, but not long term due to side effects and risk of dependance (3). If the patient is unable to tolerate these medications, tricyclic antidepressants and Monoamine oxidase inhibitors (MAOIs) are available as alternative treatments but are not preferred (3).

## 2.2 Background of Anxiety Disorders

Greek and Roman philosophers indicate that the concept of anxiety has been recognized throughout history, although not fully understood and identified until recent years (2). The Hippocratic corpus, a collection of ancient Greek medical texts, has one of the first indications of a case of phobia demonstrated through Nicanor's fear of a "flute girl" (2). A Roman statesman, named Cicero, completed a publication called *Tusculan Disputations* in 45 B.C. that discussed psychological uncertainties being studied by Greek philosophers during that era (2). The text identifies many clinical indications of mental illness or disorders referred to as *aegritudo* (2). These include *molestia, sollicitudo,* and *angor* that indicate a troubled mind and diseased body (2). *Angor* was identified as a constricting disorder, *molestia* as more permanent, and *sollicitudo* as ruminative (2). Further study of these texts has lead philosophers and scientists to identify them as *anxiety (angor), affliction (molestia), and worry (sollicitudo)* (2).

As time progressed, philosophers began to gain a deeper understanding of how individuals were demonstrating these symptoms and the term melancholia was coined (2). The *Anatomy of Melancholy* was published in 1621 by author Robert Burton and described melancholia as a condition characterized by markedly depressed mood, bodily complaints, and hallucinations/delusions with a key criterion of the patient being quiet (2). This clinical diagnosis included qualities of both depression and anxiety described in current manuals, like the DSM-5, that we use for classification today (2). Symptoms of panic attacks were noted as well and connected to both melancholia and a condition referred to as "vapors," which was a nervous disorder (2). Before the 18th century, most treatment for mental illness was in "lunatic asylums" with a barbaric approach of chained restraint and physical punishment (5). Dr Philippe Pinel revolutionized the outlook by introducing the concept of moral treatment and is known for removing the chains from patients (5).

Dr Philippe Pinel was strongly influenced by French philosopher François Boissier de Sauvages de Lacroix's *Nosologia Methodica* which explained his formulation of the nosology for diseases (5). The term *vesaniae*, referring to the eighth class of diseases encompassing mental disorders, was divided into four orders: Hallucinations, Morositates, Deliria, and Folies Anomales (2). Panophobia, defined as panic terror, falls under the category of Morositates and is highly associated with the current definition of anxiety (2). The remaining disorders in the Morositates category include Bulimi, Polydipsia, Pica, and Nostalgia (2). Subtypes of Panophobia, *panophobia hysterica* and *panophobia phrontis*, are analogous to modern concepts of anxiety, including fright from being startled and constant worrying respectively (2).

The introduction of the Country Asylum Act, the Commissioners in Lunacy, and the Lunacy Act in the early 19th century promoted an increase in safer public mental institutions with improved oversight due to recognition of the harsh conditions at Bethlem Hospital (5). At this point in time, physicians began reconsidering mentally ill patients as individuals that were able to receive treatment and reformers, such as Dorothea Dix, advocated for the first state asylum to be constructed (5). With the understanding that psychiatric conditions may have a biological basis, medical case reports on schizophrenia and bipolar disorder were published by Benedict Morel and Jules Falret respectively (5). Dr Benedict Morel described a condition similar to schizophrenia that started at a young age, using the term *démence précoce*, but Eugene Bleuler later coined the term deriving it from the Greek words for "I split" and "mind" (5). The studies Morel conducted led him to believe that individuals inherited mental degeneration that worsened throughout generations, causing these symptoms (5).

Emil Krapelin built on Morel's work in psychiatric disorders, leading to his declaration of psychiatric disorders having a biological basis and the translation of *démence précoce* to dementia praecox (5). This updated term focused on the long-term change in cognition beginning at an early stage in life, which included hallucinations and delusions (5). Patients who experienced alternating periods of normal functioning in the absence of a long-term deterioration were considered as having manic-depressive psychosis, and patients without either who experienced delusions were identified as having paranoia (5). Bleuler's introduction of the updated term schizophrenia emphasized that the condition did not necessitate a deteriorating course, but instead needed specific symptoms she termed "the four A's" (5). These indications for schizophrenia included associations (disturbances of thought), affect, autism, and ambivalence (5). Hallucinations were considered a secondary symptom along with delusions (5).

During the 20th century, World War II influenced many physicians to focus on treating veterans and other individuals impacted by the severe trauma of this period (5). Psychobiology was founded by Swiss psychiatrist Adolf Meyer and introduced the concept that mental health was not only biological but influenced by the changes in our surrounding environment as well (5). A consideration of both prompted other physicians, including Walter Menninger, to develop a psychosocial model for treating patients and recognizing that an underlying cause may be attributed to a failure to adapt (5). Research following this model led to discoveries in medicine related to neurotransmitters, electrical stimulation, neuroimaging, and advancement in medications to treat the biological component (5).

The *Diagnostic and Statistical Manual of Mental Disorders*, first published in 1952 by the American Psychiatric Association, is the main reference book used by mental health-care providers for all psychiatric and brain-related conditions (1). With almost 300 individual diagnoses in the DSM-5, the publication covers all classifications, symptoms, criteria for diagnosis, and statistical information regarding risk and prognostic factors (6). The first two editions were considered preliminary works as they discussed main approaches from psychiatrists, but the update to DSM-3 represented a specific advancement in medicine with its multiaxial approach for diagnosis (6). The National Institute of Mental Health developed the Research Diagnostic Criteria in the 1970s, based off the works of the Feighner Criteria, to remove any biases or assumptions for the origin of diseases that the prior two editions of the DSM contained (6). A multiaxial approach considers the five DSM "axes" that need to be considered during the evaluation and diagnosis of a patient (6).

Axis I focused on clinical syndromes that included psychological or substance abuse disorders that impaired individuals from living their daily lives, which covered mood, anxiety, and eating disorders (7). Disorders that impaired the ability to relate to the surrounding community or environment, including personality disorders or mental retardation, were discussed in Axis II (7). Medical impairments, like HIV/AIDS and brain injuries, were discussed in Axis III and had the ability to worsen the former two axes (7). Major stressors or life-altering events that may be a temporary situation were covered in Axis IV and a global assessment of functioning to better understand the initial four axes was concluded in Axis V (7). These five categories encompassed a biological, environmental, and psychological approach to properly evaluate a patient while considering the multiple influences on mental health (7).

The latest edition, the DSM-5, was updated in 2013 with the primary goal of improving the usability in clinical and research settings while incorporating updated data and statistics to provide the highest quality of care (6). More than seventy established diagnoses were updated with an addition of prolonged grief disorder and verbiage regarding gender dysphoria, intellectual disability, and race was revised (6). Prior editions of the text included many gaps in cultural factors, so when assembling the work groups in the DSM-5 Task Force each group was required to have an international participant (6). Compared to the International Classification of Diseases (ICD) that is managed by the World Health Organization, the DSM-5 is a US classification system that correlates to the ICD statistical codes and has a more detailed classification for each disease (6).

## 2.3 Types of Anxiety Disorders

The DSM-5 has divided the category of anxiety disorders into eleven subtypes: Separation Anxiety Disorder, Selective Mutism, Specific Phobia, Social Anxiety Disorder, Panic Disorder, Agoraphobia, Generalized Anxiety Disorder, Substance/Medication-Induced Anxiety Disorder, Anxiety Disorder Due to Another Medical Condition, Other Specified Anxiety Disorder, and Unspecified Anxiety Disorder (8). Each specific disorder has an individual set of diagnostic criteria, prevalence, course, risks, and comorbidities (8). For younger children, the presence of separation anxiety is frequently seen, but when it continues past a developmental milestone or interferes with daily living, it can be classified as a disorder (8).

Separation Anxiety Disorder (SAD) is classified as an excessive amount of fear or anxiety related to being separated from an individual with a strong emotional attachment (9). This may be expressed as the inability to leave a location without that person, trouble with sleeping, a fear of serious harm to themselves or a loved one, or even physical symptoms (headaches, nausea, vomiting, palpitations) (9). Consistent symptoms need to be present for a minimum of 4 weeks in children and 6 months in adults but must not be attributed to another disorder that is present (9). An attachment to a parent that leads to crying at a younger age is commonly seen, but individuals with SAD may display aggression, have trouble in social situations, struggle with academic work, report seeing figures in the dark, and require constant need for attention (9).This condition is most prevalent in children under 12 years old and may develop following high periods of stress, with GAD (generalized anxiety disorder) and specific phobias being highly comorbid (9).

Selective Mutism presents commonly in children before the age of 5 with a fear of communicating with individuals in a public location, not including their immediate family (10). This disorder interferes with the child's ability to function in a school setting and may lead them to develop a set of nonverbal communication methods due to their anxiety around speaking (10). The inability to interact with others is not due to a lack of understanding the words spoken to them or knowledge about language (10). Children with this disorder may appear isolated from society, excessively attached to a parent, compulsive, show temper tantrums, or even mild oppositional actions (10). Although Selective Mutism is not a common disorder, over 70% of these children meet the diagnosis for Social Anxiety Disorder and other common comorbidities are specific phobias or separation anxiety (10).

Specific phobias are classified as an intense fear for an object or situation, which leads to an out of proportion behavioral response including avoidance, crying, severe distress, and panic (8). An individual may have multiple phobias that will be individually diagnosed as separate disorders to properly treat each directly (8). A stimulus or thought of the phobia may trigger a response, even when the phobia is not currently present (8). Active avoidance is common and may cause an interference with daily routines or social events (not attending family gatherings or taking another route to a location that adds a significant amount of time) (8). In most settings, the behavioral response is overexaggerated for the actual danger the person is currently in and the individual recognizes that after the panic subsides (8). Studies have indicated that around 7–9% of the population in the United States experience this disorder, while African or Asian countries may only have a prevalence of 2–4% of the population (8). Development of this disorder is commonly attributed to experience with a traumatic event, including witnessing or hearing about it in detail (8).

Social Anxiety Disorder is characterized by fear or anxiety related to social situations that could lead to the possibility of being humiliated or judged by others (11). Most social situations are avoided, or symptoms of physical distress may be shown while enduring the event (sweating, trembling, blushing) (11). The fear is commonly exaggerated beyond the actual chance of judgement or embarrassment, and these symptoms last 6 months or more (11). Individuals diagnosed with this disorder may be submissive, withdrawn, avoid eye contact, and soft-spoken (11). The prevalence in the United States is estimated to be around 7% and is commonly associated with an onset in males ranging from the ages of 8, 10, and 15 years old (11). Substance abuse is frequently seen in these individuals as well as major depressive disorder (MDD) and other anxiety disorders (11).

Panic attacks are described as unexpected episodes of intense fear or discomfort that last for a few minutes (12). Four or more physical symptoms need to be present for the validity of the diagnosis which include: palpitations, sweating, trembling, shortness of breath, chest pain, nausea, dizziness, chills, and paresthesias (12). This episode will be followed by at least 1 month of the individual having extreme concern that they will experience a second panic attack, leading to a change in behavior to avoid situations that might cause a reoccurrence (12). Panic attacks are frequently associated with an additional subtype of anxiety disorder, MDD or Post-traumatic stress disorder (PTSD), and are classified as either expected (with a cue or trigger) or unexpected (12). Nocturnal episodes, panic attacks that wake someone from their sleep in a state of terror, may happen to up to a third of patients with this diagnosis (12). Studies show that 2–3% of the population in the United States currently experience this, with a predominance in females (12). Unlike the previous subtypes discussed, the onset for this disorder is 20–24 years old and rarely starts during childhood (12).

Agoraphobia is classified as a panic-like disorder with fear or anxiety around being in a situation where escape would be difficult or help may not be available, including open, crowded, or closed spaces away from one's home (13). Standing in a line to order something, taking public transportation, or even just being outside the house alone causes severe distress for these individuals (13). The symptoms are similar to those of other panic disorders or phobias and the presence of active avoidance is a significant contributor to the diagnosis (13). Cultural aspects and age may influence presentation of symptoms or how the patient justifies their actions (older individuals attributing not leaving the house to constraints instead of fears) (13). Severe forms of this disorder include homebound individuals who will not step outside their residence or complete simple tasks (walking to the mailbox) (13). It is estimated that less than 2% of people in the United States experience this with the average onset being 17 years with panic attacks and 25–29 years without panic attacks (13).

Generalized anxiety disorder is classified as persistent fear or anxiety regarding multiple situations for a period of 6 months or more (8). These individuals present with restlessness, fatigue, irritability, tension, trouble focusing, and complications with sleep (8). Symptoms cause severe impairment of daily activities, including educational and occupational, and is not attributed to any other physiological conditions (8). The situations that trigger this worry are not cohesive and may range from the health of themselves or loved ones to simple daily activities like cleaning the house (8). Almost 15% of the population may experience GAD at some point in their lives according to a study done by the CDC (Centers for Disease Control) and the median onset is around 30 years old (14).

The following subtypes are attributed to substance abuse or other medical conditions and include Substance/Medication-Induced Anxiety Disorder, Anxiety Disorder Due to Another Medical Condition, Other Specified Anxiety Disorder, and Unspecified Anxiety Disorder (8). Substance or medication-induced anxiety is not common in the general population and includes any symptoms experienced during use of the substance, but also during the withdrawal period (8). Medical conditions, like hyperthyroidism or cardiovascular complications, can increase an individual's heart rate or blood pressure leading to symptoms or anxiety (8). The fear of an illness progressing to a terminal state may also provoke the onset of panic attacks or generalized anxiety (8). Other anxiety symptoms that do not meet the criteria of other diagnoses due to the time requirements or number of symptoms are placed in the final two categories (8).

## 2.4 Anatomy of Anxiety Disorders

The area of the brain responsible for modulating fear and anxiety is known as the amygdala, which is part of the limbic system along with the hippocampus, thalamus, hypothalamus, basal ganglia, and cingulate gyrus (15). It is a round mass of gray matter, located in each of the cerebral hemispheres, that plays a role in learning, emotion, behavior, and processing fearful and threatening stimuli (15). Thirteen nuclei make up the amygdala and are divided into the basolateral, corticomedial, and centromedial groups (15). The basolateral group mainly manages stress, feeding, and drinking, while the corticomedial group is only involved in the hunger and eating aspects (15). When experiencing fear or other emotions that may increase your heart rate, the centromedial group of nuclei are responsible for coordinating the information with other areas of the brain that regulate respiratory and cardiovascular functions (15).

When generating a behavior or emotion, the amygdala receives information about the external stimuli from the prefrontal cortex, temporal lobe, limbic structures, and posterior association area (15). After the information is processed, it departs through two possible pathways: the dorsal route and the ventral route (15). The stria terminalis conduct the information from the centromedial nucleus via the dorsal route to the septal area and the ventromedial nucleus of the hypothalamus (15). A second pathway, the ventral amygdalofugal pathway, transports information from the basolateral and centromedial groups of nuclei to major areas of the brain stem and forebrain (15).

The stria terminalis pathway connects with the bed nucleus of stria terminalis (BNST) to regulate autonomic functions that are associated with behavioral changes (16). During high levels of stress, the BNST signals the paraventricular nucleus to release corticotropin releasing hormone (CRH) to activate the hypothalamus-pituitary-adrenal axis (16). CRH signals the anterior pituitary to produce adrenocorticotropic hormone (ACTH) leading to the activation of the adrenal glands to produce cortisol, the stress hormone (16). Cortisol releases stored glucose to raise blood sugar levels while the hypothalamus sends signals to raise heart rate and blood pressure (16).

The neurotransmitters associated with this condition are part of the monoaminergic signaling pathway, which include norepinephrine, Gamma-aminobutyric-acid (GABA), serotonin, and dopamine, while dysregulation of corticotrophin-releasing factor and cholecystokinin may also play a role (17). Norepinephrine is released from the locus coeruleus, which serves as the alarm center, when activated by pain or stress to increase the sympathetic nervous system response (18). Serotonin is produced by the raphe nuclei and low levels are seen in both anxiety and depression (18). Neuroimaging studies report that the insula, amygdala, anterior cingulate cortex, and raphe nucleus all have decreased binding of serotonin to receptors in numerous types of anxiety disorders (18). Dopamine is released from the substantia nigra and ventral tegmental area during activities that we experience as pleasurable (18). This neurotransmitter is associated with reward, concentration, motivation, and enjoyment, while lower levels may lead to depressive symptoms (18).

Norepinephrine can stimulate the release of serotonin by binding to the α α receptor on neuronal cell bodies, while also inhibiting the release when binding to α2α receptors on axon terminals (18). Serotonin has the ability to provide negative feedback by interacting with 5-HT2A and 5-HT2C receptors (18). Levels of dopamine can also be influenced by the 5-HT system, with 5-HT1 receptors increasing and 5-HT2 receptors decreasing release (18). When secreted in the central nervous system, neurotransmitters are frequently released with neuropeptides that include cholecystokinin, galanin, neuropeptide Y, vasopressin, oxytocin, and corticotropin-releasing factor (17). This pairing can help modulate the effects of the neurotransmitters to control the strength (17).

GABA is an inhibitory neurotransmitter that synthesized from the precursor glutamate, which is an excitatory neurotransmitter (19). The amygdala contains GABAergic neurons that deactivate potassium conductance to modulate the activity of the central and basolateral nucleus (19). There are two types of GABA receptors: ionotropic GABA$_A$ receptors for rapid inhibition and metabotropic GABA$_B$ receptors for slow and prolonged inhibition (19). Increased levels of GABA during an episode of anxiety create a calming effect to balance the increase in norepinephrine (19).

## 2.5 Pathophysiology of Anxiety Disorders

Although the etiology of anxiety disorders has not been proven, there are many studied theories including the noradrenergic, GABA receptor, and serotonin models (20). The noradrenergic model explores the concept of overactivation of the autonomic nervous system due to hypersensitivity (20). The locus coeruleus produces noradrenergic norepinephrine that projects to the basolateral amygdala (BLA) (20). This interaction drives the development of anxiety and fear in stressful situations (20). The three main G-coupled protein receptors that norepinephrine binds to are alpha 1, alpha 2, and beta receptors, with the alpha receptors being more prominent in the amygdala, thalamus, and hippocampus (21). Alpha 1 and 2 receptors are associated with working memory, attention, and fear and spatial learning, while beta receptors modulate auditory fear, spatial reference and fear memory, and memory retrieval

(21). The multiple receptor types assist in balancing the effects through excitatory action of alpha 1 and beta receptors and inhibitory action of alpha 2 receptors (21). Serotonin-norepinephrine reuptake inhibitors (SNRIs), including venlafaxine and duloxetine, are frequently used in treatment of anxiety disorders by blocking the uptake of both serotonin and norepinephrine (22).

The GABA receptor model focuses on the lack of inhibition on excitatory states caused by 5-HT, NE, and DA that Gamma-aminobutyric acid would usually provide during periods of stress or worry (21). When higher levels of GABA are produced, the individual will experience sedation, amnesia, and ataxia if the balance is not controlled (21). Low levels of GABA lead to restlessness, insomnia, arousal, and anxiety (21). A major class of pharmaceuticals used to treat anxiety, benzodiazepines, targets GABA receptors to increase the inhibitory reaction (21). GABA produced by the body interacts with the two beta subunits of the receptor, while benzodiazepines bind to the two alpha subunits present (22). As the benzodiazepines connect with the alpha subunits, they enhance the binding of natural GABA to its own receptor (22). The binding of GABA to the receptor causes an influx of chloride into the neuron to hyperpolarize and lower the excitability (21). Other medications that interact with GABA include gabapentin, pregabalin, valproate, and vigabatrin (22).

The major excitatory neurotransmitter in the central nervous system is glutamate, which opposes the action of GABA (23). Glutamate has two types of receptors in the brain, ionotropic and metabotropic, which act in a voltage gated and ligand gated manner respectively (23). One of the main ionotropic receptors is N-methyl D-aspartate (NMDA) (23). It is only permeable to calcium when glutamate is bound and the neuron is already depolarized (23). If not depolarized, the channel would be blocked by magnesium and unable to let calcium pass (23). The metabotropic receptors are much slower acting through gene expression and protein synthesis (23). Group II and III of the receptors have shown an association with anxiety when dysregulated due to their location on the presynaptic membrane (23). Studies show that high levels of stress can cause neuronal death or damage from glutamate excitotoxicity when either overproduced or underregulated by lack of glutamate (23).

The serotonergic model describes the imbalance of serotonin (5-hydroxytryptamine, 5-HT) causing an overactivation of the amygdala circuit (24). Serotonin-1A (5-HT$_{1A}$) receptors are the specific major inhibitory subtype linked to anxiety or depression and are coupled to two G protein effector systems (24). When bound, they inhibit adenylyl cyclase activity and open potassium channels for hyperpolarization of the neuron (24). The dorsal and median raphe of the brain stem is the main location for serotonergic neurons, which contain the 5-HT$_{1A}$ autoreceptors on their soma and dendrites (25). Postsynaptic 5-HT$_{1A}$ heteroreceptors, or receptors that can respond to neurotransmitters from other cells, are located on pyramidal neurons or GABAergic interneurons (25).

Tryptophan hydroxylase-2 (TPH2) is the rate-limiting enzyme in the brain for the conversion of tryptophan to serotonin (26). The transcription factor Pet-1 is responsible for activating the TPH2 gene leading to the differentiation of the progenitors (26). Serotonin release from the raphe is then triggered and projects to areas throughout the brain, which is then picked up by 5-HT transporters (26). Excess amounts of serotonin can lead to the development of a condition referred to as serotonin syndrome, with symptoms of shivering, diarrhea, muscle rigidity, fever, and seizures (26). Low amounts of serotonin in the body cause changes in mood (depression, anxiety, and mania), memory complications, difficulty with sleep, and appetite issues (26). The first-line treatments for many anxiety disorders target the 5-HT transporters and are known as selective serotonin reuptake inhibitors (26).

Dopamine is the neurotransmitter responsible for the sensations of pleasure and satisfaction as well as motivation (27). There are five different G protein coupled receptors that are classified as either D1-like (increase Cyclic Adenosine mono phosphate (cAMP)) or D2-like (no effect or prevents cAMP) (27). Both classes of receptors are implicated in mediating anxiety or depression, as a low level of dopamine may lead to either condition (27). Monoamine oxidase converts dopamine to 3,4-dihydroxyphenylacetic acid (DOPAC) in the terminal of synapses and mitochondria and this ratio can be monitored to determine an imbalance (27). The mesolimbic pathway that connects the ventral tegmental area to the prefrontal cortex and limbic structures is the mechanism by which dopamine influences motivation and reward (27). Stress can activate this pathway and can cause large amounts of dopamine to collect in the synaptic cleft through lack of reuptake (27).

Excess dopamine projected to the amygdala may cause BLA nucleus hypertrophy and a reduction in size leads to decreased anxiety (27). The BLA nucleus is normally suppressed by the median prefrontal cortex, but anxiety-like behaviors develop when the suppression is lifted during a high stress environment (27). The amygdaloid D2 dopamine receptor in the central nucleus is frequently studied for its regulatory role in anxiety disorders (27). Bupropion is a noradrenaline and dopamine reuptake inhibitor used in the treatment of anxiety and depression by increasing the amount of neurotransmitters in the synaptic cleft (28). This medication has also been used in smoking cessation for its activity with mimicking the reward pathway (28).

## 2.6 Conclusion

Since the 20th century, anxiety has been considered a psychological disorder displaying excessive fear and worry for an extended period of time. Physical symptoms may include trembling, sweating, chest pain, shortness of breath, fatigue, and restlessness. The DSM-5 has classified anxiety disorders into twelve separate types ranging from agoraphobia to generalized anxiety disorder. Generalized anxiety disorder is the most prevalent in the United States, as 15% of people may experience this at some point of their life, and has an average age of onset of around 30 years old. Specific types of anxiety are more common in children, including separation anxiety and Selective Mutism, while others are more common in adults (agoraphobia and GAD).

With one in five Americans experiencing anxiety throughout their life, many studies have been conducted to discover the etiology behind the disease. Genetic factors may play a role in inheritance, but social interactions during developmental milestones in early ages and an imbalance in neurotransmitters seem to play a vital role in how these disorders come upon us.

The main neurotransmitters associated with anxiety disorders are norepinephrine, serotonin, dopamine, GABA, and glutamate. Imaging studies have indicated amygdala hyperactivity in many subtypes of anxiety disorders. This area of the brain, along with the remaining components of the limbic system, is responsible for modulating emotional responses and behavior, including fear and anger.

Three main models of the pathophysiology of anxiety are the noradrenergic model, the serotonin model, and the GABA receptor model. Norepinephrine is the "fight or flight" neurotransmitter released from the locus coeruleus that increases wakefulness and alertness. The noradrenergic model focuses on the hypersensitivity of the amygdala and overstimulation. GABA is the inhibitory neurotransmitter that balances the other excitatory components, and the model is centered around a lack of inhibition. Serotonin helps with regulation of behavior, attention, and body temperature and low amounts can lead to anxiety and depression. Large amounts of serotonin can cause "serotonin syndrome" with fever, chills, and muscle rigidity. Glutamate is the main excitatory neurotransmitter that opposes GABA. Dopamine is the neurotransmitter associated with pleasure, satisfaction, and motivation.

## 2.7 Future Trends

Currently research surrounding anxiety disorders is mainly focused on therapeutic agents and other treatment methods (27). Studies have shown that only 60–80% of individuals see improvement with treatments, with around half of those patients reaching a point of recovery with minimal symptoms (27). A nasal spray called Aloradine is currently being developed and studied for its use in Social Anxiety Disorder (27). Trials have included public-speaking challenges producing promising results (27). SRX246 is undergoing trials for treatment of PTSD, generalized anxiety disorder, and aggressive behavior as a vasopressin V1A receptor antagonist (27).

The Mayo Clinic is focusing on other non-pharmaceutical treatments with a video game study for children with social anxiety and a stress management and resilience training (SMART) program for health-care employees (28). This SMART program is also being studied in populations of family caregivers and students to assess their overall wellness, physical education, and nutrition (28). Holistic approaches, including massage therapy or aromatherapy, are increasingly gaining popularity throughout many communities due to lack of side effects and other health risks (28).

## References

1. Crocq MA. A History of Anxiety: From Hippocrates to DSM. *Dialogues in Clinical Neuroscience.* 2015; 17(3): 319–325. doi: 10.31887/DCNS.2015.17.3/macrocq
2. Bhatt NV & Baker MJ. Anxiety Disorders. *Medscape.* 2019. https://emedicine.medscape.com/article/286227-overview
3. Boland R, Verduin M, & Ruiz P. A Brief History of Psychiatry. *Kaplan & Sadock's Synopsis of Psychiatry.* 2021; 12: 1097–1134.
4. Gottschalk MG & Domschke K. Novel Developments in Genetic and Epigenetic Mechanisms of Anxiety. *Current Opinion in Psychiatry.* 2016; 29(1): 32–38. doi: 10.1097/YCO.0000000000000219
5. Suris A, Holiday R, & North CS. The Evolution of the Classification of Psychiatric Disorders. *Behavioral Sciences.* 2016; 6(1): 5. doi: 10.3390/bs6010005
6. Redier DA, Kuhl EA, & Kupfer DJ. The DSM-5: Classification and Criteria Changes. *World Psychiatry.* 2013; 12: 2.
7. Johnstone EC & Lawrie SM. An Introduction to Psychiatry. *Companion to Psychiatric Studies.* 2010; 8: 1–15.
8. American Psychiatric Association. *Diagnostic and statistical manual of mental disorders.* 2013; 5. doi: 10.1176/appi.books.9780890425596
9. Feriante J & Bernstein B. Separation Anxiety. *StatPearls.* 2022. https://www.ncbi.nlm.nih.gov/books/NBK560793/
10. Shipon-Blum E. Selective Mutism - A Comprehensive Overview. *Selective Mutism, Anxiety, and Related Disorders Treatment Center.* https://selectivemutismcenter.org/whatisselectivemutism/
11. Schneier F & Goldmark J. Social Anxiety Disorder. In D. J. Stein & B. Vythilingum (Eds.), *Anxiety Disorders and Gender.* 2015: 49–67. Springer International Publishing/ Springer Nature. https://doi.org/10.1007/978-3-319-13060-6_3
12. Locke AB, Kirst N, & Shultz CG. Diagnosis and Management of Generalized Anxiety Disorder and Panic Disorder in Adults. *American Family Physicians.* 2015; 91(9): 617–624.
13. Balaram K & Marwaha R. Agoraphobia. *StatPearls.* 2022. https://www.ncbi.nlm.nih.gov/books/NBK560793/
14. Terlizzi EP & Villarroel MA. *Symptoms of Generalized Anxiety Disorder Among Adults: United States, 2019.* Centers for Disease Control and Prevention. 2020.
15. Rajmohan V & Mohandas E. The Limbic System. *Indian Journal of Psychiatry.* 2007; 49(2): 132–139.
16. Crestani CC, Alves FH, Gomes FV, Resstel LBM, Correa FMA, & Herman JP. Mechanisms in the Bed Nucleus of the Stria Terminalis Involved in Control of Autonomic and Neuroendocrine Functions: A Review. *Current Neuropharmacology.* 2013; 11(2): 141–159.
17. Martin EI, Ressler KJ, Binder E, & Nemeroff CB. The Neurobiology of Anxiety Disorders: Brain Imaging, Genetics, and Psychoneuroendocrinology. *Psychiatric Clinics of North America.* 2009; 32(3): 549–575.

18. Liu Y, Zhao J, & Guo W. Emotional Roles of Mono-Aminergic Neurotransmitters in Major Depressive Disorder and Anxiety Disorders. *Frontiers in Psychology*. 2018; 9: 2201.
19. Nuss P. Anxiety Disorders and GABA Neurotransmission: A Disturbance of Modulation. *Neuropsychiatry in Disease and Treatment*. 2015; 11: 165–175.
20. McCall JG, Siuda ER, Bhatti DL, Lawson LA, McElligott ZA, Stuber GD, & Bruchas MR. Locus Coeruleus to Basolateral Amygdala Noradrenergic Projections Promote Anxiety-Like Behavior. *eLife*. 2017; 6: e18247.
21. Hussain LS, Reddy V, & Maani CV. Physiology, Noradrenergic Synapse. *StatPearls*. 2022. https://www.ncbi.nlm.nih.gov/books/NBK560793/
22. Stahl S, Grady M, Moret C, & Briley M. SNRIs: The Pharmacology, Clinical Efficacy, and Tolerability in Comparison with Other Classes of Antidepressants. *CNS Spectrums*. 2005; 10(9): 732–747.
23. Kaur S & Singh R. Role of Different Neurotransmitters in Anxiety: A Systemic Review. *International Journal of Pharmaceutical Sciences and Research*. 2017; 8(2): 411–421.
24. Michel TC. Intravenous Anesthetics and Benzodiazepines. *Anesthesia Secrets*. 2011; 4: 90–94.
25. Institute of Medicine (US) Forum on Neuroscience and Nervous System Disorders. Overview of the Glutamatergic System. *Glutamate-Related Biomarkers in Drug Development for Disorders of the Nervous System: Workshop Summary*. 2011; 2. https://pubmed.ncbi.nlm.nih.gov/21977546/
26. Frazer A & Hensler J. Serotonin Receptors. *Basic Neurochemistry: Molecular, Cellular and Medical Aspects*. 1999; 6. https://www.ncbi.nlm.nih.gov/books/NBK28234/
27. Garcia-Garcia A, Newman-Tancredi A, & Leonardo ED. 5-HT1A Receptors in Mood and Anxiety: Recent Insights into Autoreceptor versus Heteroreceptor Function. *Psychopharmacology*. 2014; 231(4): 623–636.
28. Albert P, Vahid-Ansari F, & Luckhart C. Serotonin-Prefrontal Cortical Circuitry in Anxiety and Depression Phenotypes: Pivotal Role of Pre- and Post-synaptic 5-HT1A Receptor Expression. *Frontiers in Behavioral Neuroscience*. 2014; 8: 199.

# 3

# Diagnosis and Management of Social Anxiety Disorder

Erik Feldtmann, Pier Pointdujour, Carlos Bellido, and Charles Preuss

## Contents

DOI: 10.1201/9781003333821-3

# 3.1 Background

Anxiety and fear may be beneficial emotions because they may make us more aware of potentially dangerous conditions and situations.

The American Psychiatric Association (APA) considers normal anxiety to be concern over future situations, and fear as a response to an imminent danger or trouble leading to the natural flight or fight response (1).

There is, however, a difference between normal levels of anxiety or fear, and anxiety disorders which leave a person with such excessive levels of these emotions that they impede their ability to interact with the world around them. The APA estimates that almost 30% of all adults in the U.S. will suffer from an anxiety disorder sometime during their life, making it the most common class of mental disorders (1).

The APA includes six different disorders as anxiety disorders, including panic disorder, various phobias, and generalized anxiety disorder. One such anxiety disorder is Social Anxiety Disorder (SAD), previously known as social phobia. The National Institute of Mental Health (NIMH), a part of the National Institute of Health (NIH), describes SAD to be displayed as a constant fear of social interactions or performance scenarios. This fear is particularly prevalent when these interactions or performances involve unknown people or where there may be some form of judgment. Typically, this fear leads those afflicted to believe they will behave poorly or display noticeable physical signs of anxiety that will cause further judgment and embarrassment. These possible situations tend to be disconcerting or mortifying to those with SAD, further leading them to avoid them (2).

Prior to the COVID-19 global pandemic, the NIMH, using data from the National Comorbidity Survey Replication (NCS-R) study, estimated that an average of 7.1% of adults in the U.S. will have been clinically diagnosed with SAD in the previous year, although those who identify as females tended to have higher rates than those who identify as male, 8.0% and 6.1% respectively

## Previous Year Prevalence of Social Anxiety Disorder Among U.S. Adults (2001-2003)

Data from NIH-NIMH National Comorbidity Survey Replication (NCS-R)

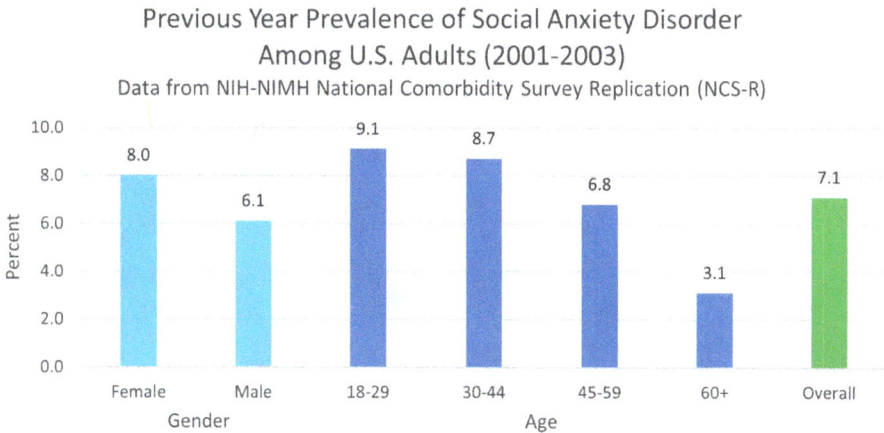

**Figure 3.1** *[Taken from www.nimh.nih.gov/health/statistics/social-anxiety-disorder.]*

(see Figure 3.1). Additionally, the study estimates that SAD will affect 12.1% of people in the U.S. over the age of 18 at some point in their life (2). Mental disorders impact people in varying degrees, leading to the APA to classify impairment as mild, moderate, or severe. Of the people surveyed in the NCS-R, the study estimated that their level of impairment rated at mild, moderate, and severe were 31.3%, 38.8%, and 29.9% respectively using the Sheehan Disability Scale (2).

People in the U.S. under the age of 18 are also not immune to mental disorders. Using the National Comorbidity Survey Adolescent Supplement (NCS-A), the study estimated that about 9.1% of teenagers ages 13 to 18.4 suffered from SAD. As with the adult population, females had a higher rate than males, at 11.2% and 7.0% respectively. The study estimated that 1.3% of the teenagers had severe impairment using the *Diagnostic and Statistical Manual of Mental Disorders*, Fourth Edition (DSM-IV) criteria (see Figure 3.2) (2). While the NCS-A only included teenagers of ages 13 to 18.4, the median age of onset of SAD in the U.S. is 13, but the age of onset for 75% of children and teens is from 8 to 15 years of age (3).

The World Mental Health (WMH) Survey Initiative, conducted by the World Health Organization (WHO), looked at mental health in 28 WHO participating countries. The socio-economic analysis showed that the highest rate of SAD was in the countries designated as high income and lowest in the low/lower-middle income (4). There are some socioeconomic and geographic parallels displayed in people with SAD around the world including prevalence in younger people who are unmarried, especially in females. In addition, the prevalence is higher in people with lower incomes and education levels.

## Lifetime Prevalence of Social Anxiety Disorder Among Adolescents (2001-2004)
### Data from NIH-NIMH National Comorbidity Survey Adolescent Supplement (NCS-A)

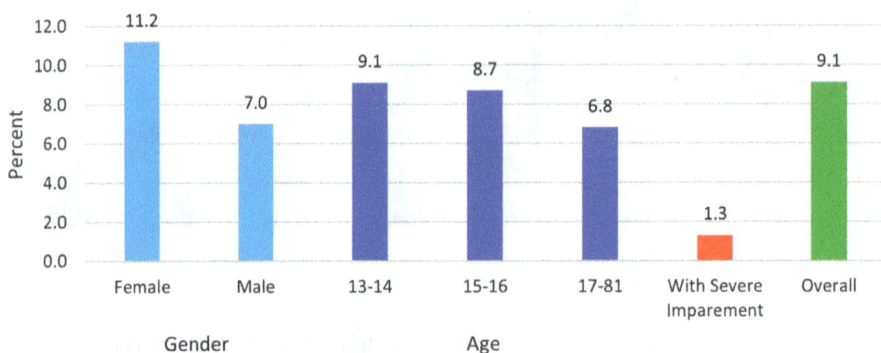

*Figure 3.2 [Taken from www.nimh.nih.gov/health/statistics/social-anxiety-disorder.]*

As mentioned before, the previous data was collected and analyzed before the outbreak of the novel COVID-19 global pandemic. With most countries instituting "lockdown" procedures at some point in 2020, it would not be surprising to have increased levels of stress, depression, and anxiety. Mental Health America (MHA) has an online screening tool for anxiety and depression, and they analyzed the data from January through September 2020 with more than 1.5 million people using both tools. While not specific to SAD, 315,220 people, or 20%, took the anxiety screening between January and September 2020, which was a 93% increase over the number of people who took the anxiety screening from January through December 2019 (5). Beyond that, the number of people who took the anxiety screen in September 2020 was 634% higher than the number who took the screening in January 2020 (6).

Of the 1.5 million people who used one of the nine screening tools, 25% identified themselves as male, 73% identified themselves as female, and 2% identified themselves as other. In April 2020, the MHA added the transgender category and between April and September 2020, 3% identified themselves as transgender. Likewise, the number of adolescents between 11 and 17 years of age who used one of the nine screening tools between January and September 2020 increased by 9% over the total amount in 2019 (See Table 3.1) (5).

At the beginning of the pandemic in the U.S., there were pockets of animosity towards Asian peoples because the spread of COVID-19 began in China. Notably, the number of Asian or Pacific Islanders who used one of the nine screening tools increased from 9% in all of 2019 to 16% in January through September 2020 (See Table 3.2) (5).

The MHA screen tool for anxiety uses the Generalized Anxiety Disorder 7-item (GAD-7) tool to screen for anxiety and to rate the severity of the symptoms.

**Table 3.1** 2019 and 2020 Use of Mental Health America Screening Tools by Age [Adapted from https://mhanational.org/sites/default/files/Spotlight%202021%20-%20COVID-19%20and%20Mental%20Health.pdf]

| Age Range | 2019 (Jan–Dec) | 2020 (Jan–Sep) |
|-----------|----------------|----------------|
| 11 to 17 | 29% | 38% |
| 18 to 24 | 32% | 32% |
| 25 to 34 | 20% | 16% |
| 35 to 44 | 9% | 7% |
| 45 to 54 | 5% | 3% |
| 55 to 64 | 3% | 2% |
| 65 and older | 1% | 1% |

*Adapted from (7)*

**Table 3.2** 2019 and 2020 Use of Mental Health America Screening Tools by Identified Ethnic Group [Adapted from https://mhanational.org/sites/default/files/Spotlight%202021%20-%20COVID-19%20and%20Mental%20Health.pdf]

| Ethnic Group | 2019 (Jan–Dec) | 2020 (Jan–Sep) |
|--------------|----------------|----------------|
| Asian or Pacific Islander | 9.13% | 15.50% |
| Black or African American (non-Hispanic) | 8.79% | 8.30% |
| Hispanic or Latina | 12.36% | 12.27% |
| More than one of the above | 5.45% | 5.03% |
| Native American or American Indian | 1.31% | 1.17% |
| Other | 3.36% | 4.70% |
| White (non-Hispanic) | 59.60% | 53.02% |

*Adapted from (8)*

In September 2020 alone, about 48% of the people who used the screening tool scored a severity rating of severe for their symptoms. Figure 3.3 shows the percentage of people who scored a severity rating of moderate to severe (5).

The MHA data from April to September 2020 showed that 70% of the people taking the screens disclosed that isolation or loneliness was the major contributor to their mental health issues (6). Studies have shown that people who expressed having feelings of loneliness developed more severe levels of social anxiety, depression, and paranoia (9).

## 3.2 Anatomy and Pathophysiology

The causes of SAD are being shown to be a complicated interaction between numerous factors. Potential causes include psychological factors, environmental

## GAD-7 Scoring Moderate to Severe Anxiety
### January - Septemeber 2020

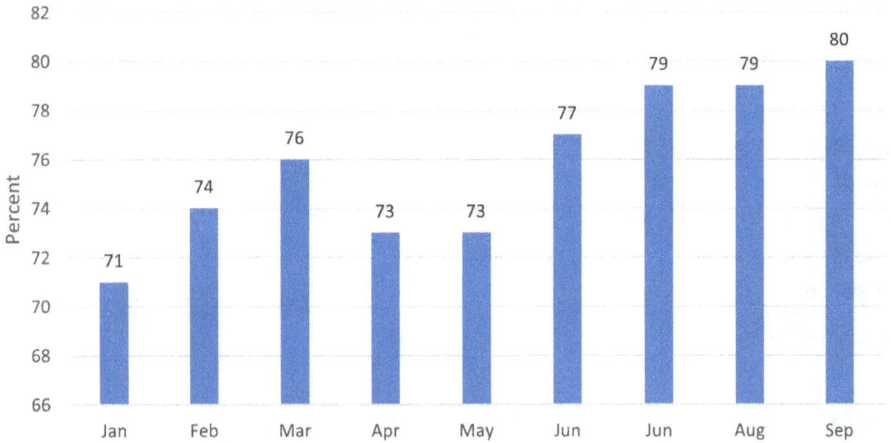

*Figure 3.3 [Data taken from the Mental Health America Generalized Anxiety Disorder 7-item (GAD-7) Tool.] Reproduced with permission from (5), please ask for permission.*

factors, developmental factors, physiological brain structure, and genetics (1). In addition, about 90% of the people suffering from SAD also suffer from other disorders. This complicates identifying the cause of SAD alone (10).

## 3.2.1 Psychological Factors

Events perceived as severely traumatic tend to have a higher potential to lead to mental health issues. A person who has been subjected to serious family conflict, physical or mental abuse, or an extremely disturbing event is more likely to develop SAD. Parents can have a huge effect on their children. There is some speculation that a person who sees or has seen their parents display anxious behavior in social circumstances may be more likely to develop the same behaviors. Also, parents who are or have been domineering or over-protective may cause their children to develop SAD signs and symptoms. Furthermore, a person whose family has SAD is more likely to develop the disorder themselves (11). SAD may be an inheritable disorder. A person whose first-degree relatives have SAD are two to six times more likely to develop the disorder (3).

## 3.2.2 Environmental Factors

People maybe more disposed to developing SAD if they have been excessively teased, bullied, rejected at home or at school, ridiculed, or otherwise humili-ated. It is also possible that new or heightened social or job-related demands may bring about initial SAD symptoms. Since the average age of onset of SAD is in adolescents, meeting new people and having more responsibilities in the academic setting could be a factor in the onset of SAD (11). Historically, racism and ethnic discrimination against African Americans and black Caribbeans has also been associated with SAD (3). As mentioned before, the onset of the COVID-19 pandemic increased discriminations against people of Asian or Pacific Islander descent resulting in a 7% increase in SAD among that group between 2019 to 2020 (5).

### 3.2.3 Developmental Factors

People who are more timid, withdrawn when dealing with novel situations, or repressed when meeting new people may be at a greater risk. Likewise, a person who has a physical appearance or condition which attracts attention, such as a person with a disfigurement, who stutters, or who has tremors, may be at a higher risk of SAD (11). It has been shown that the traits of low levels of gregariousness or high levels of negative affectivity (negative emotions and poor self-identity) are common among people with SAD. Similarly, the trait of fearing negative appraisals, and the reluctance to participate in certain behaviors may lead to a higher risk of developing SAD (3).

### 3.2.4 Brain Structure

If a person has an overactive amygdala, they may experience higher levels of fear and anxiety (11). A study published by Zhang, Suo, Yang et al. in early 2022 used high-resolution structural magnetic resonance imaging (MRI), resting-state functional MRI images, whole-brain voxel-based morphometry (VBM) analysis, and correlation and mediation analyses to look at structural and functional deficits in people with SAD as opposed to healthy people. The VBM analysis study showed that people clinically diagnosed with SAD had significant reductions in gray matter volume (GMV) in the bilateral putamen versus the people in the healthy control (HC) group. Both the putamen and amygdala are part of the basal ganglia, located in the subcortex of the brain. A large amount of evidence has been presented to document that the putamen is involved in motor and cognitive control, cognitive and emotional regulation, social learning, and more importantly for people with SAD, reward processing (reward versus punishment) which may largely influence anxiety and decision-making. (10)

### 3.2.5 Genetic Factors

Inheritable changes in DNA that do not change the DNA sequence are called epigenetics. There are many operations of epigenetics including DNA methylation (DNAm), which can inhibit the expression of some genes (8).

The origination and development of SAD has been linked to both genetic and environmental factors. One of the more common risk factors is early life adversity (ELA). Children who are abused or suffer neglect may develop long-lasting behavioral and neurobiological issues which increase their risk of developing SAD. Studies have also shown differential DNAm configurations associated with SAD. Similarly, multiple studies have linked long-lasting variances in DNAm levels with ELA (8).

In early 2021, Wiegand, Kreifelts, Munk, et al. published an epigenome-wide study which looked at DNA methylation assemblages from samples of whole blood from people suffering from SAD and ELA. The study looked at epigenetic links situations: SAD without ELA, ELA without SAD, SAD and ELA, and the severity of SAD and ELA (8).

### 3.2.5.1 Epigenetic links to SAD without ELA

The Wiegand, Kreifelts, Munk et al. study found two differentially methylated regions (DMRs) associated with SAD without ELA. The first was the coding region of the *TNXB* gene, and the second was in an intron of the *SLC43A2* gene, which is part of the solute carrier (SLC) family and encodes the essential amino acid transporter LAT4. Both genes have already been linked to panic disorder, which is another anxiety disorder. Additionally, there has been documentation showing increases in the DNAm of the *SLC43A2* gene in people suffering from panic disorder because of cognitive-behavioral therapy (CBT) treatment (8).

### 3.2.5.2 Epigenetic links to ELA without SAD

The study by Wiegand, Kreifelts, Munk et al. identified the *SLC17A3* promoter region and the *SIAH3* gene as DMRs which showed differential DNAm related to ELA without SAD by comparing people with high and low ELA. The promoter region of *SLC17A3* encodes the sodium-phosphate transporter NPT4 as part of the SLC family. The groups also performed a correlation analysis which showed a nominally significant methylation of *SLC17A3* connection with physical abuse which was not there with emotional abuse or neglect. However, the analysis did not show any relationship between methylation of *SIAH3* and emotional, physical, or sexual abuse, but did show a nominally significant relationship with emotional neglect (8).

### 3.2.5.3 Epigenetic links to SAD and ELA

The Wiegand, Kreifelts, Munk et al. study identified multiple DMRs in people with SAD and ELA, of which the two largest were on genes *MRPL28* and *C2CD2L*. *C2CD2L* encodes the transmembrane protein 24 (TMEM24), which concentrates in the endoplasmic reticulum, and has already been related to substance abuse both genetically and with DNAm levels. Even so, the team only found hypermethylation of *C2CD2L* in people diagnosed with SAD and high levels of ELA. On the other hand, control patients with high levels of ELA without SAD were the only groups to show hypermethylation of the *MRP28L* gene (8).

### 3.2.5.4 Epigenetic links to the severity of SAD and ELA

The study by Wiegand, Kreifelts, Munk et al. detected two DMRs related to severity of both SAD and ELA which were located upstream of the *ADAMTS16* and *GALR1* genes. *ADAMTS16* encodes a member of the disintegrin and metalloproteinase with thrombospondin motifs (ADAMTS) family of multidomain extracellular protease enzymes, while *GALR1* encodes the galanin receptor type 1. Research has linked *ADAMTS16* with hypertension, which has been associated with ELA and early-onset SAD. The group performed a mediation analysis on the *ADAMTS16* and *GALR1* genes and found that there was no statistical proof for a mediation of the elevated risk of ELA or SAD because of the effect of DNAm of these genes (8).

## 3.3 Diagnosis

In 2022, the APA published a list of ten criteria (A-J) to use in the diagnosis of SAD.

### 3.3.1 Criterion A

Pronounced fear or anxiety related to social events which may lead to scrutiny by others. (3)

Scrutiny in this case typically means being thought of in a negative way, having the patient's imperfections or the faults of his or her actions being assessed in a negative light, and/or being embarrassed. People with SAD display fear and anxiety in the following situations:

- Meeting or being with unfamiliar people,
- Going to parties or social events,
- Going on a date,
- Going to a store to return a purchase,
- Having to begin talking to someone,
- Making eye contact with people (11).

It should be noted that many children have anxiety when dealing with adults or children considerably older than themselves. To be diagnosed with SAD, children must experience *significant* fear or anxiety around children about their own age (3).

Some people with SAD experience extreme fear and anxiety only when they are speaking or performing in front of people. This is known as performance-only

SAD. This version of SAD may impact people in their careers, such as with musicians, dancers, or athletes, or in work or academic situations where there is a need to present information in front of others. Conversely, people who suffer with this specific subtype of SAD have no issues with typical social situations unrelated to performances (3).

## 3.3.2 Criterion B

Fears about being negatively evaluated because of how his or her anxiety symptoms will be evident. (3)

Most people have blushed when they are embarrassed or have had sweaty palms when they are nervous, but they are not particularly anxious or fearful of these times. People with SAD, however, are worried about humiliating themselves in most social situations or they are afraid that their anxiety will be noticed. People with SAD fear that their symptoms of anxiety, including blushing, sweating, trembling, or having a shaky voice, will embarrass them (11). Some people with SAD are afraid of offending other people by their actions. This alone does not result in a diagnosis of SAD. Cultural differences in social interactions may play a role in what is considered abnormal. Some cultures demonstrate some anxiety or avoidance actions as a sign of respect, for example not looking an elder directly in the eyes (3).

## 3.3.3 Criterion C

Fear and anxiety consistently occur in social situations. (3)

Under normal circumstances, some people are extroverts who have less problems in social situations, while others are introverts who naturally have more anxiety during them. On the other hand, people with SAD experience fear or anxiety in *most* social situations. In some cases, just being seen by or making eye contact with others can cause anxiety and fear that they will be seen in a negative light, such as when:

- Dining or drinking in places where there are other people,
- Using a public restroom,
- Entering a room, especially when the people there are seated (11).

## 3.3.4 Criterion D

Social situations are routinely avoided or experienced with deep fear or anxiety. (3)

People with more severe symptoms of SAD will avoid social situations whenever possible, especially if they are going to be the center of attention (11). In the case of avoidance, some people with SAD will have broad avoidance patterns while others may have more indirect avoidance, for example shifting the attention to someone else, avoiding eye contact, or redoing their speech an irrational number of times (3).

### 3.3.5 Criterion E

Fear or anxiety is disproportionate to the real threat of the social situation. (3)

Most people get anxious over certain situations, such as making a major life decision or deciding to change careers, and that is a normal reaction. People with SAD may begin feeling anxious and fearful well before the time of the social situation. In addition, the people will believe that the social situation will lead to a negative contact with the worst possible results (11). It is important to take cultural beliefs and practices into account when judging a person's anxiety before a social event because, in some cultures, anxiety related to a social event may be considered correct in certain situations and may even be considered a sign of respect (3).

### 3.3.6 Criterion F

Fear, anxiety, or avoidance last continually for 6 months or more. (3)

People with SAD may experience changes in their symptoms over time or increased symptoms related to a specific event (11). However, if the fear or anxiety is transitory, it is considered normal social fears and not SAD (3).

### 3.3.7 Criterion G

Fear, anxiety, or avoidance result in clinically considerable distress or impairment in social, occupational, or other important areas of life. (3)

People with SAD have so much fear and anxiety about social situations that they avoid normal social situations such as relationships, work, school, or even daily routines (11). It is important to remember that this criterion applies to anxiety about social occurrences that occur regularly in the person's job or school, or in their relationships. If the social situation a person is afraid of or anxious about does not occur regularly, this criterion is not met. On the other hand, if a person loses a job or is skipped over for a raise or promotion because they cannot perform in a social setting, then this criterion is met (3).

### 3.3.8 Criterion H

Fear, anxiety, or avoidance is not the result of the physiological effects of a substance or a medical condition (3).

The use or abuse of legal medications or illegal drugs may induce anxiety or worsen existing fears and anxiety. Even ingesting caffeine or smoking/vaping nicotine may cause or worsen anxiety. Similarly, trying to quit any addictive substance may produce abnormal levels of anxiety, but this does not mean that the person has SAD, based on the absence of other criteria (11).

## 3.3.9 Criterion I

Fear, anxiety, or avoidance is not more appropriately attributed as a symptom of another mental disorder, such as panic disorder, body dysmorphic disorder, or autism spectrum disorder. (3)

## 3.3.10 Criterion J

The fear, anxiety, or avoidance is not related to another medical condition (e.g., Parkinson's disease, obesity, disfigurement from burns or injury) or is excessive with another medical condition. (3)

A person suffering from SAD may experience physical symptoms although they may not always be present. Possible signs of SAD may include, but are not limited to blushing, muscle tension, tachycardia, shaking, sweating, nausea or vomiting, dyspnea, or faintness or disequilibrium. For children, the fear or anxiety about interacting with adults may be shown by, but is not limited to: continuous crying, having temper tantrums, clinging to parents, freezing completely, shrinking back, or refusing to speak at all. It is important to point out that, when dealing with children, shyness, uneasiness, and even alarm are not necessarily indicative of SAD (11).

The World Mental Health (WMH) Survey Initiative, conducted by the World Health Organization (WHO), identified that there can be some differences between the patterns of impairment in countries around the world. There were, however, several similarities around the world including, onset and young age, persistence, and impairment. The study further revealed that the threshold for diagnosis is very close irrespective of geography or income levels in a country (4).

In addition to the physical symptoms, people suffering from SAD can have the following complications:

- Low self-esteem,
- An inability to be assertive,
- Speaking negatively about oneself,
- Being oversensitive to criticism,
- Inadequate social skills,
- Excessive tendency to withdraw from society,
- Difficulty with social relationships,
- Low scholarly and/or employment accomplishments,
- Substance abuse (11).

Additionally, reports indicate that SAD increases the risk of suicidal thoughts and suicide attempts among U.S. teenagers of white Hispanics, regardless of family income and the presence of major depression. This higher risk is not prevalent for U.S. white non-Hispanic teenagers (3).

People suffering from SAD may also be suffering with other disorders such as major depressive disorder (especially from chronic isolation), other anxiety disorders, substance abuse disorder, schizophrenia, and some eating disorders which cause the person to avoid eating in front of others. SAD will typically develop before other disorders, except for individual phobias and separation anxiety disorder (3).

There are some tendencies related to gender, although age of onset is not one of them. Women report having a larger number of social fears than men, more prevalence of major depressive disorder, and other anxiety disorders. Instead, men report that they are afraid of dating more than women, have oppositional defiant disorders, conduct disorder or antisocial personality disorder, and have paruresis (difficulty urinating in the presence of others). Men also tend to use alcohol or drugs to relieve the symptoms of SAD more often than women (3).

Prior to giving a diagnosis of SAD, clinicians should review disorders which may present symptoms similar to SAD and rule them out. These include, but are not limited to the following:

- Acute stress disorder,
- Agoraphobia,
- Delusional disorder (previously known as paranoid disorder),
- Generalized anxiety disorder,
- Panic disorder,
- Posttraumatic stress disorder,
- Separation anxiety disorder,
- Specific phobias (3).

## 3.4 Current Management

Many people may not realize that there are safe and effective treatments available for SAD (1). The results of the 2007 survey conducted by the Anxiety and Depression Association of America (ADAA) show that 36% of people with SAD stated they had signs and symptoms of the disorder for 10 years or more before attempting to get help (12).

After the onset of the global COVID-19 pandemic, Mental Health America reported that between January and September 2020, only 43% of adults with mental illnesses obtained treatment, and only 40% of teenagers obtained treatment for depression. In addition, almost 11% of the people in the U.S. with mental health disorders were uninsured, which is the first time the percentage has increased since the passage of the Affordable Care Act (ACA) (6).

People suffering from almost all types of anxiety disorders, including SAD, improve from two types of treatment either separately or in conjunction with each other. The first treatment method is psychotherapy, which is talk therapy designed to change the way people think and act, so they do not feel as anxious or fearful (1).

The second is the use of medications to relieve the symptoms of anxiety disorders and may include antianxiety drugs (used only for a short time) and antidepressants. In some cases, a beta-blocker may be used to relieve heart-related symptoms (1). Treatment of symptoms of anxiety with medications is predominantly safe and effective, although it sometimes can take trying several different drugs to identify the best one for the patient. The Medical Expenditure Panel Survey (MEPS) of 2013 collected data on the expense and utilization of health care in the U.S. and found that more than one in six people take a psychiatric medication (antidepressant or antianxiety). In fact, the survey found that 12% of adults stated that they filled a prescription for antidepressants, making this type of drug the most common psychiatric drug used. National survey data from the Centers for Disease Control and Prevention (CDC) reported that between 2011 and 2014, almost one in nine people of all ages in the U.S. stated that they had taken at least one antidepressant in the previous month (13).

## 3.4.1 Psychotherapy Treatment Methods

### 3.4.1.1 Cognitive Behavioral Therapy (CBT)

Cognitive behavioral therapy (CBT) is a very effective, long-lasting evidence-based treatment method designed so that people can understand and learn to change their patterns of behavior and thinking, often to reduce anxiety or negative thoughts. A typical program of CBT will run for 12 to 16 weeks during which time the person owns part of the process of recovery, has personal control over their future, and masters the skills needed to participate in a social world. The usual content for a CBT program includes having the person read about their disorder, keeping records of issues and thoughts between appointments, and finishing homework assignments by practicing techniques learned in the clinician-led therapy sessions (14).

The COVID-19 global pandemic forced most governments to impose mandatory lockdown periods where there were limits on in-person social interactions. Increased mental health issues related to anxiety and stress as well as fear of contracting COVID-19 were reported in the general population, especially in students, during lockdown periods. In addition, there were widespread concerns that people with preexisting mental health issues might fare worse than those without pre-existing issues (15).

### 3.4.1.2 Internet Delivered Cognitive Behavioral Therapy (ICBT)

Many times, people suffering from SAD do not receive treatment because the standard treatment involves repeated social contact. In addition, barriers to treatment may include the expense, especially for the uninsured, and distance, as treatment locations may be far away. The widespread use of the internet allows for online cognitive-behavioral therapy treatments, making therapy more readily accessible. In a 2017–2018 study in Sweden, internet-delivered cognitive behavioral therapy (ICBT) for SAD in young people ages 10 to 17 and their parents was studied versus active comparators, using internet-delivered supportive therapy (ISUPPORT). Both forms of treatment included ten online modules for the youth, five separate modules for the parents, and three video call sessions with a therapist. The results showed that ICBT was substantially more effective in reducing symptom severity than ISUPPORT (16).

### 3.4.1.3 Exposure Therapy

Exposure therapy, which is a form of cognitive behavioral therapy, exposes people to situations they are afraid of a little at a time. The goal is to desensitize them to these situations to reduce their fear and anxiety (14).

### 3.4.1.4 Virtual Reality Exposure Therapy (VRET)

The most common and most efficacious treatment for SAD has been shown to be CBT in conjunction with exposure therapy, either in individual or group sessions. However, with high levels in the safety and ease of use, virtual reality (VR) is being used in exposure therapy (VRET). Likewise, VR's use of multiple sensory stimulation and elimination of real-world sensory input allows people to perceive they are being exposed to real or almost real social situations, and to become completely immersed in the experience. Studies on the use of VR in exposure therapy showed that self-guided VRET produced reductions in SAD severity, job interview anxiety, and trait worry when used as an independent treatment as compared to people who had no treatment. Yet some clinicians avoid in-vivo exposure therapy because it is hard to control and difficult to assess the effects of the therapy at the time. Also, patients may reject this form of therapy because they find the exposure intolerable. Arnfred et al. are conducting a study of the use of VRET versus *in vivo* in group exposure therapy in Denmark. The study was started in February 2019 with a standard 14-week cognitive behavior therapy program with eight exposure therapy sessions. The subjects were randomly placed in either *in vivo* or VR programs with concealed placement sequences. The study is expected to end in June 2023 after follow-up assessments of the treatment (17). In another study in 2021, Zainal et al. compared the use of self-guided virtual reality exposure therapy (VRET) and people on the waiting list for therapy in patients with SAD and related comorbidities. The results showed that the self-guided VRET had no effect on depression (18).

### 3.4.1.5 Acceptance and Commitment Therapy (ACT)

Acceptance and commitment therapy combined acceptance and mindfulness approaches with commitment and behavior changes to teach people with SAD to cope with their negative thoughts and feelings and to deal with their unwanted sensations. Mindfulness is the practice of purposely focusing on the present moment and experiencing life without evaluation. The goal of ACT is to have a person develop the tools needed to accept their experiences and put them in an alternate context, to get greater clarity about personal values, and to follow through with essential behavioral changes (14).

### 3.4.1.6 Dialectical Behavioral Therapy (DBT)

Using a combination of approaches taken from cognitive behavior, meditation, and mindfulness, dialectical behavioral therapy (DBT) helps a person accept situations and make necessary changes to their life. DBT is usually a combination of individual and group therapy to teach people interpersonal effectiveness, how to deal with distress, and how to regulate their emotions (14).

## 3.4.2 Medication Treatments

There are varying classes of medications that can be used to treat SAD: selective serotonin reuptake inhibitors (SSRIs), serotonin-norepinephrine reuptake inhibitors (SNRIs), benzodiazepines, and tricyclic antidepressants (13).

### 3.4.2.1 Selective Serotonin Reuptake Inhibitors (SSRIs)

To alleviate symptoms, selective serotonin reuptake inhibitors (SSRIs) block the reuptake of serotonin by specific nerve cells in the brain. As a result, more serotonin is available in the body, which helps to improve mood. SSRIs are regarded as efficacious treatment for all anxiety disorders. SSRIs include drugs such as citalopram, escitalopram, fluoxetine, paroxetine, and sertraline, and have been shown to have less side effects than tricyclic antidepressants. The most frequently experienced side effects of SSRIs are insomnia or sleepiness, sexual dysfunction, and increases in weight (13).

### 3.4.2.2 Serotonin-Norepinephrine Reuptake Inhibitors (SNRIs)

The serotonin-norepinephrine reuptake inhibitors (SNRIs) are noteworthy because they increase serotonin and norepinephrine by inhibiting their reuptake into cells in the brain. SNRIs, such as venlafaxine and duloxetine, are considered equally as effective as SSRIs and are usually one of the first medications to be tried for treating anxiety disorders. Common side effects associated with SNRIs are stomach upset, insomnia, headache, sexual dysfunction, increases in weight, and small increase in blood pressure (13).

### 3.4.2.3 Benzodiazepines

Benzodiazepines are extremely effective in facilitating relaxation and decreasing muscle tension and other common physical symptoms of anxiety. Benzodiazepines include alprazolam, clonazepam, diazepam, and lorazepam, and are usually used for short-term management of anxiety. However, benzodiazepines are not recommended for use in the treatment of post-traumatic stress disorder. Problems with benzodiazepines have been associated with long-term use because the dosage may need to be increased over time to stay effective, which could result in tolerance, dependency issues, and increased risk for respiratory compromise (13).

### 3.4.2.4 Tricyclic Antidepressants

While tricyclic antidepressants may be efficacious for some anxiety disorders, they are not effective for Social Anxiety Disorder (SAD). Tricyclic antidepressants, including amitriptyline, imipramine, and nortriptyline, may cause significant side effects such as orthostatic hypotension (drop in blood pressure on standing), constipation, urinary retention, dry mouth, and blurred vision. Due to their side effect profile and narrow therapeutic index, TCAs are often avoided in several populations or comorbid conditions (13). Table 3.3 is a summary of SAD pharmacological treatments.

**Table 3.3** Pharmacologic Treatments of SAD

| Class | Examples | Mechanism of Action | Adverse Effects |
|---|---|---|---|
| Selective serotonin reuptake inhibitors (SSRIs) | Fluoxetine, sertraline, paroxetine, citalopram, escitalopram | Inhibition of serotonin reuptake in the neuronal synaptic cleft | Headache, Sexual dysfunction, SIADH, Serotonin syndrome, Diarrhea, Nausea |
| Serotonin and norepinephrine reuptake inhibitors (SNRIs) | Venlafaxine, duloxetine | Inhibition of serotonin and norepinephrine reuptake in the neuronal synaptic cleft | Similar to SSRIs, Increased blood pressure, Insomnia, Stimulant effect |
| Monoamine oxidase inhibitors | Isocarboxazid, moclobemide, phenelzine, selegiline, tranylcypromine | Unclear, hypothesis is that MAOIs increase dopaminergic, noradrenergic, and serotonergic neurotransmission | Serotonin syndrome, Hypertensive crisis, Overdose |
| Benzodiazepines | Lorazepam, alprazolam, diazepam | GABA$_A$ receptor agonist | Drowsiness, Respiratory depression, Addictive potential |
| GABA analogues | Gabapentin, pregabalin | Interacts with an auxiliary subunit of voltage-sensitive Ca2+ channels in nerves | Central Nervous System (CNS) depression, Dizziness, Drowsiness, Respiratory depression |

### 3.4.3 Complementary and Alternative Treatments

The use of complementary and alternative medicine (CAM) is expanding among patients and clinicians who seek added ways to treat anxiety, depression, and other mental health disorders. Complementary health care is used alongside conventional medicine, while alternative health care is used instead of conventional medicine (20).

#### 3.4.3.1 Relaxation Techniques and Meditation

Relaxation techniques may result in some amount of short-term reduction of anxiety in some people, especially for older adults (20). With repetitive use and training, such techniques can be beneficial in reducing levels of anxiety when used in conjunction with cognitive behavioral therapy (CBT) or medication. Meditation is another similar practice that can help to improve mindfulness, which can be helpful to reduce symptoms of anxiety and depression in adults (20).

#### 3.4.3.2 Yoga

Yoga uses physical postures, breathing exercises, meditation, and a distinct philosophy to improve overall health of the body. It is one of the top ten practices of complementary and alternative medicine today. It may also aid in reducing symptoms of anxiety and depression (20)

Other ways of managing the anxiety of SAD may be through support groups, education about the disorder itself, and avoidance of aggravating medications or substances such as caffeine. Support groups, whether in-person or online, may give a person a chance to share experiences and coping techniques with others (1).

#### 3.4.3.3 Logging or Journaling

Keeping a log or journal is a typical part of CBT, but can help before and after CBT treatment as well. Writing about what situations cause stress or anxiety, and what things seem to improve symptoms, may help the patient better understand their condition, as well as the clinician.

Identifying and making time for the things a person enjoys doing can further assist in the reduction of stress and anxiety. Setting priorities and carefully managing time can afford a person more time and the energy to do the things they enjoy (11).

## 3.5 Conclusion

People with SAD fear public events or encounters which leads to avoidance of social situations or causes them to endure intense feelings of anxiety. This impedes their ability to interact with the world around them. Research into what triggers the disorder is still developing, but the current body of evidence suggests a multitude of potential causes ranging from psychological factors such as negative experiences, to environmental factors, or even genetic or anatomical variances. Thankfully, there have also been advancements in management and treatment of the disorder, with options such as psychotherapy and medication available. Many find alternative methods of treatment like relaxation techniques and yoga to further be beneficial in managing SAD when used in conjunction with the conventional treatments. In light of the recent global pandemic, combating Social Anxiety Disorder is now more important than ever. As the medical field becomes more attuned to this disorder, there have been great strides towards alleviating symptoms and improving the lives of those affected.

# References

1. American Psychiatric Association. (n.d.). *What are anxiety disorders?* Psychiatry.org. Retrieved May 19, 2022, from https://psychiatry.org/patients-families/anxiety-disorders/what-are-anxiety-disorders
2. U.S. Department of Health and Human Services. (n.d.). *Social anxiety disorder.* National Institute of Mental Health. Retrieved May 21, 2022, from https://www.nimh .nih.gov/health/statistics/social-anxiety-disorder
3. American Psychiatric Association Publishing. (2022). Social Anxiety Disorder. In *Diagnostic and Statistical Manual of Mental Disorders* (5th Edition, Text Revisions, pp. 229–235).
4. Stein, D. J., Lim, C. C. W., Roest, A. M., de Jonge, P., Aguilar-Gaxiola, S., Al-Hamzawi, A., Alonso, J., Benjet, C., Bromet, E. J., Bruffaerts, R., de Girolamo, G., Florescu, S., Gureje, O., Haro, J. M., Harris, M. G., He, Y., Hinkov, H., Horiguchi, I., Hu, C., & WHO World Mental Health Survey Collaborators. (2017, July 31). *The cross-national epidemiology of Social Anxiety Disorder: Data from the World Mental Health Survey Initiative.* National Library of Medicine. Retrieved May 20, 2022, from https://www .ncbi.nlm.nih.gov/pmc/articles/PMC5535284/
5. Mental Health America. (2021). *2021 Covid-19 and Mental Health: A Growing Crisis.* Mental Health America. Retrieved May 21, 2022, from https://mhanational.org/sites/ default/files/Spotlight%202021%20-%20COVID-19%20and%20Mental%20Health.pdf
6. Mental Health America. (2020, October 20). *Number of people reporting anxiety and depression nationwide since start of pandemic hits all-time high in September, hitting young people hardest.* www.mhanational.org. Retrieved May 23, 2022, from https:// www.mhanational.org/number-people-reporting-anxiety-and-depression-nationwide -start-pandemic-hits-all-time-high
7. U.S. Department of Health and Human Services. (2022, June 2). *First degree relative.* National Human Genome Research Institute. Retrieved June 2, 2022, from https:// www.genome.gov/genetics-glossary/First-Degree-Relative
8. Wiegand, A., Kreifelts, B., Munk, M.H.J., & Nieratschker, V. (2021, February 4). *DNA methylation differences associated with social anxiety disorder and early life adversity.* National Library of Medicine. Retrieved May 23, 2022, from https://pubmed.ncbi .nlm.nih.gov/33542190/
9. Eres, R., Lim, M. H., Lanjam, S., Jillard, C., & Bates, G. (2021, April 7). *Loneliness and emotion regulation: implications of having social anxiety disorder.* Taylor and Francis Online. Retrieved May 21, 2022, from https://doi.org/10.1080/00049530.2021.1904498

10. Zhang, X., Suo, X., Yang, X., et al. (2022, January 21). *Structural and functional deficits and couplings in the cortico-striato-thalamo-cerebellar circuitry in social anxiety disorder*. National Library of Medicine. Retrieved May 23, 2022, from https://pubmed.ncbi.nlm.nih.gov/35064097/

11. Mayo Clinic Staff. (n.d.). *Social anxiety disorder (social phobia)*. Mayo Clinic. Retrieved May 21, 2022, from https://www.mayoclinic.org/diseases-conditions/social-anxiety-disorder/symptoms-causes/syc-20353561?p=1

12. Anxiety and Depression Association of America, ADAA. (n.d.). *Did You Know?* Anxiety and Depression Association of America, ADAA. Retrieved May 21, 2022, from https://adaa.org/understanding-anxiety/facts-statistics

13. Anxiety and Depression Association of America, ADAA. (n.d.). *Medication options*. Anxiety and Depression Association of America, ADAA. Retrieved May 30, 2022, from https://adaa.org/find-help/treatment-help/medication-options

14. Anxiety and Depression Association of America, ADAA. (n.d.). *Types of therapy*. Anxiety and Depression Association of America, ADAA. Retrieved May 30, 2022, from https://adaa.org/find-help/treatment-help/types-of-therapy

15. Samantaray, N. N., Kar, N., & Mishra, S. R. (2022, February 12). *A follow-up study on treatment effects of cognitive-behavioral therapy on Social Anxiety Disorder: Impact of covid-19 fear during post-lockdown period*. National Institute of Mental Health. Retrieved May 31, 2022, from https://www.ncbi.nlm.nih.gov/pmc/articles/PMC8840826/

16. Nordh, M., Wahlund, T., Jolstedt, M., Sahlin, H., Bjureberg, J., Ahlen, J., & Serlachius, E. (2021, May 21). *Therapist-guided internet-delivered cognitive behavioral therapy vs internet-delivered supportive therapy for children and adolescents with social anxiety disorder: A randomized clinical trial*. National Library of Medicine. Retrieved May 21, 2022, from https://pubmed.ncbi.nlm.nih.gov/33978699/

17. Arnfred, B., Bang, P., Hjorthøj, C., Christensen, C. W., Moeller, K. S., Hvenegaard, M., & Nordentoft, M. (2022). Group cognitive behavioural therapy with virtual reality exposure versus group cognitive behavioural therapy with in vivo exposure for social anxiety disorder and agoraphobia: A protocol for a randomised clinical trial. *BMJ open*, *12*(2), e051147. https://doi.org/10.1136/bmjopen-2021-051147

18. Zainal, N. H., Chan, W. W., Saxena, A. P., Taylor, C. B., & Newman, M. G. (2021, October 6). *Pilot randomized trial of self-guided virtual reality exposure therapy for Social Anxiety Disorder*. National Library of Medicine. Retrieved May 23, 2022, from https://www.ncbi.nlm.nih.gov/pmc/articles/PMC8759454/

19. American Psychological Association. (2017, July 31). *Eye movement desensitization and reprocessing (EMDR) therapy*. Clinical Practice Guideline for the Treatment of Posttraumatic Stress Disorder. Retrieved June 3, 2022, from https://www.apa.org/ptsd-guideline/treatments/eye-movement-reprocessing

20. Anxiety and Depression Association of America, ADAA. (n.d.). *Integrative behavioral health*. Anxiety and Depression Association of America, ADAA. Retrieved May 30, 2022, from https://adaa.org/find-help/treatment-help/integrative-behavioral-health

# Anxiety Disorders
## Symptoms and Causes

Rena Jiang, Katherine Tsay, Steven Herd-Bond,
Carlos Bellido, and Charles Preuss

## Contents

## 4.1 Introduction

Panic disorder (PD) is an anxiety disorder characterized by recurrent panic attacks. Panic disorder is described in the American Psychiatric Association's *Diagnostic and Statistical Manual of Mental Disorders*, Fifth Edition (DSM-V) (1) as recurrent panic attacks greater than or equal to one panic attack with one or more of the following: greater than one month of preoccupation with another panic attack, or significant maladaptive behavior related to the panic attacks. Traditionally, panic attacks are defined in the DSM-V as "a discrete period of intense fear with four or more of the required symptoms developing abruptly and reaching a peak within 10 minutes." The symptoms are described in further detail in the *Symptoms* section of this chapter.

A panic attack with more than four of the required symptoms can be classified as a full-symptom panic attack. An attack consisting of fewer than four symptoms is called a limited-symptom attack. Panic attacks can happen both within and outside the context of diagnosed panic disorder and can be either provoked or unprovoked. Triggers for provoked attacks may vary from person to person and may also be culturally dependent. Unexpected attacks may feel like they happen out of nowhere and the individual may not notice a cause

DOI: 10.1201/9781003333821-4

or a trigger, whereas expected panic attacks occur after exposure to a known trigger or stressor for that person (e.g., public speaking, large crowds). Panic attacks may also vary widely in terms of severity and symptoms.

Panic disorder is often associated with agoraphobia, but the two disorders can occur separately. This chapter will focus on panic disorder.

## 4.2  Etiology and Pathogenesis

In order to understand the etiology of PD, it is important to understand that the fight-or-flight response that is experienced during a panic attack, as well as fear and anxiety, is an evolutionary adaptive response developed to deal with danger (2). These responses are important in dealing with real dangers and would never want to be completely eliminated. However, the unwanted overactivation of these systems can cause great distress in modern living and can be a hindrance to daily living when not appropriately managed. The fight-or flight response that is typically overactivated during a panic attack provides a series of adaptations that would usually help an individual to either attack or evade a dangerous situation. These manifestations can include increased heart rate, faster respirations, and increased blood flow to muscles. One model that has been helpful to describe how evolutionary responses to danger correlate to current threats responses is the Threat Imminence Model by Fanselow and colleagues (3,4). Recognizing the role these systems play in responding to threats can help increase understanding of the susceptibility of an individual to developing a pathological panic disorder.

Although the precise etiology has yet to be elucidated, scientists hypothesize a neurobiological basis of PD that involves gene–environment interactions that contribute to the dysfunctional processing of emotions (5). Several elements of the neurobiological basis of PD include genetic vulnerability, epigenetic mechanisms, temperament, autonomic reactivity, neurotransmitter functioning, and psychosocial factors (Figure 4.1).

The current body of evidence does not suggest biological determinism. PD may run in families, but it does not necessarily mean an individual will develop the disorder. However, there is strong evidence of a genetic component to PD, including higher rates of PD in first-degree relatives of patients with PD compared to relatives of healthy subjects (6). Additionally, a twin study by Torgersen in 1983 showed higher concordance for monozygotic compared to dizygotic twins (31% and 0% respectively) (7). Genome-wide association studies (GWAS) have identified many potential loci of genetic vulnerability. Because neurotransmitter systems have been successfully targeted in the treatment of PD, it has been hypothesized that genetic vulnerability in these systems may underpin the etiology of PD. Indeed, the Val158Met polymorphism of catechol-O-methyltransferase (COMT)—a gene involved in prefrontal cortex dopamine neurotransmission—confers susceptibility to PD (8).

# Pathogenesis of Panic Disorder

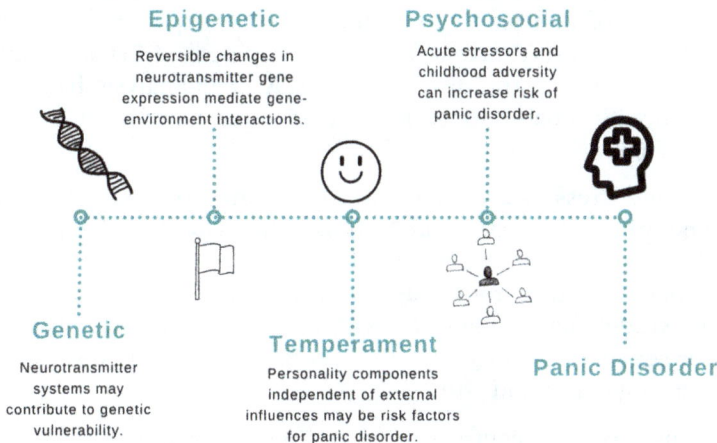

**Epigenetic**

Reversible changes in neurotransmitter gene expression mediate gene-environment interactions.

**Psychosocial**

Acute stressors and childhood adversity can increase risk of panic disorder.

**Genetic**

Neurotransmitter systems may contribute to genetic vulnerability.

**Temperament**

Personality components independent of external influences may be risk factors for panic disorder.

**Panic Disorder**

*Figure 4.1 Pathogenesis of panic disorder.*

The orexin 2 receptor gene—which is involved in arousal regulation—also appears to confer susceptibility (9).

Epigenetic mechanisms, which refer to reversible changes in gene expression that preserve the DNA sequence, serve as a mediator in gene–environment interactions. Hypomethylation of the gene that encodes MAO-A, an enzyme that metabolizes neurotransmitters, is associated with PD in women and can be normalized with cognitive behavioral therapy (CBT) (10). In addition, negative life events that increase risk of developing PD are linked to glutamate decarboxylase 1 (GAD1) gene hypomethylation (8). GAD1 is an enzyme that catalyzes synthesis of gamma-aminobutyric acid (GABA), an inhibitory neurotransmitter that is deficient in anxiety disorders.

A look at fear and anxiety at the neuroanatomical level shows a number of neural structures and mechanisms involved in a fear network that have been shown to contribute to fear responses in animals. These same mechanisms have been hypothesized to contribute to fear and anxiety in humans and may have a role in development of panic disorder. The neuroanatomical hypothesis by Gorman (5,11) focuses on the amygdala and its projections to the hypothalamus, hippocampus, and prefrontal cortex, showing that these areas are responsible for responses similar to those seen in panic attacks.

Temperament is a component of personality that determines behaviors related to emotionality and is relatively independent of external influences or learning. High behavioral inhibition (i.e., neophobic tendencies) is a weak childhood predictor of later development of anxiety disorders such as PD (12).

According to a systematic review of PD and major depressive disorder, harm avoidance and low self-directedness are also associated with mood and anxiety symptoms (13). Neuroticism, a personality trait characterized by poor stress resilience and increased reactivity to stressors, and anxiety sensitivity, which is a fear of behaviors associated with the experience of anxiety, are both reported to be risk factors for the development of PD and may even be early manifestations of the disease (14,15). A meta-analysis has also shown that children with separation anxiety are 3.5 times more likely to develop PD in adulthood (16).

Although acute stressors are known to trigger onset of PD, such as the loss of a loved one, physical threats, and illnesses, the evidence related to the effect of chronic stress on PD remains largely preclinical. It has been shown, however, that people with chronic pain often have a comorbid anxiety disorder (17). Other studies have shown that childhood adversity such as a history of physical or sexual abuse increases the risk of PD in adulthood (18), as well as smoking during childhood (19).

However, there is some controversy regarding how much of this is still due to biological influence. Some of this controversy comes from studies looking at laboratory provocation of panic attacks. Given that it can be difficult to observe a panic attack happening under natural circumstances, panic attacks can be provoked by researchers. This can consist of having participants breathe carbon dioxide rich air (20). These studies have shown heightened physiological responses in most people including increased heart rate and rapid breathing. However, only certain participants experienced panic attacks, mainly those vulnerable to or previously diagnosed with PD. It has been suggested that the laboratory provocation triggers an underlying biological dysfunction, but this idea is controversial. While there appears to be a greater likelihood of a panic attack in response to provocation among those with PD versus those without, it is not clear that this is from underlying biological dysfunction.

Learning processes during development have also been theorized to play a role in the etiology of PD. Early learning experiences may heighten future susceptibility to PD and are thought to be involved in the transition from an initial panic attack to developing full-blown PD. Evidence suggests that those who go on to develop PD are more likely than those who do not develop PD to have experienced caregivers in their youth who either modeled or reinforced sick role behaviors in response to anxiety (21). Barlow's integrated model (as well as later updates based on a modern learning theory perspective by Bouton and colleagues) considers a myriad of factors that interact to lead to the development of PD from both distal and proximal perspectives (2,22,23). These models have been highly influential in describing and bringing together many of the vulnerability areas seen in PD development. These models assume that genetic susceptibility combined with early learning experiences suggesting that the environment is uncontrollable and unpredictable combine to increase an individual's susceptibility to PD.

## 4.3 Diagnosis

The 12-month prevalence of PD in adults has been placed at 1–3%. The life-time prevalence has been placed at 3–7%, with women on the higher end and men on the lower end of the spectrum (24,25). PD is diagnosed via criteria outlined by the DSM-V, as described below (1):

A. Recurrent unexpected panic attack
B. At least one of the attacks has been followed by a month or more of one or both of the following:
   a. Persistent concern or worry about additional panic attacks or their consequences (e.g., losing control, having a heart attack, "going crazy").
   b. A significant maladaptive change in behavior related to the attacks (e.g., behaviors designed to avoid having panic attacks, such as avoidance of exercise or unfamiliar situations).
C. The disturbance is not attributable to the physiological effects of a substance (e.g., medication or illicit drug) or another medical condition (e.g., hyperthyroidism, cardiopulmonary disorders).
D. The disturbance is not better explained by another mental disorder. For example, the panic attacks do not occur only in response to:
   a. Feared social situations, as in social anxiety disorder
   b. Circumscribed phobic objects or situations, as in specific phobia
   c. Obsessions, as in obsessive-compulsive disorder (OCD)
   d. Reminders of traumatic events, as in post-traumatic stress disorder (PTSD)
   e. Separation from attachment figures, as in separation anxiety disorder

The Severity Measure for PD Adult from the DSM-V is a scale that can accompany clinical assessment for individuals 18 years and older (1). It involves the patient filling out a ten-item questionnaire about their thoughts, feelings, and behaviors regarding panic attacks. Each item on the measure is rated on a 5-point scale (0=Never, 1=Occasionally, 2=Half of the time, 3=Most of the time, 4=All of the time). The total score ranges from 0–40 points, with a higher score corresponding to a higher severity of panic disorder. This measure was created to help diagnose PD during the initial patient encounter, as well as a marker to monitor treatment progression.

Unfortunately, there are high rates of missed diagnoses or misdiagnoses. This is partially due to the high prevalence of comorbidity with other mental health conditions (24). The diagnosis of PD is differentiated from other causes of panic attacks or anxiety disorders by the symptom course, precipitating factors, and a thorough review of prior psychiatric and medical history. The differentials for PD often include 1) other mental health disorders: social anxiety disorder, specific phobias, obsessive compulsive disorder, post-traumatic stress disorder, separation anxiety disorder, 2) substances: caffeine, albuterol, drug withdrawal, and 3) physical causes: heart conditions, thyroid disorders.

*Post-traumatic stress disorder* (PTSD): panic attacks may occur in both PTSD and PD; the differentiating factor is that the panic attacks in PTSD are precipitated by exposure to or a recollection of a traumatic event, whereas the panic attacks in PD occur spontaneously.

*Specific phobia and social anxiety disorder:* panic attacks are also a common feature shared among specific phobia disorder, social anxiety disorder, and PD. However, in specific phobia and social anxiety disorder, the panic attacks are triggered by exposure to a feared object or social situation respectively.

*Substance use disorder:* substance intoxication or withdrawal can precipitate sudden onset anxiety or panic symptoms. For example, intoxication of stimulant drugs like cocaine and amphetamines, or withdrawal from narcotics or alcohol may result in panic attacks. To differentiate these from PD, it is important to look for a temporal association between the substance use/withdrawal and the onset of symptoms.

*Cardiovascular disease:* panic attacks or anxiety may also be associated with anginal events or other cardiac etiologies like arrhythmias. These may be differentiated from PD by obtaining an electrocardiogram.

*Thyroid disorder:* hyperthyroidism can present with anxiety and other associated symptoms like restlessness or irritability. These conditions can be evaluated with thyroid function tests.


## 4.4 Symptoms

PD is characterized by recurrent episodic panic attacks. A panic attack is the rapid onset of intense fear that peaks within minutes and resolves within an hour. These panic attacks may or may not have a trigger, but a diagnosis of PD requires that some of the attacks be untriggered or unexpected. The DSM-V criteria for a panic attack include at least four of the following symptoms occurring during the attack (Figure 4.2):

1. Palpitations, pounding heart, or accelerated heart rate
2. Sweating
3. Trembling or shaking
4. Sensations of shortness of breath or smothering
5. Feelings of choking
6. Chest pain or discomfort
7. Nausea or abdominal distress
8. Feeling dizzy, unsteady, light-headed, or faint
9. Chills or heat sensations

# Symptoms of Panic Attacks

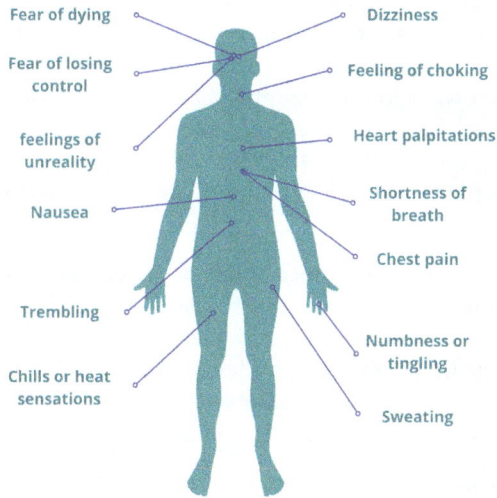

Fear of dying

Fear of losing control

feelings of unreality

Nausea

Trembling

Chills or heat sensations

Dizziness

Feeling of choking

Heart palpitations

Shortness of breath

Chest pain

Numbness or tingling

Sweating

**Figure 4.2** *Symptoms of panic attacks.*

10. Paresthesias (numbness or tingling sensations)
11. Derealization (feelings of unreality) or depersonalization (being detached from oneself)
12. Fear of losing control or "going crazy"
13. Fear of dying

Following at least one panic attack, patients experience at least one month of persistent worry about having more panic attacks or will have maladaptive changes in behavior to avoid having panic attacks. Less commonly, patients may actually experience "nonfearful" panic attacks, which are panic attacks that do not involve immense fear (26). This makes the diagnosis of a panic attack more difficult in these individuals. Other patients may also experience culture-specific symptoms such as neck pain, headache, tinnitus, or uncontrollable crying that do not count toward the four symptoms. Other possible symptoms include acute fear, chronic anxiety, and interoceptive sensation sensitivity.

30 to 50% of patients also report agoraphobia, or the fear or avoidance of situations where escape may be difficult if things go wrong (24). The lifetime prevalence of PD with agoraphobia is reported to be around 1.1%, whereas the prevalence of PD without agoraphobia is around 3.7% (27). While agoraphobia is commonly associated with PD, it is also a separate diagnosis on its

own with criteria listed in the DSM-V. The presence of agoraphobia along with PD is associated with higher functional impairment, degree of disability, and level of unemployment due to the life limitations associated with the avoidant behavior classically seen in this population (28).

PD is also frequently associated with substance abuse. Individuals may turn to substances such as alcohol or sedative hypnotics to self-medicate their panic symptoms, but prolonged use or withdrawal from substances may actually precipitate or even worsen their symptoms. Over time, prolonged use of alcohol may have an anxiogenic effect and lead to a worsening of the PD disease course. One study showed that after controlling for cannabis use, abuse, alcohol use, and polysubstance use, lifetime history of cannabis dependence was associated with a higher risk of panic attacks (29).

Individuals with PD are also more likely to attempt suicide as compared to individuals without PD. Risk factors for suicide attempts include comorbid depression, depressive symptoms, older age, younger age of panic disorder onset, and history of alcohol dependence. Risk factors for suicide ideation include depressive symptoms, anxiety symptoms, longer illness duration, comorbid depressive disorder, agoraphobia, and younger age of onset (30).

There is also an increased use of healthcare utilization in this population. Individuals tend to seek healthcare from a general medical clinician rather than a mental health clinician, and are often dissatisfied by a negative medical workup, particularly if they have ongoing symptoms of PD. These patients end up repeatedly seeking medical care, resulting in frequent medical evaluations, emergency department visits, use of medications, and frequent tests. For example, cardiac testing is often done for unexplained chest pain, pulmonary function tests for shortness of breath, endoscopy for abdominal pain, and MRI scans for dizziness (31).

Panic disorder is a chronic, recurrent disease that rarely achieves full remission despite extensive treatment. In a large, longitudinal study following individuals with PD, 64% of subjects achieved remission within two years, but symptoms recurred in 21% of those patients (32).

It is important to recognize that a panic attack is a symptom and not a diagnosis. Panic attacks may be seen in the context of many other psychiatric or medical conditions, such as post-traumatic stress disorder, mood disorders, anxiety disorders, cardiovascular disorders, or pulmonary disorders. Differentiation between panic disorder and other differential diagnoses requires careful history taking and a thorough physical exam.

## 4.5 Management

The combination of psychotherapy and pharmacological intervention is considered an effective first-line treatment for panic disorder (PD). In particular, this combination may be more effective for moderate to severe symptoms (33) and may reduce risk of relapse (34). First-line pharmacologic therapy is often an selective serotonin reuptake inhibitor (SSRI) or serotonin and norepinephrine reuptake inhibitor (SNRI) antidepressant (35).

To properly assess the effect of psychotherapy, patients should receive psychotherapy once per week for at least eight weeks (24). Mindfulness-based stress reduction, which is based on meditation, has been shown to be similarly effective compared to the more established cognitive behavioral therapy (CBT) (36,37). CBT is a form of talk therapy that helps patients become aware of their negative or inaccurate thoughts and respond to difficult situations more effectively. CBT is the preferred form of psychotherapy in panic disorder specifically as it has been the most studied and has the most robust evidence to support its efficacy. Based on a 2017 meta-analysis of 41 randomized placebo-controlled trials, CBT has a small to moderate effect size for PD and a larger effect size for other anxiety disorders such as obsessive-compulsive disorder and generalized anxiety disorder (38). In light of the COVID-19 pandemic, a meta-analysis from 2021 also looked at remote CBT for PD. CBT conducted online was found to be more effective than the passive control and is similarly effective as in-person CBT (39).

Patient education and compassionate listening are important elements of forming a therapeutic alliance between physicians and patients. Such an alliance can help mitigate fears of intervention and improve outcomes (40). It is critical to include the patient in clinical decision-making in regard to PD as compliance with both medications and psychotherapy plays an important role in successful therapy. Conversations with the patient should center around expectations for what improvement feels like and the timeline for noticeable improvements.

Socioeconomic factors affecting patient access should also be considered when making recommendations. A 2006 survey of psychotherapy training in psychiatry, psychology, and social work graduate programs found that only 28.1% of psychiatry training programs have required didactic and clinical course work in evidence-based therapies (EBT) with CBT being the most frequently required form of EBT (41). This shortage of qualified mental health professionals able to provide CBT can have a significant negative impact on the ability for patients to access care. It is also important to keep financial limits in mind as costs of psychotherapy can be prohibitively high. Open and frank discussions with patients regarding treatment options allow clinicians to select the best treatment options for each individual.

The role of lifestyle in PD management should not be underestimated. Triggers of panic attacks can include caffeine, stimulants, nicotine, stress, and certain dietary choices. Some patients with PD are more sensitive to caffeine due to differences in adenosine receptor genes (42). A link between PD and both sleep quality and quantity has been established, although the causality is unclear (43). Physical activity at 60–90% of maximum heart rate for 20 minutes three times weekly has also been shown to improve symptoms.

Acute therapy for panic attacks is often warranted while initiating long-term pharmacotherapy or psychotherapy. Benzodiazepines such as clonazepam are an effective first-line treatment for acute symptoms of a panic attack in patients without a history of substance use disorder (SUD). A 2001 double-blind randomized controlled trial (RCT) showed significant improvement in early panic symptoms with coadministration of sertraline (an SSRI) and clonazepam versus sertraline with placebo (44).

Special considerations must be taken for those with acute symptoms of PD who also have a history of SUD. Benzodiazepines are known to be highly addictive and should be used with caution. When considering adjuvant treatment for individuals with active or historical SUD there are alternatives that have evidence that back their use. A 2000 placebo-controlled trial showed that gabapentin is an effective choice for adjuvant therapy (45). Pregabalin can be considered as an alternative, but its status as a controlled substance may indicate a higher risk for misuse, and further studies on abuse potential in this population is needed. As such, gabapentin should be trialed before pregabalin. Another potential adjuvant is the atypical antidepressant mirtazapine. A case report from 2007 showed that treatment-resistant PD showed improvement after addition of mirtazapine to paroxetine (an SSRI) therapy (46).

Many patients with PD first present to the healthcare system in emergency departments with chief complaints of chest pain or shortness of breath. This leads to workup for myocardial infarction. A small 2012 study compared the efficacy of the usual care for PD versus either single session CBT-based intervention or seven session CBT-based therapy initiated within two weeks of presentation to the emergency department with PD symptoms (47). While the significance of this study is limited by small population the evidence indicates that early intervention with CBT-based therapy effectively lowers self-reported PD symptom severity. Early intervention with CBT-based therapy after initial presentation warrants further study.

## 4.6 Pharmacology

Medications (Table 4.1), especially in combination with other interventions, are an effective approach to treating PD. Because of individual variability in PD etiology and presentation, medications should be titrated to the highest dose and continued for four weeks before being declared ineffective. Furthermore, medications should be used for at least 12 months after symptoms improve, then tapered off slowly to reduce the risk of relapse (24).

Selective serotonin reuptake inhibitors (SSRIs) are commonly used as a first-line medication. SSRIs work by selectively inhibiting 5-HT1A and 5-HT2A transport

**Table 4.1** Pharmacologic Treatment of Panic Disorder

| Drug Class | Drug Examples | Mechanism of Action | Adverse Effects |
|---|---|---|---|
| Selective serotonin reuptake inhibitors (SSRIs) | Fluoxetine, paroxetine, sertraline, citalopram, escitalopram | Inhibition of serotonin reuptake in the synaptic cleft | Early: headache, diarrhea, nausea<br>Late: sexual dysfunction, Syndrome of inappropriate antidiuretic hormone secretion (SIADH), serotonin syndrome |
| Selective serotonin and norepinephrine reuptake inhibitors (SNRIs) | Venlafaxine, duloxetine | Inhibition of serotonin and norepinephrine reuptake in the synaptic cleft | Similar to SSRIs<br>Increased blood pressure, insomnia, stimulant effect |
| Tricyclic antidepressants (TCAs) | Amitriptyline, nortriptyline, clomipramine, imipramine | Inhibition of serotonin and norepinephrine reuptake in the synaptic cleft | Prolonged QTc, orthostatic hypotension, anticholinergic effects |
| Benzodiazepines | Lorazepam, alprazolam, diazepam | $GABA_A$ receptor agonist | Drowsiness, respiratory depression, addictive potential |
| Second-generation (atypical) antipsychotics | Olanzapine, quetiapine, clozapine, risperidone | $D_2$ receptor antagonist | Metabolic effects (weight gain, hyperglycemia), prolonged QTc, hyperprolactinemia, anticholinergic effects |

pumps in the presynaptic membrane (Figure 4.3). This thereby increases the synaptic concentration of serotonin (48,49). The current clinically approved SSRIs have known differences in their selectivity for serotonin transporters and their potency of serotonin reuptake inhibition. These differences have not been shown to provide any significant differences in efficacy (50).

There are certain adverse effects that must be considered in patients starting an SSRI. It is well established that SSRIs, with the exception of paroxetine, have a small but statistically significant prolonging effect on the QTc interval (51). In patients with hereditary long QT or those taking multiple medications that prolong the QTc interval, caution should be used when prescribing SSRIs. Additionally, SSRI use has been associated with precipitation of manic and hypomanic episodes in patients with bipolar disorder. As such, thorough screening for family history of bipolar disorder or history of manic symptoms is critical before initiating SSRI therapy.

In addition to SSRIs, serotonin norepinephrine reuptake inhibitors (SNRIs) have been proven in multiple RCTs as an effective treatment for anxiety disorders (Figure 4.3). The use of SNRIs for PD has only been studied in venlafaxine, which was shown to be efficacious. As such, venlafaxine is the only

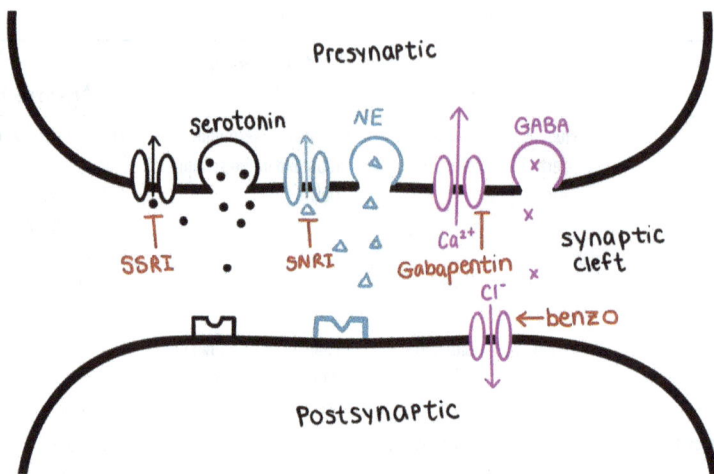

**Figure 4.3** *Mechanism of action of SSRI, SNRI, gabapentin, and benzodiazepines.*

SNRI currently approved for PD (52). The use of SNRIs carries many of the same risks as SSRIs. One of the additional considerations for SNRIs is its hypertensive properties; inhibition of norepinephrine will lead to increased sympathetic tone and therefore increased blood pressure.

Tricyclic antidepressants (TCAs) are equally effective for PD but can have more adverse effects (53). The main mechanism of action of TCAs is to inhibit the reuptake of norepinephrine and serotonin, but they also exert effects on a wide array of neurotransmitter systems. The relatively wide range of neurotransmitter alterations is the cause for this class of medications' poor safety and tolerability profile (48). As such, TCAs have fallen out of favor with clinicians to treat PD and other psychiatric illnesses.

Benzodiazepines are recommended for short-term crisis situations, but they do not improve long-term outcomes (40). Benzodiazepines should be used carefully because they appear to have a dose–response association with sedation, confusion, tolerance, and mortality (54). Benzodiazepines exert their effect by binding to a specific allosteric site on the gamma-aminobutyric acid (GABA) receptor and potentiating the inhibitory effect of the GABA neurotransmitter. Benzodiazepines have the advantage of rapid onset of action, but this contributes to the increased rates of abuse of this class of drugs. Higher doses of these medications can also produce serious unwanted side effects including sedation, physical dependence, and impaired concentration (48).

Azapirones such as buspirone are ineffective for treating PD specifically but can treat other anxiety disorders (55). Bupropion is often used to treat comorbid depression and other conditions, but its potential anxiogenic properties may render it unsuitable for PD patients (56). There is limited research on the use of other anxiolytics medications: pregabalin, gabapentin, and hydroxyzine for treating PD specifically (24). Gabapentin and pregabalin are structural analogs of GABA and bind to voltage-gated calcium channels in the CNS (central nervous system). The anxiolytic effect is achieved by increasing relative concentration of inhibitory neurotransmitter GABA in the CNS. Hydroxyzine is a first-generation antihistamine that exerts effects on H1 receptors both centrally and peripherally. The central antihistamine effects lead to lower arousal levels, thereby achieving the anxiolytic effect. Hydroxyzine may be used as an acute treatment for panic symptoms or as an adjuvant therapy while initiating long-term therapy with an SSRI or SNRI (57).

The role of anticonvulsants and antipsychotics in treating PD has been evaluated mainly in the context of comorbid psychiatric disorders (58). Generally, these drugs are well tolerated and can benefit treatment-resistant PD. Second-generation antipsychotics, such as quetiapine, are known to modulate dopaminergic and serotonergic systems in the CNS, though the exact mechanism of action has not been fully elucidated. Patients with bipolar disorder and PD who took valproate or quetiapine-XR (extended release) showed an improvement in PD symptoms, but these effects were not observed using the antipsychotics risperidone or ziprasidone (58). Other antipsychotics like clozapine, haloperidol, and olanzapine, and the anticonvulsant topiramate may actually cause new onset of panic symptoms (58). Overall, the use of anticonvulsants and antipsychotics for PD needs further clinical studies due to the small sample sizes and lack of long-term studies.

## 4.7 Conclusion

Panic disorder is an anxiety disorder characterized by recurrent panic attacks. Because PD is often missed or misdiagnosed, the development of a more sensitive and specific diagnostic workup would be largely beneficial. Although the etiology of PD is complex and not fully understood, there are diverse combinations of treatments that can help patients manage the disorder. Future studies may aim to 1) focus clinical trials on PD, rather than targeting several anxiety disorders at once and 2) optimize treatment plans for patients with comorbidities.

## References

1. American Psychiatric Association. Committee on nomenclature and S. Anxiety disorders. *Diagn Stat Man Ment Disord* 2022; 189–234.
2. Bouton ME, Mineka S, Barlow DH. A modern learning theory perspective on the etiology of panic disorder. *Psychol Rev* 2001;108(1):4–32.
3. Fanselow MS, Lester LS. A functional behavioristic approach to aversively motivated behavior: Predatory imminence as a determinant of the topography of defensive behavior. In: *Evolution and learning*. Hillsdale, NJ: Lawrence Erlbaum Associates, Inc; 1988. pp. 185–212.

4. Rau V, Fanselow MS. Neurobiological and neuroethological perspectives on fear and anxiety. In: *Understanding trauma: Integrating biological, clinical, and cultural perspectives.* New York: Cambridge University Press; 2007. pp. 27–40.

5. Dresler T, Guhn A, Tupak SV, Ehlis AC, Herrmann MJ, Fallgatter AJ, et al. Revise the revised? New dimensions of the neuroanatomical hypothesis of panic disorder. *J Neural Transm Vienna Austria* 2013;120(1):3–29.

6. Goldstein RB, Weissman MM, Adams PB, Horwath E, Lish JD, Charney D, et al. Psychiatric disorders in relatives of probands with panic disorder and/or major depression. *Arch Gen Psychiatry* 1994;51(5):383–94.

7. Torgersen S. Genetic factors in anxiety disorders. *Arch Gen Psychiatry* 1983;40(10):1085–9.

8. Domschke K, Deckert J, O'Donovan MC, Glatt SJ. Meta-analysis of COMT val158met in panic disorder: Ethnic heterogeneity and gender specificity. *Am J Med Genet B Neuropsychiatr Genet* 2007;144B(5):667–73.

9. Annerbrink K, Westberg L, Olsson M, Andersch S, Sjödin I, Holm G, et al. Panic disorder is associated with the Val308Iso polymorphism in the hypocretin receptor gene. *Psychiatr Genet* 2011;21(2):85–9.

10. Ziegler C, Richter J, Mahr M, Gajewska A, Schiele MA, Gehrmann A, et al. MAOA gene hypomethylation in panic disorder-reversibility of an epigenetic risk pattern by psychotherapy. *Transl Psychiatry* 2016;6(4):e773.

11. Gorman JM, Kent JM, Sullivan GM, Coplan JD. Neuroanatomical hypothesis of panic disorder, revised. *Am J Psychiatry* 2000;157(4):493–505.

12. Kagan J, Reznick JS, Snidman N. The physiology and psychology of behavioral inhibition in children. *Child Dev* 1987;58(6):1459.

13. Moscovitch DA, Gavric DL, Senn JM, Santesso DL, Miskovic V, Schmidt LA, et al. Changes in judgment biases and use of emotion regulation strategies during cognitive-behavioral therapy for social anxiety disorder: Distinguishing treatment responders from nonresponders. *Cognit Ther Res* 2012;36(4):261–71.

14. Hettema JM, Neale MC, Myers JM, Prescott CA, Kendler KS. A population-based twin study of the relationship between neuroticism and internalizing disorders. *Am J Psychiatry* 2006;163(5):857–64.

15. Schmidt NB, Lerew DR, Jackson RJ. The role of anxiety sensitivity in the pathogenesis of panic: Prospective evaluation of spontaneous panic attacks during acute stress. *J Abnorm Psychol* 1997;106(3):355–64.

16. Kossowsky J, Pfaltz MC, Schneider S, Taeymans J, Locher C, Gaab J. The separation anxiety hypothesis of panic disorder revisited: A meta-analysis. *Am J Psychiatry* 2013;170(7):768–81.

17. Kroenke K, Outcalt S, Krebs E, Bair MJ, Wu J, Chumbler N, et al. Association between anxiety, health-related quality of life and functional impairment in primary care patients with chronic pain. *Gen Hosp Psychiatry* 2013;35(4):359–65.

18. Kessler RC, Davis CG, Kendler KS. Childhood adversity and adult psychiatric disorder in the US National comorbidity Survey. *Psychol Med* 1997;27(5):1101–19.

19. Cosci F, Knuts IJE, Abrams K, Griez EJL, Schruers KRJ. Cigarette smoking and panic: A critical review of the literature. *J Clin Psychiatry* 2010;71(5):606–15.

20. Roberson-Nay R, Gorlin EI, Beadel JR, Cash T, Vrana S, Teachman BA. Temporal stability of multiple response systems to 7.5% carbon dioxide challenge. *Biol Psychol* 2017;124:111–8.

21. Ehlers A. Somatic symptoms and panic attacks: A retrospective study of learning experiences. *Behav Res Ther* 1993;31(3):269–78.

22. Barlow DH. *Anxiety and its disorders: The nature and treatment of anxiety and panic.* New York: The Guilford Press; 1988. xvii, 698 p.

23. Barlow DH. *Anxiety and its disorders: The nature and treatment of anxiety and panic*, 2nd ed. New York: The Guilford Press; 2002. xvi, 704 p.

24. Locke AB, Kirst N, Shultz CG. Diagnosis and management of generalized anxiety disorder and panic disorder in adults. *Am Fam Phys* 2015;91(9):617–24.
25. Goddard AW. The neurobiology of panic: A chronic stress disorder. *Chronic Stress Thousand Oaks Calif* 2017; 1:2470547017736038.
26. Fleet RP, Martel JP, Lavoie KL, Dupuis G, Beitman BD. Non-fearful panic disorder: A variant of panic in medical patients? *Psychosomatics* 2000;41(4):311–20.
27. Kessler RC, Chiu WT, Jin R, Ruscio AM, Shear K, Walters EE. The epidemiology of panic attacks, panic disorder, and agoraphobia in the national comorbidity survey replication. *Arch Gen Psychiatry* 2006;63(4):415–24.
28. Wittchen HU, Gloster AT, Beesdo-Baum K, Fava GA, Craske MG. Agoraphobia: A review of the diagnostic classificatory position and criteria. *Depress Anxiety* 2010;27(2):113–33.
29. Zvolensky MJ, Bernstein A, Sachs-Ericsson N, Schmidt NB, Buckner JD, Bonn-Miller MO. Lifetime associations between cannabis, use, abuse, and dependence and panic attacks in a representative sample. *J Psychiatr Res* 2006;40(6):477–86.
30. Tietbohl-Santos B, Chiamenti P, Librenza-Garcia D, Cassidy R, Zimerman A, Manfro GG, et al. Risk factors for suicidality in patients with panic disorder: A systematic review and meta-analysis. *Neurosci Biobehav Rev* 2019;105:34–8.
31. Klerman GL, Weissman MM, Ouellette R, Johnson J, Greenwald S. Panic attacks in the community: Social morbidity and health care utilization. *JAMA* 1991;265(6):742–6.
32. Batelaan NM, de Graaf R, Penninx BWJH, van Balkom AJLM, Vollebergh W a. M, Beekman ATF. The 2-year prognosis of panic episodes in the general population. *Psychol Med* 2010;40(1):147–57.
33. Van Apeldoorn FJ, Van Hout WJPJ, Timmerman ME, Mersch PPA, den Boer JA. Rate of improvement during and across three treatments for panic disorder with or without agoraphobia: Cognitive behavioral therapy, selective serotonin reuptake inhibitor or both combined. *J Affect Disord* 2013;150(2):313–9.
34. Pull CB, Damsa C. Pharmacotherapy of panic disorder. *Neuropsychiatr Dis Treat* 2008;4(4):779–95.
35. Stein MB, Goin MK, Pollack MH, Roy-Byrne P, Sareen J, Simon NM, et al. Guideline for the treatment of patients with panic disorder: Second edition. *Am J Psychiatry* 2009; 166(2):1.
36. Marchand WR. Mindfulness-based stress reduction, mindfulness-based cognitive therapy, and zen meditation for depression, anxiety, pain, and psychological distress. *J Psychiatr Pract* 2012;18(4):233–52.
37. Khoury B, Lecomte T, Fortin G, Masse M, Therien P, Bouchard V, et al. Mindfulness-based therapy: A comprehensive meta-analysis. *Clin Psychol Rev* 2013;33(6):763–71.
38. Carpenter JK, Andrews LA, Witcraft SM, Powers MB, Smits JAJ, Hofmann SG. Cognitive behavioral therapy for anxiety and related disorders: A meta-analysis of randomized placebo-controlled trials. *Depress Anxiety* 2018;35(6):502–14.
39. Efron G, Wootton BM. Remote cognitive behavioral therapy for panic disorder: A meta-analysis. *J Anxiety Disord* 2021;79:102385.
40. Generalised anxiety disorder and panic disorder in adults: Management. In: NICE Clinical Guidelines, No 113. National Institute for Health and Care Excellence; 2011.
41. Weissman MM, Verdeli H, Gameroff MJ, Bledsoe SE, Betts K, Mufson L, et al. National survey of psychotherapy training in psychiatry, psychology, and social work. *Arch Gen Psychiatry* 2006;63(8):925–34.
42. Charney DS, Heninger GR, Jatlow PI. Increased anxiogenic effects of caffeine in panic disorders. *Arch Gen Psychiatry* 1985;42(3):233–43.
43. Chapman DP, Presley-Cantrell LR, Liu Y, Perry GS, Wheaton AG, Croft JB. Frequent insufficient sleep and anxiety and depressive disorders among U.S. community dwellers in 20 states, 2010. *Psychiatr Serv J Am Psychiatr Assoc* 2013;64(4):385–7.

44. Goddard AW, Brouette T, Almai A, Jetty P, Woods SW, Charney D. Early coadministration of clonazepam with sertraline for panic disorder. *Arch Gen Psychiatry* 2001;58(7):681–6.
45. Pande AC, Pollack MH, Crockatt J, Greiner M, Chouinard G, Lydiard RB, et al. Placebo-controlled study of gabapentin treatment of panic disorder. *J Clin Psychopharmacol* 2000;20(4):467–71.
46. Milan Pavlovic Z. Remission of panic disorder with mirtazapine augmentation of paroxetine: A case report. *Prim Care Companion J Clin Psychiatry* 2007;9(5):396.
47. Lessard MJ, Marchand A, Pelland MÈ, Belleville G, Vadeboncoeur A, Chauny JM, et al. Comparing two brief psychological interventions to usual care in panic disorder patients presenting to the emergency department with chest pain. *Behav Cogn Psychother* 2012;40(2):129–47.
48. Koen N, Stein DJ. Pharmacotherapy of anxiety disorders: A critical review. *Dial Clin Neurosci* 2011;13(4):423–37.
49. Celada P, Puig MV, Amargós-Bosch M, Adell A, Artigas F. The therapeutic role of 5-HT1A and 5-HT2A receptors in depression. *J Psychiatry Neurosci* 2004;29(4):252–65.
50. Cipriani A, Furukawa TA, Salanti G, Geddes JR, Higgins JP, Churchill R, et al. Comparative efficacy and acceptability of 12 new-generation antidepressants: A multiple-treatments meta-analysis. *Lancet Lond Engl* 2009;373(9665):746–58.
51. Funk KA, Bostwick JR. A comparison of the risk of QT prolongation among SSRIs. *Ann Pharmacother* 2013;47(10):1330–41.
52. Katzman MA, Jacobs L. Venlafaxine in the treatment of panic disorder. *Neuropsychiatr Dis Treat* 2007;3(1):59–67.
53. Ravindran LN, Stein MB. The pharmacologic treatment of anxiety disorders: A review of progress. *J Clin Psychiatry* 2010;71(7):839–54.
54. Weich S, Pearce HL, Croft P, Singh S, Crome I, Bashford J, et al. Effect of anxiolytic and hypnotic drug prescriptions on mortality hazards: Retrospective cohort study. *BMJ* 2014;348:g1996.
55. Imai H, Tajika A, Chen P, Pompoli A, Guaiana G, Castellazzi M, et al. Azapirones versus placebo for panic disorder in adults. *Cochrane Database Syst Rev* 2014;9:CD010828.
56. Wiseman CN, Gören JL. Does bupropion exacerbate anxiety? :*Current Psychiatry*. 2012;11(6):E3–4.
57. Iskandar JW, Griffeth B, Rubio-Cespedes C. Successful treatment with hydroxyzine of acute exacerbation of panic disorder in a healthy man: A case report. *Prim Care Companion CNS Disord*. 2011;13(3):PCC.10l01126.
58. Masdrakis VG, Baldwin DS. Anticonvulsant and antipsychotic medications in the pharmacotherapy of panic disorder: A structured review. *Ther Adv Psychopharmacol* 2021;11:20451253211 0023.

# 5

# Pharmacology of Human Anxiety

Carrie Wang, Jonathan Charles, Grant Morrison,
Thomas Wotherspoon, and Charles Preuss

## Contents

## 5.1 Introduction

Generalized anxiety disorder (GAD) is a prevalent mental illness with a variety of consequences for sufferers, including an increased risk of hypertensive disease (1), strong associations with substance use disorders (2), and an overall decreased quality of life (3). With the advent of the COVID-19 pandemic and ensuing restrictions on socializing, as well as the loss of employment for millions, anxiety disorders have increased dramatically in prevalence worldwide (4).

The *Diagnostic and Statistical Manual of Mental Disorders*, commonly known as the DSM, is the standard text by which mental health professionals in the United States define and classify various disorders. Its first iteration, the DSM-1, was published in 1952 and listed anxiety only as a symptom of "neurotic" disorders or other "nervous" dispositions (5). It was not until the publication

DOI: 10.1201/9781003333821-5

of the DSM-III in 1980 that "generalized anxiety disorder" as a separate diagnosis finally came to fruition (6). By the publication of the DSM-IV in 1994, the definition of generalized anxiety disorder had coalesced into "excessive anxiety and worry (apprehensive expectation), occurring more days than not for at least 6 months, about a number of events or activities (such as work or school performance)" with several other qualifying symptoms including that the:

> focus of the anxiety and worry is not confined to features of an Axis I disorder (e.g., the anxiety or worry is not about having a panic attack [as in panic disorder], being embarrassed in public [as in social phobia], being contaminated [as in obsessive-compulsive disorder] being away from home or close relatives [as in separation anxiety disorder], gaining weight [as in anorexia nervosa], or having a serious illness [as in hypochondriasis]), and the anxiety and worry do not occur exclusively during posttraumatic stress disorder.
>
> (7)

In the latest iteration of the DSM-5, GAD's definition expanded. In this latest text, GAD is characterized by "excessive anxiety and worry" the patient struggles to control which occurs "more days than not for at least 6 months" (8) and is present in a variety of contexts (i.e., work, school, social situations) as opposed to being associated with one discrete activity, which may suggest a specific phobia rather than a generalized anxiety disorder. The patient should also experience at least three of the following six symptoms for a majority of days in the past 6 months: restlessness, feeling fatigued, difficulty concentrating, irritability, muscle tension, or a sleep disturbance. Unlike the DSM-IV, however, the DSM-V does not specify that the anxiety must not be confined to the symptoms of an Axis I disorder such as hypochondriasis, anorexia nervosa, obsessive-compulsive disorder, or separation anxiety disorder. Instead, the DSM-V broadly states that if the anxiety is not "better explained" by a "different disorder" or substance abuse, the sufferer may qualify for generalized anxiety disorder (8). The separation of generalized anxiety disorder from the symptoms experienced by individuals suffering from a substance abuse disorder was a meaningful and important deviation of the DSM-V from previous editions, marking a novel recognition of withdrawal and its ensuing symptoms as separate from clinical anxiety (9).

An estimated 2.7% of U.S. adults reported fulfilling the requirements for clinical GAD in the past year, while an estimated 5.7% will experience GAD at some point in their lifetime. Rates were higher among women compared to men, with 3.9% of U.S. women and 1.9% of U.S. men experiencing GAD in the past year. This gender skew stays consistent among various age cohorts, with prevalence doubled amongst adolescent females compared to their male counterparts. Rates were also highest among those in the 30–59 years of age cohort, more than doubling rates in the 60+ cohort (3.4–3.5% to 1.5%, respectively). Young adults from age 17 to 18 had the second highest prevalence, with 3.0% reporting experiencing GAD in the past year (10). This suggests that older age is a protective factor against GAD, while adolescents are at greatest risk when transitioning into adulthood.

GAD is also more prevalent in those of lower socioeconomic status, suggesting financial stressors may contribute to the development of the disorder (11–13). Previous research has suggested those with an annual income of less than $20,000 USD are twice as likely as those with an annual income of $70,000 USD or higher to develop GAD. Similarly, patients who have not completed a high school degree are *over* twice as likely to develop GAD as their college-educated counterparts (14). That being said, it is important to note that anxiety is a natural response to stressful life situations such as poverty. A 2012 analysis by Baer et al. noted that due to the extensive changes which the definition of GAD has received over the years, more individuals are being diagnosed with the disorder. The authors cautioned clinicians to be aware of life context; although those in poverty may be more likely to develop an anxiety disorder, not all anxiety in these situations is pathological, and may instead be protective and adaptive responses to imminent threats such as loss of housing or inability to clothe or feed oneself (15). The astute clinician must treat each patient in regard to their unique life circumstance. These epidemiological factors suggest GAD is a complex disorder, evolving in response to the patient's environment, individual stressors, and life experience.

The healthcare costs associated with a diagnosis of GAD are a burden both to the system and the individual patient. According to a 2020 editorial published in *The Lancet*, anxiety and depression cost the global economy $1 trillion USD annually as a result of lost productivity (16). Individual patients with GAD may also experience financial strain as a result of their diagnosis. A 2012 review by Revicki et al. found that patients with a diagnosis of GAD had an average annual medical cost of $2,375 USD, compared to just $1,448 USD for patients who did not have GAD. Furthermore, the review found that the mean annual medical cost of GAD was $2,138 USD higher than that of other anxiety disorders, suggesting that GAD may be particularly burdensome for patients (17). Selective serotonin reuptake inhibitors, or SSRIs, and Cognitive Behavioral Therapy, or CBT, are often considered first-line treatment for GAD (18). Despite this, the cost of Cognitive Behavioral Therapy is often a prohibitive barrier to patients receiving treatment. As previously discussed, Americans in poverty are some of the highest risk individuals to develop GAD, yet lack of health insurance may prove detrimental, as even diagnosed patients may suffer to receive adequate therapy and medication.

Aside from the financial impacts of treating GAD, patients suffer decreased quality of life (QoL) from uncontrolled symptoms. Quality of life is defined by the World Health Organization as an individual's perception of "their position in life in the context of the culture and value systems in which they live and in relation to their goals, expectations, standards, and concerns" (19). Previous research has consistently shown decreased quality of life scores associated with anxiety disorders (20, 21), with newer research exploring the effect of COVID-19 lockdowns, resultant anxiety, and decreased QoL. A 2021 study by Wilmer et al. found that females, unemployed individuals, the elderly, and those with a chronic medical condition requiring a caretaker experienced the greatest anxiety-related decrease in QoL. This decrease was driven by maladaptive coping strategies individuals adopted to subvert their anxiety, including substance abuse, denial of anxiety, and avoidance of anxiety-provoking situations (22). This suggests that anxiety-associated decreases in QoL are subject to a variety of factors, including non-modifiable factors such as age and sex, and more modifiable factors such as coping mechanisms. It is difficult to precisely quantify a decrease in QoL associated with generalized anxiety disorder, as QoL is by nature a subjective measure defined by each individual; that being said, the consistency of the research suggests GAD has a significant impact on sufferers' ability to function in professional, academic, and personal environments.

Part of GAD's significant impact on the sufferer's QoL may be mediated by an increased likelihood to develop a substance abuse disorder. Alcohol use disorder is one of the most prevalent substance abuse disorders in the United States, with an estimated 14.5 million individuals diagnosed with an alcohol use disorder in 2019. In youth aged 12 to 17, a full 1.7%, or 414,000 adolescents, qualified for an alcohol use disorder that same year (23). Furthermore, diagnosis with an independent mood or anxiety disorder is *significantly* positively associated with suffering from a simultaneous substance abuse disorder (24). Diagnosing anxiety in an individual suffering from a substance abuse disorder can represent a challenge to the clinician, as symptoms of withdrawal can mimic symptoms of anxiety, and vice versa. Withdrawal from alcohol, for example, can present with agitation, insomnia, and tachycardia. These symptoms can further complicate the clinical picture, as tachycardia may be experienced subjectively by the individual as an anxious mood (25). Conversely, individuals with anxiety may self-medicate with alcohol, putting them at increased risk of subsequent development of an alcohol use disorder. Clinicians treating either GAD or substance abuse disorders should be aware of the increased risk of co-occurrence. Specifically, in individuals with substance use disorder, treatment of any co-occurring anxiety or mood disorder should become a priority, as continuing anxiety may increase the difficulty of treating the coexisting substance use disorder.

Both the consequences and root causes of anxiety are a rapidly expanding field of study. For example, emerging research regarding the brain-gut axis and the effect of the gut microbiome on mental health disorders such as anxiety has increased in recent years, with several studies suggesting gut interventions may be able to alleviate the burden of anxiety for some patients. A 2021 meta-analysis by Simpson et al. found that patients with anxiety, depression, or a confluence of the two had a higher abundance of pro-inflammatory bacterial species (such as Enterobacteriaceae and Desulfovibrio). Similarly, short-chain fatty acid producing bacteria, thought to be anti-inflammatory, were found in *lower* abundance in these patients (26). The effect of supplements such as pro- and prebiotics on anxiety is still being explored, with conflicting research necessitating larger scale studies. Although many studies have reported a decrease in anxiety symptoms with the supplementation of probiotics for sufferers (27–30), the role of prebiotics and their interaction with probiotics has yet to be clarified (31).

GAD is a multifaceted mental disorder which is experienced in a unique manner by each individual patient. Epidemiological factors such as age, gender, and income level, comorbidities such as substance abuse, and even individually differing gut microbiomes can make every patient a different challenge for the astute clinician. This chapter aims to help define and identify the symptomatology of generalized anxiety disorder, explore the underlying pathophysiology, examine the current literature and status of the field, discuss the emerging research regarding GAD, and provide clinicians with a solid foundation of knowledge with which to approach these patients. Although it can be a challenging diagnosis to make, and its etiology is not yet fully understood, GAD is a condition which can be skillfully managed and is within the scope of a well-rounded clinician's practice.

## 5.2  Pathophysiology of Generalized Anxiety Disorder

The pathophysiology of generalized anxiety disorder (GAD) is one that is simultaneously complex and actively being researched, with many findings suggesting a high-level of intersection between inborn genetics and neurological structures of the central nervous system. Although the exact mechanism of the disorder is an ongoing area of research and ultimately relatively little is known about the biological and psychological mechanisms underlying the condition, data suggests that the disorder has been linked to changes in the functional connectivity and mechanisms of the amygdala, and the process through which it handles fear and anxiety (32). Through the nuclei of the basolateral complex, which is comprised of the basal, accessory, and lateral basal nuclei, sensory information begins its journey into the amygdala. This complex carries the responsibility of processing sensory-related fear memories and consequently communicates information relating to the assignment of threat levels to other areas in the brain dealing with memory and sensory processing, such as the medial prefrontal cortex and other sensory cortices (32). It is postulated that changes to the amygdala, as well as the insula and orbitofrontal cortex, allow for a heightened amygdala response to emotional stimuli. These changes may have a higher prevalence in individuals with GAD as compared to those who do not meet the diagnostic criteria for GAD (33). These individuals are believed to have a greater medial prefrontal cortex and amygdala response to fearful or anxiety-provoking stimuli than those who do not suffer from GAD. However, studies have demonstrated increased OR decreased activity in the prefrontal cortex can be found in individuals with clinical GAD (33). Therefore, researchers are unable at this time to parse out whether individuals who have GAD possess an amygdala that is more sensitive to stimuli than those individuals without GAD, or whether prefrontal cortex hyperactivity is majorly responsible for changes in the responsiveness of the amygdala to stimuli (33), and a full understanding of the relationship between the amygdala and the medial prefrontal cortex/orbitofrontal cortex remains to be elucidated.

Neurobiological mechanisms involved in GAD remain predominantly unexplored, however existing evidence does support that GAD is associated with dysregulations in γ-aminobutyric acid (GABA), serotonin, corticotropin-releasing factor, and norepinephrine. Given the normal stress responses are accompanied by increases in autonomic activity, such as heart rate and blood pressure, and stress-hormone production, and that GAD is commonly thought of as a disorder with a lower threshold for stress responses, it would be inferred that individuals with GAD would display heightened autonomic and stress-hormone responses. However, current literature has demonstrated that GAD patients do not significantly differ from healthy controls in terms of resting heart rate, blood pressure, respiration, or skin conductance (34). Even individuals with GAD exhibit hyporesponsiveness to stress challenges. The same study found that when women with GAD were exposed to stress, they were found to have an accentuated skin conductance response as well as a slower return to baseline (34). Norepinephrine has been suggested to play a role in chronic anxiety and GAD as it becomes activated during periods of anxiety and stress (35). Some data suggest that baseline plasma catecholamine levels do not differ between healthy controls and those with GAD (36). Other data have shown a difference when measuring indirect methods of norepinephrine levels, such as a blunted growth hormone response to clonidine administration, suggesting increased baseline norepinephrine activity (37).

GABA is another neurotransmitter that may be implicated in GAD development, given that benzodiazepines are effective as a therapy. It is speculated that GABA is deficient in people with GAD. Evidence has pointed towards reduced lymphocyte and platelet benzodiazepine receptors in patients with GAD that was effectively reversed with benzodiazepine treatment (38, 39). Further work has suggested that patients with GAD have a reduced sensitivity of central GABA-benzodiazepine receptors (40). A study utilizing single-photon emission computed tomography imaging and analysis found that individuals with GAD demonstrated significantly decreased binding of a benzodiazepine receptor ligand in the left temporal lobe when compared to healthy control (41). These findings point towards decreased inhibitory response, through GABA and its respective receptors, can be found in patients who suffer from GAD when compared to healthy individuals.

In the same light as benzodiazepines, pharmaceutical serotonin agents are effective in the treatment of a spectrum of anxiety-related conditions, including GAD. Therefore, there has been a growing focus on the role that the neurotransmitter serotonin plays in manifestations of GAD. Neurobiological models have proposed that serotonergic pathways starting in the raphe nucleus project into brain areas classically associated with anxiety regulation, such as the amygdala (42). Further studies have found that reduced serotonin levels correlate with GAD. One study found reduced levels of serotonin in the cerebrospinal fluid of GAD patients relative to healthy controls (43). Administration of m-chlorophenylpiperazine, a 5-HT1 and 5-HT2 receptor agonist, was shown to increase anxiety and anger in people with GAD but had no effect on controls (44). Another study also reported that paroxetine, a selective serotonin reuptake inhibitor, demonstrated reduced platelet binding when compared to controls, however other research failed to find any differences between controls and GAD patients in relation to platelet binding of imipramine, a tricyclic antidepressant with high serotonergic characteristics (45).

The hypothalamic-pituitary-adrenal (HPA) axis plays an integral role in homeostasis and regulating anxiety and stress-related responses, with increased cortisol levels central to this response. Many studies have reported that cortisol levels are at baseline values in GAD patients compared to non-anxious controls (46). However, most recent studies utilizing dexamethasone as an HPA axis suppressant have found that some GAD patients displayed nonsuppression, suggesting that their HPA axes functioned at a higher level, and one study even reported that this nonsuppression diminished after treatment for GAD was initiated (47). Taken together, these potential differences in neurotransmitter function evidenced by an increasing body of data implicate a potential dysregulation of neurobiological systems and adaptive response to stress in patients with GAD.

Approaching a more thorough understanding of GAD through a genetic lens has produced data that suggests that GAD is at least partially inherited. A review of twin studies estimated that approximately 32% of the variance in manifesting GAD can be explained by genetic factors. Further data from family studies support this claim of a partial genetic transmission of GAD. One study found that first-degree relatives of individuals with GAD had an increased risk of developing GAD themselves but had no increased risk of developing panic disorder when compared to controls (48). Another, larger female twin study found that major depressive disorder and GAD were largely influenced by the same genetic factors (49). Additionally, further work has also demonstrated that anxiety, depression, and neuroticism contain considerable overlaps in manifestation and underlying pathophysiology (50). These genetic studies and results taken as a whole suggest that there exists a general predisposition towards heightened anxiety in select individuals rather than a cut-and-dry specific heritability mechanism for GAD, with the ever-present environmental factors conferring an increased risk towards development of anxiety disorders. And although the environment has been hypothesized to be a crucial factor in the pathophysiology of GAD, there are relatively few studies that have directly examined its contribution to the development of GAD specifically. It seems that the majority of these studies have worked to evaluate how the environment plays a role in the development of anxiety disorders as a whole. Although they share many features, more work is needed to elucidate the effects on GAD specifically.

On the other hand, similarities between GAD and other anxiety disorders, such as social anxiety disorder, have been highlighted through developmental models, shining light onto the importance of specific parenting behaviors on the manifestation of the disorder (51). Behaviors such as the modeling of avoidant or anxious behavior (52), overinvolvement or overprotection (53), or the encouragement of avoidance behaviors (54) have been shown to play a role. More contemporary models suggest that a dynamic interaction of both child effects (where the child's behavior elicits a certain behavior from the parents) and parental effects (intrinsic parental anxiety and behavior) plays a part in the development of GAD and other anxiety disorders (51).

Furthermore, there are a collection of studies that suggest that stressful life events can play a role in the development of GAD. A study showed that individuals with GAD were more likely to report exposure to a potentially traumatic event than non-anxious controls (55). Additionally, it is notable that early stressful life events can lead to long-term changes in the HPA axis, thereby increasing one's sensitivity to stress which places a person at a greater risk of developing anxiety-related problems (56). One explanatory model delineates that early experiences with intrusive and controlling parents in combination with an inborn disposition towards anxiety may lead to a diminished perception of control over one's life and environment, leading to an increased predisposition to frequent worry and anxiety (57).

In exploring the potential avenues of pathophysiology of GAD, numerous psychopathological models have been developed in attempts to explain GAD. Some theories have postulated that self-generating worry is a form of cognitive and emotional avoidance (58), designed to avoid the occurrence of distressing thought, future catastrophe, and emotions. If assumed to be true, people with GAD are more likely to assert that worry is an effective strategy in distracting themselves from potentially deep emotional topics (58). More in-depth research has shown that worry results in immediate suppression of sympathetic responses to anxiety-provoking material (59). However, it must be noted that worry, as is the case with other methods of avoidance, prevents thorough mental processing of emotional content, preventing extinction from occurring.

Another set of models focuses on the potential information-processing biases that may be playing a key role in GAD. Research has shown that people with

GAD selectively pay attention to threatening stimuli and are more prone to interpret a neutral piece of information as a negative one (60). This preferential processing of threat-based stimuli may play a role in GAD since patterns of selective negative processing have been demonstrated to predict and precede negative emotional responses to stressful events (61). Some cognitive behavioral models of GAD propose that a central cognitive process of worry and GAD is an intolerance of uncertainty (62). These individuals react negatively on a multi-level basis to uncertain events and may begin to believe that the possibility of a future negative outcome, despite a small probability value, is unacceptable and avoided at all costs. These feelings towards uncertainty may even evolve into a positive belief about the utility of worry, in that worrying helps these individuals discover solutions or protect from negative emotions, cognitive avoidance, or poor problem orientation (where a focus on uncertain aspects of problems and appraisal of them as a threat is enhanced), all of which have been linked to GAD (63). A prolonged sequence of worry activates negative meta-cognitive beliefs about worry, leading to beliefs about the uncontrollability and unpredictability of worry and the mental, social, and physical consequences of worry. These negative beliefs motivate safety-seeking behaviors, such as distraction and double-checking, which can disrupt emotional processing and ultimately maintain the excessive worry. A variety of cognitive and behavioral processes have been implicated in GAD, designed to circumvent potential negative future outcomes and distressing thoughts and emotions.

## 5.3 Symptoms and Diagnosis

The diagnosis of GAD is largely dependent on clinical findings. Currently, lab work and imaging, such as computerized tomography (CT) or magnetic resonance imaging (MRI), does not have an established role in detecting this condition. Instead, GAD is in large part diagnosed by taking a thorough medical history, performing a mental status exam, and utilizing screening tools. Even with these tools, diagnosis can be difficult. In a study focused on physician diagnosis of GAD, 72.5% of patients with GAD were recognized as having a "clinically significant mental disorder," however only 34.4% of patients were properly diagnosed with GAD (63). In this section, we will discuss the signs and symptoms of GAD, the recommended criteria for its diagnosis, common challenges in distinguishing GAD from other conditions, and methods for screening, diagnosing, and monitoring the severity of GAD.

People with GAD frequently describe having an overwhelming feeling of anxiousness, causing significant distress. Unlike conditions such as specific phobia (fear of a specific object or situation), the anxiety is not limited to any one matter. Patients with GAD report that their anxiety relates to a wide range of situations. Despite this, only 13% of patients with GAD list anxiety as their primary complaint when seeking health care (64). GAD may manifest as vague somatic symptoms, such as fatigue, dizziness, shortness of breath, or palpitations (65). Additionally, patients may report developing insomnia because of their anxiety. As a result, the presentation of GAD may mimic other conditions associated with these symptoms, potentially delaying diagnosis and treatment.

The *Diagnostic and Statistical Manual of Mental Disorders*, Fifth Edition (DSM-V) establishes a standardized criteria for diagnosis of GAD. These guidelines aid clinicians in differentiating GAD from non-pathologic causes and other conditions associated with anxiety. To be diagnosed with GAD, an individual must meet all the criteria listed in Table 5.1.

A key aspect of setting a diagnostic criterion for GAD is the ability to differentiate pathological anxiety, caused by an underlying anxiety disorder, and physiologic anxiety, which is an expected response to a stressor. While stressful life events (such as an upcoming exam or deadline) are understandably associated with anxiety, an individual responding to a particular stressor with what is deemed to be a reasonable level of anxiety would not meet criteria for diagnosis of GAD.

As recognized by the DSM-V criteria, individuals presenting with a substance use disorder or taking medications known to cause anxiety can often resemble individuals with GAD. Thus, clinicians must be sure to differentiate these situations by taking a thorough medical and social history. Stimulants, whether prescribed (e.g., methylphenidate) or used recreationally (e.g.,

**Table 5.1** (66) DSM-V Criteria for Diagnosis of GAD

A) Excessive anxiety and worry (apprehensive expectation), occurring more days than not for at least 6 months, about a number of events or activities (such as work or school performance)

B) The person finds it difficult to control the worry

C) The anxiety and worry are associated with three or more of the following six symptoms (with at least some symptoms present for more days than not for the past 6 months)
  1. Restlessness or feeling keyed up or on edge
  2. Being easily fatigued
  3. Difficulty concentrating or mind going blank
  4. Irritability
  5. Muscle tension
  6. Sleep disturbance (difficulty falling or staying asleep, or restless unsatisfying sleep)

D) The anxiety, worry, or physical symptoms cause clinically significant distress or impairment in social, occupational, or other important areas of functioning

E) The disturbance is not attributable to the physiological effects of a substance (e.g., a drug of abuse, a medication) or another medical condition (e.g., hyperthyroidism)

F) The disturbance is not better explained by another mental disorder (e.g., anxiety or worry about having panic attacks in panic disorder, negative evaluation in social anxiety disorder [social phobia], contamination or other obsessions in obsessive-compulsive disorder, separation from attachment figures in separation anxiety disorder, reminders of traumatic events in post-traumatic stress disorder, gaining weight in anorexia nervosa, physical complaints in somatic symptom disorder, perceived appearance flaws in body dysmorphic disorder, having a serious illness in illness anxiety disorder, or the content of delusional beliefs in schizophrenia or delusional disorder) cocaine, methamphetamine) are commonly associated with feelings of agitation and anxiety. Thus, sustained use can appear similarly to GAD, despite not meeting diagnosis due to Criterion E of the DSM-V. In individuals with a substance dependence who suddenly abstain from use, withdrawal symptoms may also produce anxiety, especially in prescriptions and recreational drugs associated with central nervous system depression (e.g., alcohol, benzodiazepines, opioids). The diagnostic picture is further blurred when considering the close association between GAD and substance use disorder. The National Epidemiologic Survey on Alcohol and Related Conditions found that individuals diagnosed with GAD were more likely to have alcohol dependence (odds ratio = 2.8) or drug dependence (odds ratio = 9.5) (67). In patients with a substance use disorder who are being assessed for anxiety, eliciting a history of anxiety symptoms prior to initial substance use or during a period of extended sobriety is useful to confidently diagnose GAD instead of substance-induced anxiety.

Patients with GAD are at an increased risk of developing symptoms of depression. In children identified as depressed or anxious, between 15.9% and 61.9% will have comorbid anxiety and depressive disorders (68). Patients who develop GAD frequently develop symptoms of depression around the same period they initially developed GAD. The results from patient responses in a national comorbidity survey demonstrated that patients who were diagnosed with GAD within the past year were 54.1 times more likely to be diagnosed with major depressive disorder (MDD) than the general population (69). Those with comorbid GAD and MDD demonstrate a significant increase in impairment relative to isolated MDD. Respondents to a survey by the World Health Organization with comorbid GAD and MDD were more likely to report severe role impairment (64.4% vs 46.0%) and suicidal ideation (19.5% vs 8.9%) than respondents with MDD alone (70). Awareness of the high rates of comorbidity of these two conditions and how they interplay is important when evaluating patients for anxiety and in forming treatment plans to mitigate associated risks.

Many primary care and mental health professionals utilize self-reporting questionnaires to screen patients for possible GAD. While a multitude of these questionnaires exist, the most used are the Generalized Anxiety Disorder Scale-7 (GAD-7) and the Generalized Anxiety Disorder Scale-2 (GAD-2). The GAD-7 consists of presenting seven problems to a patient and asking them how frequently they have experienced these problems in the past 2 weeks (71) These problems include 1) "feeling nervous, anxious or on edge," 2) "not being able to stop or control worrying," 3) "worrying too much about different things," 4) "trouble relaxing," 5) "being so restless that it is hard to sit still," 6) "becoming easily annoyed or irritable," and 7) "feeling afraid as if something awful might happen" (71). For each problem, the patient can answer with one of four possible options, with each one assigned a point value between 0 and 3. A response of "not at all" earns a point value of 0, "several days" a point value of 1, more than half the days a point value of 2, and nearly every day a point value of 3. Scores for each response are added up, giving an overall

**Table 5.2** A Summary of Mainline GAD Pharmacology (74, 84, 85, 93, 94)

| Drug or Drug Class | Role and Indications | Method of Action |
|---|---|---|
| SSRIs | First-line option, Comorbid depression | Inhibition of serotonin re-uptake |
| SNRIs | First-line option, Comorbid depression | Inhibition of serotonin and norepinephrine reuptake |
| Hydroxyzine | Second-line, Augmentation, acute flares, insomnia | First-generation $H_1$ receptor antagonist |
| Buspirone | Second-line, Augmentation, long-term | $5\text{-HT}_{1A}$ receptor stimulation |
| Pregabalin | Third-line, Augmentation | Binds to alpha-delta subunit of voltage-gated calcium channels, reduces neurotransmitter release |
| Quetiapine | Third-line, Augmentation | $5\text{-HT}_{2A}$ receptor antagonist, $D_2$receptor antagonist |
| Benzodiazepines | Treatment refractory GAD, acute flares | Indirect $GABA_A$ agonists |

score. When setting a cutoff point at an overall score of greater than or equal to 10, the GAD-7 demonstrates a sensitivity of 89% and a specificity of 82% for GAD (72). GAD-7's strong sensitivity for GAD makes it a useful screening tool, and positive results indicate the need for further evaluation and possible treatment for GAD (see Table 5.2).

In addition to its utility in screening for GAD, the GAD-7 can also be used to measure symptom severity. The GAD-7 rates scores between 0 and 4 as minimal anxiety, 5 and 9 as mild anxiety, 10 and14 as moderate anxiety and 15 or greater as severe anxiety (72). By having patients retake the GAD-7 in subsequent visits, clinicians can gauge the change in severity of symptoms over time and modify treatment plans accordingly.

The GAD-2 is a truncated version of the GAD-7 and allows for quicker screening of patients. Using the same scoring system as the GAD-7, the GAD-2 only asks patients to rate their frequency of feeling nervous, anxious, or on edge and not being able to stop or control worrying. A meta-analysis of studies analyzing the GAD-2 demonstrated a sensitivity of 76% and specificity of 81% for GAD using a cutoff score of 3 (73). Thus, this tool provides a time-efficient, albeit less sensitive, method for screening for GAD, and highlights patients who may require a more in-depth workup.

## 5.4 Initial Management of GAD

Managing generalized anxiety disorder (GAD) initially involves making the decision of whether to treat. Patients with mild GAD and manageable symptoms that do not impair daily functioning may be adequately managed with lifestyle modifications (74). If clinical assessment of a patient's symptoms determines a significant level of functional impairment or symptoms are worsening, treatment is generally recommended. Treatment of GAD is centered on pharmacotherapy, Cognitive Behavioral Therapy (CBT), or a combination of both (74).

Lifestyle modifications are a low-risk initial intervention for subclinical, mild GAD (74). Recommended adjustments to lifestyle for alleviation of GAD symptoms include maintaining proper sleep hygiene (to improve duration and quality of sleep), committing to regular exercise (common methods include aerobic exercise or yoga), reducing alcohol and caffeine use, and reducing nicotine or illicit drug use (74–76). Additional low-intensity interventions include self-help, stress education, and group therapy (75, 76). Follow-up with patients undergoing lifestyle modification is beneficial for providing regular assessment of symptom severity and monitoring for progression to moderate or severe GAD (74).

## 5.5 A Treatment Decision; CBT or Pharmacotherapy

Initiation of treatment for moderate to severe GAD generally begins with either CBT or pharmacotherapy with combination therapy for those whose symptoms persist on monotherapy (74). It is difficult to elucidate a difference in the efficacy of CBT and pharmacotherapy given a relative scarcity of literature involving their direct comparison. When compared indirectly in a meta-analysis of 79 randomized controlled trials (RCTs), CBT alone was demonstrated to have a larger effect size than pharmacotherapy alone (77). An important limitation to this meta-analysis and most indirect comparisons made between pharmacotherapy and psychotherapy is that the pharmacotherapy studies are more likely to have a placebo control condition, thus limiting the value of indirect comparisons made between effect sizes (77).

Given an unclear difference in efficacy between the two treatment modalities for GAD, selection of therapy often involves shared decision-making with the patient and careful consideration of a patient's comorbid factors. Starting with either psychotherapy or pharmacotherapy are both reasonable courses of action, as evidence supports their individual efficacies in the treatment of GAD (78, 79). Guideline-based indications for an initial CBT approach include patient hesitance with medications, pediatric patients, and concern for drug side effects (75, 80). Guideline-based indications for an initial pharmacological approach include limited access to trained psychotherapists, limited patient availability, and comorbid depression (75, 80).

## 5.6 CBT in Treating GAD

Cognitive Behavioral Therapy for GAD is generally delivered in person, individually, in 12 to 16 sessions that are each 1 hour long (74). Evidence supports the efficacy of alternative modes of delivery that include group sessions, computer delivery with assistance from a therapist, and telephone therapy (74). CBT for GAD centers on changing pathological worries into normal worries through functional analysis, psychoeducation, an emotional and behavioral approach, and a cognitive approach (81). Functional analysis identifies circumstances of triggers and evaluates their intensity (81). Psychoeducation follows functional analysis and provides the patient with an understanding of the tools used to facilitate change; this is a crucial step in the motivation of patients (81). The emotional, behavioral, and cognitive approaches then aid the patient in creating relaxation, increasing fear tolerance, and utilizing mindfulness to evaluate their biases and negative thought patterns.

The body of evidence supporting the efficacy of CBT in treating GAD is robust. CBT provides moderate benefits to patients with GAD in the acute phase and maintains these gains in longer term follow-up (77, 82). Response rates for CBT in GAD are as high as 50% in both immediate and long-term follow-up (83). In addition to providing benefits to GAD symptoms, CBT has proven effective in improving symptoms of secondary depression, a common comorbid disorder (77).

## 5.7 Introduction to Pharmacology of GAD

Pharmacotherapy for GAD is broad, and several drugs can be used to manage the symptoms of GAD. The generally accepted first-line pharmacological treatment of GAD is selective serotonin reuptake inhibitors (SSRIs) (74, 84). However, serotonin-norepinephrine reuptake inhibitors (SNRIs) are another first-line option, with recent data showing them to have a similar efficacy to the SSRIs (74). Other drugs have proven beneficial in modulation therapy secondary to an SSRI or SNRI and serve to augment the partial response to the serotonin modulators or reduce anxiety in the 4 to 6 weeks before for serotonin modulators to begin to take effect, they include hydroxyzine, benzodiazepines, buspirone, pregabalin, gabapentin, and quetiapine.

## 5.8 Selective Serotonin Reuptake Inhibitors

When selecting a serotonin modulating agent, it is important to understand that not all serotonin modulators are equal in efficacy or tolerability. There is data that demonstrates support for and ranks the efficacy of many different SSRIs and SNRIs in treating GAD. Among the SSRIs, escitalopram is shown to have the largest abundance of data demonstrating efficacy and tolerability (85). Paroxetine has a similar efficacy to escitalopram, but is noted to have worse tolerability, with increased discontinuation when compared to placebo (85). Sertraline and fluoxetine have also proven efficacious and well tolerated in RCTs but have less evidence when compared to escitalopram and paroxetine (85). Among the SNRIs, duloxetine and venlafaxine have the strongest evidence, and neither is associated with increased discontinuation when compared to placebo (85).

Despite the differences demonstrated in meta-analysis, most SSRIs or SNRIs have demonstrated efficacy when compared to placebo. Switching to a different serotonin modulator based on side-effect profiles, previous patient response, or other factors would be a reasonable decision (74). Length of treatment is mired in uncertainty, with limited data on maintenance therapy. Clinical practice findings recommend pharmacological treatment for at least 12 months and literature evidence demonstrates that SSRIs remain efficacious in preventing relapse for at least 6 months (74, 86).

## 5.9 A Neurobiological Basis for Serotonin Modulation

An earlier section of this chapter established the general pathophysiology of GAD and the role played by serotonin. Modulation of serotonin by SSRIs or SNRIs can reverse much of the neurostructural changes found in GAD in addition to ameliorating clinical symptoms of GAD (87, 88). This structural change begins with the concept of neuroplasticity, the brain's ability to form new connections and reorganize existing ones (89). Selective serotonin reuptake inhibitors have been found to act at the molecular level, increasing molecules that promote plasticity like Neural Cell Adhesion Molecules (NCAMs) (89). Increasing NCAMs are associated with changes in neurons that allow for improved neuronal connectivity through changes in cellular dendrites and axonal structures (89). The neuroplastic changes induced by serotonin modulators target specific portions of the brain that play a role in the pathophysiology of GAD like the structures of the limbic system (87).

The Prefrontal Cortex (PFC) is an important structure for providing top-down regulation of the amygdala and other limbic system structures (90). The use of serotonin modulators increases activation of a specific part of the PFC called the ventrolateral Prefrontal Cortex (vlPFC). Increased activation of the vlPFC in response to emotional stimuli demonstrates increased top-down control of the limbic system (90). The idea of increased top-down control from enhancing the vlPFC is further solidified by evidence of increased specific connectivity between the vlPFC and the amygdala (87). Increasing connectivity to the amygdala drives inhibition of a strong emotional response to stress stimuli via a reduction in the neuronal activity of the amygdala, insula, and limbic system in general (91). Increased specific connections from the basolateral amygdala to the vlPFC even indicate an improved prognosis in GAD patients (87). Literature suggests serotonin modulators increase this functional connectivity to the amygdala in as early as 2 weeks of treatment and that normalizing functional connectivity can have beneficial effects in reversing the pathophysiology of GAD (87). Other areas implicated to play a role in improved emotional regulation following serotonin modulation include the rostral Anterior Cingulate Cortex (rACC) and the median frontal gyrus, however, more research is needed to understand their specific roles (92).

In summary, serotonin modulation increases neuroplasticity in fear circuits to improve regulation of the limbic system by the PFC. This increased functional connectivity is believed to better attenuate the emotional or anxiety response in GAD patients.

## 5.10 Augmentation Therapy

There are options for augmenting serotonin modulation that can be used to improve management of GAD symptoms. Hydroxyzine is a first-generation antihistamine with moderate efficacy in managing anxiety over short periods of time and is often used in the lag period of serotonin modulators, in acute flare-ups of anxiety, and as a sleep aid for comorbid insomnia (because of its sedative effects) (74, 85). Buspirone is an azapirone recommended to augment a partial response to first-line treatment with an SSRI or SNRI and can be used in the long term because it is not sedating (84, 85). Buspirone is often the augmentative agent of choice for long-term management of GAD (74).

Pregabalin has limited data in support of its use in anxiety disorders (93). However, there are some data that suggest it is both superior to placebo in managing GAD and it has a similar efficacy to that of benzodiazepines (94). In addition to maintaining a similar efficacy to benzodiazepines, pregabalin is safer than benzodiazepines and has demonstrated lower dropout rates when compared to benzodiazepines (93, 94). Pregabalin also benefits from a faster onset of action and faster improvement to symptoms than SSRIs or SNRIs (94). However, there remains a risk for abuse and dependence with pregabalin, resulting in a significant limitation for its widespread use (93). As such, pregabalin is reserved for use as augmentation in refractory patients and is not a first or second-line treatment option (74).

Another unique augmentation option includes atypical antipsychotics. The antipsychotic with the most evidence to support reduction in anxiety symptoms and efficacy in treating GAD is quetiapine (74). Quetiapine has a major advantage in that it may have the largest effect on reducing anxiety in GAD of all the commonly used treatment options (85). This reduction in anxiety is significant, possibly greater than benzodiazepines (85). More head-to-head clinical trials are necessary to solidify these claims and elucidate the magnitude of the difference. However, quetiapine is poorly tolerated with the highest discontinuation rate compared to placebo (85). An additional challenge with the use of quetiapine involves required regular monitoring of a patient's lipid levels, HbA1C, and weight to watch for development of a metabolic syndrome (74). Poor tolerance of quetiapine plagues its usefulness in a clinical setting, and it is reserved as a tertiary option in the treatment of GAD.

## 5.11 A Limited Role for Benzodiazepines

Benzodiazepines are an efficacious treatment for GAD but no longer a recommended first-line agent in its management (74). Risk for dependance, misuse, and withdrawal are all concerns that contribute to hesitancy in using benzodiazepines (74). Despite their drawbacks, the high efficacy and quick onset of benzodiazepines preserve a limited role for benzodiazepines (93). Benzodiazepines remain an option as a short-term agent that can be used in the lag period before SSRI or SNRI onset, in acute exacerbation, and in GAD that is refractory to multiple serotonin modulators and multiple augmentative therapies (84, 93). Benzodiazepines are not recommended for time periods greater than 3 to 6 months (74). However, it is important to assess for a history of substance abuse, medication use, or comorbid mood disorder before utilizing benzodiazepines in a treatment plan (74, 93).

## 5.12 Natural and Alternative Treatments for GAD

Kava is a phytoextract with a history of use in herbal remedies that dates back over 200 years in the South Pacific Islands as a part of ceremonial and social activities (95). Kava has a more recent history of use as a general anxiolytic or psychoactive substance (95). The method of action in kava is uncertain but it is hypothesized to act on calcium or sodium channels, and likely acts on GABA-A receptors in a similar manner to benzodiazepines (93, 95). Data on the efficacy of kava is more substantial than data associated with most other herbal compounds (96). Review of multiple RCTs demonstrates a significant anxiolytic effect when compared to placebo (96). Kava is generally well tolerated, however, there are reported cases of severe hepatotoxicity associated with kava consumption and data to suggest a causal link between the two (95). In spite of rare instances of hepatotoxicity, kava has promising efficacy that warrants cautious exploration.

Chamomile is an additional substance with a history of use as a medicinal herb and anxiolytic (97). Chamomile is suggested to act as an anxiolytic and sedative via binding of flavonoid and apigenin components to GABA-A receptors in the brain (97). The data concerning efficacy for chamomile use in GAD is similarly sparse to kava. Review of existing trials on chamomile in GAD demonstrates that there is some support for mild reduction in GAD symptoms after 2 to 4 weeks of chamomile use (97). In addition to a mild improvement in general symptoms, chamomile has a significant effect on improving sleep quality and resolving insomnia. Chamomile's benefits as a sleep aid could be very valuable in managing GAD given the prevalence of insomnia in GAD patients (74, 97).

Lavender and saffron have both demonstrated some efficacy in reducing general symptoms of anxiety and depression (98). Lavender was even shown to have a similar reduction in anxiety to pharmacologic anxiolytics in a small number of RCTs (98). Additional data suggest a possible modulating effect of lavender on the activity of citalopram (98). However, neither saffron nor lavender have been sufficiently tested for efficacy in managing GAD. Other natural compounds explored as anxiolytics with minimal or mixed data include black cohosh, chasteberry, passionflower, ginkgo, lemon balm, and echinacea (93, 98).

## 5.13 Conclusion

After this thorough review of GAD and the respective exploration of its pathophysiology, diagnosis, and current and novel treatments, it can be concluded that GAD is a pathology that requires extensive continued research surrounding the optimization of its care and the treatments thereof. Despite being documented in the literature for several decades now, a pure neurobiological mechanistic model of the underlying pathophysiology of the disorder has yet to be fully elucidated. Along that same vein, current therapies are effective but are not yet infallible, and future research into developing more efficacious treatments is warranted. Later sections of this textbook will explore the mechanisms and implications of the gut microbiome on the development and course of GAD and other anxiety pathologies.

## References

1. Lim LF, Solmi M, Cortese S. Association between anxiety and hypertension in adults: A systematic review and meta-analysis. *Neurosci Biobehav Rev.* 2021;131:96–119. doi:10.1016/j.neubiorev.2021.08.031.
2. Brady KT, Haynes LF, Hartwell KJ, Killeen TK. Substance use disorders and anxiety: A treatment challenge for social workers. *Soc Work Public Health.* 2013;28(3–4):407–423. doi:10.1080/19371918.2013.774675.
3. Wilmer MT, Anderson K, Reynolds M. Correlates of quality of life in anxiety disorders: Review of recent research. *Curr Psychiatry Rep.* 2021;23(11):77. doi:10.1007/s11920-021-01290-4.
4. Covid-19 pandemic triggers 25% increase in prevalence of anxiety and depression worldwide. World Health Organization. https://www.who.int/news/item/02-03-2022-covid-19-pandemic-triggers-25-increase-in-prevalence-of-anxiety-and-depression-worldwide#:~:text=In%20the%20first%20year%20of,Health%20Organization%20(WHO)%20today. Published March 2, 2022. Accessed October 16, 2022.
5. *Diagnostic and Statistical Manual: Mental Disorders.* Washington, DC: American Psychiatric Association, Mental Hospital Service; 1952.
6. *Diagnostic and Statistical Manual of Mental Disorders. III.* Washington, DC: American Psychiatric Association; 1980.
7. Substance Abuse and Mental Health Services Administration. Impact of the DSM-IV to DSM-5 changes on the National survey on drug use and health [Internet]. Rockville, MD: Substance Abuse and Mental Health Services Administration (US); 2016 Jun. Table 3.15, DSM-IV to DSM-5 Generalized Anxiety Disorder Comparison. Available from: https://www.ncbi.nlm.nih.gov/books/NBK519704/table/ch3.t15/.

8. Glasheen C, Batts K, Karg R, Bose J, Hedden S, Piscopo K. *Impact of the DSM-IV to DSM-5 Changes on the National Survey on Drug Use and Health*. Rockville, MD: Substance Abuse and Mental Health Services Administration; 2016.

9. Grant BF, Stinson FS, Dawson DA, et al. Prevalence and co-occurrence of substance use disorders and independent mood and anxiety disorders: Results from the national epidemiologic survey on alcohol and related conditions. *Arch Gen Psychiatry*. 2004;61(8):807–816. doi:10.1001/archpsyc.61.8.807.

10. Generalized anxiety disorder. National Institute of Mental Health. https://www.nimh .nih.gov/health/statistics/generalized-anxiety-disorder#part_2652. Accessed October 16, 2022.

11. Nunes JC, Carroll MK, Mahaffey KW, et al. General anxiety disorder-7 questionnaire as a marker of low socioeconomic status and inequity. *J Affect Disord*. 2022;317:287–297. doi:10.1016/j.jad.2022.08.085.

12. Kessler RC, Chiu WT, Demler O, Merikangas KR, Walters EE. Prevalence, severity, and comorbidity of 12-month DSM-IV disorders in the national comorbidity survey replication. [published correction appears in *Arch Gen Psychiatry*. 2005;62(7):709. Merikangas, Kathleen R [added]]. *Arch Gen Psychiatry*. 2005;62(6):617–627. doi:10.1001/archpsyc.62.6.617.

13. Kessler RC, McGonagle KA, Zhao S, et al. Lifetime and 12-month prevalence of DSM-III-R psychiatric disorders in the United States: Results from the national comorbidity survey. *Arch Gen Psychiatry*. 1994;51(1):8–19. doi:10.1001/archpsyc.1994.03950010008002.

14. Budhwani H, Hearld KR, Chavez-Yenter D. Generalized anxiety disorder in racial and ethnic minorities: A case of nativity and contextual factors. *J Affect Disord*. 2015;175:275–280. doi:10.1016/j.jad.2015.01.035.

15. Baer JC, Kim M, Wilkenfeld B. Is it generalized anxiety disorder or poverty? An examination of poor mothers and their children. *Child Adolesc Soc Work J*. 2012;29(4):345–355. doi:10.1007/s10560-012-0263-3.

16. Mental health matters. *Lancet Glob Health*. 2020;8(11). doi:10.1016/s2214-109x(20)30432-0.

17. Revicki DA, Travers K, Wyrwich KW, et al. Humanistic and economic burden of generalized anxiety disorder in North America and Europe. *J Affect Disord*. 2012;140(2):103–112. doi:10.1016/j.jad.2011.11.014.

18. Bandelow B, Michaelis S, Wedekind D. Treatment of anxiety disorders. *Dial Clin Neurosci*. 2017;19(2):93–107. doi:10.31887/DCNS.2017.19.2/bbandelow.

19. *The World Health Organization Quality of Life User Manual*. The World Health Organization; 1998.

20. Rapaport MH, Clary C, Fayyad R, Endicott J. Quality-of-life impairment in depressive and anxiety disorders. *Am J Psychiatry*. 2005;162(6):1171–1178. doi:10.1176/appi.ajp.162.6.1171.

21. Barrera TL, Norton PJ. Quality of life impairment in generalized anxiety disorder, social phobia, and panic disorder. *J Anxiety Disord*. 2009;23(8):1086–1090. doi:10.1016/j.janxdis.2009.07.011.

22. Wilmer MT, Anderson K, Reynolds M. Correlates of quality of life in anxiety disorders: Review of recent research. *Curr Psychiatry Rep*. 2021;23(11):77. doi:10.1007/s11920-021-01290-4.

23. Alcohol facts and statistics. National Institute on Alcohol Abuse and Alcoholism. https://www.niaaa.nih.gov/publications/brochures-and-fact-sheets/alcohol-facts-and-statistics. Accessed November 24, 2022.

24. Grant BF, Stinson FS, Dawson DA, et al. Prevalence and co-occurrence of substance use disorders and IndependentMood and anxiety disorders: Results from the National epidemiologic survey on alcohol and RelatedConditions. *Arch Gen Psychiatry*. 2004;61(8):807–816. doi:10.1001/archpsyc.61.8.807.

25. Attilia F, Perciballi R, Rotondo C, et al. Alcohol withdrawal syndrome: Diagnostic and therapeutic methods. *Riv Psichiatr.* 2018;53(3):118–122. doi:10.1708/2925.29413.

26. Simpson CA, Diaz-Arteche C, Eliby D, Schwartz OS, Simmons JG, Cowan CSM. The gut microbiota in anxiety and depression - A systematic review. *Clin Psychol Rev.* 2021;83:101943. doi:10.1016/j.cpr.2020.101943.

27. Slykerman RF, Hood F, Wickens K, et al. Effect of Lactobacillus rhamnosus HN001 in pregnancy on postpartum symptoms of depression and anxiety: A randomised double-blind placebo-controlled trial. *EBiomedicine.* 2017;24:159–165. doi:10.1016/j.ebiom.2017.09.013.

28. Tran N, Zhebrak M, Yacoub C, Pelletier J, Hawley D. The gut-brain relationship: Investigating the effect of multispecies probiotics on anxiety in a randomized placebo-controlled trial of healthy young adults. *J Affect Disord.* 2019;252:271–277. doi:10.1016/j.jad.2019.04.043.

29. Nishida K, Sawada D, Kuwano Y, Tanaka H, Rokutan K. Health benefits of *Lactobacillus gasseri* CP2305 tablets in young adults exposed to chronic stress: A randomized, double-blind, placebo-controlled study. *Nutrients.* 2019;11(8):1859. doi:10.3390/nu11081859.

30. Lee HJ, Hong JK, Kim JK, et al. Effects of probiotic NVP-1704 on mental health and sleep in healthy adults: An 8-week randomized, double-blind, placebo-controlled trial. *Nutrients.* 2021;13(8):2660. doi:10.3390/nu13082660.

31. Liu RT, Walsh RFL, Sheehan AE. Prebiotics and probiotics for depression and anxiety: A systematic review and meta-analysis of controlled clinical trials. *Neurosci Biobehav Rev.* 2019;102:13–23. doi:10.1016/j.neubiorev.2019.03.023.

32. Etkin, A, Prater, KE, Schatzberg, AF, Menon, V, Greicius, MD. Disrupted amygdalar subregion functional connectivity and evidence of a compensatory network in generalized anxiety disorder. *Arch Gen Psychiatry.* 2009;66(12):1361–1372. doi:10.1001/archgenpsychiatry.2009.10.

33. Stern, TA. Anxiety disorders (chapter 32). Massachusetts General Hospital Comprehensive Clinical Psychiatry, 2nd ed. London: Massachusetts General Hospital; 2015. ISBN 978-0-323-32899-9. OCLC 905232521.

34. Hoehn-Saric R, McLeod DR, Zimmerli WD. Somatic manifestations in women with generalized anxiety disorder. Psychophysiological responses to psychological stress. *Arch Gen Psychiatry.* 1989;46(12):1113–1119.

35. Brawman-Mintzer O, Lydiard RB. Biological basis of generalized anxiety disorder. *J Clin Psychiatry.* 1997;58(Suppl 3):16–25, discussion 26.

36. Munjack DJ, Baltazar PL, DeQuattro V, et al. Generalized anxiety disorder: Some biochemical aspects. *Psychiatry Res.* 1990;32(1):35–43.

37. Abelson JL, Glitz D, Cameron OG, Lee MA, Bronzo M, Curtis GC. Blunted growth hormone response to clonidine in patients with generalized anxiety disorder. *Arch Gen Psychiatry.* 1991;48(2):157–162.

38. Weizman R, Tanne Z, Greanek M. Peripheral benzodiazepine binding sites on platelet membranes are increased during diazepam treatment of anxious patients. *Eur J Pharmacol.* 1987;129:123–130.

39. Ferrarese C, Appollonio I, Frigo M, et al. Decreased density of benzodiazepine receptors in lymphocytes of anxious patients: Reversal after chronic diazepam treatment. *Acta Psychiatr Scand.* 1990;82(2):169–173.

40. Roy-Byrne PP, Cowley DS, Greenblatt DJ, Shader RI, Hommer D. Reduced benzodiazepine sensitivity in panic disorder. *Arch Gen Psychiatry.* 1990;47(6):534–538.

41. Tiihonen J, Kuikka J, Rasanen P, et al. Cerebral benzodiazepine receptor binding and distribution in generalized anxiety disorder: A fractal analysis. *Mol Psychiatry.* 1997;2(6):463–471.

42. Deakin JFW, Graeff FG. 5-HT and mechanisms of defence. *J Psychopharmacol.* 1991;5(4):305–315.

43. Brewerton T, Lydiard RB, Johnson MR, et al. CSF serotonin: Diagnostic and seasonal differences. Paper presented at the annual meeting of the American Psychiatric Association, Miami, FL; 1995.

44. Germine M, Goddard AW, Woods SW, Charney DS, Heninger GR. Anger and anxiety responses to m-chlorophenylpiperazine in generalized anxiety disorder. *Biol Psychiatry*. 1992;32(5):457–461.

45. Schneider LS, Munjack D, Severson JA, Palmer R. Platelet [3H]imipramine binding in generalized anxiety disorder, panic disorder, and agoraphobia with panic attacks. *Biol Psychiatry*. 1987;22(1):59–66.

46. Fossey MD, Lydiard RB, Ballenger JC, Laraia MT, Bissette G, Nemeroff CB. Cerebrospinal fluid corticotropin-releasing factor concentrations in patients with anxiety disorders and normal comparison subjects. *Biol Psychiatry*. 1996;39(8):703–707.

47. Tiller JW, Biddle N, Maguire KP, Davies BM. The dexamethasone suppression test and plasma dexamethasone in generalized anxiety disorder. *Biol Psychiatry*. 1988;23(3):261–270.

48. Noyes R Jr, Clarkson C, Crowe RR, Yates WR, McChesney CM. A family study of generalized anxiety disorder. *Am J Psychiatry*. 1987;144(8):1019–1024.

49. Kendler KS, Walters EE, Neale MC, Kessler RC, Heath AC, Eaves LJ. The structure of the genetic and environmental risk factors for six major psychiatric disorders in women. Phobia, generalized anxiety disorder, panic disorder, bulimia, major depression, and alcoholism. *Arch Gen Psychiatry*. 1995;52(5):374–383.

50. Hettema JM, Neale MC, Myers JM, Prescott CA, Kendler KS. A population-based twin study of the relationship between neuroticism and internalizing disorders. *Am J Psychiatry*. 2006;163(5):857–864.

51. Hudson JL, Rapee RM. From anxious temperament to disorder: An etiological model. In: Heimberg RG, Turk CL, Mennin DS, editors: *Generalized anxiety disorder: Advances in research and practice*. New York: Guilford Press; 2004.

52. Gerull FC, Rapee RM. Mother knows best: Effects of maternal modelling on the acquisition of fear and avoidance behaviour in toddlers. *Behav Res Ther*. 2002;40(3):279–287.

53. Hudson JL, Rapee RM. Parent-child interactions and anxiety disorders: An observational study. *Behav Res Ther*. 2001;39(12):1411–1427.

54. Barrett PM, Rapee RM, Dadds MM, Ryan SM. Family enhancement of cognitive style in anxious and aggressive children. *J Abnorm Child Psychol*. 1996;24(2):187–203.

55. Roemer L, Molina S, Borkovec TD. An investigation of worry content among generally anxious individuals. *J Nerv Ment Dis*. 1997;185(5):314–319.

56. Heim C, Nemeroff CB. The impact of early adverse experiences on brain systems involved in the pathophysiology of anxiety and affective disorders. *Biol Psychiatry*. 1999;46(11):1509–1522.

57. Chorpita BF, Barlow DH. The development of anxiety: The role of control in the early environment. *Psychol Bull*. 1998;124(1):3–21.

58. Borkovec TD, Roemer L. Perceived functions of worry among generalized anxiety disorder subjects: Distraction from more emotionally distressing topics? *J Behav Ther Exp Psychiatry*. 1995;26(1):25–30.

59. Lyonfields JD, Borkovec TD, Thayer JF. Vagal tone in generalized anxiety disorder and the effects of aversive imagery and worrisome thinking. *Behav Ther*. 1995;26:457–466.

60. MacLeod C, Rutherford E. Information-processing approaches: Assessing the selective functioning of attention, interpretation, and retrieval. In: Heimberg RG, Turk CL, Mennin DS, editors: *Generalized anxiety disorder: Advances in research and practice*. New York: Guilford Press; 2004.

61. MacLeod C, Hagan R. Individual differences in the selective processing of threatening information, and emotional responses to a stressful life event. *Behav Res Ther*. 1992;30(2):151–161.

62. Dugas MJ, Buhr K, Ladouceur R. The role of intolerance and uncertainty in etiology and maintenance. In: Heimberg RG, Turk CL, Mennin DS, editors: *Generalized anxiety disorder: Advances in research and practice.* New York: Guilford Press; 2004.

63. Dugas MJ, Gagnon F, Ladouceur R, Freeston MH. Generalized anxiety disorder: A preliminary test of a conceptual model. *Behav Res Ther.* 1998;36(2):215–226.

64. Hoge EA, Ivkovic A, Fricchione GL. Generalized anxiety disorder: Diagnosis and treatment. *BMJ.* 2012;345:e7500. doi:10.1136/bmj.e7500.

65. Munir S, Takov V. Generalized anxiety disorder. [Updated 2022 Jan 9]. In: StatPearls [Internet]. Treasure Island, FL: StatPearls Publishing. https://www.ncbi.nlm.nih.gov/books/NBK441870/.

66. American Psychiatric Association. *Diagnostic and Statistical Manual of Mental Disorders*, 5th ed.; 2013. doi:10.1176/appi.books.9780890425596.

67. Smith JP, Book SW. Anxiety and substance use disorders: A review. *Psychiatr Times.* 2008;25(10):19–23.

68. Brady EU, Kendall PC. Comorbidity of anxiety and depression in children and adolescents. *Psychol Bull.* 1992;111(2):244–255. doi:10.1037/0033-2909.111.2.244.

69. Kessler RC, Gruber M, Hettema JM, Hwang I, Sampson N, Yonkers KA. Co-morbid major depression and generalized anxiety disorders in the national comorbidity survey follow-up. *Psychol Med.* 2008;38(3):365–374. doi:10.1017/S0033291707002012.

70. Kessler RC, Sampson NA, Berglund P, et al. Anxious and non-anxious major depressive disorder in the World Health Organization World Mental Health Surveys. *Epidemiol Psychiatr Sci.* 2015;24(3):210–226. doi:10.1017/s2045796015000189.

71. Spitzer RL, Kroenke K, Williams JB, Löwe B. A brief measure for assessing generalized anxiety disorder: The GAD-7. *Arch Intern Med.* 2006;166(10):1092. doi:10.1001/archinte.166.10.1092.

72. Sapra A, Bhandari P, Sharma S, Chanpura T, Lopp L. Using generalized anxiety disorder-2 (GAD-2) and GAD-7 in a primary care setting. *Cureus.* 2020. doi:10.7759/cureus.8224.

73. Plummer F, Manea L, Trepel D, McMillan D. Screening for anxiety disorders with the GAD-7 and GAD-2: A systematic review and diagnostic metaanalysis. *Gen Hosp Psychiatry.* 2016;39:24–31. doi:10.1016/j.genhosppsych.2015.11.005.

74. Stein MB, Sareen J. Clinical practice: Generalized anxiety disorder. *N Engl J Med.* 2015;373(21):2059–2068.

75. Bandelow B, Sher L, Bunevicus R, et al. Guidelines for the pharmacological treatment of anxiety disorders, obsessive-compulsive disorder and posttraumatic stress disorder in primary care. *Int J Psychiatry Clin Pract.* 2012;16(2):77–84.

76. Simon NM, Hofmann SG, Rosenfield D, et al. Efficacy of yoga vs cognitive behavioral therapy vs stress education for the treatment of generalized anxiety disorder: A randomized clinical trial. *JAMA Psychiatry.* 2021;78(1):13–20.

77. Carl E, Witcraft SM, Kauffman BY, et al. Psychological and pharmacological treatments for generalized anxiety disorder (GAD): A meta-analysis of randomized controlled trials. *Cogn Behav Ther.* 2020;49(1):1–21.

78. Mitte K. Meta-analysis of cognitive-behavioral treatments for generalized anxiety disorder: A comparison with pharmacotherapy. *Psychol Bull.* 2005;131(5):785–795.

79. DeMartini J, Patel G, Fancher TL. Generalized anxiety disorder. *Ann Intern Med.* 2019;170(7):49–64.

80. Baldwin DS, Anderson IM, Nutt DJ et al. Evidence-based pharmacological treatment of anxiety disorders, post-traumatic stress disorder and obsessive-compulsive disorder: A revision of the 2005 guidelines from the British association for psychopharmacology. *J Psychopharmacol (Oxford).* 2014;28(5):403–439.

81. Borza L. Cognitive-behavioral therapy for generalized anxiety. *Dial Clin Neurosci.* 2017;19(2):203–208.

82. Carpenter JK, Andrews LA, Witcraft SM, Powers MB, Smits JAJ, Hofmann SG. Cognitive behavioral therapy for anxiety and related disorders: A meta-analysis of randomized placebo-controlled trials. *Depress Anxiety.* 2018;35(6):502–514.

83. Loerinc AG, Meuret AE, Twohig MP, Rosenfield D, Bluett EJ, Craske MG. Response rates for CBT for anxiety disorders: Need for standardized criteria. *MG Clin Psychol Rev.* 2015;42:72–78.

84. Abejuela HR, Osser DN. The psychopharmacology algorithm project at the Harvard south shore program: An algorithm for generalized anxiety disorder. *Harv Rev Psychiatry.* 2016;24(4):243–256.

85. Slee A, Nazareth I, Bondaronek P, Liu Y, Cheng Z, Freemantle N. Pharmacological treatments for generalised anxiety disorder: A systematic review and network meta-analysis. *Lancet.* 2019;393(10173):768–777.

86. Rickels K, Rynn M, Iyengar M, Duff D. Remission of generalized anxiety disorder: A review of the paroxetine clinical trials database. *J Clin Psychiatry.* 2006;67(1):41.

87. Lu L, Mills JA, Hailong L, et al. Acute neurofunctional effects of escitalopram in pediatric anxiety: A double-blind, placebo-controlled trial. *J Am Acad Child Adolesc Psychiatry.* 2021;60(10):1309–1318.

88. Whalen PJ, Johnstone T, Somerville LH, et al. A functional magnetic resonance imaging predictor of treatment response to venlafaxine in generalized anxiety disorder. *Biol Psychiatry.* 2008;63(9):858–863.

89. Carceller H, Perez-Rando M, Castren E, Nacher J, Guirado R. Effects of the antidepressant fluoxetine on the somatostatin interneurons in the basolateral amygdala. *Neuroscience.* 2018;386:205–213.

90. Maslowsky J, Mogg K, Bradley BP, et al. A preliminary investigation of neural correlates of treatment in adolescents with generalized anxiety disorder. *J Child Adolesc Psycho Pharmacol.* 2010;20:105–111.

91. Gorka SM, Young CB, Klumpp H, et al. Emotion-based brain mechanisms and predictors for SSRI and CBT treatment of anxiety and depression: A randomized trial. *Neuropsychopharmacology.* 2019;44(9):1639–1648.

92. Burkhouse KL, Kujawa A, Hosseini B, et al. Anterior cingulate activation to implicit threat before and after treatment for pediatric anxiety disorders. *Prog Neuro Psycho Pharmacol.* 2018;84:250–256.

93. Garakani A, Murrough JW, Freire RC, et al. Pharmacotherapy of anxiety disorders: Current and emerging treatment options. *Front Psychiatry.* 2020;11:584–595.

94. Generoso MB, Trevisol AP, Kasper S, Cho HJ, Cordeiro Q, Shiozawa P. Pregabalin for generalized anxiety disorder: An updated systematic review and meta-analysis. *Int Clin Psychopharmacol.* 2017;32(1):49–55.

95. Teschke R, Genthner A, Wolff A. Kava hepatotoxicity: Comparison of aqueous, ethanolic, acetonic kava extracts and kava–herbs mixtures. *J Ethnopharmacol.* 2009;123(3):378–384.

96. Savage K, Firth J, Stough C, Sarris J. GABA-modulating phytomedicines for anxiety: A systematic review of preclinical and clinical evidence. *Phytother Res.* 2018;32(1):3–18.

97. Hieu TH, Dibas M, Surya Dila KA, et al. Therapeutic efficacy and safety of chamomile for state anxiety, generalized anxiety disorder, insomnia, and sleep quality: A systematic review and meta-analysis of randomized trials and quasi-randomized trials. *Phytother Res.* 2019;33(6):1604–1615.

98. Yeung KS, Hernandez M, Mao JJ, Haviland I, Gubili J. Herbal medicine for depression and anxiety: A systematic review with assessment of potential psycho-oncologic relevance. *Phytother Res.* 2018;32(5):865–891.

6

# Gut Microbiota and Mental Health

## The Gut–Brain Axis

Ashley Oake, Nicole Nesto, and Yashwant V. Pathak

## Contents

## 6.1 Introduction

The gut–brain axis is the connection between the central nervous system (CNS) and enteric nervous system (ENS) that allows the brain and gastrointestinal tract to influence each other (1). Over 500 million neurons are present in the ENS, which is five times the amount contained in the CNS (1). There are many nerves running between these systems, but the largest is the vagus nerve (cranial nerve ten) that originates from the medulla and connects to the esophagus and stomach as it gives off branches, terminating at the left splenic flexure (1). The vagus nerve transmits sensory and motor information between these systems in both an efferent and afferent manner (1). Information from the stomach and composition of GI (gastrointestinal) contents is sent to the CNS, which processes this and sends signals back to the stomach to produce acid and subsequently stimulate contractions (1). Reflex circuits in the ENS also allow the gut to act in an independent manner to process food (1).

DOI: 10.1201/9781003333821-6

Generally, four pathways are used to communicate information: vagal and spinal afferent neurons, cytokines, endocrine hormones, and microbial factors (2). This connection is needed to determine hunger and satiety, distinguish dangerous food, and maintain homeostasis (2). Endocrine cells in the gut are in close approximation to the microbiome, which activates these cells to produce hormones (2). Bacteria in the microbiome produce necessary metabolites and vitamins and other compounds including lipopolysaccharides, peptides, and microbe-associated molecular patterns (2). These metabolites are recognized by the innate immune system and activate toll-like receptors at several levels of the body (2).

The connection between the mind and gastrointestinal tract was initially discussed during the year 1765 when Dr Robert Whytt coined the term "nervous sympathy" while observing the vast nervous supply throughout the gut (3). He sparked a community-wide interest in the concept that the stomach has a strong influence on an individual's mental and emotional well-being (3). In the year 1811, a doctor in London named John Abernethy became fascinated by the connection and went on to publish 11 editions of a book titled *Surgical Observations on the Constitutional Origin and Treatment of Local Diseases* followed by another publication titled *The Abernethian Code of Health and Longevity* (3). Throughout these texts he aimed to connect all mental and bodily disorders to the composition and dysfunction of the gastrointestinal tract (3). A physician's main concern during this time period was to protect the nerves, not the microbiome, by eating natural foods that were not refined or processed (3). If a patient had a poor diet or an issue with alcohol, the thought process was then focused on "disorder of the nerves" which was the resultant ailment (3).

During the late 1800s, most women lived off a diet of white bread and tea in attempts to save nutritious food for their children and husbands (3). Physicians determined that tea was a nervous stimulant that was causing women to experience high levels of anxiety (3). The Dean of Bangor claimed that overconsumption of tea was creating the nervousness, hysterical behavior, and discontent that women were experiencing, and it would eventually lead to dangerous and rebellious behavior (3). Dyspepsia, a term used for an upset stomach without an obvious cause, was thought to be caused by large amounts of tea and determined to be the precursor for emotional distress (3).

The use of the term "gut–brain axis" started in the 1960s and 1970s when scientists discovered that there are several peptides that occur in both the gastrointestinal system and the brain (2). This connection was termed the amine precursor uptake and decarboxylation hypothesis which indicated that peptide-producing cells contained in both areas shared the common origin of neural crest cells (2). Neuropeptides are short chains of polypeptides that have the ability to act as neurotransmitters throughout our system (2). Common neuropeptides studied in association with the gut–brain axis are substance P, calcitonin gene-related peptide and neuropeptide Y (NPY), vasoactive intestinal polypeptide, somatostatin, and corticotropin-releasing factor (2). Later studies did disprove this theory, but the knowledge gained from experiments contributed further to our understanding of the composition of the GI tract vastly (2).

This bidirectional pathway has been studied in the pathophysiology of both gastrointestinal and brain-related disorders, which include irritable bowel syndrome, autism spectrum disorders, Parkinson's, and mood disorders (4). Studies have shown that the microbiota has influence on behaviors, stress, emotion, pain response, and even the biochemistry of the brain (4). Many individuals have invested in prebiotics or probiotics to promote the overall health of their GI system, while studies have shown taking certain antibiotics can dysregulate homeostasis of this system specifically (4). The connection between the two systems is clear, but there is not a definite answer as to whether the primary alteration is in the brain (top-down effects) or in the gastrointestinal system (bottom-up effects) (4).

A properly regulated microbiome may be crucial for early-stage development of the inhibitory response to hypothalamic-pituitary-adrenal (HPA) axis activation in the neuroendocrine system (5). With over $10^{14}$ bacteria colonizing the gastrointestinal tract, maturation of the immune system and efficient absorption of macromolecules require a functional population of microbes to produce the necessary metabolites and vitamins (5). Activation of the HPA axis by the limbic system leads to excess cortisol production and a consequent increased level of anxiety (5). Early exposure to microbes is required for development of the inhibitory response to the HPA axis during stress and some studies have indicated that the introduction of healthy bacterium during certain developmental stages may help control these responses (5). Dysregulation for an extended period of time can lead to mood disorders including anxiety and depression and exposure too late during development increases the chances of lacking a functional inhibitory component (5).

## 6.2 Anatomy of the Gastrointestinal System

The gastrointestinal tract is composed of a series of hollow organs that run from the mouth to the anus (6). Namely, this tract includes the pharynx, esophagus, stomach, small intestine, large intestine, and rectum (6). The small intestine can be further divided into the duodenum, jejunum, and ileum; and the large intestine, also known as the colon, can be divided into the cecum, ascending, transverse, descending, and sigmoid colon (6). The large intestine also includes the appendix, which is a blind pouch composed predominantly of lymphoid tissue and attached to the cecum (6). In addition to these hollow GI viscera, there are accessory solid organs of the digestive system which include the liver, the pancreas, and the gallbladder (6). All of these organs play a specific and vital role in the function of the GI tract (7).

If we further examine the GI tract via cross section, there are several readily apparent layers consistently seen throughout the entire tract (7). These layers from outward to inward consist of (i) the serosa, (ii) a longitudinal smooth muscle layer, (iii) a circular smooth muscle layer, (iv) the submucosa, and (v) the mucosa (7). The serosa or adventitia is the outermost layer composed of loose connective tissue and lined by visceral peritoneum; the serosa also contains blood vessels, nerves, and lymphatics (8). Both the longitudinal and circular smooth muscle layers are the primary driving force of peristalsis which propels food along the length of the GI tract (8). The submucosa is another layer of loose connective tissue that contains an array of larger blood vessels, nerves, and lymphatics as well as some mucous glands (8). Lastly, the innermost layer, or the mucosa, is comprised of a thin layer of longitudinal smooth muscle called the muscularis mucosae, a thin layer of connective tissue called the lamina propria which provides vascular support for the epithelium and contains mucous glands as well as lymphoid follicles, and lastly, the epithelium (8).

The oral cavity functions to mechanically process food via mastication, to lubricate food by mixing chewed contents with saliva, and to initiate the digestion process of carbohydrates and lipids via the actions of amylase and lipase respectively (9). The principal glands of salivation located in the oral cavity are the parotid, submandibular, and sublingual glands (10). The parotid gland secretes almost entirely a serous secretion (predominantly composed of amylase and lipase) whereas the submandibular and sublingual glands secrete both a serous and a mucous secretion (10). Aside from the production of saliva, the salivary glands also aid in defense against the numerous microbes present in the oral cavity (11). Plasma cells reside in the salivary glands which secrete the antibody IgA, which then binds to the mucous layer that covers the epithelial lining of the oral cavity, thus providing a barrier against potentially dangerous pathogens (11). The oral cavity is primarily lined by both keratinized stratified squamous and nonkeratinized stratified squamous epithelium (12).

The pharynx serves as a passageway of food from the oral cavity to the esophagus although it also serves a respiratory function (9). To accomplish this purpose, during swallowing, closure of the nasopharynx and larynx occurs to maintain the patency of the airway (9). The esophagus's primary function is to empty food into the stomach via peristalsis (9). The upper third of the esophagus is composed of (voluntary) skeletal muscle, the middle third is composed of a mixture of skeletal and smooth muscle, and the lower third is composed of (involuntary) smooth muscle (9). The pharynx and esophagus are lined with stratified squamous epithelium which serves as a protective barrier against injury from the swallowed food bolus (12).

Once the food arrives in the stomach, it serves as a storage site where the food can then be further mechanically and chemically broken down (9). In contradistinction to other segments in the GI tract, the stomach possesses three muscular layers: an inner oblique layer, a middle circular layer, and an outer longitudinal layer (9). The consistent contraction and relaxation of these muscle layers makes the stomach especially suited to mix and churn food to produce chyme (9). Additional digestion occurs via the production of digestive enzymes from the parietal and chief cells (9). The parietal cells elaborate hydrochloric acid, and the chief cells produce a zymogen called pepsinogen which is activated at a pH between 1.5 and 2 to become the enzyme pepsin (a protein-digesting enzyme) (9).The acidic environment of the stomach brought about by hydrochloric acid destroys most of the microorganisms ingested with food, denatures protein, breaks down plant cell walls, and, as already mentioned, is essential for the activation and function of pepsin (9). The mucosal surface of the stomach consists of simple columnar epithelium which contains additional mucous-secreting cells essential for the protection against acidic corrosion of the stomach wall (12).

Unlike the stomach, which has minor absorptive properties, 90% of food absorption takes place in the small intestine (9). The epithelium of the small intestine is typified by simple columnar epithelium with microvilli which is highly specialized to aid in absorption (12). There are numerous adaptations present in the mucosa of the small intestine designed to increase the surface area available for absorption (13). The folds of Kerckring increase the absorptive area threefold, the villi enhance the surface area another tenfold and, lastly, the microvilli further increase the surface area another twentyfold (13). Thus, the entire absorptive area of the small intestine is amplified a thousand-fold—creating a surface area of almost 250 or more square meters which is analogous to the size of a tennis court (13). Before the food can be absorbed into the hepatic circulation, it must be broken down into its most basic constituents via the action of numerous digestive enzymes (9). The enzymes produced by the small intestine include lipase for fat digestion, peptidase for peptide breakdown and sucrase, maltase, and lactase for sucrose, maltose, and lactose breakdown, respectively (9).

As discussed earlier, the small intestine can be further classified into segments such as the duodenum, the jejunum, and the ileum (6). The duodenum receives acidic chyme from the stomach as well as secretions from the pancreas and the liver that aid in the digestion process (9). The secretion from the pancreas contains mainly digestive enzymes as well as bicarbonate which then combines with bile secreted from the liver in the common bile duct (9). The pancreatic enzymes are produced as zymogens, which includes trypsinogen, chymotrypsinogen, and procarboxypeptidase, which are then activated by enteropeptidase when they reach the brush border of the small intestine (9). Others include alpha-amylase; lipase and colipase, which act on triglycerides and phospholipids; and several other enzymes like ribonuclease, elastase, and collagenase (9). The bile produced from the liver and stored in the gallbladder emulsifies fat and aids in the digestion of lipids (9). The combined secretions then enter the proximal duodenum through the ampulla of Vater (9). In order to prevent damage to the lining of the duodenum from the acidic chyme, the secretions also contain bicarbonate (9). Additionally, the duodenum contains a specialized mucosal adaption called Brunner's glands that secrete an alkaline solution to further neutralize the acidity of the chyme from the stomach (9). Moving past the duodenum, the jejunum is where the bulk of chemical digestion and absorption occur (9). Although the jejunum lacks true defining characteristics, it is notable for possessing long arterial arcades adapted for maximizing circulation through the small intestine (12). The ileum is the terminal portion of the small intestine which opens into the cecum (the first portion of the large intestine) (9). Although nutrients continue to be absorbed in the ileum, the bulk of absorption occurs in the more proximal duodenum and jejunum (9). A defining characteristic of the ileum is the presence of Peyer's patches (9). Peyer's patches are collections of mucosal-associated lymphoid tissue (MALT) that constitute an important component of the gut immune system (9). The surface epithelium of Peyer's patches is formed by low cuboidal M-cells, specialized enterocytes which facilitate the interaction between antigen and lymphocytes in order to initiate a competent immune response to foreign invaders (9).

The remaining unabsorbed and undigested food material progresses into the cecum of the large intestine; at this point, the material is referred to as feces (9). The primary function of the large intestine is to reabsorb water and electrolytes in order to create solid feces (9). This is further accomplished via the action of goblet cells, which produce copious amounts of mucous that helps to bind the feces together in a solid mass (12). While the small intestine also possesses goblet cells, the large intestine contains a much greater number of these cells (12). Most of the absorption in the large intestine occurs in the proximal colon (the cecum, ascending and transverse colon), giving this portion the name absorbing colon, whereas the distal colon (the descending and sigmoid colon), functions principally for feces storage until a convenient time for excretion and is therefore referred to as the storage colon (13). The peristaltic movement of the large intestine (accomplished by longitudinal muscle bands called taeniae coli) moves the feces into the rectum (9). In the rectum, stretch receptors signal for the defecation process to start, which includes a reflexive relaxation of internal anal sphincter smooth muscle and conscious relaxation of the external anal sphincter skeletal muscle (9). While the rectum is lined by nonkeratinized stratified squamous epithelium, the remainder of the large intestine is lined with simple columnar epithelium that lacks the microvilli seen in the small intestine portion of the GI tract (12).

In summary, the gastrointestinal tract supplies the body with the necessary water, electrolytes, vitamins, and nutrients which requires the following: movement of food through the GI tract, secretion of digestive juices into food, absorption of water, electrolytes, and vitamins, circulation of blood through the GI viscera to carry away necessary nutrients and, lastly, control of all these functions via local, nervous, and hormonal systems (7).

## 6.2.1 The Microbiome

Up until the time of birth, the human fetus lives in a protected and mostly sterile environment, however this rapidly begins to change as the newborn infant is exposed to bacteria, archaea, fungi, and viruses from the parents, close contacts, and the environment (14). Over the next few years, communities of organisms, also known as microbiota, form on the surfaces of the infant's skin, nares, oral cavity, intestines, and genitourinary tract (14). Upon the completion of this colonization, it is estimated that bacterial cells outnumber human cells in the host by 10:1 and the bacterial population contributes an additional three-hundredfold more unique protein genes than the host alone (14). The Human Microbiome Project collected samples from the nose, mouth, skin, gut, and vagina of volunteers (15). Their analyses demonstrated that there is substantial variation in the species and gene composition for individuals and at different body sites (15). For example, there is a unique microbiome profile in each of the tested locations, i.e., the bacteria colonizing the gut are significantly different from those colonizing the mouth, skin, and other body sites (15). The body site among participants that exhibited the greatest diversity in its microbiome composition was the intestine; in contrast, the vagina exhibited the least diverse microbiome profile among participants (14). The symbiotic relationship of the microbiome with the host is essential in providing needed metabolic functions, stimulating innate immunity, and preventing colonization with unwanted pathogens (14).

Most individuals share a core microbiome which can be defined as a specific profile of species that are present at a specific site in 95% or more of individuals (14). Typically, it is the species that make up the core microbiome that are the most numerous in a sample; the remaining species profile is referred to as the secondary microbiome (14). Based on this observation, it can be hypothesized that the species present in the core microbiome are critical in providing functions in the host essential to retaining homeostatic metabolic and immunologic activities (14). The secondary microbiome, in contrast, is more diverse, and therefore, it can be hypothesized that these organisms are responsible for a broader niche that can be filled by a variety of different organisms (14). In other words, although the genomic diversity between any two individuals may be great, there is functional redundancy (14). The sample sites in individuals most likely to constitute a core microbiome are the mouth, followed by the nose, intestine, and skin (14). The fewest shared species among individuals, i.e., the least likely site to constitute a core microbiome is the vagina (14).

There are many factors that determine the diversity of the host microbiome: the pH or salt in a given environment, the ability to use oxygen or lack thereof, and the relative availability of minerals or nutrients in a given location (16). For example, many sites in the body contain little to no oxygen, such as the mouth, intestine, and genitourinary tract and, as such, these sites are mainly inhabited by anaerobic or facultative anaerobic bacteria (16). Additionally, the microbiome is also influenced by personal hygiene, diet, water source, medicine, and exposure to environmental toxins (16).

Because humans and their intestinal microbiomes have coevolved together, the microbiome has been shown to have a profound influence on the immune system (17). Commensal organisms in the intestines induce and regulate both innate and adaptive immune responses locally in the gut as well as systemically (17). Studies in mice have shown that commensal bacteria are actually necessary for the repair and proliferation of the epithelial barrier after injury (17). Additionally, commensal bacteria are essential in stimulating Th17 immune responses and in driving the development of T-regulatory immune responses (17).

Although the gut microbiome is incredibly diverse, the dominant species are members of just three groups: Actinobacteria (e.g., *Bifidobacterium*), Bacteroidetes (e.g., *Bacteroides*), and Firmicutes (e.g., *Eubacterium, Ruminococcus, Faecalibacterium, Blautia*) (18). These species produce bacteriocins and other antibacterial metabolites that can deter competitor species from colonizing (18). Bacteria in the gut are responsible for metabolizing complex carbohydrates (cellulose, pectin, and xylan) into short chain fatty acids that can be readily transported across the intestinal wall and utilized by the rest of the body (18). Additionally, the acids also limit the growth of pathogenic bacteria by dampening the neutrophil inflammatory response in the gut (17). Bacteroidetes and Firmicutes are more efficient than other species at breaking down these complex carbohydrates into fatty acids and, as such, excess increases in these bacteria in the gut can lead to a higher efficiency in storage of metabolic products (17). This has been postulated to be of benefit to malnourished patients or patients with wasting syndromes seen in AIDS or cancer patients (14).

## 6.3 The Enteric Nervous System

The gastrointestinal system is surrounded by its own organized network consisting of thousands of small ganglia called the enteric nervous system (ENS) (18). These ganglia lie within the walls of the entire digestive tract, starting from the esophagus and following through to the colon, making the ENS the largest section of the ANS (autonomic nervous system) (18). Stemming from the peripheral nervous system, the ENS has the ability to modulate autonomous functions independently of the other nervous systems (18). This systematic approach instructs the GI system to hold contents in specific locations, allowing each section of the stomach and bowel to complete their individual tasks before moving onto the next (18). Churning, segmentation, haustration, and all secretory functions are tightly regulated to ensure proper pH balance, absorption of nutrients, and expulsion of waste products (18).

In contrast to the CNS, the enteric nervous system lacks a blood-enteric nervous system barrier, but it does contain supportive glial cells throughout (19).

The ganglia are separated into two sets: the external myenteric plexus and the internal submucosal ganglia (19). Also known as the Auerbach plexus, the myenteric plexus is positioned between the two muscularis externa layers (the inner circular muscle layer and the outer longitudinal muscle) (19). Myenteric ganglia are continuous throughout the entire GI system and are responsible for peristaltic movement of the bowel (19). Dysfunction of this set of neurons specifically can lead to Hirschsprung disease, achalasia, and gastroparesis (20). Inhibitory neurotransmitters involved in GI motility that allow relaxation are vasoactive intestinal peptide (VIP), nitric oxide, pituitary adenylate cyclase-activating peptide, and purine (20). Neurotransmitters that are excitatory and stimulate contraction are mainly tachykinins and acetylcholine (20). In the inner circular layer of muscle, spindle-shaped cells called interstitial cells of Cajal act as pacemaker cells to initiate activity within the myenteric plexus (20).

The submucosal plexus is only present in the small and large intestine with very few ganglia present in the stomach and consists of two layers: the outermost Schabadasch's plexus and the Meissner's plexus (19). Schabadasch's plexus projects to the motor neurons in the circular smooth layer while the Messiner's plexus (or inner layer) innervates the submucosal glands and lies next to the muscularis mucosa (21). Collectively, the layers of the submucosal plexus are responsible for modulating blood flow, increasing digestive and protective secretions, and aiding in absorption of essential nutrients (21). Dysregulation of this plexus is involved with conditions such as inflammatory bowel disease (21).

Control of the movement of water and electrolytes between tissues involves the activity of secretomotor neurons that are under the control of vasoactive intestinal peptide (VIP) and acetylcholine (19). Fluid influx and outflux is influenced by sympathetic pathways responding to the change in blood pressure and volume (19). Vasodilation accompanies secretion to ensure proper fluid outflux and concentration of secretory products (19). Cholinergic neurons in the stomach receive input from the vagus nerve to initiate gastric acid secretion (19). HCl, pepsinogen, and other enzymes are controlled mainly by the vago-vagal reflex of the ENS (19). Endocrine cells in the GI tract secrete gastrin-releasing peptide and serotonin to communicate internally as well (19).

The enteric nervous system contains a bidirectional connection with the CNS to transmit information regarding satiety, nausea, and hunger (23). Originating from the vagal, truncal, and sacral neural crest cells, intrinsic primary afferent neurons predominate indicating that a majority of this pathway is in the direction of the CNS (23). Interneurons and motor neurons constitute the remaining portion of the ENS to regulate independent reflex control (23). A large majority of information sent to the brain is received unconsciously but may influence an individual's emotional state (23). Due to the connection favoring the majority of signals being sent to the CNS, dysregulation in the gastrointestinal system can lead to pathological affects throughout the brain (23).

## 6.4 Pathways of the Gut–Brain Axis

Research has shown that several prevalent mood disorders have been linked to disruptions in gut microbiome and overall diet may additionally play a role in cognitive function (22). The four major pathways that are involved in the gut–brain axis are the neurologic, endocrine, humoral/metabolic, and immune (22). Each pathway works in conjunction with the other three in order to achieve a synergistic effect (22).

### 6.4.1 The Neurologic Pathway

The neurologic pathway involves the production of neurotransmitters (GABA, serotonin, histamine, acetylcholine) and the association with cranial nerve ten (22). In the late 1990s, the connection between the microbiome and the gut–brain axis was identified and studies began to shift towards balancing the ratio of bacteria in the gut (22). A study with the administration of *Campylobacter jejuni* into rats demonstrated an increase in anxiety-like behavior along with activation of corresponding areas in the brain through the vagus nerve (22). Other studies have shown that treatment with *Lactobacillus rhamnosus* can decrease anxiety and depression by activation of $GABA_{A\alpha2}$ and $GABA_{B1b}$ receptor mRNA in the CNS (2).

Depending on the composition of the microbiome, the contractions controlling motility and mucous production supplying the epithelial barrier are modulated by the ANS (4). An overgrowth of bacteria in the GI tract can lead to a reduction in migrating contracts causing constipation and irritable bowel syndrome (4). Mucous produced by intestinal cells creates a biofilm for bacteria to colonize which is increased or decreased depending on parasympathetic or sympathetic stimulation (4). A reduction in the mucous barrier increases permeability to the epithelium and organisms may pass through to activate the immune system (4). Catecholamines are widely studied for their host to microbe signaling abilities and stressors can increase the levels in the plasma and lumen (25). Excess amounts of norepinephrine can activate the virulent properties of *Campylobacter jejuni* (25). Studies have shown that enterohemorrhagic Escherichia coli (EHEC) increases in virulence, motility, and chemotaxis when catecholamines interact with the QseC receptor (25).

### 6.4.2 The Endocrine Pathway

The endocrine pathway involves the formation of peptides from the enteroendocrine cells and the activation of the HPA axis (22). Galanin is a major peptide released from the GI tract during chemical stimulation of mucosa and intestinal distension (23). It stimulates the activity of the central branch of the HPA axis to release corticotropin-releasing factor and ACTH (adrenocorticotropic hormone), leading to an increased release of cortisol and norepinephrine (23).

This neuropeptide is involved in modulating feeding, mood, blood pressure, sleep, and behavior (23).

In 2004, the connection between the microbiome and the development of the neural system was studied using rodents by monitoring the hypothalamic-pituitary-adrenal reaction to stress (5). The mice were separated into three groups: germ-free (GF), specific pathogen-free (SPF) and gnotobiotic mice with a full microbiome (5). When exposed to stressful situations, ACTH and corticosterone levels were significantly higher in the germ-free mice while brain-derived neurotrophic factor levels were reduced (5). Researchers introduced *Bifidobacterium infantis*, considered a healthy bacterium, to the germ-free mice and the excess HPA stress response was reduced (5). When SPF feces was cultured into GF mice at an early stage rather than later stage in life, the HPA stress response was able to become regulated (5). This study indicated that exposure to bacteria at an early age is crucial for the proper development of inhibitory control of the HPA system which is necessary during stressful environments (5).

### 6.4.3 The Humoral/Metabolic Pathway

Metabolites, including short chain fatty acids, are produced when bacteria ferment indigestible polysaccharides (24). These end products are taken up by transporters and receptors to be distributed across the body and effect various cellular processes, comprising the humoral/metabolic pathway of the gut–brain axis (24). Hydrogen or sodium dependent monocarboxylate transporters interact with metabolites to transfer them into the epithelial cells of the colon to then be further transported into the portal circulation (24). These SCFAs (short chain fatty acids) can act as hormones and stimulate the sympathetic aspect of the ANS, while also having the ability to cross the blood-brain barrier to interact with microglia (24). Studies show that they play an important role in maintaining the blood-brain barrier by ensuring expression of tight junction proteins, including claudin and occludin (24). Regulation of the microglia is necessary for proper brain development and a lack of SCFAs is studied for their association with autism (24). Microglia refine circuits and synaptic connection by eliminating unnecessary or faulty areas for appropriate brain maturation.

Binding to G protein coupled receptors throughout the GI, nervous, and immune system can initiate the production of peptides and enzymes (24). Enteroendocrine cells secrete glucagon-like peptide 1 and peptide YY to signal the release of insulin during meals in order to distribute and store nutrients (24). The gut provides almost 95% of the serotonin in the body and enteroendocrine cells are responsible for regulating the release from enterochromaffin cells in the gut when interacting with SCFAs (24). SCFAs play a role in maintaining the amount of tryptophan 5-hydroxylase 1, which converts tryptophan to serotonin, and tyrosine hydroxylase, which produces catecholamines (24).

Gram negative bacteria contain surface glycolipids, called lipopolysaccharides (LPS), that act as proinflammatory components in the gut microbiota and gut-associated lymphoid tissue (25). They are comprised of three components (lipid A, a core oligosaccharide, and O antigen) and act as a protective agent against antibiotics for the bacteria (25). When the permeability of the epithelial barrier is increased, the LPS can enter the circulation and lead to septic shock, disruption of the immune system, and irritable bowel disease (25). LPS can increase the permeability of tight junctions in the gut epithelium directly by inducing enterocyte membrane expression and localization of TLR-4 and CD14 to further worsen conditions (25). The inflammatory changes in the GALT (gut-associated lymphoid tissue) and microbiota are associated with further development to ulcerative colitis and Crohn's disease (25).

## 6.4.4 The Immune Pathway

The immune pathway is engaged when the microbiome is dysregulated and the innate immune system releases cytokines (IL-10 or IL-4) and other inflammatory mediators to destroy the suspected invader (26) Lipopolysaccharides, which are involved in humoral and metabolic pathways, trigger the immune system when they enter into the blood stream (26). An overactive innate immune response for an extended time can increase an individual's risk for disorders including depression, dementia, and schizophrenia (26). Cases of depression show increases in IL-1β, IL-6, tumor necrosis factor-α, as well as interferon gamma, and C-reactive protein (26).

The methods used to study the connection between the microbiome and CNS are currently germ-free models, antibiotics, fecal microbiota transplant (FMT), prebiotics/fermented foods, probiotics, and brain imaging (27). Germ-free models lack all microorganisms and are under tight control to prevent contamination in order to have a reliable control group (27). Antibiotics are titrated to determine an ideal dosage for absorption and minimal side effects (27). The main concerns for antibiotics are depletion of the normal flora leading to dysregulation of homeostasis (27). FMT involves transplanting the microbiota from one patient into another that lacks a proper microbiota (27). This procedure is common in *Clostridium difficile* infections (27). Prebiotics are high fiber supplements that feed the microbiome and probiotics are live microorganisms used to maintain the "good" bacteria (27). MRI studies to determine structure and function of the brain became frequently used in the 2000s to study the connection with microbiota development (27).

## 6.5 Conclusion

The gut–brain axis is the neurological connection between the central nervous system and the enteric nervous system that allows the brain and the GI tract to influence one another. Studies have shown that composition of the microbiota has influence in both GI diseases, such as IBD (inflammatory bowel disease) and IBS (irritable bowel syndrome), and neurological conditions, including but not limited to Parkinson's, Alzheimer's, anxiety, and depression. Starting from birth, a community of organisms develop on the skin and epithelial tissue throughout the GI tract. Human cells are outnumbered 10:1 by bacteria which show a unique variation in species and gene composition across different locations in the body. The intestine is the site in the body that shows the largest diversity, and the vagina shows the least variation of bacteria.

The enteric nervous system, which is a subset of the PNS, is composed of over 500 million neurons starting at the esophagus and continuing all the way down to the anus. Motility, secretion, and other digestive functions are all independently controlled by the ENS, but four pathways have the ability to transfer this information to the CNS. Neurotransmitters, along with the vagus nerve, are involved in the neurologic pathway of the gut–brain axis. The autonomic nervous system works through this pathway to influence motility and produce gastric acid, but also to alert the brain of pain, hunger, and satiety. Peptide hormones released from enteroendocrine cells that activate the HPA axis are involved in the endocrine pathway. Galanin is one of the major peptides released from the gut and it modulates the contractions and secretions throughout the GI tract.

During digestion, small chain fatty acids and other metabolites are produced from the epithelial cells of the small and large intestines to regulate other systems in the body as part of the humoral/metabolic pathway. These SCFAs can influence the production of serotonin and GABA, along with increasing peptides to signal the release of insulin during a meal. Lipopolysaccharides are present in gram negative bacteria and when they come in contact with the epithelium they increase the permeability for entrance into the bloodstream, leading to shock. This interaction activates the innate immune system to release cytokines and other inflammatory mediators to signal the body of an invader through the immune pathway of the gut–brain axis.

## 6.6 Future Trends

Current research regarding the gut–brain axis is mainly focused on the pathways connecting the CNS to the GI tract, the composition of bacteria, and the pharmacological treatments for microbiome dysregulation (28). Researchers are interested in the possibility of the structure of the microbiome controlling the feeding and appetite center (28). This regulatory pathway could be used to control weight and other metabolic disorders including diabetes and obesity (28). Nod2 receptors play a role in modulating the metabolism in individuals by the interaction with short chain fatty acids from the metabolic pathway (28). These receptors are located on GABA inhibitory neurons and show a connection with the neurologic pathway as well (28).

New proposed ideas with translational microbiome research are interested in investigating metabolites and other compounds to understand their impact on neurological disorders, mainly Alzheimer's (29). Most current studies are completed with the use of rodents, which give us an idea of the impact, but scientists are looking to a closer biological model to properly reflect pathology of the disease (29). Another barrier that has been presented is the fact that lab animals are too far removed from the natural environment to demonstrate the course of disease in the natural world (29). Prior research has given us tremendous insight up until this point, but without an improved model, there are concerns that future studies will be limited (29).

## Bibliography

1. Furness B, Callaghan BP, Rivera LR, & Cho HJ. The Enteric Nervous System and Gastrointestinal Innervation: Integrated Local and Central Control. *Advances in Experimental Medicine and Biology*. 2014; 817: 39–71.
2. Holzer P, & Farzi A. Neuropeptides and the Microbiota-Gut-Brain Axis. *Advances in Experimental Medicine and Biology*. 2014; 817: 195–219.
3. Miller I. The Gut–Brain Axis: Historical Reflections. *Microbial Ecology in Health and Disease*. 2014 Nov; 29: 154292.
4. Mayer EA, Tillisch K, & Gupta A. Gut/Brain Axis and the Microbiota. *The Journal of Clinical Investigation*. 2015 Feb; 125(3): 926–938.
5. Sudo N, Chida Y, Aiba Y, et al. Postnatal Microbial Colonization Programs the Hypothalamic–Pituitary–Adrenal System for Stress Response in Mice. *The Journal of Physiology*. 2004 Jul; 558(1): 263–275.
6. National Institure of Diabetes, Digestive, and Kidney Disease. Your Digestive System & How It Works. NIDDK. [Online]. 2017.
7. Hall JE, & Hall ME. Chapter 63. General Principles of Gastrointestinal Function-Motility, Nervous Control, and Blood Circulation. *Guyton and Hall Textbook of Medical Physiology*. 2021; 14: 787–796.
8. University of Leeds. Oral: Four Layers of the G.I. Tract. *University of LEEDS - The Histology Guide*. [Online]. 2022.
9. Ogobuiro I, Gonzales J, & Tuma F. Physiology, Gastrointestinal. *StatPearls*. 2022 Apr.
10. Hall JE, & Hall ME. Chapter 65. Secretory Functions of the Alimentary Tract. *Guyton and Hall Textbook of Medical Physiology*. 2021; 14: 807–822.
11. Humphreys I. Immunity in the Salivary Gland. *British Society for Immunology*. [Online]. 2022.
12. King D. Study Guide Histology of the Gastrointestinal System. *Southern Illinois University* [Online]. 2022 Jun.
13. Hall JE, & Hall ME. Chapter 66. Digestion and Absorption in the Gastrointestinal Tract. *Guyton and Hall Textbook of Medical Physiology*. 2021; 14: 823–832.
14. Murray PR. Chapter 2. Human Microbiome in Health and Disease. *Medical Microbiology*. 2020; 9-: 25
15. NIH Human Microbiome Portfolio Analysis Team. A Review of 10 Years of Human Microbiome Research Activities at the US National Institutes of Health, Fiscal Years 2007–2016. *Microbiome*. 2019 Feb; 7(31): 7–31.
16. Hasan N, & Yang H. Factors Affecting the Composition of the Gut Microbiota, and Its Modulation. *PeerJ: Life and Environment*. 2019 Aug; 7: e7502.
17. Abbas AK, Lichtman AH, Pillai S, & Baker DL. Chapter 14. Specialized Immunity at Epithelial Barriers and in Immune Priviledged Tissues. *Cellular and Molecular Immunology*. 2020; 10: 10–35.

18. Siezen RJ, & Kleerebezem M. The Human Gut Microbiome: Are We Our Enterotypes? *Microbial Biotechnology*. 2011 Sept; 4(5): 550–553.
19. Rao M, & Gershon MD. The Bowel and beyond: The Enteric Nervous System in Neurological Disorders. *Nature Reviews. Gastroenterology and Hepatology*. 2016 Jul; 13(9): 517–528.
20. Furness JB. Enteric Nervous System. *Scholarpedia*. 2007; 2(10): 4064.
21. Shahrestani J, & Das JM. Neuroanatomy, Auerbach Plexus. *StatPearls*. 2022 Jan.
22. Loukopoulou C. Submucosal Plexus (Meissner Plexus). *Kenhub*. [Online]. 2022.
23. Mittal R, Debs LH, Patel AP, et al. Neurotransmitters: The Critical Modulators Regulating Gut–Brain Axis. *Journal of Cellular Physiology*. 2016 Aug; 232(9): 2359–2372.
24. Appleton J. The Gut-Brain Axis: Influence of Microbiota on Mood and Mental Health. *Integrative Medicine: A Clinician's Journal*. 2018 Aug; 17(4): 28–32.
25. Asano Y, Hiramoto T, Nishino R, et al. Critical Role of Gut Microbiota in the Production of Biologically Active, Free Catecholamines in the Gut Lumen of Mice. *American Journal of Physiology: Gastrointestinal and Liver Physiology*. 2012 Dec; 303(11): G1288–G1295.
26. Tortorella C, Neri G, & Nussdorfer GG. Galanin in the Regulation of the Hypothalamic-Pituitary-Adrenal Axis (Review). *International Journal of Molecular Medicine*. 2007 Apr; 19(4): 639–647.
27. Silva YP, Bernardi A, & Frozza RL. The Role of Short-Chain Fatty Acids From Gut Microbiota in Gut-Brain Communication. *Frontiers in Endocrinology*. 2020 Jan; 11: 11–37.
28. Candelli M, Franza L, Pignataro G, et al. Interaction between Lipopolysaccharide and Gut Microbiota in Inflammatory Bowel Diseases. *International Journal of Molecular Sciences*. 2021 Jun; 22(6242): 6242–6256.
29. Rutsch A, Kantsjo JB, & Ronchi F. The Gut-Brain Axis: How Microbiota and Host Inflammasome Influence Brain Physiology and Pathology. *Frontiers in Immunology*. 2020 Dec; 11: 604179.

# Inflammation and the Gut Microbiome in Depression and Anxiety

Komal Parmar, Sai Patel, and Jayvadan Patel

## Contents

## 7.1 Introduction

### 7.1.1 Focus on Depression and Anxiety

The prevalence of common mental diseases including depression and anxiety has increased over the past few decades, raising concerns about mental health on a global scale (Friedrich 2017, Tariku Seboka et al. 2022). The prevalence of depression in the world increased significantly after the 2020 Covid-19 pandemic (Abbott 2021), markedly even in children and adolescents (Wang et al. 2022). There are considerable negative effects on health due to the growing burden of mental diseases. Up to 25% of patients in general practice have co-occurring depression and anxiety disorders. Approximately 85% of people with depression experience considerable anxiety, and 90% of people with anxiety disorders experience depression (Tiller 2013). Depression is characterized by short-term emotional reactions that hinder daily functioning and are accompanied by symptoms including sadness and frustration, guilt-related sensations, numbness, and loss of interest (Wahed and Hassan 2017). The term "anxiety disorders" refers to a set of mental disorders that are characterized by unpleasant feelings of unease, worry about the future, or

DOI: 10.1201/9781003333821-7

the dread of reacting to the present. It could happen without a clear inciting factor (Penninx et al. 2021). Therefore, a fresh approach to treatment, which might involve microbiome-mediated techniques, is urgently needed given the increased prevalence of mental illnesses worldwide.

## 7.1.2 Gut Microbiota

"All disease begins in the gut"—Hippocrates, a Greek physician who is commonly credited as the founder of modern medicine, is said to have made this declaration more than 2,000 years ago. Even if the citation to Hippocrates has been debated, its intrinsic wisdom remains to have an impact on scholars and practitioners across the medical field.

The human gastrointestinal (GI) tract is the largest organ for any foreign material to come in contact with the body. The gastrointestinal (GI) tract of the human is home to a diverse variety of microorganisms, primarily bacteria, which are vital for human health. The collection of bacteria-dominated microbes that live in the human host's gastrointestinal tract is known as the gut microbiome (Thursby and Juge 2017, Neish 2009). An estimated 60 tonnes of food travel through the human GI tract in a lifetime, along with numerous environmental bacteria. More than $10^{14}$ microorganisms are thought to reside in the GI tract, which has about ten times as many bacterial cells as human cells and more than 100 times as much genomic information as the human genome. The microbiota provides the host with numerous advantages through a variety of physiological processes, including preserving gut integrity or forming the intestinal epithelium, generating energy, warding off pathogens, and controlling host immunity (Natividad and Verdu 2013, den Besten et al. 2013, Bäumler and Sperandio 2016, Gensollen et al. 2016). This chapter summarizes our existing knowledge of the makeup, growth, and effects of the human GI microbiota on depression and anxiety.

## 7.1.3 Composition and Structure of the Human GI Microbiota

Due to the development of culture-independent techniques like high-throughput and affordable sequencing tools, our capacity to survey the breadth of the gut microbiota has significantly increased recently. A common strategy is to target the bacterial 16S ribosomal RNA (rRNA) gene, which is present in all bacteria and archaea and has nine highly variable sections (V1–V9) that make it easy to identify between different species (Matsumoto and Sugano 2013, Zheng et al. 2015, Hassler et al. 2022). Whole-genome sequencing metagenomics may offer more accurate estimates of microbiota composition and diversity due to its better resolution and sensitivity. The Human Microbiome Project and MetaHIT data combined have given researchers the most complete understanding of the microbial diversity associated with humans to date (NIH HMP Working Group et al. 2009, Aagaard et al. 2013). Data from these investigations were combined to identify 2,172 human-isolated species that were divided into

12 different phyla and 93.5% of which belonged to Proteobacteria, Firmicutes, Actinobacteria, and Bacteroidetes (Hugon et al. 2015). According to a different study, the human gut contains thousands of different bacterial species. The most prevalent genera include Bacteroides, Clostridium, Fusobacterium, Eubacterium, Ruminococcus, Peptococcus, Peptostreptococcus, Lactobacillus, and Bifidobacterium (Guarner and Malagelada 2003, Tomova et al. 2019).

Although there have been a small number of studies where microorganisms have been found in womb organs like the placenta that cast doubt on the conventional wisdom that the formation of the microbiota begins at birth (Walker et al. 2017). The GI tract is quickly colonized after birth, and changes in food, sickness, and antibiotic use, all cause erratic shifts in the microbiota (Bull and Plummer 2014). Infants born vaginally presented a high abundance of Lactobacilli for the first few days, reflecting the high load of Bacteroides, Bifidobacteria, and Lactobacilli in the vaginal flora. This suggests that the mode of delivery may also have an impact on the microbiota's makeup (Coelho et al. 2021). Even while the composition of the gut microbiota is largely constant in maturity, life experiences can nevertheless cause it to change. In contrast to the younger population, where cluster XIVa is more prominent, the microbial community changes in older adults, with an increasing abundance of the Bacteroidetes phylum and Clostridium cluster IV.

## 7.1.4 Gut Microbiome: Influence on Depression and Anxiety

With the development of better molecular and metagenomic technologies, human and animal research has offered growing data pointing to a significant relationship between the neuroendocrine system and the gut microbiome (Clapp et al. 2017, Yang et al. 2019, Dong et al. 2021). Due to the negative effects of dysbiosis on brain function, the relationship between the gut microbiota and the central nervous system has drawn more attention recently. It is believed that this biochemical signaling network, sometimes referred to as the gut–brain axis (Figure 7.1), affects mood and cognitive function through neuronal, metabolic, hormonal, and immune-mediated pathways (Carabotti et al. 2015). Gut microbes communicate with the central nervous system by producing neurotransmitters like glutamate, acetylcholine, gamma-aminobutyric acid, serotonin, and dopamine, as well as in response to hormones.

Changes in diet may result in an unbalanced level of microbial variety and richness (alpha-diversity), which lowers the number of gut Firmicutes and raises the number of Bacteroides phyla (Rinninella et al. 2019). Short-chain fatty acids, including acetate, propionate, and butyrate, are produced by the colon microbiota's fermentation of indigestible carbohydrates and are linked to the maintenance of homeostasis, the control of hunger, and anti-inflammatory actions (Gill et al. 2018). Under dysbiosis, an increase in bacterial lipopolysaccharides causes the intrinsic immune system to become active. Through the subdiaphragmatic ambiguous nerve, these endotoxins produce pro-inflammatory cytokines such as interleukin-6 and tumor necrosis factor-alpha and

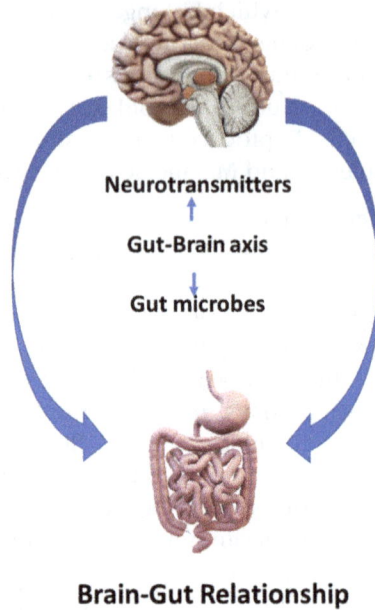

**Brain-Gut Relationship**

*Figure 7.1* Brain–gut relationship.

downregulate synaptic proteins (Navarro-Tapia et al. 2021). Furthermore, current research indicates that the gut microbiome regulates the Hypothalamic-Pituitary-Adrenal Axis responsiveness, which affects the endocrine pathway. Consequently, its imbalance can result in aberrant glucocorticoid levels and urge behavioral abnormalities (Rosin et al. 2021, Huo et al. 2017).

It is reported that the fecal microbiota of patients with major depressive disorder was found to be different when compared to healthy controls (Chen et al. 2018). A recent study revealed age-specific differences in the composition of the gut microbiome in people with severe depressive illness (Chen et al. 2020). In another study, sex differences in gut microbiota in patients with major depressive disorder was observed. Female and male major depressive disorder patients, respectively, had higher Actinobacteria and lower Bacteroidetes counts when compared to their healthy counterparts (Chen et al. 2018a). However, biological material transfer in the neonatal stage might influence the mental health of the child at a later age. Recent research revealed that stress during pregnancy in mice causes neuroinflammation, decreased oxytocin receptors, and decreased serotonin metabolism in their cortex in adulthood, all of which are connected to impaired social behavior (Gur et al. 2019). Additionally, a transfer of the vaginal microbiota from stressed mothers to progeny who was not stressed led to greater corticosterone levels and changed gene expression in the paraventricular nucleus of the hypothalamus (Jašarević et al. 2018). Investigational models demonstrate the correlation between anxiety-like behaviors and disruptions in the gut microbiota caused by antibiotics, delivery methods, or fecal microbiota transplantation from anorexic nervosa patients (Hata et al. 2019, Zhao et al. 2020, Lach et al. 2020, Mosaferi et al. 2021, Li et al. 2022). In another study, general anxiety disorder patients had lower levels of microbial diversity and richness, a different metagenomic composition with fewer bacteria that produce short-chain fatty acids, which are indicative of health, and an overgrowth of bacteria like Escherichia coli, Fusobacterium, and Ruminococcus gnavus, as compared to healthy controls (Jiang et al. 2018).

## 7.1.5 Inflammation and Changes in the Central Nervous System (CNS)

The immune system of humans provides defense against pathogens and a variety of harmful shocks. Inflammation, also known as an inflammatory response, is the result of the immune system being activated and frequently appears as a localized reaction to itchiness, damage, or infections. It is characterized by heat, redness, swelling, and pain, as well as occasionally by fever. Researchers have been examining the consequences of peripheral inflammation on the CNS since it plays a part in depression and anxiety. Low-grade anxiety, for instance, is demonstrated in depression. About 21–34% of patients had systemic inflammation as measured by increased levels of C-reactive protein (CRP) (CRP >3 mg/L) (Osimo et al. 2019), along with elevated concentrations of interleukin-6 (IL)-6 and other inflammatory cytokines in blood and in cerebrospinal fluid (CSF) (Köhler et al. 2017, Orlovska-Waast et al. 2019). A few modifications might be taking place at the blood-brain barrier (BBB), which divides the CNS parenchyma from peripheral blood flow.

Since innate immune myeloid cells, such as macrophages/monocytes and dendritic cells, as well as lymphoid cells, such as natural killer cells, constantly probe the circulation to give quick responses, the innate immunity system serves as the first line of defense (Marshall et al. 2018). Microglia, which make up between 5 and 10% of all brain cells and perform tasks similar to those of macrophages and other specialized immune cells, are found in the brain. Recent research has demonstrated the significance of microglia for synaptic regulation, including synapse pruning and neurogenesis (Cornell et al. 2022). Microglia are also active in many neurodegenerative and neuropsychiatric illnesses, where they contribute to pathogenesis by encouraging neuroinflammation. Cytokines are tiny proteins that influence how cells interact and function. They can either promote or suppress inflammation. The CNS's microglia and other immune cells are the main producers of cytokines (Figure 7.2). Interleukin (IL)-6, tumor necrosis factor (TNF), IL-1, and interferons (IFNs) on the inflammatory side and IL-10 on the alleviating side are the most investigated cytokines in the context of psychoneuroimmunology.

Multiple meta-analyses have conclusively shown that MDD (major depressive disorder) patients have higher levels of acute phase proteins and

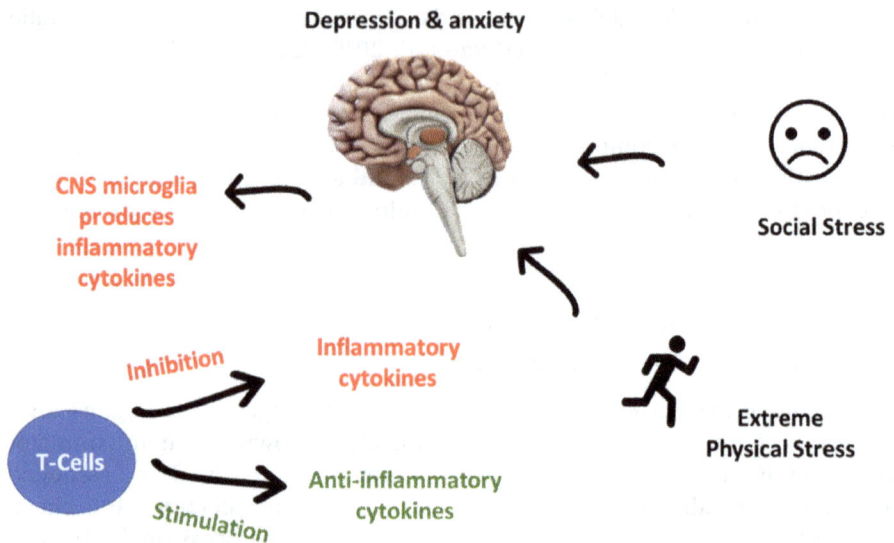

**Figure 7.2** *Inflammation–CNS relationship.*

proinflammatory cytokines (Köhler et al. 2017, Köhler et al. 2018). The levels of IL-6, TNF, IL-10, sIL-2, C-C motif ligand (CCL)2, IL-13, IL-18, IL-12, and soluble TNF receptor (sTNFR)2 are higher in MDD patients than in healthy controls, according to a recent meta-analysis of 82 studies that included 3,212 MDD patients and 2,798 healthy controls. In contrast, the level of interferon (IFN) is lower in these patients (Köhler et al. 2017). Stress-induced interleukin (IL)-6 activity has been found to change gene expression in monocytes and result in anxiety-like behavior in mice on a molecular level (Niraula et al. 2019). By repeatedly activating the neuroendocrine and autonomic systems, psychosocial stress is capable of producing immunological dysregulation and increased neuroinflammatory signaling, which may contribute to the emergence of anxiety and depression (Ramirez et al. 2017). Overall, neuroinflammation fosters an environment that is toxic, unsuited for normal brain function, and possibly damaging to mental health.

## 7.2 Conclusion

It is critical to deepen our understanding of the causes of depression and anxiety as well as the underlying mechanisms because these conditions have symptoms that have a considerable negative impact on those who experience them. However, our comprehension of the mechanisms underlying nervous system disorders including depression and anxiety is being revolutionized by research on the gut microbiome-brain axis and inflammation. Further research into this connection between gut microbiome and inflammation with psychological systems will help us better understand the causes of disease and guide the development of more effective therapies for those suffering from depression and anxiety.

# References

Aagaard K, Petrosino J, Keitel W, Watson M, Katancik J, Garcia N, Patel S, Cutting M, Madden T, Hamilton H, Harris E, Gevers D, Simone G, McInnes P, Versalovic J. The Human microbiome Project strategy for comprehensive sampling of the human microbiome and why it matters. *FASEB J* 2013;27(3):1012–1022. doi: 10.1096/fj.12-220806.

Abbott A. COVID's mental-health toll: How scientists are tracking a surge in depression. *Nature* 2021;590(7845):194–195. doi: 10.1038/d41586-021-00175-z.

Bäumler AJ, Sperandio V. Interactions between the microbiota and pathogenic bacteria in the gut. *Nature* 2016;535(7610):85–93. doi: 10.1038/nature18849.

Bull MJ, Plummer NT. Part 1: The human gut microbiome in health and disease. *Integr Med (Encinitas)* 2014;13(6):17–22.

Carabotti M, Scirocco A, Maselli MA, Severi C. The gut-brain axis: Interactions between enteric microbiota, central and enteric nervous systems. *Ann Gastroenterol* 2015;28(2):203–209.

Chen JJ, He S, Fang L, Wang B, Bai SJ, Xie J, Zhou CJ, Wang W, Xie P. Age-specific differential changes on gut microbiota composition in patients with major depressive disorder. *Aging (Albany NY)* 2020;12(3):2764–2776. doi: 10.18632/aging.102775.

Chen JJ, Zheng P, Liu YY, Zhong XG, Wang HY, Guo YJ, Xie P. Sex differences in gut microbiota in patients with major depressive disorder. *Neuropsychiatr Dis Treat* 2018a;14:647–655. doi: 10.2147/NDT.S159322.

Chen Z, Li J, Gui S, Zhou C, Chen J, Yang C, Hu Z, Wang H, Zhong X, Zeng L, Chen K, Li P, Xie P. Comparative metaproteomics analysis shows altered fecal microbiota signatures in patients with major depressive disorder. *NeuroReport* 2018;29(5):417–425. doi: 10.1097/WNR.0000000000000985.

Clapp M, Aurora N, Herrera L, Bhatia M, Wilen E, Wakefield S. Gut microbiota's effect on mental health: The gut-brain axis. *Clin Pract* 2017;7(4):987. doi: 10.4081/cp.2017.987.

Coelho GDP, Ayres LFA, Barreto DS, Henriques BD, Prado MRMC, Passos CMD. Acquisition of microbiota according to the type of birth: An integrative review. *Rev Lat Am Enferm* 2021;29:e3446. doi: 10.1590/1518.8345.4466.3446.

Cornell J, Salinas S, Huang HY, Zhou M. Microglia regulation of synaptic plasticity and learning and memory. *Neural Regen Res* 2022;17(4):705–716. doi: 10.4103/1673-5374.322423.

den Besten G, van Eunen K, Groen AK, Venema K, Reijngoud DJ, Bakker BM. The role of short-chain fatty acids in the interplay between diet, gut microbiota, and host energy metabolism. *J Lipid Res* 2013;54(9):2325–2340. doi: 10.1194/jlr.R036012.

Dong Z, Shen X, Hao Y, Li J, Li H, Xu H, Yin L, Kuang W. Gut microbiome: A potential indicator for differential diagnosis of major depressive disorder and general anxiety disorder. *Front Psychiatry* 2021;12:651536. doi: 10.3389/fpsyt.2021.651536.

Friedrich MJ. Depression is the leading cause of disability around the world. *JAMA* 2017;317(15):1517. doi: 10.1001/jama.2017.3826.

Gensollen T, Iyer SS, Kasper DL, Blumberg RS. How colonization by microbiota in early life shapes the immune system. *Science* 2016;352(6285):539–544. doi: 10.1126/science.aad9378.

Gill PA, van Zelm MC, Muir JG, Gibson PR. Review article: Short chain fatty acids as potential therapeutic agents in human gastrointestinal and inflammatory disorders. *Aliment Pharmacol Ther* 2018;48(1):15–34. doi: 10.1111/apt.14689.

Guarner F, Malagelada JR. Gut flora in health and disease. *Lancet* 2003;361(9356):512–519. doi: 10.1016/S0140-6736(03)12489-0.

Gur TL, Palkar AV, Rajasekera T, Allen J, Niraula A, Godbout J, Bailey MT. Prenatal stress disrupts social behavior, cortical neurobiology and commensal microbes in adult male offspring. *Behav Brain Res* 2019;359:886–894. doi: 10.1016/j. bbr.2018.06.025.

Hassler HB, Probert B, Moore C, Lawson E, Jackson RW, Russell BT, Richards VP. Phylogenies of the 16S rRNA gene and its hypervariable regions lack concordance with core genome phylogenies. *Microbiome* 2022;10(1):104. doi: 10.1186/ s40168-022-01295-y.

Hata T, Miyata N, Takakura S, Yoshihara K, Asano Y, Kimura-Todani T, Yamashita M, Zhang XT, Watanabe N, Mikami K, Koga Y, Sudo N. The gut microbiome derived from anorexia nervosa patients impairs weight gain and behavioral performance in female mice. *Endocrinology* 2019;160(10):2441–2452. doi: 10.1210/en.2019-00408.

Hugon P, Dufour JC, Colson P, Fournier PE, Sallah K, Raoult D. A comprehensive repertoire of prokaryotic species identified in human beings. *Lancet Infect Dis* 2015;15(10):1211–1219. doi: 10.1016/S1473-3099(15)00293-5.

Huo R, Zeng B, Zeng L, Cheng K, Li B, Luo Y, Wang H, Zhou C, Fang L, Li W, Niu R, Wei H, Xie P. Microbiota modulate anxiety-like behavior and endocrine abnormalities in hypothalamic-pituitary-adrenal axis. *Front Cell Infect Microbiol* 2017;7:489. doi: 10.3389/fcimb.2017.00489.

Jašarević E, Howard CD, Morrison K, Misic A, Weinkopff T, Scott P, Hunter C, Beiting D, Bale TL. The maternal vaginal microbiome partially mediates the effects of prenatal stress on offspring gut and hypothalamus. *Nat Neurosci* 2018;21(8):1061–1071. doi: 10.1038/s41593-018-0182-5.

Jiang HY, Zhang X, Yu ZH, Zhang Z, Deng M, Zhao JH, Ruan B. Altered gut microbiota profile in patients with generalized anxiety disorder. *J Psychiatr Res* 2018;104:130–136. doi: 10.1016/j.jpsychires.2018.07.007.

Köhler CA, Freitas TH, Maes M, de Andrade NQ, Liu CS, Fernandes BS, Stubbs B, Solmi M, Veronese N, Herrmann N, Raison CL, Miller BJ, Lanctôt KL, Carvalho AF. Peripheral cytokine and chemokine alterations in depression: A meta-analysis of 82 studies. *Acta Psychiatr Scand* 2017;135(5):373–387. doi: 10.1111/acps.12698.

Köhler CA, Freitas TH, Stubbs B, Maes M, Solmi M, Veronese N, de Andrade NQ, Morris G, Fernandes BS, Brunoni AR, Herrmann N, Raison CL, Miller BJ, Lanctôt KL, Carvalho AF. Peripheral alterations in cytokine and chemokine levels after antidepressant drug treatment for major depressive disorder: Systematic review and meta-analysis. *Mol Neurobiol* 2018;55(5):4195–4206. doi: 10.1007/s12035-017-0632-1.

Lach G, Fülling C, Bastiaanssen TFS, Fouhy F, Donovan ANO, Ventura-Silva AP, Stanton C, Dinan TG, Cryan JF. Enduring neurobehavioral effects induced by microbiota depletion during the adolescent period. *Transl Psychiatry* 2020;10(1):382. doi: 10.1038/ s41398-020-01073-0.

Li J, Pu F, Peng C, Wang Y, Zhang Y, Wu S, Wang S, Shen X, Li Y, Cheng R, He F. Antibiotic cocktail-induced gut microbiota depletion in different stages could cause host cognitive impairment and emotional disorders in adulthood in different manners. *Neurobiol Dis* 2022;170:105757. doi: 10.1016/j.nbd.2022.105757.

Marshall JS, Warrington R, Watson W, Kim HL. An introduction to immunology and immunopathology. *Allergy Asthma Clin Immunol* 2018;14(Suppl 2):49. doi: 10.1186/ s13223-018-0278-1.

Matsumoto T, Sugano M. 16S rRNA gene sequence analysis for bacterial identification in the clinical laboratory. *Rinsho Byori* 2013;61(12):1107–1115. Japanese.

Mosaferi B, Jand Y, Salari AA. Gut microbiota depletion from early adolescence alters anxiety and depression-related behaviours in male mice with Alzheimer-like disease. *Sci Rep* 2021;11(1):22941. doi: 10.1038/s41598-021-02231-0.

Natividad JM, Verdu EF. Modulation of intestinal barrier by intestinal microbiota: Pathological and therapeutic implications. *Pharmacol Res* 2013;69(1):42–51. doi: 10.1016/j.phrs.2012.10.007.

Navarro-Tapia E, Almeida-Toledano L, Sebastiani G, Serra-Delgado M, García-Algar Ó, Andreu-Fernández V. Effects of microbiota imbalance in anxiety and eating disorders: Probiotics as novel therapeutic approaches. *Int J Mol Sci* 2021;22(5):2351. doi: 10.3390/ijms22052351.

Neish AS. Microbes in gastrointestinal health and disease. *Gastroenterology* 2009;136(1):65–80. doi: 10.1053/j.gastro.2008.10.080.

NIH HMP Working Group, Peterson J, Garges S, Giovanni M, McInnes P, Wang L, Schloss JA, Bonazzi V, McEwen JE, Wetterstrand KA, Deal C, Baker CC, Di Francesco V, Howcroft TK, Karp RW, Lunsford RD, Wellington CR, Belachew T, Wright M, Giblin C, David H, Mills M, Salomon R, Mullins C, Akolkar B, Begg L, Davis C, Grandison L, Humble M, Khalsa J, Little AR, Peavy H, Pontzer C, Portnoy M, Sayre MH, Starke-Reed P, Zakhari S, Read J, Watson B, Guyer M. The NIH human microbiome project. *Genome Res* 2009;19(12):2317–2323. doi: 10.1101/gr.096651.109.

Niraula A, Witcher KG, Sheridan JF, Godbout JP. Interleukin-6 induced by social stress promotes a unique transcriptional signature in the monocytes that facilitate anxiety. *Biol Psychiatry* 2019;85(8):679–689. doi: 10.1016/j.biopsych.2018.09.030.

Orlovska-Waast S, Köhler-Forsberg O, Brix SW, Nordentoft M, Kondziella D, Krogh J, Benros ME. Cerebrospinal fluid markers of inflammation and infections in schizophrenia and affective disorders: A systematic review and meta-analysis. *Mol Psychiatry* 2019;24(6):869–887. doi: 10.1038/s41380-018-0220-4.

Osimo EF, Baxter LJ, Lewis G, Jones PB, Khandaker GM. Prevalence of low-grade inflammation in depression: A systematic review and meta-analysis of CRP levels. *Psychol Med* 2019;49(12):1958–1970. doi: 10.1017/S0033291719001454.

Penninx BW, Pine DS, Holmes EA, Reif A. Anxiety disorders. *Lancet* 2021;397(10277):914–927. doi: 10.1016/S0140-6736(21)00359-7. Epub 2021 Feb 11. Erratum in: *Lancet* 2021;397(10277):880.

Ramirez K, Fornaguera-Trías J, Sheridan JF. Stress-induced microglia activation and monocyte trafficking to the brain underlie the development of anxiety and depression. *Curr Top Behav Neurosci* 2017;31:155–172. doi: 10.1007/7854_2016_25.

Rinninella E, Raoul P, Cintoni M, Franceschi F, Miggiano GAD, Gasbarrini A, Mele MC. What is the healthy gut microbiota composition? A changing ecosystem across age, environment, diet, and diseases. *Microorganisms* 2019;7(1):14. doi: 10.3390/microorganisms7010014.

Rosin S, Xia K, Azcarate-Peril MA, Carlson AL, Propper CB, Thompson AL, Grewen K, Knickmeyer RC. A preliminary study of gut microbiome variation and HPA axis reactivity in healthy infants. *Psychoneuroendocrinology* 2021;124:105046. doi: 10.1016/j.psyneuen.2020.105046.

Tariku Seboka B, Hailegebreal S, Negash M, Mamo TT, Ali Ewune H, Gilano G, Yehualashet DE, Gizachew G, Demeke AD, Worku A, Endashaw H, Kassawe C, Amede ES, Kassa R, Tesfa GA. Predictors of mental health literacy and information seeking behavior toward mental health among university students in resource-limited settings. *Int J Gen Med* 2022;15:8159–8172. doi: 10.2147/IJGM.S377791.

Thursby E, Juge N. Introduction to the human gut microbiota. *Biochem J* 2017;474(11):1823–1836. doi: 10.1042/BCJ20160510.

Tiller JW. Depression and anxiety. *Med J Aust* 2013;199(S6):S28–S31. doi: 10.5694/mja12.10628.

Tomova A, Bukovsky I, Rembert E, Yonas W, Alwarith J, Barnard ND, Kahleova H. The effects of vegetarian and vegan diets on gut microbiota. *Front Nutr* 2019;6:47. doi: 10.3389/fnut.2019.00047.

Wahed WYA, Hassan SK. Prevalence and associated factors of stress, anxiety and depression among medical Fayoum University students. *Alex J Med* 2017;53(1):77–84.

Walker RW, Clemente JC, Peter I, Loos RJF. The prenatal gut microbiome: Are we colonized with bacteria in utero? *Pediatr Obes* 2017;12(Suppl 1):3–17. doi: 10.1111/ijpo.12217.

Wang S, Chen L, Ran H, Che Y, Fang D, Sun H, Peng J, Liang X, Xiao Y. Depression and anxiety among children and adolescents pre and post COVID-19: A comparative meta-analysis. *Front Psychiatry* 2022;13:917552. doi: 10.3389/fpsyt.2022.917552.

Yang B, Wei J, Ju P, Chen J. Effects of regulating intestinal microbiota on anxiety symptoms: A systematic review. *Gen Psychiatr* 2019;32(2):e100056. doi: 10.1136/gpsych-2019-100056.

Zhao Z, Wang B, Mu L, Wang H, Luo J, Yang Y, Yang H, Li M, Zhou L, Tao C. Long-term exposure to ceftriaxone sodium induces alteration of gut microbiota accompanied by abnormal behaviors in mice. *Front Cell Infect Microbiol* 2020;10:258. doi: 10.3389/fcimb.2020.00258.

Zheng W, Tsompana M, Ruscitto A, Sharma A, Genco R, Sun Y, Buck MJ. An accurate and efficient experimental approach for characterization of the complex oral microbiota. *Microbiome* 2015;3:48. doi: 10.1186/s40168-015-0110-9.

# 8

# Stress, Depression, Diet, and the Gut Microbiota

*Human–Bacteria Interactions at the Core of Psychoneuroimmunology and Nutrition*

Malcolm Padgett, Jad Mouslle, and Dr Yashwant V. Pathak

## Contents

## 8.1 Introduction

Diet, stress, and depression are interconnected factors that can substantially impact an individual's health and well-being. One of the most pressing issues is the increased prevalence of poor mental health in the context of cardio-metabolic disease (Dietary inflammation score is associated with perceived stress, depression, and cardiometabolic health risk factors among a young adult cohort of women). Although there are connections between nutrition, obesity, metabolic syndrome (MetS), stress, and mental illnesses, causal pathways have not been demonstrated (Diet, stress and mental health).

Recent research has indicated that the gut microbiota, or community of bacteria residing in the digestive tract, plays an essential role in these interactions—changes in the microbiome influence the pathophysiology of depression, including emotions, behavior, and stress response. Depression and anxiety are usually associated with dysbiosis and inflammatory bowel disease (Gut

DOI: 10.1201/9781003333821-8

microbiome as a therapeutic target in the treatment of depression and anxiety). This causes stress and reduces the quality of the microbiome.

Stress and depression are two of the most prevalent mental health conditions worldwide. An increasing body of studies has connected anxiety and depression to unfavorable health consequences, including cardiovascular disease, immunological dysfunction, and gastrointestinal issues. Neurological and psychiatric disorders, a category of pervasive chronic diseases, generate significant mental and physical health difficulties in persons (Diet and depression: Exploring the biological mechanisms of action). The case for the involvement of the complex, bidirectional communication axis between the brain and the gastrointestinal tract in neuropsychiatric disorders such as depression is growing (The effects of stress and diet on the "brain-gut" and "gut–brain" pathways in animal models of stress and depression).

Anxiety and inadequate diet quality are linked (Anxiety is more related to inadequate eating habits in inactive than in physically active adults during COVID-19 quarantine). With a poor diet and rising anxiety, depression can develop and damage individuals' mental states. Anxiety and depression are linked to several adverse health outcomes, including gastrointestinal issues, immunological dysfunction, and cardiovascular disease. Both may have substantial effects on physical health.

Stress, a normal response to demanding or dangerous circumstances, can be beneficial in moderation. However, chronic stress can negatively affect mental health, resulting in symptoms such as anxiety, depression, and attention deficits. Stress can disrupt sleep, which can exacerbate mental health issues.

In addition to its effects on mental health, stress can negatively affect physical health. Chronic stress has been related to numerous adverse health impacts, including immune system dysfunction, gastrointestinal issues, and cardiovascular disease. In addition to raising the chance of unhealthy behaviors such as overeating and lack of exercise, stress can also be a component in developing these undesirable practices.

Stress and depression have a reciprocal, complex relationship. Chronic stress has also been related to structural and functional changes in the brain that may increase the risk of depression. Both depression and anxiety have an inverse relationship in terms of occurrence probability. According to the study, the greater the stress level, the greater the likelihood of emotional eating (Evaluation of perceived depression, anxiety, stress levels and emotional eating behaviors and their predictors among adults during the COVID-19 pandemic).

## 8.2 Stress and the Microbiota of the Gut

The gut microbiota is a diversified bacterial population with rapid growth. It is an adaptive immunity that varies based on human habits, environmental conditions, and diet (Is the gut microbiota a neglected aspect of gut and brain disorders?). According to a study, variations in gut flora are linked to changes in stress and anxiety levels. The gut microbiota is crucial for the stress response system of the body. Studies have revealed, for instance, that individuals with a more significant number of specific types of bacteria in their gut microbiota experience less stress and anxiety than individuals with absence of these bacteria.

Although the specific methods by which the gut microbiota influences the stress response system remain unknown, evidence suggests that the gut microbiota may connect with the brain via the gut–brain axis. The neurological system, immunological system, and endocrine system are also included in this communication channel. Neurotransmitters and hormones are just two of the compounds that the gut flora is capable of producing.

Diet and stress are interrelated, with pressure influencing food habits. Due to the complex bidirectional connections between the brain, the gut, and the gut microbiota, nutritional interventions may be able to prevent mental health decline (The effects of walnuts and academic stress on mental health, general well-being and the gut microbiota in a sample of university students: A randomised clinical trial). Several potential medicines could alter the gut flora and influence our stress and anxiety levels. These include dietary adjustments, probiotic supplementation, and transplantation of fecal microbiota. Like the beneficial bacteria in the stomach, live microorganisms known as probiotics have been shown to provide numerous health benefits, including reducing stress and anxiety. The transplantation of feces microbiota is effective in treating a variety of gastrointestinal disorders. This approach involves transplanting the gut microbiota of a healthy individual into the gut of an individual whose microbiota has been disturbed. The gut microbiota is significantly influenced by diet. Some diets are connected with healthy gut flora and a reduced risk of adverse health outcomes, while others may raise the risk. Psychological stress and depression increase the consumption of beautiful meals, influencing which gut bacteria thrive (Stress, depression, diet, and the gut microbiota: human–bacteria interactions at the core of psychoneuroimmunology and nutrition). Macronutrient profiles predict unique gut microbiota populations. Recent emphasis on the impact of macronutrients on the gut microbiota has attracted attention to the nutrition field's increasing convergence.

## 8.3 The Intestinal Flora and Depression

Gut microbiota is crucial to human health and well-being. Studies have shown that the host's genetics, nutrition, and other environmental exposures influence the microbiota's composition and diversity, which has implications for the host organism's immune and nervous system development (Microbe-immune-stress interactions impact behaviour during postnatal development).

Diet is a crucial factor that influences the composition and function of the gut microbiota. Abuse of refined, simple, and low-quality carbohydrates affects the pathophysiology of the body and mind in a direct manner (The burden of carbohydrates in health and disease).

In addition to general eating patterns, specific dietary components have been shown to influence gut flora. Studies have indicated, for instance, that diets high in fiber, particularly soluble fiber, may promote the growth of beneficial bacteria in the gut and improve gut health. Conversely, diets high in saturated fats and processed carbohydrates have been related to poor gut flora and an increased risk of unfavorable health impacts. Due to the imbalance of the brain-gut-microbiota axis, the hypothalamic-pituitary-adrenal (HPA) axis is dysregulated. This imbalance substantially impacts the etiology of depression (Role of brain-gut-microbiota axis in depression: Emerging therapeutic avenues).

Multiple gastrointestinal ailments, metabolic disorders, and obesity have all been linked to gut microbiota. According to research, specific diets may alter the gut microbiota in ways that increase the risk of various diseases, whereas others may reduce this. For instance, research has shown that diets high in fat and sugar are associated with an increased risk of obesity and metabolic diseases. A sample of socio-health and commercial services companies investigated the association between headaches and lifestyle, metabolic, and employment-related factors. Employees with headaches reported having a higher body mass index (Headache in workers: A matched case-control study). In contrast, fiber-rich and plant-based diets have been linked to a reduced risk of these illnesses.

Depression has also been linked to poor metabolic responses, weight gain, and an increased risk of metabolic disorders, including diabetes and cardiovascular disease. Adults with type 2 diabetes (T2D) typically experience anxiety and depression symptoms connected to their condition (Self-efficacy mediates the associations of diabetes distress and depressive symptoms with type 2 diabetes management and glycemic control). Depression may damage metabolic responses by altering hormone levels, interfering with hunger management, and influencing physical activity levels.

In addition to gastroenterological illnesses, the gut microbiota may be associated with psychiatric conditions (The microbiota-gut–brain axis in psychiatric disorders). Similar to the association between stress and gut microbiota, research suggests that gut microbiota may be implicated in the onset and management of depression. According to studies, the types and concentrations of bacteria in the gut microbiota of depressed individuals differ from those of healthy individuals. These microbiome changes may be associated with the severity of a person's depression symptoms. In addition, research suggests altering the gut microbiota with probiotic supplements or fecal microbiota transplantation could have antidepressant effects.

## 8.4 Impact of Gut Microbiota on Food Cravings

Gut flora may influence food cravings and appetite, according to a study. Studies have revealed, for instance, that individuals with higher numbers of specific types of bacteria in their gut microbiota have a more significant desire for fiber-rich, healthful meals. People with fewer amounts of these bacteria have a more incredible selection of unhealthy, high-fat, and high-sugar diets.

The gut microbiome may alter food consumption and eating patterns. Some research suggests that gut flora may influence satiety and appetite. People with good gut microbiota are more likely to feel pleased and full after a meal, whereas those with poor gut microbiota may feel hungrier.

Numerous hypotheses have been advanced to explain the occurrence of the metabolically healthy obese phenotype, particularly those including a healthy lifestyle and diet (Cross-sectional study about nutritional risk factors of metabolically unhealthy obesity). Various potential therapies may alter gut flora and influence appetite and food desires. These include dietary adjustments, probiotic supplementation, and transplantation of fecal microbiota. Live microorganisms known as probiotics, comparable to the beneficial bacteria in the stomach, have been shown to offer numerous health benefits, such as reducing food cravings and improving eating habits. The transplantation of feces microbiota is effective in treating a variety of gastrointestinal disorders. This approach involves transplanting the gut microbiota of a healthy individual into the gut of an individual whose microbiota has been disturbed. Some diets have been associated with more extraordinarily beneficial gut flora and a decreased risk of adverse health outcomes.

The development of TDR (Total Diet Replacement) programs is to encourage healthy eating habits and improve microbiomes programs replace every nutritional need with formula foods rich in nutrients. They are commonly used to induce rapid weight loss (Effects of total diet replacement programs on mental well-being: A systematic review with meta-analyses). These lifestyle modifications have a substantial impact on overall mental and physical health. Lifestyle changes can enhance psychological and quality of life indicators in people with metabolic syndrome (A randomized controlled trial of fasting and lifestyle modification in patients with metabolic syndrome: Effects on patient-reported outcomes).

## 8.5 Diet and Depression

Nutrition is an essential factor that can affect physical and mental health, and accumulating data suggests that diet may reduce depression and stress reactivity. The gut microbiota is a crucial target for depression's influence via the gut–brain axis (Gut microbiota mediates the pharmacokinetics of Zhi-Zi-chi decoction for the personalized treatment of depression). Stress reactivity is a person's physiological, behavioral, and emotional responses to stress. Depression is a common mental health illness characterized by persistent feelings of melancholy, a loss of interest or pleasure, and difficulty accomplishing daily chores. Several possible mechanisms exist through which nutrition may affect mental health. Several pathways can be altered, including inflammation, oxidative stress, epigenetics, mitochondrial dysfunction, the gut microbiome, tryptophan-kynurenine metabolism, the HPA axis, neurogenesis and BDNF (brain-derived neurotrophic factor), epigenetics, and obesity (Diet and depression: Exploring the biological mechanisms of action).

Diet can influence the structure and function of the brain via these brain-gut-microbiota (BGM) communication pathways and has a crucial role in shaping the gut microbiome (Role of diet and its effects on the gut microbiome in the pathophysiology of mental disorders). According to a study, eating may influence the body's stress response system and stress reactivity. Research has shown, for instance, that those who consume a diet high in fruits, vegetables, and other plant-based foods are less responsive to stress than those who consume a diet heavy in processed and refined foods. In addition, specific dietary components, such as omega-3 fatty acids, have been associated with a decreased risk of stress-related disorders and enhanced stress reactivity.

The onset and treatment of depression may be influenced by nutrition. According to some research, consuming an abundance of fruits, vegetables, and other plant-based foods may help prevent depression, whereas consuming a quantity of processed and refined foods may increase the likelihood of depression. Moreover, many dietary components, such as probiotics and omega-3 fatty acids, have been linked to a lower prevalence of depression and may be helpful as an adjunctive treatment for the illness. Other evidence-based therapies may be added or used in conjunction with lifestyle-based interventions for individuals with Major Depressive Disorder (Clinical guidelines for the use of lifestyle-based mental health care in major depressive disorder: World Federation of Societies for Biological Psychiatry (WFSBP) and Australasian Society of Lifestyle Medicine (ASLM) taskforce).

## 8.6 Lack of Diet and Research Progress

Diet is an essential aspect of general health and well-being. Nonetheless, despite its relevance, the effect of nutrition on many health outcomes remains to be investigated. This lack of advancement in research is most likely due to several variables, including the complexity of analyzing dietary patterns and their impact on health and the difficulties of conducting long-term dietary intervention studies.

Some diets, such as the Western diet, have been shown to have negative mental and physical impacts. The Western diet (WD) is characterized by a high daily intake of refined carbohydrates and saturated fats, which has been related to cognitive decline and emotional disorders in animal models and humans (Western diet: Implications for brain function and behavior). Other diets and foods have been shown to help treat and prevent depression and neurological illnesses. The tryptophan-rich proteins in sunflower seeds may be able to prevent depression (The antidepressant effect of deoiled sunflower seeds on chronic unpredictable mild stress in mice through regulation of microbiota-gut–brain axis).

Many people are damaged by high blood pressure, which can seriously harm the body. Despite medical and preventive advances, less than one in every five hypertensive persons has the illness under control (Examining the role of psychosocial stressors in hypertension). Overall, the present food and health research is constrained by the necessity for long-term dietary intervention trials with high sample sizes. Because of the lack of research advances, it is difficult to entirely understand the role of diet in various health outcomes and to develop focused interventions to improve well-being. More research is needed to fill these information gaps and find the best dietary patterns for overall health and well-being.

## 8.7 Conclusion

In conclusion, the gut microbiota plays an essential role in the relationship between stress, depression, diet, and human health. The gut microbiota is regulated by anxiety and depression, and its impacts on brain function and behavior can influence the development and severity of both diseases. A diet rich in plant-based foods and fiber promotes a more diversified and advantageous gut microbiome. These connections are central to the burgeoning area of psychoneuroimmunology, which focuses on the intricate interplay of psychological, neurological, and immunological processes. To completely comprehend the mechanisms underlying these human–bacteria interactions and to design targeted interventions for enhancing well-being regarding the involvement of the gut microbiota in the onset and severity of stress and depression, additional research is required.

For instance, stress and depression are connected with alterations in the quantities of specific bacteria in the gut, such as decreases in the good bacteria Bifidobacterium and Lactobacillus. These alterations may lead to dysbiosis, an imbalance in the gut microbiota associated with inflammation, and other adverse health effects.

In addition, the gut microbiota can influence brain function by synthesizing mood-regulating neurotransmitters such as serotonin and dopamine. Changes in the gut microbiota, especially those caused by stress or depression, might interfere with the production of these neurotransmitters and contribute to the development and severity of these diseases.

Overall, the gut microbiota appears to be intimately connected to stress and depression and may be a viable therapeutic target for enhancing mental health.

Additional research is required to ultimately comprehend the mechanisms behind these human–bacteria interactions and to design targeted therapies for improving health.

# References

Balan, Y., Gaur, A., Sakthivadivel, V., Kamble, B., & Sundaramurthy, R. (2021). Is the gut microbiota a neglected aspect of gut and brain disorders? *Cureus, 13*(11), e19740. https://doi.org/10.7759/cureus.19740

Ben Othman, R., Berriche, O., Gamoudi, A., Mizouri, R., Jerab, D., Ben Amor, N., Mahjoub, F., & Jamoussi, H. (2022). Cross-sectional study about nutritional risk factors of metabolically unhealthy obesity. *Rom J Intern Med*. https://doi.org/10.2478/rjim-2022-0023

Bhatt, S., Kanoujia, J., Mohana Lakshmi, S., Patil, C. R., Gupta, G., Chellappan, D. K., & Dua, K. (2023). Role of brain-gut-microbiota axis in depression: Emerging therapeutic avenues. *CNS Neurol Disord Drug Targets, 22*(2), 276–288. https://doi.org/10.2174/187 1527321666220329140804

Bremner, J. D., Moazzami, K., Wittbrodt, M. T., Nye, J. A., Lima, B. B., Gillespie, C. F., Rapaport, M. H., Pearce, B. D., Shah, A. J., & Vaccarino, V. (2020). Diet, stress and mental health. *Nutrients, 12*(8). https://doi.org/10.3390/nu12082428

Christofaro, D. G. D., Tebar, W. R., Silva, G. C. R., Lofrano-Prado, M. C., Botero, J. P., Cucato, G. G., Malik, N., Hollands, K., Correia, M. A., Ritti-Dias, R. M., & Prado, W. L. (2022). Anxiety is more related to inadequate eating habits in inactive than in physically active adults during COVID-19 quarantine. *Clin Nutr ESPEN, 51*, 301–306. https://doi .org/10.1016/j.clnesp.2022.08.010

Clemente-Suárez, V. J., Mielgo-Ayuso, J., Martín-Rodríguez, A., Ramos-Campo, D. J., Redondo-Flórez, L., & Tornero-Aguilera, J. F. (2022). The burden of carbohydrates in health and disease. *Nutrients, 14*(18). https://doi.org/10.3390/nu14183809

Di Prinzio, R. R., Arnesano, G., Meraglia, I., & Magnavita, N. (2022). Headache in workers: A matched case-control study. *Eur J Investig Health Psychol Educ, 12*(12), 1852–1866. https://doi.org/10.3390/ejihpe12120130

Francella, C., Green, M., Caspani, G., Lai, J. K. Y., Rilett, K. C., & Foster, J. A. (2022). Microbe-immune-stress interactions impact behaviour during postnatal development. *Int J Mol Sci, 23*(23). https://doi.org/10.3390/ijms232315064

Gao, F. Y., Chen, X. F., Cui, L. X., Zhai, Y. J., Liu, J. L., Gao, C. C., Fang, Y. C., Huang, T. H., Wen, J., & Zhou, T. T. (2023). Gut microbiota mediates the pharmacokinetics of Zhi-Zi-chi decoction for the personalized treatment of depression. *J Ethnopharmacol, 302*(B), 115934. https://doi.org/10.1016/j.jep.2022.115934

Gao, Y., Xiao, J., Han, Y., Ji, J., Jin, H., Mawen, D. G., Zhong, Y., Lu, Q., Zhuang, X., & Ma, Q. (2022). Self-efficacy mediates the associations of diabetes distress and depressive symptoms with type 2 diabetes management and glycemic control. *Gen Hosp Psychiatry, 78*, 87–95. https://doi.org/10.1016/j.genhosppsych.2022.06.003

Góralczyk-Bińkowska, A., Szmajda-Krygier, D., & Kozłowska, E. (2022). The microbiota-gut-brain axis in psychiatric disorders. *Int J Mol Sci, 23*(19). https://doi.org/10.3390/ijms231911245

Harris, R. A., Fernando, H. A., Seimon, R. V., da Luz, F. Q., Gibson, A. A., Touyz, S. W., & Sainsbury, A. (2022). Effects of total diet replacement programs on mental well-being: A systematic review with meta-analyses. *Obes Rev, 23*(11), e13465. https://doi.org/10 .1111/obr.13465

Herselman, M. F., Bailey, S., & Bobrovskaya, L. (2022). The effects of stress and diet on the "brain-gut" and "gut-brain" pathways in animal models of stress and depression. *Int J Mol Sci, 23*(4). https://doi.org/10.3390/ijms23042013

Herselman, M. F., Bailey, S., Deo, P., Zhou, X. F., Gunn, K. M., & Bobrovskaya, L. (2022). The effects of walnuts and academic stress on mental health, general well-being and the gut microbiota in a sample of university students: A randomised clinical trial. *Nutrients*, *14*(22). https://doi.org/10.3390/nu14224776

Horn, J., Mayer, D. E., Chen, S., & Mayer, E. A. (2022). Role of diet and its effects on the gut microbiome in the pathophysiology of mental disorders. *Transl Psychiatry*, *12*(1), 164. https://doi.org/10.1038/s41398-022-01922-0

Jeitler, M., Lauche, R., Hohmann, C., Choi, K. A., Schneider, N., Steckhan, N., Rathjens, F., Anheyer, D., Paul, A., von Scheidt, C., Ostermann, T., Schneider, E., Koppold-Liebscher, D., Kessler, C. S., Dobos, G., Michalsen, A., & Cramer, H. (2022). A randomized controlled trial of fasting and lifestyle modification in patients with metabolic syndrome: Effects on patient-reported outcomes. *Nutrients*, *14*(17). https://doi.org/10.3390/nu14173559

Kaner, G., Yurtdaş-Depboylu, G., Çalık, G., Yalçın, T., & Nalçakan, T. (2022). Evaluation of perceived depression, anxiety, stress levels and emotional eating behaviours and their predictors among adults during the COVID-19 pandemic. *Public Health Nutr*, 1–10. https://doi.org/10.1017/S1368980022002579

Katasonov, A. B. (2021). Gut microbiome as a therapeutic target in the treatment of depression and anxiety. *Zh Nevrol Psikhiatr S S Korsakova*, *121*(11), 129–135. https://doi.org/10.17116/jnevro2021121111129

Knight, R., Cedillo, Y., Judd, S., Tison, S., Baker, E., & Moellering, D. (2022). Dietary inflammation score is associated with perceived stress, depression, and cardiometabolic health risk factors among a young adult cohort of women. *Clin Nutr ESPEN*, *51*, 470–477. https://doi.org/10.1016/j.clnesp.2022.06.013

López-Taboada, I., González-Pardo, H., & Conejo, N. M. (2020). Western diet: Implications for brain function and behavior. *Front Psychol*, *11*, 564413. https://doi.org/10.3389/fpsyg.2020.564413

Lu, X., Qi, C., Zheng, J., Sun, M., Jin, L., & Sun, J. (2022). The antidepressant effect of deoiled sunflower seeds on chronic unpredictable mild stress in mice through regulation of microbiota-gut-brain axis. *Front Nutr*, *9*, 908297. https://doi.org/10.3389/fnut.2022.908297

Madison, A., & Kiecolt-Glaser, J. K. (2019). Stress, depression, diet, and the gut microbiota: Human-bacteria interactions at the core of psychoneuroimmunology and nutrition. *Curr Opin Behav Sci*, *28*, 105–110. https://doi.org/10.1016/j.cobeha.2019.01.011

Marwaha, K. (2022). Examining the role of psychosocial stressors in hypertension. *J Prev Med Public Health*, *55*(6), 499–505. https://doi.org/10.3961/jpmph.21.266

Marx, W., Lanc, M., Hockey, M., Aslam, H., Berk, M., Walder, K., Borsini, A., Firth, J., Pariante, C. M., Berding, K., Cryan, J. F., Clarke, G., Craig, J. M., Su, K. P., Mischoulon, D., Gomez-Pinilla, F., Foster, J. A., Cani, P. D., Thuret, S., Staudacher, H. M., Sánchez-Villegas, A., Arshad, H., Akbaraly, T., O'Neil, A., Segasby, T., & Jacka, F. N. (2021). Diet and depression: Exploring the biological mechanisms of action. *Mol Psychiatry*, *26*(1), 134–150. https://doi.org/10.1038/s41380-020-00925-x

Marx, W., Manger, S. H., Blencowe, M., Murray, G., Ho, F. Y., Lawn, S., Blumenthal, J. A., Schuch, F., Stubbs, B., Ruusunen, A., Desyibelew, H. D., Dinan, T. G., Jacka, F., Ravindran, A., Berk, M., & O'Neil, A. (2022). Clinical guidelines for the use of lifestyle-based mental health care in major depressive disorder: World Federation of Societies for Biological Psychiatry (WFSBP) and Australasian Society of Lifestyle Medicine (ASLM) taskforce. *World J Biol Psychiatry*, 1–54. https://doi.org/10.1080/15622975.2022.2112074

Miller, L., Déchelotte, P., Ladner, J., & Tavolacci, M. P. (2022). Effect of the COVID-19 pandemic on healthy components of diet and factors associated with unfavorable changes among university students in France. *Nutrients*, *14*(18). https://doi.org/10.3390/nu14183862

Nguyen, S. A., Oughli, H. A., & Lavretsky, H. (2022). Complementary and integrative medicine for neurocognitive disorders and caregiver health. *Curr Psychiatry Rep, 24*(9), 469–480. https://doi.org/10.1007/s11920-022-01355-y

Pepe, R. B., Coelho, G. S. M. A., Miguel, F. D. S., Gualassi, A. C., Sarvas, M. M., Cercato, C., Mancini, M. C., & de Melo, M. E. (2022). Mindful eating for weight loss in women with obesity: A randomized controlled trial. *Br J Nutr*, 1–28. https://doi.org/10.1017/S0007114522003932

Ram, B., Foley, K. A., van Sluijs, E., Hargreaves, D. S., Viner, R. M., & Saxena, S. (2022). Developing a core outcome set for physical activity interventions in primary schools: A modified-Delphi study. *BMJ Open, 12*(9), e061335. https://doi.org/10.1136/bmjopen-2022-061335

Ravikumar, D., Vaughan, E., & Kelly, C. (2022). Diet quality, health, and wellbeing within the Irish homeless sector: A qualitative exploration. *Int J Environ Res Public Health, 19*(23). https://doi.org/10.3390/ijerph192315976

Reemst, K., Broos, J. Y., Abbink, M. R., Cimetti, C., Giera, M., Kooij, G., & Korosi, A. (2022). Early-life stress and dietary fatty acids impact the brain lipid/oxylipin profile into adulthood, basally and in response to LPS. *Front Immunol, 13*, 967437. https://doi.org/10.3389/fimmu.2022.967437

Ricci, A., Idzikowski, M. A., Soares, C. N., & Brietzke, E. (2020). Exploring the mechanisms of action of the antidepressant effect of the ketogenic diet. *Rev Neurosci, 31*(6), 637–648. https://doi.org/10.1515/revneuro-2019-0073

Seifollahi, A., Sardari, L., Yarizadeh, H., Mirzababaei, A., Shiraseb, F., Clark, C. C., & Mirzaei, K. (2022). Associations between adherence to the MIND diet and prevalence of psychological disorders, and sleep disorders severity among obese and overweight women: A cross-sectional study. *Nutr Health*, 2601060221127461. https://doi.org/10.1177/02601060221127461

Sharma, H., & Bajwa, J. (2021). Approach of probiotics in mental health as a psychobiotics. *Arch Microbiol, 204*(1), 30. https://doi.org/10.1007/s00203-021-02622-x

Shiri, R., Väänänen, A., Mattila-Holappa, P., Kauppi, K., & Borg, P. (2022). The effect of healthy lifestyle changes on work ability and mental health symptoms: A randomized controlled trial. *Int J Environ Res Public Health, 19*(20). https://doi.org/10.3390/ijerph192013206

Solomou, S., Logue, J., Reilly, S., & Perez-Algorta, G. (2022). A systematic review of the association of diet quality with the mental health of university students: Implications in health education practice. *Health Educ Res*. https://doi.org/10.1093/her/cyac035

Takahashi, E., & Ono, E. (2022). Differential effects of different diets on depressive-like phenotypes in C57BL/JJmsSLc mice. *Physiol Behav, 243*, 113623. https://doi.org/10.1016/j.physbeh.2021.113623

Thangaleela, S., Sivamaruthi, B. S., Kesika, P., & Chaiyasut, C. (2022). Role of probiotics and diet in the management of neurological diseases and mood states: A review. *Microorganisms, 10*(11). https://doi.org/10.3390/microorganisms10112268

Tokarchuk, A., Abenavoli, L., Kobyliak, N., Khomenko, M., Revun, M., Dolgaia, N., Molochek, N., Tsyryuk, O., Garnytska, A., Konakh, V., Pellicano, R., Fagoonee, S., Ostapchenko, L., & Falalyeyeva, T. (2022). Nutrition program, physical activity and gut microbiota modulation: A randomized controlled trial to promote a healthy lifestyle in students with vitamin D3 deficiency. *Minerva Med, 113*(4), 683–694. https://doi.org/10.23736/S0026-4806.22.07992-7

Trzeciak, P., & Herbet, M. (2021). Role of the intestinal microbiome, intestinal barrier and psychobiotics in depression. *Nutrients, 13*(3). https://doi.org/10.3390/nu13030927

Tyagi, R., Vaidya, B., & Sharma, S. S. (2022). Crosstalk between neurological, cardiovascular, and lifestyle disorders: Insulin and lipoproteins in the lead role. *Pharmacol Rep, 74*(5), 790–817. https://doi.org/10.1007/s43440-022-00417-5

Vujanovic, S., Vujanovic, J., & Vujanovic, V. (2022). Microbiome-driven proline biogenesis in plants under stress: Perspectives for balanced diet to minimize depression disorders in humans. *Microorganisms, 10*(11). https://doi.org/10.3390/microorganisms10112264

Yao, Z., Xie, X., Bai, R., Li, L., Zhang, X., Li, S., Ma, Y., Hui, Z., & Chen, J. (2022). The impact of eating behaviors during COVID-19 in health-care workers: A conditional process analysis of eating, affective disorders, and PTSD. *Heliyon, 8*(10), e10892. https://doi .org/10.1016/j.heliyon.2022.e10892

Zagórska, A., Marcinkowska, M., Jamrozik, M., Wiśniowska, B., & Paśko, P. (2020). From probiotics to psychobiotics - The gut-brain axis in psychiatric disorders. *Benef Microbes, 11*(8), 717–732. https://doi.org/10.3920/BM2020.0063

Zhang, L., Xie, Y., Li, B., Weng, F., Zhang, F., & Xia, J. (2022). Psychiatric symptoms and frequency of eating out among commuters in Beijing: A bidirectional association? *Nutrients, 14*(20). https://doi.org/10.3390/nu14204221

Zohrabi, T., Ziaee, A., Salehi-Abargouei, A., Ferns, G. A., Ghayour-Mobarhan, M., & Khayyatzadeh, S. S. (2022). Dietary total anti-oxidant capacity is inversely related to the prevalence of depression in adolescent girls. *BMC Pediatr, 22*(1), 535. https://doi .org/10.1186/s12887-022-03589-4

# 9

# Effects of Psychological, Environmental, and Physical Stressors on the Gut Microbiota

Abdullah Abdelkawi, Diban Sabbagh, Muhamed Hobi,
and Yashwant V. Pathak

## Contents

## 9.1 Psychological Stressors

Psychological stress is a common and often inevitable feature of modern living. It is a condition of mental or emotional strain or stress caused by harsh or difficult conditions. Psychological stressors may include work-related stress, family and marital problems, financial hardship, and other life situations that are seen as threatening or demanding.

Several research studies have examined the impact of psychological stress on the gut microbiome, with varied results. Some studies have indicated that psychological stress is connected with alterations in the gut microbiota, including reductions in the variety and richness of the microbiota as well as alterations in the relative abundance of particular bacterial taxa. For instance, a study by

DOI: 10.1201/9781003333821-9

Desbonnet et al. (2014) indicated that persistent psychological stress was associated with decreased abundance of Bifidobacterium and Lactobacillus species in mice. Other research has discovered that psychological stress is connected with increases in pro-inflammatory bacterial taxa, including Escherichia coli and Enterobacteriaceae (Bailey et al., 2011; Desbonnet et al., 2014).

There are multiple potential mechanisms via which psychological stress may alter the gut microbiome. Stress may stimulate the hypothalamic-pituitary-adrenal (HPA) axis, resulting in increased production of corticosteroids such as cortisol. Cortisol has been found to modify the gut microbiota of animals (Bailey et al., 2011), and it may potentially have an effect on the gut microbiota of people. Additionally, psychological stress may disrupt gut motility and digestion, which can have an effect on the gut microbiota (Desbonnet et al., 2014).

Alterations in gut motility and digestion may also be a potential method by which psychological stress influences the microbiota of the stomach. Stress has been proven to change gut motility and digestion in both animals and humans, which can have a substantial effect on the gut microbiota (Desbonnet et al., 2014). For instance, stress may modify the velocity of transit in the gut, resulting in changes in the amount of time different bacterial species are exposed to the gut environment. Stress may also influence the synthesis of digestive enzymes, which can affect digestion and absorption of nutrients and lead to alterations in the gut microbiome.

It is also plausible that psychological stress may influence the microbiota of the gastrointestinal tract through altering the immune system. It has been demonstrated that stress alters immunological function, including the generation of cytokines and other chemicals related to inflammation. These alterations in immune function may have repercussions on the gut microbiome.

Notably, the effects of psychological stress on the gut microbiota may be complex and variable depending on the exact nature and degree of the stressor as well as the individual's baseline microbiota composition. Further study is required to completely comprehend the processes by which psychological stressors affect the gut microbiota and how these effects may contribute to the development or worsening of a variety of health disorders.

## 9.2 Environmental Stressors

Environmental stressors are external environmental factors that may affect the gut microbiota. These stressors may include food, exposure to chemicals, and contact with infections.

Diet is an important environmental stressor that can have a substantial effect on the gut flora. The types and quantities of nutrients and other chemicals present in the diet, as well as the frequency and timing of meals, shape the gut microbiota. Diets high in processed and refined foods, as well as diets high in animal protein and fat, have been linked to alterations in the gut microbiota that may contribute to the development of obesity, metabolic syndrome, and inflammatory bowel disease (IBD) (David et al., 2014). Alternatively, diets rich in fruits, vegetables, and whole grains have been linked to a more diversified and healthier gut flora.

## 9.2.1 Diet

Diet is a significant environmental component that can influence the makeup and function of gut microbiota. The gut microbiota, also known as the gut microbiome, is a diverse community of bacteria that reside in the gastrointestinal system and play a crucial role in human health. Certain mechanisms of production, including the breakdown of essential nutrients, can also play an important role in the metabolism of the gut microbiota (Zmora et al., 2019; Conlon and Bird, 2014). The gut microbiota is regulated by numerous factors, including genetics, drug usage, and, most significantly, food.

The types of nutrients and food components consumed can have an effect on the gut flora. Different types of nutrients and food components can have varying effects on the growth and activity of various gut bacteria. Fiber, a type of carbohydrate present in plant-based diets, is fermented by the gut microbiota and can encourage the growth of beneficial bacteria such as Bifidobacteria and Lactobacilli. In contrast, diets high in refined carbohydrates and saturated fats have been linked to a gut microbial composition that is less diverse and less healthy.

Through the presence of particular dietary additives and toxins, diet can also influence the gut flora. In animal and human research, it has been shown that artificial sweeteners, which are routinely employed in low-calorie and sugar-free diets, change the gut microbiome. Exposure to environmental toxins such as pesticides and heavy metals, which may be found in some foods, has also been related to alterations in the gut microbiota.

Dietary influences on the gut microbiota can have significant effects on human health. The gut microbiota plays a crucial role in numerous physiological processes, such as digestion and absorption of nutrients, generation of short-chain fatty acids and other metabolites, and control of the immune system. A range of health issues, including obesity, inflammatory bowel disease, and digestive diseases, has been linked to gut microbiota disruptions, such as those generated by an improper diet.

In conclusion, food is a significant environmental component that can influence the gut microbiota and, in turn, human health. To support the health of the gut microbiota, it is essential to have a balanced and diverse diet consisting of a wide variety of unprocessed, whole foods.

Environmental toxins and contaminants can also alter the gut microbiome. Certain pesticides, herbicides, and other chemicals have been associated with alterations in the gut microbiota that may contribute to the development of inflammatory bowel disease (IBD). Additionally, human gut microbiome changes have been connected to air pollution.

## 9.2.2 Pollutants

Environmental toxins and contaminants can have a major effect on the gut microbiota, the colony of bacteria that inhabits the digestive system. The gut microbiota is a complex and dynamic ecology that is vital for general health and wellness. Exposure to chemicals and pollutants can affect the composition and function of the gut microbiota, resulting in a decrease in helpful bacteria and an increase in pathogenic bacteria, according to scientific research. This can result in a variety of gastrointestinal issues, including irritable bowel syndrome (IBS) and inflammatory bowel disease (IBD). Heavy metals are an example of a hazardous material that might influence the gut microbiota. Heavy metals, including lead, mercury, and cadmium, are poisonous to the body and can accumulate in the gut microbiome, causing a decrease in beneficial bacteria and an increase in pathogenic bacteria. The toxicity of heavy metals has been related to a variety of gastrointestinal and systemic issues, such as abdominal pain, diarrhea, and immunological dysfunction.

Pesticides are another example of a harmful agent that might disrupt the gut microbiome. Pesticides are chemicals typically found in the environment that are used to control pests. Pesticide exposure has been related to a variety of health issues, including gastrointestinal issues such abdominal pain, diarrhea, and nausea. Additionally, pesticides can affect the composition and function of the gut microbiome, resulting in a decrease in beneficial bacteria and an increase in pathogenic bacteria. In addition to heavy metals and pesticides, the environment contains numerous additional chemicals and contaminants that can damage the gut flora. Air pollution, for instance, has been related to a variety of health issues, such as respiratory and cardiovascular disorders, and research indicates that it can also influence the gut flora. Air pollution can affect the composition and function of the gut microbiome, leading to an increase in pathogenic bacteria and a decrease in beneficial bacteria. Overall, environmental chemicals and contaminants can have a considerable impact on the gut flora. These chemicals can change the content and function of the gut microbiome, resulting in a variety of gastrointestinal and systemic disorders. In order to maintain a healthy gut microbiota and general health and wellness, it is essential to limit exposure to toxins and contaminants.

Pathogens, such as viruses and bacteria, can potentially affect the microbiota of the stomach. Infection with certain viruses, such as norovirus, has been related to alterations in the gut microbiota, which may contribute to the development of gastrointestinal illnesses. Exposure to certain bacterial pathogens, such as Salmonella, has been associated to alterations in the gut microbiota that may contribute to the development of disorders such as inflammatory bowel disease (IBD).

## 9.2.3 Pathogens

Pathogens can have an effect on the gut microbiota by directly killing or suppressing the proliferation of bacteria. Bacterial infections such as Salmonella and Escherichia coli, for instance, can cause diarrhea and other gastrointestinal symptoms by destroying helpful bacteria and increasing the number of dangerous bacteria in the gut. Pathogens can also influence the gut microbiota by affecting the immune system. The immune system is essential for maintaining the balance of the gut microbiota and defending against illnesses. Pathogen exposure can activate the immune system and cause inflammation, which can affect the microbiome's makeup and function. This can lead to a drop in good bacteria and an increase in harmful bacteria, which can result in a variety of gastrointestinal issues such as irritable bowel syndrome (IBS) and inflammatory bowel disease (IBD). In addition, pathogen exposure can have long-lasting consequences on the gut microbiome. Exposure to the bacterium Helicobacter pylori, a major cause of stomach ulcers, has been found to modify the gut microbiota and increase the risk of gastrointestinal disorders such as IBD. Viruses such as the common cold and influenza can also alter the microbiota of the gut. These infections can cause gastrointestinal symptoms including diarrhea and vomiting, which might affect the microbiome's composition and function. In addition, certain viruses, such as the norovirus, can directly attack and destroy gut bacteria, resulting in a disruption in the microbiological equilibrium. Overall, pathogen exposure can have a substantial effect on the gut microbiome. It is essential to decrease pathogen exposure in order to maintain a healthy gut microbiota and general health and wellness.

Notably, the impact of environmental stressors on the gut microbiota may differ based on the kind and degree of the stressor, as well as the microbiota composition of the individual at baseline. Due to genetics, lifestyle, and food, certain individuals may be more susceptible to the harmful effects of environmental stresses on the gut microbiota. Others, however, may be more resistant to these effects. In addition, it is essential to recognize that the gut microbiota is a dynamic and complex ecosystem that is influenced by a range of factors, and that the impact of any one stressor may be influenced by the presence of additional stressors. Understanding the individual and combined effects of environmental stresses on the gut microbiota can help us better comprehend how they contribute to general health and well-being. To completely comprehend the processes by which environmental stressors alter the gut microbiota and how these changes may contribute to the development or worsening of various health disorders, additional study is required.

## 9.3 Physical Stressors

Physical stressors are external physical stimuli that can influence the microbiota of the gut. Included among these stressors are physical injury, surgery, and physical activity.

Both physical injuries and surgery can have major effects on the microbiome of the gut. Injuries and surgical procedures can affect the normal function of the gastrointestinal tract, resulting in altered gut motility and digestion, as well as increased inflammation and oxidative stress. These modifications can alter the gut microbiota, which may contribute to the development or worsening of a variety of diseases. Both physical injuries and surgery can have major effects on the gut microbiota, the colony of microorganisms that inhabit the digestive system. The gut microbiota is a complex and dynamic ecology that is vital for general health and wellness. In numerous ways, a physical injury might influence the gut microbiome. First, injuries can cause inflammation and changes in blood flow, which can alter the makeup and function of the microbiome in the gut. For instance, research has demonstrated that damage can lead to a drop in beneficial bacteria and an increase in harmful bacteria in the gut, resulting in a variety of gastrointestinal disorders such as irritable bowel syndrome (IBS) and inflammatory bowel disease (IBD). Second, physical trauma can disturb the normal functioning of the gastrointestinal system, resulting in alterations to the gut flora. For instance, damage might result in altered gut motility and secretions, which can impact the growth and survival of gut bacteria. Additionally, surgery can have profound effects on the gut microbiome. During surgery, the immune system is engaged to aid in tissue repair and defense against infection. This immune reaction can result in inflammation, which can affect the microbiome's makeup and function. Moreover, surgery can affect the normal functioning of the gastrointestinal system, resulting in alterations to the gut flora. For instance, surgery can cause changes in gut motility and secretions, and the use of antibiotics can impact the growth and survival of gut bacteria. Injuries and surgical procedures can have major effects on the gut microbiome. To maintain a healthy gut microbiota and general health and well-being, it is necessary to examine the potential effects of these stresses on the gut microbiome and to take actions to mitigate their negative effects.

Exercise is another physical stressor that might impact the microbiome of the stomach. It has been demonstrated that exercise alters the gut microbiota of both humans and animals. The specific effects of exercise on the gut microbiota may vary on the intensity and duration of the activity as well as the microbiome composition of the individual at baseline. Some studies have revealed that severe and sustained exercise is connected with alterations in the gut microbiota that may contribute to the development of gastrointestinal illnesses like IBD (Gleeson et al., 2011). In contrast, moderate physical exercise has been linked to a more diversified and healthier gut flora.

## 9.4 Mechanisms of Action

The methods by which psychological, environmental, and physical stressors may affect the gut microbiota are incompletely known. Nevertheless, other plausible processes have been presented.

## 9.4.1  HPA Axis

An example of a possible mechanism is the HPA axis. As previously stated, psychological stress activates the HPA axis, resulting in increased cortisol and other stress hormone production. In addition to altering gut motility and digestion, these hormones can also increase inflammation and oxidative stress (Bailey et al., 2011). The hypothalamic-pituitary-adrenal (HPA) axis is a complicated physiological system that regulates stress and maintains homeostasis. The HPA axis consists of the hypothalamus, pituitary gland, and adrenal gland. The hypothalamus is a tiny brain area that serves as the HPA axis' control center. It causes the pituitary gland to secrete adrenocorticotropic hormone (ACTH) by releasing corticotropin-releasing hormone (CRH). The ACTH then travels through the bloodstream to the adrenal gland, where it stimulates cortisol production and release. Cortisol is a stress hormone that enables the body to adapt to stress by increasing blood sugar levels, boosting energy, and decreasing nonessential processes including digestion and immunological function. The HPA axis is also involved in the regulation of the gut microbiome, the community of bacteria that reside in the digestive tract. The microbiome of the gut is a complex and dynamic system that is vital for maintaining overall health and well-being. Chronic stress alters the composition and function of the gut microbiome, resulting in a drop in beneficial bacteria and an increase in dangerous bacteria, according to research. This can result in a variety of gastrointestinal issues, including irritable bowel syndrome (IBS) and inflammatory bowel disease (IBD). In addition, the HPA axis can influence the gut–brain axis, a bidirectional communication link between the gut and the brain that regulates a number of physiological processes. Dysregulation of the HPA axis can result in alterations in the gut–brain axis, which can contribute to gastrointestinal symptoms. The HPA axis is essential for controlling stress and maintaining homeostasis in the body. It also has a substantial effect on the gut flora and the gut–brain axis, which can have knock-on consequences on the health and well-being of the individual.

## 9.4.2  Immune System

The immune system is an additional possible mechanism. Stressors can change the immune system, which can have an effect on the gut microbiome. For instance, stress-induced immunological alterations can lead to increased inflammation and oxidative stress, which might affect the gut microbiota.

The immune system plays a key role in maintaining the gut microbiome, the community of bacteria that reside in the digestive tract. The gut microbiome is a complex and dynamic ecology that is vital for general health and wellness. According to research, the immune system and the gut microbiome have a two-way influence on one another. The gut microbiome serves to educate and regulate the immune system, while the immune system can also influence the microbiome's composition and function. For instance, the gut microbiota aids in the early stimulation and maintenance of the immune system, which is essential for preventing autoimmune disorders and allergies. Certain bacteria in the microbiome of the gut generate compounds that can stimulate the formation of immune cells, while others create substances that serve to suppress the immunological response. The immune system can also regulate the gut microbiome by secreting cytokines and other signaling molecules that affect the growth and survival of gut bacteria. For instance, inflammation and the activation of the immune system can reduce the diversity and abundance of beneficial bacteria in the gut microbiome, resulting in a shift in the balance of microorganisms and possibly contributing to gastrointestinal problems such as irritable bowel syndrome (IBS) and inflammatory bowel disease (IBD). Overall, the interaction between the immune system and the gut microbiome is intricate and interrelated. This interaction can help us better understand how the immune system and gut microbiome contribute to general health and wellness.

### 9.4.3 Gut–Brain Axis

The gut–brain axis is a putative third pathway. The gut microbiota can affect the brain by multiple mechanisms, including the generation of neurotransmitters and other signaling molecules, as well as the activation of the immune system. Through the release of stress hormones and other signaling molecules, the brain can in turn alter the gut flora. The gut–brain axis is a two-way communication connection between the gut and the brain that regulates numerous physiological processes. It consists of a network of neurons, hormones, and immune cells that connects the gut to the brain and enables communication between them. The gut microbiome, the community of bacteria that reside in the digestive tract, plays a crucial function in the gut–brain axis. The gut microbiome is a complex and dynamic ecology that is vital for general health and wellness. Recent research suggests that the gut microbiota plays an imperative role in neural regulation and development (Chen et al., 2013). The gut microbiota regulates the development and operation of the neural system in the gut, particularly the enteric nervous system, which controls gastrointestinal motility and secretions. Second, the gut microbiota creates signaling chemicals, such as neurotransmitters and cytokines, that can influence the neurological system and brain function. Certain bacteria in the gut microbiome, for instance, create serotonin, a neurotransmitter that influences mood and behavior. Thirdly, the gut microbiota can have an effect on the immune system, which is intimately linked to the gut–brain axis. The immune system can create cytokines and other signaling molecules that can influence brain function, while the gut microbiome can influence the immune system by producing numerous chemicals. The gut–brain axis is a dynamic, complex system that is regulated by the gut bacteria. The gut–brain axis has been found to be impacted by common early-stage actions, such as bacterial infection and the counter-use of antibiotics (Cryan et al., 2019). Several gastrointestinal and neurological illnesses, such as irritable bowel syndrome (IBS), inflammatory bowel disease (IBD), anxiety, and depression, have been related to dysregulation of the gut–brain axis. Furthermore, the relationship between the gut–brain axis and gut microbiota has been linked to the development of obesity and its effects (Bliss and Whiteside, 2018). Understanding the link between the gut microbiota and the gut–brain axis can enhance our knowledge of how the gut microbiome contributes to overall health and well-being. It may also shed light on prospective therapeutic techniques for treating digestive and neurological diseases.

## 9.5 Conclusion

Psychological, environmental, and physical stressors can all influence the gut microbiota, the community of bacteria that inhabit the gastrointestinal system. The gut microbiota is a complex and dynamic ecology that is vital for general health and wellness. Thus, psychological stresses such as stress, anxiety, and depression can influence the gut microbiota via several methods.

For instance, psychological stress can modify gut motility and secretions, resulting in alterations to the microbiome of the stomach. Additionally, psychological stress can impact the immune system, causing inflammation and alterations to the gut flora. Environmental stresses, such as environmental chemicals and contaminants, can also impact the gut microbiota. These chemicals can change the content and function of the gut microbiome, resulting in a variety of gastrointestinal and systemic disorders.

Additionally, physical stressors, such as physical damage and surgery, can have major effects on the gut microbiome. These stressors can cause inflammation and alterations in the normal functioning of the gastrointestinal tract, which can alter the microbiome of the gut. In order to maintain a healthy gut microbiome and overall health and well-being, it is essential to examine the potential effects of psychological, environmental, and physical stressors on the gut microbiota and to take actions to reduce their negative consequences. The specific impacts of various stressors on the gut microbiota may vary on the stressor's nature and degree, as well as the individual's microbiota makeup at baseline. To completely comprehend the processes by which stresses alter the gut microbiota and how these changes may contribute to the development or worsening of various health disorders, additional study is required.

## Bibliography

Bailey, M. T., Dowd, S. E., Galley, J. D., Hufnagle, A. R., Allen, R. G., & Lyte, M. (2011). Exposure to a social stressor alters the structure of the intestinal microbiota: Implications for stressor-induced immunomodulation. *Brain Behav Immun*, *25*(3), 397–407.

Bercik, P., Park, A. J., Sinclair, D., & Verdu, E. F. (2011). The anxiolytic effect of Bifidobacterium longum NCC3001 involves vagal pathways for gut-brain communication. *Neurogastroenterol Motil, 23*(12), 1132–1139.

Bliss, E. S., & Whiteside, E. (2018). The gut-brain axis, the human gut microbiota and their integration in the development of obesity. *Front Physiol, 9*, 900.

Canakis, A., Haroon, M., & Weber, H. C. (2020). Irritable bowel syndrome and gut microbiota. *Curr Opin Endocrinol Diabetes Obes, 27*(1), 28–35. doi:10.1097/med .0000000000000523.

Cenit, M. C., Sanz, Y., & Codoñer-Franch, P. (2017). Influence of gut microbiota on neuropsychiatric disorders. *World J Gastroenterol, 23*(30), 5486–5498. doi:10.3748/wjg.v23.i30.5486.

Chen, X., D'Souza, R., & Hong, S.-T. (2013). The role of gut microbiota in the gut-brain axis: Current challenges and perspectives. *Protein Cell, 4*(6), 403–414.

Collins, S. M., Surette, M., & Bercik, P. (2012). The interplay between the intestinal microbiota and the brain. *Nat Rev Microbiol, 10*(11), 735–742.

Conlon, M. A., & Bird, A. R. (2014). The impact of diet and lifestyle on gut microbiota and human health. *Nutrients, 7*(1), 17–44.

Cryan, J. F., & Dinan, T. G. (2012). Mind-altering microorganisms: The impact of the gut microbiota on brain and behaviour. *Nat Rev Neurosci, 13*(10), 701–712.

Cryan, J. F., O'Riordan, K. J., Cowan, C. S. M., Sandhu, K. V., Bastiaanssen, T. F. S., Boehme, M., Codagnone, M. G., Cussotto, S., Fulling, C., Golubeva, A. V., Guzzetta, K. E. et al. (2019). The microbiota-gut-brain axis. *Physiol Rev.* 2019 Oct 1; *99*(4), 1877–2013. doi: 10.1152/physrev.00018.2018. PMID: 31460832.

Dalile, B., Van Oudenhove, L., Vervliet, B., & Verbeke, K. (2019). The role of short-chain fatty acids in microbiota-gut-brain communication. *Nat Rev Gastroenterol Hepatol, 16*(8), 461–478. doi:10.1038/s41575-019-0157-3.

Dalton, A., Mermier, C., & Zuhl, M. (2019). Exercise influence on the microbiome-gut-brain axis. *Gut Microbes, 10*(5), 555–568. doi:10.1080/19490976.2018.1562268.

David, L. A., Maurice, C. F., Carmody, R. N., Gootenberg, D. B., Button, J. E., Wolfe, B. E., … Turnbaugh, P. J. (2014). Diet rapidly and reproducibly alters the human gut microbiome. *Nature, 505*(7484), 559–563.

Davidson, G. L., Cooke, A. C., Johnson, C. N., & Quinn, J. L. (2018). The gut microbiome as a driver of individual variation in cognition and functional behaviour. *Philos Trans R Soc Lond B, 373*(1756). doi:10.1098/rstb.2017.0286.

Desbonnet, L., Clarke, G., Shanahan, F. et al. (2014). Microbiota is essential for social development in the mouse. *Mol Psychiatry, 19*, 146–148. https://doi.org/10.1038/mp.2013.65

Dinan, T. G., Stanton, C., Cryan, J. F., & Ross, R. P. (2013). Psychobiotics: A novel class of psychotropic. *Biol Psychiatry, 74*(10), 720–726.

D'Souza, A. L., Rajkumar, C., Cooke, J., Bulpitt, K. J., & Yaqoob, P. (2015). The impact of surgery and injury on the gut microbiota. *Front Microbiol, 6*, 879.

Farzi, A., Fröhlich, E. E., & Holzer, P. (2018). Gut microbiota and the neuroendocrine system. *Neurotherapeutics, 15*(1), 5–22. doi:10.1007/s13311-017-0600-5.

Frank, J., Gupta, A., Osadchiy, V., & Mayer, E. A. (2021). Brain-gut-microbiome interactions and intermittent fasting in obesity. *Nutrients, 13*(2). doi:10.3390/nu13020584.

Frankiensztajn, L. M., Elliott, E., & Koren, O. (2020). The microbiota and the hypothalamus-pituitary-adrenocortical (HPA) axis, implications for anxiety and stress disorders. *Curr Opin Neurobiol, 62*, 76–82. doi:10.1016/j.conb.2019.12.003.

Freimer, D., Yang, T. T., Ho, T. C., Tymofiyeva, O., & Leung, C. (2022). The gut microbiota, HPA axis, and brain in adolescent-onset depression: Probiotics as a novel treatment. *Brain Behav Immun Health, 26*, 100541. doi:10.1016/j.bbih.2022.100541.

Gibson, G. R., & Hutkins, R. (2016). Food, gut and the microbiome. *Curr Opin Biotechnol, 37*, 1–6.

Giridharan, V. V., Barichello De Quevedo, C. E., & Petronilho, F. (2022). Microbiota-gut-brain axis in the Alzheimer's disease pathology - An overview. *Neurosci Res, 181*, 17–21. doi:10.1016/j.neures.2022.05.003.

Halverson, T., & Alagiakrishnan, K. (2020). Gut microbes in neurocognitive and mental health disorders. *Ann Med*, *52*(8), 423–443. doi:10.1080/07853890.2020.1808239.

Hantsoo, L., & Zemel, B. S. (2021). Stress gets into the belly: Early life stress and the gut microbiome. *Behav Brain Res*, *414*, 113474. doi:10.1016/j.bbr.2021.113474.

Hantsoo, L., Jašarević, E., Criniti, S., McGeehan, B., Tanes, C., Sammel, M. D., ... Epperson, C. N. (2019). Childhood adversity impact on gut microbiota and inflammatory response to stress during pregnancy. *Brain Behav Immun*, *75*, 240–250. doi:10.1016/j.bbi.2018.11.005.

Hatton-Jones, K. M., du Toit, E. F., & Cox, A. J. (2022). Effect of chronic restraint stress and western-diet feeding on colonic regulatory gene expression in mice. *Neurogastroenterol Motil*, *34*(4), e14300. doi:10.1111/nmo.14300.

Holscher, H. D. (2017). Fiber and prebiotics: Mechanisms and health benefits. *Nutrients*, *9*(4), 430.

Househam, A. M., Peterson, C. T., Mills, P. J., & Chopra, D. (2017). The effects of stress and meditation on the immune system, human microbiota, and epigenetics. *Adv Mind Body Med*, *31*(4), 10–25.

Jahnke, J. R., Roach, J., Azcarate-Peril, M. A., & Thompson, A. L. (2021). Maternal precarity and HPA axis functioning shape infant gut microbiota and HPA axis development in humans. *PLOS ONE*, *16*(5), e0251782. doi:10.1371/journal.pone.0251782.

Karl, J. P., Hatch, A. M., Arcidiacono, S. M., Pearce, S. C., Pantoja-Feliciano, I. G., Doherty, L. A., & Soares, J. W. (2018). Effects of psychological, environmental and physical stressors on the gut microbiota. *Front Microbiol*, *9*, 2013. doi:10.3389/fmicb.2018.02013.

Konturek, P. C., Brzozowski, T., & Konturek, S. J. (2011). Stress and the gut: Pathophysiology, clinical consequences, diagnostic approach and treatment options. *J Physiol Pharmacol*, *62*(6), 591–599.

Lobionda, S., Sittipo, P., Kwon, H. Y., & Lee, Y. K. (2019). The role of gut microbiota in intestinal inflammation with respect to diet and extrinsic stressors. *Microorganisms*, *7*(8). doi:10.3390/microorganisms7080271.

Malan-Muller, S., Valles-Colomer, M., Raes, J., Lowry, C. A., Seedat, S., & Hemmings, S. M. J. (2018). The gut microbiome and mental health: Implications for anxiety- and trauma-related disorders. *Omics*, *22*(2), 90–107. doi:10.1089/omi.2017.0077.

Matenchuk, B. A., Mandhane, P. J., & Kozyrskyj, A. L. (2020). Sleep, circadian rhythm, and gut microbiota. *Sleep Med Rev*, *53*, 101340. doi:10.1016/j.smrv.2020.101340.

Mayer, E. A., Knight, R., Mazmanian, S. K., Cryan, J. F., & Tillisch, K. (2014). Gut microbes and the brain: Paradigm shift in neuroscience. *J Neurosci*, *34*(46), 15490–15496. doi:10.1523/jneurosci.3299-14.2014.

Misiak, B., Łoniewski, I., Marlicz, W., Frydecka, D., Szulc, A., Rudzki, L., & Samochowiec, J. (2020). The HPA axis dysregulation in severe mental illness: Can we shift the blame to gut microbiota? *Prog Neuropsychopharmacol Biol Psychiatry*, *102*, 109951. doi:10.1016/j.pnpbp.2020.109951.

Młynarska, E., Gadzinowska, J., Tokarek, J., Forycka, J., Szuman, A., Franczyk, B., & Rysz, J. (2022). The role of the microbiome-brain-gut axis in the pathogenesis of depressive disorder. *Nutrients*, *14*(9). doi:10.3390/nu14091921.

Mohajeri, M. H., La Fata, G., Steinert, R. E., & Weber, P. (2018). Relationship between the gut microbiome and brain function. *Nutr Rev*, *76*(7), 481–496. doi:10.1093/nutrit/nuy009.

Mohr, A. E., Jäger, R., Carpenter, K. C., Kerksick, C. M., Purpura, M., Townsend, J. R., ... Antonio, J. (2020). The athletic gut microbiota. *J Int Soc Sports Nutr*, *17*(1), 24. doi:10.1186/s12970-020-00353-w.

Rea, K., Dinan, T. G., & Cryan, J. F. (2016). The microbiome: A key regulator of stress and neuroinflammation. *Neurobiol Stress*, *4*, 23–33. doi:10.1016/j.ynstr.2016.03.001.

Redpath, N., Rackers, H. S., & Kimmel, M. C. (2019). The relationship between perinatal mental health and stress: A review of the microbiome. *Curr Psychiatry Rep*, *21*(3), 18. doi:10.1007/s11920-019-0998-z.

Rieder, R., Wisniewski, P. J., Alderman, B. L., & Campbell, S. C. (2017). Microbes and mental health: A review. *Brain Behav Immun, 66*, 9–17. doi:10.1016/j.bbi.2017.01.016.

Rook, G. A., Lowry, C. A., & Raison, C. L. (2015). Hygiene and other early childhood influences on the subsequent function of the immune system. *Brain Res, 1617*, 47–62. doi:10.1016/j.brainres.2014.04.004.

Rosin, S., Xia, K., Azcarate-Peril, M. A., Carlson, A. L., Propper, C. B., Thompson, A. L., … Knickmeyer, R. C. (2021). A preliminary study of gut microbiome variation and HPA axis reactivity in healthy infants. *Psychoneuroendocrinology, 124*, 105046. doi:10.1016/j.psyneuen.2020.105046.

Simkin, D. R. (2019). Microbiome and mental health, specifically as it relates to adolescents. *Curr Psychiatry Rep, 21*(9), 93. doi:10.1007/s11920-019-1075-3.

Singh, S., Sharma, P., Pal, N., Kumawat, M., Shubham, S., Sarma, D. K., … Nagpal, R. (2022). Impact of environmental pollutants on gut microbiome and mental health via the gut-brain axis. *Microorganisms, 10*(7). doi:10.3390/microorganisms10071457.

Sudo, N. (2014). Microbiome, HPA axis and production of endocrine hormones in the gut. *Adv Exp Med Biol, 817*, 177–194. doi:10.1007/978-1-4939-0897-4_8.

Suez, J., Korem, T., Zeevi, D., Zilberman-Schapira, G., Thaiss, C. A., Maza, O., … Elinav, E. (2014). Artificial sweeteners induce glucose intolerance by altering the gut microbiota. *Nature, 514*(7521), 181–186.

Vafadari, B. (2021). Stress and the role of the gut-brain axis in the pathogenesis of schizophrenia: A literature review. *Int J Mol Sci, 22*(18). doi:10.3390/ijms22189747.

Vagnerová, K., Vodička, M., Hermanová, P., Ergang, P., Šrůtková, D., Klusoňová, P., … Pácha, J. (2019). Interactions between gut microbiota and acute restraint stress in peripheral structures of the hypothalamic-pituitary-adrenal axis and the intestine of male mice. *Front Immunol, 10*, 2655. doi:10.3389/fimmu.2019.02655.

Wang, J., Li, L., Huang, X., & Chen, X. (2017). The impact of diet on the gut microbiome and its relation to health and disease. *Front Microbiol, 8*, 1053.

Xu, C., Lee, S. K., Zhang, D., & Frenette, P. S. (2020). The gut microbiome regulates psychological-stress-induced inflammation. *Immunity, 53*(2), 417–428.e414. doi:10.1016/j.immuni.2020.06.025.

Yaklai, K., Pattanakuhar, S., Chattipakorn, N., & Chattipakorn, S. C. (2021). The role of acupuncture on the gut-brain-microbiota axis in irritable bowel syndrome. *Am J Chin Med, 49*(2), 285–314. doi:10.1142/s0192415x21500154.

Zmora, N., Suez, J., & Elinav, E. (2019). You are what you eat: Diet, health and the gut microbiota. *Nat Rev Gastroenterol Hepatol, 16*(1), 35–56.

# 10

# Translating Evidence to Real-World Reproducibility and Specific Evidence for Nutraceuticals

Emily Evangelista, Patrick Chan, Thomas Shen, and Rahul Mhaskar

## Contents

DOI: 10.1201/9781003333821-10

## 10.1 Introduction

"Nutraceutical" is a portmanteau of "nutrition" and "pharmaceuticals" coined by Dr Stephen DeFelice in 1989. Nutraceutical is defined as a food or supplement that "provides medical and or health benefits" and must also "aid in the prevention and treatment of disease and or disorder" [1]. This concept dates back to Hippocrates, but modern products that fall under this category arose in the late 20th century. According to Grand View Research, nutraceuticals have a market cap of 111.9 billion USD in 2021 in the United States and 454.6 billion USD globally. It is estimated to rise 7.5% annually from 2021–2030 [2]. Big categories of nutraceuticals on the market include vitamins, fibers, omega fatty acids, minerals, prebiotics, and probiotics. This chapter primarily focuses on nutraceuticals that affect anxiety, related psychiatric conditions, and the gut microbiome. We have highlighted evidence from the currently published literature examining the efficacy/effectiveness of these nutraceuticals.

## 10.2 Nutraceuticals and Anxiety

According to the Anxiety and Depression Association of America, as of 2022, anxiety affects 40 million adults or around 9.1% of those 18 or older in the United States. Many Americans report anxiety as challenging to treat, with as many as 50% of those with generalized anxiety disorder not responding to allopathic treatment. Many people have turned to nutraceuticals to alleviate anxiety, and the industry has been rising in the production and availability of nutraceuticals to cater to these increasing demands. While the popular saying "you are what you eat" may sound flippant, there's some truth to it from a clinical perspective, especially regarding relief from anxiety. In simple terms, people eat well to feel well. With the right nutraceuticals, research shows that people with anxiety may find improvement in their symptoms. This section examines some of the most studied and popular nutraceuticals with anxiety-relieving effects.

## 10.2.1 Cannabidiol (CBD)

Cannabidiol (CBD) is a Phyto cannabinoid that has been of interest in recent years. Concurrent with the increasing legalization of cannabis globally, we have seen a burgeoning of CBD edibles and supplements over the past decade. An extensive marketing point for CBD has been its health benefits without the psychoactive and harmful health effects of tetrahydrocannabinol, the active ingredient in cannabis. Recent literature on the efficacy of CBD revealed three systematic reviews addressing CBD's effect on anxiety and sleep. The current evidence suggests that CBD may reduce anxiety disorders without affecting sleep [3, 4], but Black et al.'s study contends that this evidence is scarce and needs further investigation [4]. All studies thus far stressed the need to investigate further the dose, method of delivery, and mechanism of action for CBD.

## 10.2.2 B Vitamins

The B vitamins are water-soluble vitamins that help cell metabolism and erythropoiesis. B vitamin complexes and individual B vitamins are frequently sold in pharmacies, health food stores, and general grocery stores. The literature mainly describes the impact of any B vitamin supplementation, and some articles focused on vitamin B as a whole, while others focused on B6 only. A meta-analysis noted that vitamin B decreases the anxiety and depression of at-risk populations suffering from poor nutrition [5]. A randomized control trial (RCT) with 478 young adults experiencing anxiety showed that a high dose of vitamin B6 explicitly increases GABAergic activity, which could have anxiolytic effects [6]. Magnesium is an ion that is sometimes given with B6, and an RCT showed that giving magnesium with B6 can lower stress and simultaneously correct hypomagnesemia [7].

## 10.2.3 Fatty Acids

Fatty acids are essential nutrients for energy and cellular function. Much research centers on Omega-3 Polyunsaturated Fatty Acids, a class of fatty acids essential in lipid metabolism, hormone synthesis, and inflammation. On average, Americans consume around 35 mg of EPA (Eicosapentaenoic acid) and 76 mg of DHA (docosahexaenoic acid), major Omega-3 fatty acids, a day, way below the World Health Organization's recommendation of 500 mg a day combined. Omega-3 supplement oils, primarily extracted from fish, have been marketed to many segments of the population, especially children and pregnant women. Two meta-analyses showed that Omega-3 supplementation could reduce anxiety symptoms. Nonetheless, similar to CBD, these studies noted the need for more research and increasing participant diversity [8, 9].

## 10.2.4 Vitamin D

It is widely known that vitamin D promotes strong bones and teeth and that the skin can create vitamin D via exposure to sunlight. However, literature shows vitamin D may also be linked with mental health. A systematic review, for example, found that most observational and interventional studies support the link between vitamin D and children's emotional well-being. Researchers learned that vitamin D might help reduce negative emotions, all while increasing quality of life by relieving anxiety and depression. While the mechanisms at play are not fully understood, researchers think they may involve vitamin D crossing the blood-brain barrier, activating receptors in the brain cells, modulating neurotrophic signaling, and regulating inflammation. More research is desired to confirm the link between vitamin D and mental health [10].

But upon a deeper dive into the published literature, we noticed that several systematic reviews had explored the link between vitamin D supplementation and mental health in adults with inflammatory bowel diseases (IBDs) and irritable bowel syndrome (IBS). Most of these studies reinforced the positive effect of vitamin D supplementation on these patients' mental health—in terms of not only anxiety and depression but the overall quality of life [11]. This is compelling information for clinicians looking to understand the latest evidence supporting supplementation.

One thing is certain at this juncture: there seems to be a positive relationship between vitamin D and anxiety. Yet more research is needed to fully understand the relationship between this key nutraceutical and mental health.

## 10.2.5 *Melissa officinalis*

Let's talk about lemon balm or *Melissa officinalis*. This perennial herb belongs to the Lamiaceae (mint) family. It features a pleasant lemon aroma and is often used in aromatherapy and herbal medicine largely due to its calming effect. But that's not all *Melissa officinalis* has to offer. The plant boasts an extensive history as a medicinal herb and has long treated a range of conditions such as insomnia, indigestion, cold sores, and anxiety.

In terms of literature supporting its use for anxiety, in an RCT investigating the effects of *Melissa officinalis* supplementation on mental health and sleep disturbance in patients with chronic stable angina (CSA), researchers concluded that eight weeks of supplementation with 3 g of *Melissa officinalis* improved symptoms [12]. But, beyond this study, there is limited literature on lemon balm's ability to alleviate anxiety. Therefore, further research is needed to investigate the efficacy, mechanism, and reliability of *Melissa officinalis* on mental health.

## 10.2.6 L-theanine

L-theanine is an amino acid found in green tea and oolong tea leaves and is known for its relaxing and calming effects. The research shows that L-theanine supplementation can reduce stress and anxiety, improve sleep quality, elevate cognitive function, and increase the activity of the neurotransmitter gamma-aminobutyric acid (GABA) [13].

A couple of noteworthy studies investigate the link between L-theanine and anxiety. In a systematic review of RCTs, the included studies investigated the potential anti-stress and anxiety-suppressing effects of L-theanine. The researchers found that a 200–400 mg daily L-theanine supplementation may offer anti-stress effects and anxiety-suppressing properties. The systematic review also noted that L-theanine might affect physiological stress biomarkers, including salivary alpha-amylase (sAA) levels, and even improve sleep quality. Since L-theanine is known to suppress excessive glutamatergic tone and bind to glutamate receptors, experts believe this, too, may contribute to its anti-stress and antianxiety effects [14].

To take things a step further from a sleep standpoint, an RCT evaluating patients with a generalized anxiety disorder (GAD) showed that adjunctive L-theanine did not significantly reduce anxiety or insomnia severity but improved self-reported sleep satisfaction. [15]. This means L-theanine seems to offer consistent improvements in sleep quality, although mixed evidence shows its benefits for people suffering from anxiety.

## 10.2.7 *Caralluma fimbriata*

*Caralluma fimbriata* is a native plant from India and is traditionally used as a hunger suppressant. It is often used in a supplement form as a weight loss aid, reducing appetite and increasing fat metabolism [16]. Yet the effects of *Caralluma fimbriata* may extend to anxiety as well. Some literature supports the use of *Caralluma fimbriata* in patients with GAD. For instance, an RCT study exploring the effects of *Caralluma fimbriata* extract (CFE) on anxiety and stress in adults found that the CFE group reduced their symptoms of anxiety and stress significantly more than the placebo group.

Also of note is that based on cortisol levels, CFE may act through the hypothalamic-pituitary-adrenal (HPA) axis—with statistically significant changes observed in men but not in women. However, this study had certain limitations, including self-reporting outcomes and a small sample size of only 49 participants [17].

## 10.2.8 Prebiotics and Probiotics

Now let's discuss prebiotics and probiotics. Prebiotics are plant fibers that promote the growth of healthy bacteria in the gut. While some research suggests that prebiotics can help lessen symptoms of anxiety and depression, a few studies did not find any notable benefit for these conditions. A systematic review and meta-analysis of controlled clinical trials found that prebiotics offered the same effect as a placebo [18]. Studies involving prebiotics and mental health disorders found no beneficial outcomes. For example, a systematic review of clinical trials and observational studies found no depression-related benefits [19]. In another study, neither prebiotics nor probiotics were found to alleviate schizophrenia symptoms [20]. Furthermore, a meta-analysis found that prebiotics did not significantly improve symptoms in patients with autism spectrum disorder (ASD) [21].

Moving on to probiotics, the mixture of live healthy bacteria and yeast in the body. While probiotics are certainly beneficial to a person's health, the current literature does not support the use of probiotics for relief from anxiety. Three systematic reviews and meta-analyses found either mixed or insignificant evidence of probiotics helping improve anxiety [22–24].

Furthermore, one study did find that probiotics reduced anxiety-like behavior in animals, but the results only applied to diseased animals, and only *Lactobacillus rhamnosus* offered any anxiolytic effect. In human studies, probiotics did not significantly reduce symptoms of anxiety.

In summary, more research is needed to determine the effects of probiotics on anxiety relief in humans, especially in clinically anxious populations [23]. One study found variability between assessment instruments and concluded that probiotics *might* alleviate anxiety symptoms. However, more research, larger sample sizes, and long-term follow-ups will be critical moving forward [24].

A final word before we conclude this section involves test-taking. Researchers believe that probiotic supplement preparation (PSP) may improve test anxiety in college students. The RCT results showed that PSP reduced symptoms of depression and anxiety in students who feel nervous taking tests—all while increasing the abundance of *Streptococcus* and *Akkermansia* in the intestinal microbiota and reducing intestinal pathogens *Fusobacterium* and *Clostridium*. In short, the authors concluded that PSP might be a promising way to decrease test anxiety and restore intestinal microbiota balance [25]. Clinicians should consider all the above information when discussing nutraceutical supplements or offering supplement recommendations.

## 10.2.9 Lavender Essential Oil (Silexan)

The National Institute of Health defines essential oils (EOs) as oils obtained through mechanical pressing or distillation, concentrated plant extracts that retain their source's natural smell and flavor [26]. EOs have been utilized in everything from perfumes and candles to cosmetics, medicine, food, and beverages [27]. Aromatherapy is the use of EOs as a complementary health approach to alleviating a variety of health conditions. Multiple studies have analyzed the use of aromatherapy to alleviate anxiety of any cause. This section will evaluate specific EOs utilized in aromatherapy targeting anxiety. Multiple meta-analyses report that aromatherapy with different essential oils alleviates anxiety significantly, no matter the cause of the anxiety [28].

Silexan is a pre-defined 80 mg preparation from Lavandula angustifolia. Silexan is derived from the fresh flowering tops of the plant by steam distillation [29]. One meta-analysis analyzed the efficacy of Silexan lavender EO in alleviating the anxiety associated with severe pain, basing the physiology of this mechanism on the (Gate) Control Theory. These findings denote a relationship between pain and psychological ailments such as anxiety [30]. The study found a significant decrease in the severity of pain and anxiety after aromatherapy induction [30]. An RCT analyzing the induction of oral lavender EO on anxiety and sleep quality of chemotherapy patients revealed a drop in anxiety severity and an improvement in PSQI (Pittsburgh Sleep Quality Index) measurements [32]. However, it is important to note that a separate meta-analysis concluded that neither lavender inhalation nor oral Silexan for six weeks was proven to significantly reduce systolic blood pressure as a physiological parameter of anxiety. Nonetheless, reported anxiety levels were decreased in both groups [32]. However, in a contrasting meta-analysis, aromatherapy using lavender EO was concluded to have favorable effects on anxiety and its physiological manifestations [33]. Utilizing the Hamilton Anxiety Scale (HAMA), Silexan was compared in a systematic review at 80 mg and 160 mg doses for anxiety disorders. A significantly greater reduction in HAMA score was found in the 160 mg group [34]. In addition to beneficial changes in HAMA scores, Silexan has also been shown to decrease bodily pain, improve general health, decrease insomnia complaints, and decrease fatigue [35]. An analysis was also completed on the best modality of lavender EO administration for the greatest anxiety reduction and found that though all study groups saw reductions in reported anxiety levels, the quickest onset of relief was found with lavender aromatherapy. The most significant relief was experienced with lavender massage and footbaths [36]. Additionally, studies on the effect of Silexan on subthreshold anxiety demonstrated improved anxiety symptoms, a beneficial effect on sleep without causing sedation, and improved health-related quality of life [37]. Future studies are recommended with an emphasis on methodological quality [32, 33].

## 10.2.10 Saffron

A singular systematic review and meta-analysis reported that saffron could be an effective intervention for anxiety symptom relief; however, evidence of publication bias and lack of regional diversity requires further trials to make any determinations [38].

## 10.2.11 Tualang Honey

Tualang honey is a wild poly-floral honey produced by *Apis dorsata* native to Malaysia that has been shown to possess neuroprotective, anti-inflammatory, and antioxidant effects [39]. More research is needed to better understand Tualang honey's bioactive components and biochemical mechanisms of action before widespread use as an anxiolytic or remedy for other neurological disorders should be advised [39].

## 10.2.12 Ashwagandha

Ashwagandha is an extract of the root of the *Withania somnifera* shrub that has been used historically as a component of Indian Ayurvedic medicine. Research has claimed Ashwagandha possesses anti-inflammatory, anticancer, anti-stress, antioxidant, immunomodulatory, hemopoietic, and rejuvenating properties [40]. A meta-analysis demonstrated decreased self-reported stress and anxiety levels with Ashwagandha supplementation but reported that the certainty of the evidence was low for both outcomes [41]. Therefore, more evidence must be acquired to conclude.

## 10.3 Nutraceuticals and the Gut Microbiome

Nutraceuticals are dietary supplements that offer health benefits beyond essential nutrition. They typically come from plants, although some nutraceuticals come from animals or other sources.

Examples of nutraceuticals include enzyme supplements, curcumin, and more. In this section, we will go into detail and explore the effects of nutraceuticals on the gut microbiome.

### 10.3.1 Enzyme Supplementation

Let's talk about enzymes. As you might know, these proteins help catalyze the body's chemical reactions and are involved in various physiological processes ranging from digestion to metabolism.

Some studies suggest that enzyme supplementation alters gut microbiota composition and influences gut health. One meta-analysis, for example, supplemented two enzyme complexes in pigs and found that the animal subjects experienced better gut health as a result [42].

That said, we still have a lot to learn about the exact mechanisms involved in how enzymes and gut microbiota interact. Their influence on gut health is not entirely understood, and more research is needed to gain fundamental knowledge of this topic.

Speaking of the nuances at play, the effects of enzyme supplementation on the gut microbiota and overall gut health may vary depending on the specific enzyme and dosage involved. It is important to keep this variability in mind.

## 10.3.2 Resistant Starch Type 2

A high-fiber diet is integral to strong digestion and good gut health. Resistant starch type 2 (RS2) is a specific dietary fiber resistant to digestion in the small intestine. In simple terms, it passes through the small intestine undigested and is fermented by the bacteria in the large intestine.

Resistant starch type 2 can be found in plant-based foods like raw potatoes, green bananas, and legumes. Resistant starch type 2 offers several health advantages, including improved digestion, reduced blood sugar and cholesterol, and better gut health. Some studies suggest that RS2 features anti-inflammatory effects that can help with weight management. Many consider RS2 fermentation by the gut microbiota to be responsible for some health benefits.

The advantages of RS2 go beyond what we've described, and some studies find that they also extend to the kidneys. A meta-analysis of RCTs evaluated the effects of RS2 on patients with end-stage renal disease undergoing maintenance hemodialysis (MHD). The study linked RS2 with a significant decrease in blood urea nitrogen and serum creatinine and a decrease in the inflammatory marker interleukin-6 in the blood. However, there was no significant difference in the levels of other markers such as uric acid, p-cresyl sulfate, indoxyl sulfate, high-sensitivity C-reactive protein, albumin, or phosphorus.

The researchers, therefore, suggest that RS2 may improve MHD patients' residual kidney function and reduce inflammation most likely by modulating the gut microbiota and increasing the production of beneficial bacteria. However, more research is needed to confirm these findings [43]. Hopefully, researchers will continue to explore the mechanisms underlying the effects of RS2 in MHD patients.

## 10.3.3 Curcumin

Turmeric is a vibrant, yellow-colored spice commonly used in cooking. The delicious spice will add both flavor and nutrients to food. But let us take a step back and discuss curcumin: the natural polyphenol compound found in turmeric that is responsible for turmeric's bright yellow color. Curcumin, it's worth noting, has an extensive history of use in Indian Ayurvedic and Chinese medicine.

In recent years, curcumin has attracted serious attention from the research community due to its potential health benefits. Studies suggest curcumin may have anti-inflammatory, antioxidant, and anticancer properties [44]. Yet the influence of curcumin on the intestinal microbiota is unclear. Researchers hypothesize that the gut microbiota can transform curcumin through various metabolic pathways, driving local and systemic effects [45, 46]. For example, an NADPH-dependent enzyme (CurA) in E. coli converts curcumin into dihydrocurcumin (DHC) and tetrahydrocurcumin (THC) [47]. Through these mechanisms, curcumin may alter the composition of the microbiota, helping to reduce pro-inflammatory bacteria and increase anti-inflammatory bacteria.

Interestingly, one RCT investigated the effects of a curcumin extract on gastrointestinal symptoms, mood, and quality of life in adults with self-reported digestive issues. The participants were randomly assigned to receive either a placebo or 500 mg of the extract called "Curcugen" once daily for eight weeks. The results were promising. Curcumin led to a significant reduction in gastrointestinal symptoms and anxiety compared to the placebo. However, it had no significant effect on the intestinal microbiota or small intestinal bowel overgrowth (SIBO) [48].

In summary, while preliminary evidence suggests that curcumin may benefit the gastrointestinal system, more research is needed to understand how it works.

## 10.3.4 Prebiotics

Prebiotics induce the growth or activity of beneficial bacteria in the body, such as in the gastrointestinal tract. Though this category is controversial, probiotics are live organisms (usually bacteria) that claim to provide health benefits by improving or restoring the gut microbiota.

According to the International Scientific Association for Probiotics and Prebiotics (ISAPP), prebiotics are substrates that host microorganisms selectively to generate health benefits [49]. These substrates can only be digested by bacterial enzymes, which allows them to offer nutrition to bacteria such as *Lactobacillus* and *Bifidobacterium*, restoring balance to the gut microbiota and producing important products like short-chain fatty acids (SCFAs).

Prebiotics, it's worth noting, are typically carbohydrate polymers, and they are found naturally in plant-based foods like whole grains, legumes, and many fruits and vegetables. Common biologically active prebiotics include galacto-oligosaccharides (GOSs), fructo-oligosaccharides (FOSs), oligofructose, chicory fiber, and inulin.

But how can prebiotics improve patients' digestive health? The studies cited in the following sections aim to uncover the effectiveness and reliability of prebiotics for various applications. Let us take an evidence-based look at prebiotics' effects on several health conditions via gut microbiome involvement.

### 10.3.4.1 Obesity

Obesity has strong ties to inflammation and prebiotics can impact a person's body weight by decreasing systemic inflammatory biomarkers such as tumor necrosis factors (TNF), C-reactive protein (CRP), endotoxins, and interleukins [50–53]. By increasing the release of glucagon-like peptide 1 (GLP-1) and reducing levels of the hunger hormone ghrelin, research shows that prebiotics can strengthen insulin resistance and glucose intolerance both of which are linked to obesity [54].

However, here's something to consider: factors involved in adiposity, like body mass index (BMI), body fat percentage, and body weight, all have fluctuating results where prebiotics are concerned. According to one meta-analysis of RCTs, there was no change in adiposity measures despite a significant decrease in inflammatory biomarkers after participants started using prebiotics [53]. Yet another meta-analysis focusing on soluble dietary fiber resulted in drastic weight reductions following the introduction of prebiotics. This illustrates the role of selectivity when recommending prebiotics to treat obesity [51].

### 10.3.4.2 Diabetes Mellitus

Multiple studies have examined how prebiotics may help patients with type 2 diabetes (T2D). A meta-analysis of RCTs examined the effect of prebiotics on the gut microbiome in T2D patients, comparing it with oral antidiabetic agents. The study found that prebiotics significantly reduced hemoglobin A1c (HbA1c) levels compared to the controls. However, the effects of prebiotics and oral antidiabetic agents did not differ significantly from the participants in the control group regarding fasting blood glucose, postprandial blood glucose, BMI, and the genera of examined gut bacteria [55]. Nevertheless, these results seem favorable and quite reliable. This is partly due to the study's focus on prebiotics without adding probiotics or synbiotics.

Another meta-analysis of RCTs investigating the effects of prebiotics on glucose homeostasis in T2D patients found that compared to a placebo or controls, prebiotic supplementation led to significant reductions in HbA1c, fasting plasma glucose (FPG), insulin, homeostasis model assessment-estimated insulin resistance (HOMA-IR), and quantitative insulin sensitivity check index (QUICKI), but not in C-peptide levels [56].

Finally, a meta-analysis of RCTs found real improvements in blood glucose profiles including fasting blood glucose (FBG), HbA1c, and HOMA-IR in diabetic patients taking prebiotics. These patients, however, were also taking probiotics and synbiotics, making the effects of prebiotics a little more ambiguous [57]. Still, the results are encouraging.

### 10.3.4.3 Liver Disease

Let's discuss the liver and specific data on the use of prebiotics for those with nonalcoholic fatty liver disease (NAFLD). A meta-analysis of RCTs examining the effects of fiber supplements on NAFLD patients' metabolism noted that prebiotic fiber supplements led to improvements in BMI, alanine aminotransferase (ALT), aspartate aminotransferase (AST), fasting insulin, and HOMA-IR.

These findings show that prebiotic fiber supplementation may have specific benefits for people with NAFLD, yet more research is needed to determine the ideal fiber type, dosage, and intervention duration [58]. Two other meta-analyses of RCTs showed similar results [59, 60].

### 10.3.4.4 Cardiovascular Disease

Research on the relationship between prebiotics and cardiovascular disease is limited. Nonetheless, a meta-analysis of RCTs in which adult end-stage renal disease patients received either hemodialysis or peritoneal dialysis explored the effects of oral prebiotic supplements.

While the results found that supplementation reduced toxic metabolites associated with cardiovascular disease and mortality, the trials were low in quality and did not limit the data to prebiotics [61]. Here again, more research is needed to come to a robust conclusion.

### 10.3.4.5 Chronic Kidney Disease

Studies evaluating the use of prebiotics in patients with chronic kidney disease (CKD) are encouraging. One meta-analysis of RCTs evaluated the effects of biotics, meaning prebiotics, probiotics, or synbiotics, on patients with CKD. The primary results showed changes in renal function, markers of inflammation, and oxidative stress; secondarily, participants revealed changes in levels of uremic toxins and variations in lipid metabolism. The studies showed that biotics had no significant effect on the estimated glomerular filtration rate or serum albumin. Prebiotics, however, reduced serum creatinine and blood urea nitrogen [62]. Two other meta-analyses confirmed that prebiotics effectively reduce the concentration of circulating p-cresyl sulfate (PCS), a protein-bound uremic toxin found in CKD patients [63, 64]. These results are encouraging.

### 10.3.4.6 Gastrointestinal Disease

Regarding gastrointestinal disease, research on the benefits of prebiotic supplements is primarily limited to IBD and irritable bowel syndrome (IBS). A meta-analysis of RCTs investigating probiotics, prebiotics, and synbiotics on individuals with IBD found that all three supplements could improve symptoms. However, the research did not explore prebiotics individually, other than citing three studies that described changes in the intestinal flora in patients with Crohn's disease when given only prebiotics [65]. Experts believe additional studies on the effects of *only* prebiotics on IBD patients will be essential moving forward.

Moving on to another meta-analysis of RCTs exploring the effects of prebiotics on patients with IBS and other functional bowel disorders (FBDs). Compared to a placebo, researchers found that prebiotics offer no significant improvements in abdominal pain or quality of life. However, they found that patients experienced relief from flatulence with specific prebiotics and higher levels of *Bifidobacteria* in the gut. Prebiotics were found to improve flatulence at doses of 6 g/day or less. Non-inulin-type fructan prebiotics improved flatulence severity, while inulin-type fructans ultimately made flatulence worse [66]. This reveals the importance of selecting the right prebiotic supplement for the symptom in question.

More research is needed to further these findings. Beyond these studies, researchers have offered either weak or insignificant data supporting the use of prebiotics in treating gastrointestinal diseases. Consider, for example, a meta-analysis of RCTs evaluating nonpharmacologic therapies in children with functional constipation. Some studies found that prebiotic and fiber mixtures improved symptoms but were not included in the meta-analysis [67]. And while *probiotics* improved symptoms, a meta-analysis of RCTs did not find significant results involving *prebiotic* supplementation in patients with lactase deficiency and lactose intolerance [68].

### 10.3.4.7 Allergies

Although research on allergic diseases and prebiotics is limited, a meta-analysis investigating oral supplements found that prebiotics and synbiotics helped significantly lower the frequency of asthma attacks in high-risk children more than probiotics [69].

### 10.3.4.8 Immunity

While the impact of prebiotics on immune function isn't entirely clear, many studies show favorable results. Two meta-analyses investigated the use of prebiotics in warding off respiratory tract infections, and one found that prebiotics may reduce respiratory tract infections (RTIs) in young children, all while increasing natural killer (NK) cell activity [70].

The second study claimed the effects of prebiotics on RTIs are still unclear [71]. Yet another meta-analysis of RCTs concluded that probiotics, prebiotics, or synbiotics leading up to surgery could reduce postoperative risk and shorten the patient's hospital stay (as well as their antibiotic use after hepatic resection) [72].

Finally, a systematic review and meta-analysis addressing the influence of biotics on the immune response to the influenza vaccination found that people who received prebiotic or probiotic supplements had higher influenza hemagglutination inhibition (HAI) antibody titers after vaccination compared to those who did not receive such supplements [73].

While additional research will be vital, the potential health benefits of nutraceuticals seem extensive. Clinicians should remember these findings when helping patients better understand their gut microbiome and overall health.

## 10.3.5 Probiotics

Among adults, probiotics or prebiotics were the third most commonly used dietary supplement behind vitamins and minerals [74]. The Food and Agriculture Organization of the United Nations (FAO) and the World Health Organization (WHO) define probiotics as "live microorganisms which, when administered in adequate amounts, confer a health benefit on the host" [75]. Probiotics regulate the gastrointestinal tract's microbiome when consumed, impacting various human systems [75–78]. Probiotics are extensively marketed and consumed worldwide, most commonly as supplements or functional foods (kombucha, kefir, sourcrout etc.), with their benefit to human health well documented [76, 78]. The common probiotics currently used are *Lactobacillus*, *Bifidobacterium*, and *Streptococcus* [79]. Mechanisms of probiosis include homeostatic balancing of intestinal microbial communities, pathogenic bacterial suppression, immune system support, stimulation of epithelial cell proliferation, and fortification of the intestinal barrier [76, 78]. The following section will outline the current literature concerning the efficacy of probiotics for various uses.

### 10.3.5.1 Obesity

Dysbiosis can occur through many of the exact mechanisms that contribute to obesity (lifestyle, diet, drugs etc.) which have been associated with decreased microbiome diversity and alteration in bacterial genes and functionality of metabolic pathways [76, 78, 80]. Four published meta-analyses supported the utility of probiotic consumption therapeutically for obesity [81–84]. Two strains of probiotics: *Lactobacillus* and *Bifidobacterium* stood out for their ability to significantly reduce a variety of physical and biochemical obesity parameters when administered as single or multispecies formulations [82, 84]. Specific factors that showed amelioration after probiotic administration included: body weight, body mass index (BMI), waist circumference (WC), fat mass, tumor necrosis factor-α, insulin, total cholesterol, and LDL (low-density lipoprotein) [81]. At a molecular level, *Lactobacillus* was shown to bind IL6 best and prevent inflammation leading to dysbiosis [82]. The dosage of probiotics required to produce such effects requires more investigation [84].

### 10.3.5.2 Diabetes Mellitus

Three published meta-analyses favor probiotics for use in diabetes mellitus [85–87]. The consensus of these studies demonstrated that supplementation with probiotics improved glucose homeostasis in diabetic patients [85, 87]. Probiotics generally reduced HbA1c levels, but not significantly [86, 87]. One analysis concluded that probiotics benefit diabetes outcomes by altering oxidative stress biomarkers such as antioxidant status, glutathione, and malondialdehyde [87]. Three other meta-analyses showed mixed evidence that gut microbiome management through probiotics decreased the risk for gestational diabetes, with one in favor, one undecided, and one against [88–90].

### 10.3.5.3 Liver Disease

The bidirectional relationship of the gut microbiome facilitates a "gut-liver axis" that involves endocrine and immunological mechanisms thought to contribute pathogenesis of numerous chronic liver diseases [91]. The treatment of liver cirrhosis and portal hypertension was analyzed in two papers. Both reported that the consumption of probiotics may have a role in amelioration but that more studies must be performed before a conclusion can be made [91, 92]. Two meta-analyses favorably considered probiotics' effect on NAFLD. The summary of studies showed a significant reduction in the levels of alanine aminotransferase (ALT), aspartate transaminase (AST), total cholesterol (TC), as well as liver stiffness, concluding probiotics may be an effective method to improve liver function and reduce blood lipid levels in NAFLD patients [93, 94]. One meta-analysis found no significant proof that modification of gut bacterial flora using probiotics affected liver enzyme levels and overall liver function [95]. One meta-analysis compiled five studies evaluating the effectiveness of probiotics in minimizing infection related to liver transplants, and all studies but one reported lower infection rates [96]. One meta-analysis analyzed 14 RCTs evaluating the effect of probiotics preventing minimal hepatic encephalopathy (MHE) [97]. Probiotics significantly decreased serum ammonia and endotoxin levels, improved MHE, and prevented overt hepatic encephalopathy development in patients with liver cirrhosis [97].

### 10.3.5.4 Cardiovascular Disease

There is an uncharacterized but present relationship between gut microbial metabolites, such as trimethylamine-N-oxide (TMAO), with major adverse cardiovascular events [98]. A literature review revealed four meta-analyses related to probiotics' effect on cardiovascular disease. One systematic review showed that probiotics did not significantly lower TMAO, which is a metabolite that increases platelet hyperactivity correlated to an increased risk for adverse cardiovascular events [99, 100]. A meta-analysis and systematic review demonstrated that in patients on dialysis, probiotic supplementation reduced toxic metabolites associated with cardiovascular disease and mortality [101]. An additional study demonstrated that probiotics could significantly reduce blood cholesterol levels which may protect against cardiovascular disease, but probiotics do not affect triglyceride levels [102]. A meta-analysis supports using *Lactobacillus plantarum* supplementation to lower systolic and diastolic blood pressure. However, it recommends more research into the topic before conclusions are drawn due to questions of the clinical relevance of the effects of lowering blood pressure [103].

### 10.3.5.5 Chronic Kidney Disease

Dysbiosis can relate to inflammation and oxidative stress rates in chronic kidney disease (CKD) [104]. Four meta-analyses were identified that evaluate probiotics' efficacy in using chronic kidney disease to preserve kidney function. Probiotic supplements had a statistically significant impact on urea levels in the non-dialysis CKD population. Still, there was no meaningful impact on uric acid, C-reactive protein, creatinine, and eGFR (estimated glomerular filtration rate) preservation [105]. A second study reported limited evidence to support the use of probiotics in CKD management for kidney function preservation [106]. However, other studies reported evidence for probiotics' potential beneficial effects of decreased oxidative stress, systemic inflammation, and the production of uremic solutes in CKD patients [104, 107].

### 10.3.5.6 Psychiatric Disorders

Thus far, the literature has identified the role of the gut microbiome and the bidirectional gut–brain axis regulation of stress and possible pathophysiology of many psychiatric disorders, i.e., depression and anxiety [108]. Multiple meta-analyses have shown that probiotic administration significantly reduced symptoms among patients with depression [108]. Probiotics can reduce subjective stress levels in healthy individuals and mitigate stress-related subthreshold anxiety/depression [109]. The same study concluded that probiotic supplementation does not affect overall cortisol levels [109]. Three meta-analyses evaluated probiotic effects on depression symptoms and generally concluded that there are quantitative decreases in symptom severity and rates [110–113]. All three meta-analyses recommended more research be done on the subject before conclusions could be made. A separate meta-analysis on the effect of probiotics on autism (ASD) demonstrated that probiotics did not significantly improve the severity of gastrointestinal problems or psychopathological comorbidities in ASD patients [114]. Two meta-analyses analyzed three studies investigating the effect of probiotic supplementation in schizophrenic patients and concluded there was no significant difference in schizophrenia symptoms with probiotic administration [115, 116].

### 10.3.5.7 Gastrointestinal Disease

Due to the nature of Crohn's disease and other IBDs, such as ulcerative colitis, being inflammatory diseases of the bowel, symbiosis of the gut microbiome through probiotic supplementation was proposed as a possible therapy. Probiotic supplements, especially those based on *Lactobacillus* and *Bifidobacterium* or composed of more than one strain at 1010–1012 CFU(colony-forming unit)/day, are likely beneficial for ulcerative colitis symptom relief and remission [117]. An analysis of two clinical trials was unable to discern the safety nor efficacy of such therapy for Crohn's disease, and more research is needed [118]. Irritable bowel syndrome (IBS) is one of the most prevalent functional gastrointestinal disorders and the pathogenesis, while not completely understood, points to the gut microbiome as having a role [119]. As such, multiple studies have analyzed the effects of probiotics on symptom relief, and the consensus is that probiotic supplementation is beneficial. However, more information on strains and dosage is needed [120]. Some studies recommended that more research be conducted to characterize which strains and combinations are most beneficial [120]. Similarly, to IBDs, celiac disease is an inflammatory autoimmune disease of the gut that was thought to be possibly ameliorated by microbiome adjustment. In a systematic review evaluating the efficacy of probiotic supplementation in celiac disease, there was no difference in gastrointestinal symptoms after probiotics [121]. Dysbiosis can alter the gastrointestinal tract's normal functioning, as seen in many patients with functional constipation. Consumption of multispecies probiotics may substantially reduce the gut transit time while increasing stool frequency and improving consistency in adults. In children, two meta-analyses show little evidence to prove that probiotics are effective in pediatric constipation, and more research needs to be performed [122, 123].

In contrast, pediatric diarrhea caused by antibiotics can be directly tied to dysbiosis. A meta-analysis analyzing RCTs that investigated the effect of probiotics on symptoms concluded high dose probiotics, especially *Lactobacillus rhamnosus* or *Saccharomyces boulardii* are beneficial. Still, they require additional studies to draw firm conclusions [124]. A meta-analysis of five studies concluded that probiotic consumption was not associated with a significant reduction in the enterocolitis risk in Hirschsprung's disease patients through normalization of the gut microbiome [124].

### 10.3.5.8 Allergies

Probiotic supplementation is a common treatment for many allergic diseases, as a healthy microbiome is thought to modify immune responses beneficially [125]. A meta-analysis of RCTs showed that only *Lactobacillus rhamnosus* probiotics played a role in asthma prevention but that larger-scale RCTs are needed for more reliable data [125]. In chronic urticaria, altered bacterial diversity in the gut is thought to disrupt the mucosal immune system [126]. A meta-analysis demonstrated that probiotics are effective adjunct therapy, but specific regimens need more research [126]. Additionally, *Lactobacillus rhamnosus* was evaluated in a meta-analysis of seven RCTs relating to childhood eczema prevention [127]. The publication concluded that the probiotic was ineffective as a therapeutic option for eczema relief [127].

### 10.3.5.9 Immunity

Probiotics are commonly utilized as adjunctive therapy to fight diseases caused by gastrointestinal dysbiosis. Still, many have recently explored their efficacy in normalizing microbiota communities in other human body areas [127, 128]. A meta-analysis demonstrated that in the oral cavity supplementation of probiotics effectively prevents and treats diseases such as halitosis and periodontitis, can slow the development of dental caries, and decrease the concentration of harmful bacteria [128]. Due to the variability of different probiotic supplements, more research should be done to characterize best practices for this use case [78, 128]. As mentioned, the diversity and composition of the gut microbiome are directly linked to genetic distribution and the functional capacity of the immune system. Therefore, immune system support may be capable via probiotics [78]. One systematic review and meta-analysis demonstrated that in elderly patients there is ample evidence that probiotic supplementation increased their immune functionality through increased polymorphonuclear phagocytic capacity and NK cell tumoricidal activity [129]. However, a second review analyzes the inflammatory response in the elderly as probiotic therapy decreases the inflammatory responses of elderly individuals [130]. This study reports no decrease in the levels of tumor necrosis factor-$\alpha$, interleukin-6, interleukin-10, C-reactive protein, interleukin-1$\beta$, or interleukin-8 [130]. In a similar review examining the effects of probiotics on respiratory viruses, the results concluded a significant decrease in viral load due to improved gut microbiota from probiotics [131]. The study reported increased anti-inflammatory markers such as interferon-$\alpha$ and interleukin-12 and decreased pro-inflammatory markers such as TNF-$\alpha$ and IL6 [131]. Gastrointestinal mucositis (GIM) is an inflammatory reaction caused by antitumor therapy, especially after chemotherapy and radiotherapy. Maintenance of intestinal homeostasis is hypothesized to be a therapeutic option [132]. A pre-treatment ($\geq$seven days before chemotherapy) with a high dose of probiotics ($\geq 10^9$ CFU/day) comprising two or more microorganism species remedied GIM most effectively in a meta-analysis of preclinical studies [132].

### 10.3.5.10 Pediatric Health

Many other use cases have been evaluated for probiotic treatment or supplementation efficacy. In one meta-analysis evaluating the efficacy of probiotics on infantile colic, the authors investigated the contribution of the microbiome in the pathogenesis of the phenotype, though they found no clear evidence that probiotics are effective at preventing colic; however, daily crying time appeared to reduce [79]. Additionally, a study evaluating the utility of probiotic supplementation to pregnant mothers at risk for preterm birth reported insufficient evidence to conclude whether there is a clinical benefit to neonates with maternal oral supplementation of probiotics [133]. Probiotics are often prescribed to promote a healthy microbiome in children, which is hypothesized to affect both height and weight [134] positively. The analysis demonstrated that there might be an appreciable small but heterogeneous effect on weight and height in healthy children under five, but only in lower- to middle-income countries [135].

## 10.3.6 Postbiotics

Postbiotics are metabolic products or byproducts of live bacteria in our bodies that provide physiological benefits to us. Unlike other nutraceuticals like probiotics, these have been less studied; thus, information is scant. The only postbiotic that we could review was "equol," created by gastrointestinal bacteria's breakdown of daidzein which is found in soybeans. A meta-analysis of how postbiotics affect obesity found that equol can bind stably on IL6, which is beneficial for treating obesity [82].

## 10.3.7 Synbiotics

Recently, synbiotics have attracted the attention of researchers as another potential way to stimulate the gut microbiome. Two meta-analyses reported that synbiotics and amino acid formulas given to the mother resulted in fewer birth defects in the baby [90, 136]. A meta-analysis of synbiotics reduces toxic metabolites that lead to cardiovascular disease [61, 117]. Synbiotics also have beneficial effects on gastrointestinal and liver pathologies. Two studies, one meta-analysis and one *in vitro* experiment, were done on synbiotics' effects on inflammatory bowel disease, and both concluded that synbiotics could benefit patients with IBD [137]. Meta-analyses have shown that synbiotics can treat nonalcoholic fatty liver and reduce infections in liver transplant surgery [96] and that controlling the gut-liver axis is important in post-liver transplant infections [138]. Chan's meta-analysis showed that synbiotics could be a nutritional strategy to prevent respiratory tract infections [139]. However, synbiotics are not relevant in psychosis, and clinical relevance must be expanded [116].

## 10.3.8 Miscellaneous

Enzyme supplementation, resistant starch type 2, and Curcugen are agents that affect the gut microbiome that do not fall under any specific category. A meta-analysis found that enzyme supplementation may promote gut health in pigs measured mainly by the *Lactobacillus:E. coli* ratio [42]. Considered a dietary fiber, resistant starch cannot be enzymatically digested and thus reaches the colon mostly unchanged. A meta-analysis found that resistant starch type 2 can benefit patients with end-stage renal disease via decreasing blood urea nitrogen, serum creatinine, and interleukin (IL)-6 levels in blood [134]. Curcugen is a branded curcumin extract that has been shown to lower digestive complaints and anxiety in a randomized control trial [48].

Overall, currently, there are many nutraceuticals that have promising beneficial effects on anxiety and gut microbiome. However, further robust research is needed regarding the efficacy, dose, method of delivery, adverse events, and mechanism of action of many of the nutraceuticals.

# References

1. Kalra, E.K., Nutraceutical-definition and introduction. *AAPS PharmSci*, 2003. 5(3): p. 27–28.
2. Grand View Research. *Nutraceuticals Market Size, Share & Trends Analysis Report by Product (Dietary Supplements, Functional Food, Functional Beverages), by Region (North America, Europe, APAC, CSA, MEA), and Segment Forecasts, 2021–2030.* [cited 2023; Available from: https://www.grandviewresearch.com/industry-analysis/nutraceuticals-market#].
3. Skelley, J.W., et al., Use of cannabidiol in anxiety and anxiety-related disorders. *Journal of the American Pharmacists Association*, 2020. 60(1): p. 253–261.
4. Black, N., et al., Cannabinoids for the treatment of mental disorders and symptoms of mental disorders: A systematic review and meta-analysis. *The Lancet Psychiatry*, 2019. 6(12): p. 995–1010.
5. Young, L.M., et al., A systematic review and meta-analysis of B vitamin supplementation on depressive symptoms, anxiety, and stress: Effects on healthy and 'at-risk' individuals. *Nutrients*, 2019. 11(9): p. 2232.
6. Field, D.T., et al., High-dose vitamin B6 supplementation reduces anxiety and strengthens visual surround suppression. *Human Psychopharmacology: Clinical and Experimental*, 2022. 37(6): p. e2852.
7. Noah, L., et al., Effect of magnesium and vitamin B6 supplementation on mental health and quality of life in stressed healthy adults: Post-hoc analysis of a randomised controlled trial. *Stress and Health: Journal of the International Society for the Investigation of Stress*, 2021. 37(5): p. 1000–1009.
8. Polokowski, A.R., et al., Omega-3 fatty acids and anxiety: A systematic review of the possible mechanisms at play. *Nutritional Neuroscience*, 2020. 23(7): p. 494–504.
9. Su, K.-P., et al., Association of use of Omega-3 polyunsaturated fatty acids with changes in severity of anxiety symptoms: A systematic review and meta-analysis. *JAMA Network Open*, 2018. 1(5): p. e182327.
10. Glabska, D., et al., The influence of vitamin D intake and status on mental health in children: A systematic review. *Nutrients*, 2021. 13(3): p. 952.
11. Glabska, D., et al., Vitamin D supplementation and mental health in inflammatory bowel diseases and irritable bowel syndrome patients: A systematic review. *Nutrients*, 2021. 13(10): p. 3662.
12. Haybar, H., et al., The effects of Melissa officinalis supplementation on depression, anxiety, stress, and sleep disorder in patients with chronic stable angina. *Clinical Nutrition ESPEN*, 2018. 26: p. 47–52.
13. Nathan, P.J., et al., The neuropharmacology of L-theanine(N-ethyl-L-glutamine): A possible neuroprotective and cognitive enhancing agent. *Journal of Herbal Pharmacotherapy*, 2006. 6(2): p. 21–30.

14. Williams, J.L., et al., The effects of green tea amino acid L-theanine consumption on the ability to manage stress and anxiety levels: A systematic review. *Plant Foods for Human Nutrition*, 2020. 75(1): p. 12–23.
15. Sarris, J., et al., L-theanine in the adjunctive treatment of generalized anxiety disorder: A double-blind, randomised, placebo-controlled trial. *Journal of Psychiatric Research*, 2019. 110: p. 31–37.
16. Jayawardena, R., et al., The use of Caralluma fimbriata as an appetite suppressant and weight loss supplement: A systematic review and meta-analysis of clinical trials. *BMC Complement med Ther*, 2021. 21(1): p. 279.
17. Kell, G., A. Rao, and M. Katsikitis, A randomised placebo controlled clinical trial on the efficacy of Caralluma fimbriata supplement for reducing anxiety and stress in healthy adults over eight weeks. *Journal of Affective Disorders*, 2019. 246: p. 619–626.
18. Liu, R.T., R.F.L. Walsh, and A.E. Sheehan, Prebiotics and probiotics for depression and anxiety: A systematic review and meta-analysis of controlled clinical trials. *Neuroscience and Biobehavioral Reviews*, 2019. 102: p. 13–23.
19. Alli, S.R., et al., The gut microbiome in depression and potential benefit of prebiotics, probiotics and Synbiotics: A systematic review of clinical trials and observational studies. *International Journal of Molecular Sciences*, 2022. 23(9)p. 4494.
20. Minichino, A., et al., The gut-microbiome as a target for the treatment of schizophrenia: A systematic review and meta-analysis of randomised controlled trials of add-on strategies. *Schizophrenia Research*, 2021. 234: p. 1–13.
21. Song, W., et al., Prebiotics and probiotics for autism spectrum disorder: A systematic review and meta-analysis of controlled clinical trials. *Journal of Medical Microbiology*, 2022. 71(4): p. 001510.
22. Liu, B., et al., Efficacy of probiotics on anxiety-A meta-analysis of randomized controlled trials. *Depression and Anxiety*, 2018. 35(10): p. 935–945.
23. Reis, D.J., S.S. Ilardi, and S.E.W. Punt, The anxiolytic effect of probiotics: A systematic review and meta-analysis of the clinical and pre-clinical literature. *PLOS ONE*, 2018. 13(6): p. e0199041.
24. El Dib, R., et al., Probiotics for the treatment of depression and anxiety: A systematic review and meta-analysis of randomized controlled trials. *Clinical Nutrition ESPEN*, 2021. 45: p. 75–90.
25. Qin, Q., et al., Probiotic supplement preparation relieves test anxiety by regulating intestinal microbiota in college students. *Disease Markers*, 2021. 2021: p. 5597401.
26. NIH, Essential oils. *Environmental Health Topics*, 2022 [cited 2022 December 28].
27. Elshafie, H.S. and I. Camele, An overview of the biological effects of some Mediterranean essential oils on human health. *BioMed Research International*, 2017. 2017: p. 1–14.
28. Gong, M., et al., Effects of aromatherapy on anxiety: A meta-analysis of randomized controlled trials. *Journal of Affective Disorders*, 2020. 274: p. 1028–1040.
29. Kasper, S., et al., Lavender oil preparation Silexan is effective in generalized anxiety disorder – A randomized, double-blind comparison to placebo and paroxetine. *International Journal of Neuropsychopharmacology*, 2014. 17(6): p. 859–869.
30. Abbasijahromi, A., et al., Compare the effect of aromatherapy using lavender and damask rose essential oils on the level of anxiety and severity of pain following C-section: A double-blinded randomized clinical trial. *Journal of Complementary and Integrative Medicine*, 2020. 17(3): p. 20190141.
31. Ozkaraman, A., et al., Aromatherapy: The effect of lavender on anxiety and sleep quality in patients treated with chemotherapy. *Clinical Journal of Oncology Nursing*, 2018. 22(2): p. 203–210.
32. Donelli, D., et al., Effects of lavender on anxiety: A systematic review and meta-analysis. *Phytomedicine: International Journal of Phytotherapy and Phytopharmacology*, 2019. 65: p. 153099.

33. Kang, H.-J., et al., How strong is the evidence for the anxiolytic efficacy of lavender?: Systematic review and meta-analysis of randomized controlled trials. *Asian Nursing Research*, 2019. 13(5): p. 295–305.

34. Yap, W.S., et al., Efficacy and safety of lavender essential oil (Silexan) capsules among patients suffering from anxiety disorders: A network meta-analysis. *Scientific Reports*, 2019. 9(1). 18042

35. Von Känel, R., et al., Therapeutic effects of Silexan on somatic symptoms and physical health in patients with anxiety disorders: A meta-analysis. *Brain and Behavior*, 2021. 11(4): p. e01997.

36. Sayed, A.M., et al., The best route of administration of lavender for anxiety: A systematic review and network meta-analysis. *General Hospital Psychiatry*, 2020. 64: p. 33–40.

37. Möller, H.-J., et al., Efficacy of Silexan in subthreshold anxiety: Meta-analysis of randomised, placebo-controlled trials. *European Archives of Psychiatry and Clinical Neuroscience*, 2019. 269(2): p. 183–193.

38. Marx, W., et al., Effect of saffron supplementation on symptoms of depression and anxiety: A systematic review and meta-analysis. *Nutrition Reviews*, 2019. 77(8): p. 557–571.

39. Azman, K.F., et al., Tualang honey: A decade of neurological research. *Molecules*, 2021. 26(17): p. 5424.

40. Singh, P., et al., Biotechnological interventions in *Withania somnifera* (L.) Dunal. *Biotechnology and Genetic Engineering Reviews*, 2015. 31(1–2): p. 1–20.

41. Akhgarjand, C., et al., Does Ashwagandha supplementation have a beneficial effect on the management of anxiety and stress? A systematic review and meta-analysis of randomized controlled trials. *Phytotherapy Research: PTR*, 2022. 36(11): p. 4115–4124.

42. Ramani, S., et al., Meta-analysis identifies the effect of dietary multi-enzyme supplementation on gut health of pigs. *Scientific Reports*, 2021. 11(1): p. 7299.

43. Jia, L., et al., Benefits of resistant starch type 2 for patients with end-stage renal disease under maintenance hemodialysis: A systematic review and meta-analysis. *International Journal of Medical Sciences*, 2021. 18(3): p. 811–820.

44. Hewlings, S.J. and D.S. Kalman, Curcumin: A review of its effects on human health. *Foods*, 2017. 6(10): p. 92.

45. Peterson, C.T., et al., Effects of turmeric and curcumin dietary supplementation on human gut microbiota: A double-blind, randomized, placebo-controlled pilot study. *Journal of Evidence-Based Integrative Medicine*, 2018. 23: p. 2515690X18790725.

46. Burapan, S., M. Kim, and J. Han, Curcuminoid demethylation as an alternative metabolism by human intestinal microbiota. *Journal of Agriculture and Food Chemistry*, 2017. 65(16): p. 3305–3310.

47. Pandey, A., et al., Reductive metabolites of curcumin and their therapeutic effects. *Heliyon*, 2020. 6(11): p. e05469.

48. Lopresti, A.L., et al., Efficacy of a curcumin extract (Curcugen) on gastrointestinal symptoms and intestinal microbiota in adults with self-reported digestive complaints: A randomised, double-blind, placebo-controlled study. *BMC Complement med Ther*, 2021. 21(1): p. 40.

49. Quigley, E.M.M., Nutraceuticals as modulators of gut microbiota: Role in therapy. *British Journal of Pharmacology*, 2020. 177(6): p. 1351–1362.

50. da Silva Borges, D., et al., Prebiotics may reduce serum concentrations of C-reactive protein and ghrelin in overweight and obese adults: A systematic review and meta-analysis. *Nutrition Reviews*, 2019. 78(3): p. 235–248.

51. Huwiler, V.V., et al., Prolonged isolated soluble dietary fibre supplementation in overweight and obese patients: A systematic review with meta-analysis of randomised controlled trials. *Nutrients*, 2022. 14(13): p. 2627.

52. Eslick, S., et al., Short-chain fatty acids as anti-inflammatory agents in overweight and obesity: A systematic review and meta-analysis. *Nutrition Reviews*, 2022. 80(4): p. 838–856.

53. Qu, H., et al., The effect of prebiotic products on decreasing adiposity parameters in overweight and obese individuals: A systematic review and meta- analysis. In: *Current Medicinal Chemistry*, 2021, Copyright© Bentham Science Publishers; For any queries, please email at epub@benthamscience.net.: United Arab Emirates. p. 419–431.

54. Fallucca, F., et al., Influence of diet on gut microbiota, inflammation and type 2 diabetes mellitus: First experience with macrobiotic Ma-Pi 2 diet. *Diabetes/Metabolism Research and Reviews*, 2014. 30(S1): p. 48–54.

55. Ojo, O., et al., The effect of prebiotics and oral anti-diabetic agents on gut microbiome in patients with Type 2 diabetes: A systematic review and network meta-analysis of randomised controlled trials. *Nutrients*, 2022. 14(23): p. 5139.

56. Paul, P., et al., The effect of microbiome-modulating probiotics, prebiotics and Synbiotics on glucose homeostasis in type 2 diabetes: A systematic review, meta-analysis, and meta-regression of clinical trials. *Pharmacological Research*, 2022. 185: p. 106520.

57. Wang, Z., et al., Effects of probiotic/prebiotic/synbiotic supplementation on blood glucose profiles: A systematic review and meta-analysis of randomized controlled trials. *Public Health*, 2022. 210: p. 149–159.

58. Stachowska, E., et al., The relationship between prebiotic supplementation and anthropometric and biochemical parameters in patients with NAFLD-A systematic review and meta-analysis of randomized controlled trials. *Nutrients*, 2020. 12(11): p. 3460.

59. Jin, H., et al., Probiotic and prebiotic interventions for non-alcoholic fatty liver disease: A systematic review and network meta-analysis. *Beneficial Microbes*, 2021. 12(6): p. 517–529.

60. Li, S., et al., The promising role of probiotics/prebiotics/Synbiotics in energy metabolism biomarkers in patients with NAFLD: A systematic review and meta-analysis. *Frontiers in Public Health*, 2022. 10: p. 862266.

61. March, D.S., et al., The efficacy of prebiotic, probiotic, and synbiotic supplementation in modulating gut-derived circulatory particles associated with cardiovascular disease in individuals receiving dialysis: A systematic review and meta-analysis of randomized controlled trials. *Journal of Renal Nutrition: The Official Journal of the Council on Renal Nutrition of the National Kidney Foundation*, 2020. 30(4): p. 347–359.

62. Liu, J., et al., Biotic supplements in patients with chronic kidney disease: Meta-analysis of randomized controlled trials. *Journal of Renal Nutrition: The Official Journal of the Council on Renal Nutrition of the National Kidney Foundation*, 2022. 32(1): p. 10–21.

63. Chen, L., et al., Effects of microbiota-driven therapy on circulating indoxyl sulfate and P-cresyl sulfate in patients with chronic kidney disease: A systematic review and meta-analysis of randomized controlled trials. *Advances in Nutrition*, 2022. 13(4): p. 1267–1278.

64. Takkavatakarn, K., et al., Protein-bound uremic toxin lowering strategies in chronic kidney disease: A systematic review and meta-analysis. *Journal of Nephrology*, 2021. 34(6): p. 1805–1817.

65. Zhang, X.F., et al., Clinical effects and gut microbiota changes of using probiotics, prebiotics or Synbiotics in inflammatory bowel disease: A systematic review and meta-analysis. *European Journal of Nutrition*, 2021. 60(5): p. 2855–2875.

66. Wilson, B., et al., Prebiotics in irritable bowel syndrome and other functional bowel disorders in adults: A systematic review and meta-analysis of randomized controlled trials. *American Journal of Clinical Nutrition*, 2019. 109(4): p. 1098–1111.

67. Wegh, C.A.M., et al., Nonpharmacologic treatment for children with functional constipation: A systematic review and meta-analysis. *Jurnalul Pediatrului*, 2022. 240: p. 136–149 e5.

68. Leis, R., et al., Effects of prebiotic and probiotic supplementation on lactase deficiency and lactose intolerance: A systematic review of controlled trials. *Nutrients*, 2020. 12(5): p. 1487.

69. Wawryk-Gawda, E., E. Markut-Miotla, and A. Emeryk, Postnatal probiotics administration does not prevent asthma in children, but using prebiotics or Synbiotics may be the effective potential strategies to decrease the frequency of asthma in high-risk children - A meta-analysis of clinical trials. *Allergologia et Immunopathologia (Madr)*, 2021. 49(4): p. 4–14.

70. Williams, L.M., et al., The effects of prebiotics, Synbiotics, and short-chain fatty acids on respiratory tract infections and immune function: A systematic review and meta-analysis. *Advances in Nutrition*, 2022. 13(1): p. 167–192.

71. Coleman, J.L., et al., Orally ingested probiotics, prebiotics, and Synbiotics as countermeasures for respiratory tract infections in nonelderly adults: A systematic review and meta-analysis. *Advances in Nutrition*, 2022. 13(6): p. 2277–2295.

72. Gan, Y., et al., Efficacy of probiotics and prebiotics in prevention of infectious complications following hepatic resections: Systematic review and meta-analysis. *Journal of Gastrointestinal and Liver Diseases: JGLD*, 2019. 28: p. 205–211.

73. Yeh, T.L., et al., The influence of prebiotic or probiotic supplementation on antibody titers after influenza vaccination: A systematic review and meta-analysis of randomized controlled trials. *Drug Design, Development and Therapy*, 2018. 12: p. 217–230.

74. CDC/NCHS. *National Health Interview Survey*. 2012 [cited 2022 December 21].

75. Hill, C., et al., Expert consensus document. The International Scientific Association for probiotics and prebiotics consensus statement on the scope and appropriate use of the term probiotic. *Nature Reviews: Gastroenterology and Hepatology*, 2014. 11(8): p. 506–514.

76. Hemarajata, P. and J. Versalovic, Effects of probiotics on gut microbiota: Mechanisms of intestinal immunomodulation and neuromodulation. *Therapeutic Advances in Gastroenterology*, 2013. 6(1): p. 39–51.

77. Wang, X., P. Zhang, and X. Zhang, Probiotics regulate gut microbiota: An effective method to improve immunity. *Molecules*, 2021. 26(19): p. 6076.

78. Valdes, A.M., et al., Role of the gut microbiota in nutrition and health. *BMJ*, 2018. 361: p. k2179.

79. Ong, T.G., et al., Probiotics to prevent infantile colic. *Cochrane Database of Systematic Reviews*, 2019. 3(3): p. CD012473.

80. Pascale, A., et al., Microbiota and metabolic diseases. *Endocrine*, 2018. 61(3): p. 357–371.

81. Pontes, K.S.D.S., et al., Effects of probiotics on body adiposity and cardiovascular risk markers in individuals with overweight and obesity: A systematic review and meta-analysis of randomized controlled trials. *Clinical Nutrition*, 2021. 40(8): p. 4915–4931.

82. Oh, K.-K., et al., Elucidation of prebiotics, probiotics, postbiotics, and target from gut microbiota to alleviate obesity via network pharmacology study. *Cells*, 2022. 11(18): p. 2903.

83. Tomé-Castro, X.M., et al., Probiotics as a therapeutic strategy in obesity and overweight: A systematic review. *Beneficial Microbes*, 2021. 12(1): p. 5–15.

84. López-Moreno, A., et al., Probiotic strains and intervention total doses for modulating obesity-related microbiota dysbiosis: A systematic review and meta-analysis. *Nutrients*, 2020. 12(7): p. 1921.

85. Paul, P., et al., The effect of microbiome-modulating probiotics, prebiotics and Synbiotics on glucose homeostasis in type 2 diabetes: A systematic review, meta-analysis, and meta-regression of clinical trials. *Pharmacological Research*, 2022. 185: p. 106520.

86. Bock, P.M., et al., The effect of probiotics, prebiotics or Synbiotics on metabolic outcomes in individuals with diabetes: A systematic review and meta-analysis. *Diabetologia*, 2021. 64(1): p. 26–41.

87. Ardeshirlarijani, E., et al., Effect of probiotics supplementation on glucose and oxidative stress in type 2 diabetes mellitus: A meta-analysis of randomized trials. *DARU: Journal of Pharmaceutical Sciences*, 2019. 27(2): p. 827–837.

88. Davidson, S.J., et al., Probiotics for preventing gestational diabetes. *The Cochrane Library*, 2021. 2021(4): p. CD009951.
89. Hasain, Z., et al., Diet and pre-intervention washout modifies the effects of probiotics on gestational diabetes mellitus: A comprehensive systematic review and meta-analysis of randomized controlled trials. *Nutrients*, 2021. 13(9): p. 3045.
90. Zhou, L., et al., Probiotics and Synbiotics show clinical efficacy in treating gestational diabetes mellitus: A meta-analysis. *Primary Care Diabetes*, 2021. 15(6): p. 937–947.
91. Milosevic, I., et al., Gut-liver axis, gut microbiota, and its modulation in the management of liver diseases: A review of the literature. *International Journal of Molecular Sciences*, 2019. 20(2): p. 395.
92. Zhang, H. and J. Gao, Antibiotics and probiotics on hepatic venous pressure gradient in cirrhosis: A systematic review and a meta-analysis. *PLOS ONE*, 2022. 17(8): p. e0273231.
93. Yang, R., et al., Effects of probiotics on non-alcoholic fatty liver disease: A systematic review and meta-analysis. *Expert Review of Gastroenterology and Hepatology*, 2021. 15(12): p. 1401–1409.
94. Sharpton, S.R., et al., Gut microbiome–targeted therapies in non-alcoholic fatty liver disease: A systematic review, meta-analysis, and meta-regression. *The American Journal of Clinical Nutrition*, 2019. 110(1): p. 139–149.
95. Khalesi, S., et al., Effect of probiotics and Synbiotics consumption on serum concentrations of liver function test enzymes: A systematic review and meta-analysis. *European Journal of Nutrition*, 2018. 57(6): p. 2037–2053.
96. Kahn, J., G. Pregartner, and P. Schemmer, Effects of both pro- and Synbiotics in liver surgery and transplantation with special focus on the gut–liver axis—A systematic review and meta-analysis. *Nutrients*, 2020. 12(8): p. 2461.
97. Cao, Q., et al., Effect of probiotic treatment on cirrhotic patients with minimal hepatic encephalopathy: A meta-analysis. *Hepatobiliary and Pancreatic Diseases International : HBPD INT*, 2018. 17(1): p. 9–16.
98. Heianza, Y., et al., Gut microbiota metabolites and risk of major adverse cardiovascular disease events and death: A systematic review and meta-analysis of prospective studies. *Journal of the American Heart Association*, 2017. 6(7): p. e004947.
99. Sohouli, M.H., et al., Impact of probiotic supplementation on trimethylamine N-oxide (TMAO) in humans: A systematic review and meta-analysis of randomized controlled trials. *Clinical Nutrition ESPEN*, 2022. 50: p. 56–62.
100. Velasquez, M., et al., Trimethylamine N-oxide: The good, the bad and the unknown. *Toxins*, 2016. 8(11): p. 326.
101. March, D.S., et al., The efficacy of prebiotic, probiotic, and synbiotic supplementation in modulating gut-derived circulatory particles associated with cardiovascular disease in individuals receiving dialysis: A systematic review and meta-analysis of randomized controlled trials. *Journal of Renal Nutrition: The Official Journal of the Council on Renal Nutrition of the National Kidney Foundation*, 2020. 30(4): p. 347–359.
102. Deng, X., et al., Effects of products designed to modulate the gut microbiota on hyperlipidaemia. *European Journal of Nutrition*, 2019. 58(7): p. 2713–2729.
103. Lewis-Mikhael, A.-M., A. Davoodvandi, and S. Jafarnejad, Effect of Lactobacillusplantarum containing probiotics on blood pressure: A systematic review and meta-analysis. *Pharmacological Research*, 2020. 153: p. 104663.
104. Lopes, R.D.C.S.O., Modulation of intestinal microbiota, control of nitrogen products and inflammation by Pre/probiotics in chronic kidney disease: A systematic review. *Nutrición Hospitalaria : Organo Oficial de la Sociedad Española de Nutrición Parenteral y Enteral*, 2017. 35(3): p. 722–730.
105. Tao, S., et al., Effects of probiotic supplements on the progression of chronic kidney disease: A meta-analysis. *Nephrology*, 2019. 24(11): p. 1122–1130.

106. Mcfarlane, C., et al., Prebiotic, probiotic, and synbiotic supplementation in chronic kidney disease: A systematic review and meta-analysis. *Journal of Renal Nutrition: The Official Journal of the Council on Renal Nutrition of the National Kidney Foundation*, 2019. 29(3): p. 209–220.
107. Thongprayoon, C., et al., Effects of probiotics on inflammation and uremic toxins among patients on dialysis: A systematic review and meta-analysis. *Digestive Diseases and Sciences*, 2019. 64(2): p. 469–479.
108. Zagórska, A., et al., From probiotics to psychobiotics – The gut-brain axis in psychiatric disorders. *Beneficial Microbes*, 2020. 11(8): p. 717–732.
109. Zhang, N., et al., Efficacy of probiotics on stress in healthy volunteers: A systematic review and meta-analysis based on randomized controlled trials. *Brain and Behavior*, 2020. 10(9): p. e01699.
110. Ng, Q.X., et al., A meta-analysis of the use of probiotics to alleviate depressive symptoms. *Journal of Affective Disorders*, 2018. 228: p. 13–19.
111. Liu, R.T., R.F.L. Walsh, and A.E. Sheehan, Prebiotics and probiotics for depression and anxiety: A systematic review and meta-analysis of controlled clinical trials. *Neuroscience and Biobehavioral Reviews*, 2019. 102: p. 13–23.
112. Goh, K.K., et al., Effect of probiotics on depressive symptoms: A meta-analysis of human studies. *Psychiatry Research*, 2019. 282: p. 112568.
113. Le Morvan De Sequeira, C., et al., Effect of probiotics on psychiatric symptoms and central nervous system functions in human health and disease: A systematic review and meta-analysis. *Nutrients*, 2022. 14(3): p. 621.
114. Song, W., et al., Prebiotics and probiotics for autism spectrum disorder: A systematic review and meta-analysis of controlled clinical trials. *Journal of Medical Microbiology*, 2022. 71(4): p. 001510.
115. Ng, X., et al., A systematic review of the effect of probiotic supplementation on schizophrenia symptoms. *Neuropsychobiology*, 2019. 78(1): p. 1–6.
116. Minichino, A., et al., The gut-microbiome as a target for the treatment of schizophrenia: A systematic review and meta-analysis of randomised controlled trials of add-on strategies. *Schizophrenia Research*, 2021. 234: p. 58–70.
117. Zhang, X.-F., et al., Clinical effects and gut microbiota changes of using probiotics, prebiotics or Synbiotics in inflammatory bowel disease: A systematic review and meta-analysis. *European Journal of Nutrition*, 2021. 60(5): p. 2855–2875.
118. Limketkai, B.N., et al., Probiotics for induction of remission in Crohn's disease. The Cochrane library, 2020. 2020(7): p. CD006634.
119. Ooi, S.L., D. Correa, and S.C. Pak, Probiotics, prebiotics, and low FODMAP diet for irritable bowel syndrome – What is the current evidence? *Complementary Therapies in Medicine*, 2019. 43: p. 73–80.
120. Ford, A.C., et al., Systematic review with meta-analysis: The efficacy of prebiotics, probiotics, Synbiotics and antibiotics in irritable bowel syndrome. *Alimentary Pharmacology and Therapeutics*, 2018. 48(10): p. 1044–1060.
121. Seiler, C.L., et al., Probiotics for celiac disease: A systematic review and meta-analysis of randomized controlled trials. *The American Journal of Gastroenterology*, 2020. 115(10): p. 1584–1595.
122. Wegh, C.A.M., et al., Nonpharmacologic treatment for children with functional constipation: A systematic review and meta-analysis. *The Journal of Pediatrics*, 2022. 240: p. 136–149.e5.
123. Gomes, D.O.V.S. and M.B.D. Morais, Gut microbiota and the use of probiotics in constipation in children and adolescents: Systematic review. *Revista Paulista de Pediatria: Orgao Oficial da Sociedade de Pediatria de Sao Paulo*, 2020. 38: p. e2018123.
124. Nakamura, H., T. Lim, and P. Puri, Probiotics for the prevention of Hirschsprung-associated enterocolitis: A systematic review and meta-analysis. *Pediatric Surgery International*, 2018. 34(2): p. 189–193.

125. Du, X., et al., Efficacy of probiotic supplementary therapy for asthma, allergic rhinitis, and wheeze: A meta-analysis of randomized controlled trials. *Allergy and Asthma Proceedings : The Official Journal of Regional and State Allergy Societies*, 2019. 40(4): p. 250–260.

126. Liu, C.W., et al., Roles of gut-microbiota and probiotics in chronic urticaria: A systematic review and meta-analysis. *Australasian Journal of Dermatology*, 2022. 63(2): p. e166–e170.

127. Szajewska, H. and A. Horvath, Lactobacillus rhamnosus G.G. in the primary prevention of eczema in children: A systematic review and meta-analysis. *Nutrients*, 2018. 10(9): p. 1319.

128. Bustamante, M., et al., Probiotics as an adjunct therapy for the treatment of halitosis, dental caries and periodontitis. *Probiotics and Antimicrobial Proteins*, 2020. 12(2): p. 325–334.

129. Miller, L.E., L. Lehtoranta, and M.J. Lehtinen, Short-term probiotic supplementation enhances cellular immune function in healthy elderly: Systematic review and meta-analysis of controlled studies. *Nutrition Research*, 2019. 64: p. 1–8.

130. Qu, H., et al., Effects of microbiota-driven therapy on inflammatory responses in elderly individuals: A systematic review and meta-analysis. *PLOS ONE*, 2019. 14(2): p. e0211233.

131. Wang, F., et al., A meta-analysis reveals the effectiveness of probiotics and prebiotics against respiratory viral infection. *Bioscience Reports*, 2021. 41(3): p. BSR20203638.

132. Lima, W.G., et al., Effect of probiotics on the maintenance of intestinal homeostasis after chemotherapy: Systematic review and meta-analysis of pre-clinical studies. *Beneficial Microbes*, 2020. 11(4): p. 305–318.

133. Grev, J., M. Berg, and R. Soll, Maternal probiotic supplementation for prevention of morbidity and mortality in preterm infants. *Cochrane Database of Systematic Reviews*, 2018. 2018(12): p. CD012519.

134. Jia, L., et al., Benefits of resistant starch type 2 for patients with end-stage renal disease under maintenance hemodialysis: A systematic review and meta-analysis. *International Journal of Medical Sciences*, 2021. 18(3): p. 811–820.

135. Catania, J., et al., Probiotic supplementation for promotion of growth in children: A systematic review and meta-analysis. *Nutrients*, 2021. 14(1): p. 83.

136. Sorensen, K., et al., Amino acid formula containing Synbiotics in infants with Cow's milk protein allergy: A systematic review and meta-analysis. *Nutrients*, 2021. 13(3): p. 935.

137. Marzorati, M., et al., Effects of combined prebiotic, probiotic, IgG and amino acid supplementation on the gut microbiome of patients with inflammatory bowel disease. *Future Microbiology*, 2022. 17(16): p. 1307–1324.

138. Loman, B.R., et al., Prebiotic and probiotic treatment of non-alcoholic fatty liver disease: A systematic review and meta-analysis. *Nutrition Reviews*, 2018. 76(11): p. 822–839.

139. Chan, C.K.Y., et al., Preventing respiratory tract infections by synbiotic interventions: A systematic review and meta-analysis of randomized controlled trials. *Advances in Nutrition*, 2020. 11(4): p. 979–988.

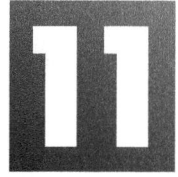

# Nutraceuticals as Modulators of Gut Microbiota

## Role in Therapy!

Rupali Joshi Panse

## Contents

DOI: 10.1201/9781003333821-11

## 11.1 Introduction

If there's one thing to understand about the human body, it's this. The human body has a ringmaster. This ringmaster controls digestion, immunity, nervous system, weight, sensitivities, and even emotional health. This ringmaster is the gut. The human gut is inhabited by a diverse range of bacterial species which grow significant metabolic and immune roles, but with a perceptible effect on the nutritional and health status of the host. The nature and the importance of the complex exchanges between the microbiome and its host are now well documented. The contributions of this commensal relationship to the health of the host increasingly appreciated. Accordingly, one can predict how any disruption of this relationship might lead to pathological consequences for the host.

Various chronic disorders like inflammatory bowel disease, metabolic syndrome, atherosclerosis, alcoholic liver disease, diabetes mellitus, nonalcoholic fatty liver disease, and cirrhosis have been linked with the human microbiota.[2] Conditions such as asthma, atopy, childhood obesity, and autism spectrum have been correlated with excess antibiotic use and a resulting alteration in the microbiome in childhood.[3] Numerous other conditions such as obesity, autoimmune disorders, cardiovascular disease, cancer, and neurological disorders have also been linked with changes in the microbiome.[4]

Dietary components play beneficial roles beyond basic nutrition, leading to the development of the functional food concept and nutraceuticals. There is growing evidence on the use of probiotics in various diseases, especially in gastrointestinal (GI) diseases. When these probiotics are combined with the appropriate nutraceuticals and herbs, this result in their improved efficacy. Ayurvedic nutraceuticals offer a broad-spectrum choice of herbs, cooking spices, and cuisine range which is in a sympathetic therapeutic relation with probiotics and may assist gut health by correction of digestive errors along with microbiome colonization.

Ayurveda science addresses the alimentary canal as the most important system in the human body. Apart from just digestion and absorption of the nutrients, Ayurveda has described the involvement of the digestive tract in other important metabolic activities like secretion of the neurotransmitters, hormones, and other vital enzymes by comparing the benefits of food to vital prana (life). Food is stated to improve strength, promote growth, nourish systems, bring joy to mind, nurture the intellect, feed the emotions, and restore the strength and immunity.[5] According to the Ayurvedic physiology, the gut is the root level of all tissue production, which it termed as "Sapta Dhatu Poshana" (seven types of tissue generation). All the tissues are nourished by the nourishing juice (Aahara Rasa) obtained in the early stage of digestion. This primitive juice undergoes the complex microscopic metabolic transformations to form every tissue in the body step by step. The ancient literature describes the role of digestion in promoting the growth, nourishment, immunity, emotional replenishment, and endurance. Anything incorrect in the digestive tract, or digestion, itself is capable of affecting the abovementioned life qualities.[5]

## 11.2 Digestion, Agni, and Their Symbiotic Association with Gut Microbiome

Agni is the invariable agent in the process of paka (digestion, transformation). The foundational theory of Agni is the supportive pillar for healthy metabolism. Agni is the functional form of energy which resides in symphony with physical physiological entities called Tridosha (Vata, Pitta, and Kapha). Agni is one of the most powerful transformative principles of Ayurveda.[6] It holds the secret to longevity, vitality, high prana or life force, good health, stable energy, clarity of mind, and wellness The major site of Agni is the gut where the digestion of food and its transformation to a bioavailable form is performed. Interestingly, Ayurveda advocates the balanced state of Agni for not only gastrointestinal functions, but also for its influence on other systems. Ayurveda considers the interdependent pathways between Agni and other systems for therapeutic goals. Just like microbiome, Agni is supposed to be the gateway for physical and mental health. Enzymes, hormones, and neurotransmitters are under the influence of Agni, according to the theories in Ayurveda.[6] The concept of gut microbiome and the theory of Agni from Ayurveda seem closely interlinked and can be used for improving gut health. Physiological Agni takes care of the gut health, metabolic processes, and can have imprints on psychological health too.

Understanding the gut through the lens of Ayurveda unlocks avenues to explore the abundant possibilities of using a broad-spectrum of herbs and food as nutraceuticals to preserve gut health in hand with probiotics and prebiotics.

## 11.3 Gut Health through the Lens of Ayurveda

To understand the role of nutraceuticals in the modulation of gut microbiota, the Ayurvedic theory of tissue generation and Agni is important. If we consider a human as a tree, Ayurveda compares the gut (digestive system/ Annavaha Srotasa) to its root. Ayurveda considers the gut is connected to every cell in the human body exactly the same way. Traditional medicine and

Ayurveda science has termed this relationship of the gut with all systems as Ashraya Ashrayi bhava (residing along with each other in harmony). Ashraya and Ashrayi are inseparable and work with each other in a synchronized manner.

Annavaha Srotasa is the site of formation of physiological Tridosha (Vata, Pitta, and Kapha). Tridosha in accordance with Agni (digestive fire) and Dhatawgni (metabolic fire) governs all the metabolic activities in the body. Being the site of formation, gut health is important in comprehensive metabolic activities like Tridosha generation and generation of various tissues in the body. The digestive system is fondly mentioned as "mahastrotasa" in all Ayurvedic ancient textbooks not because of its complex structure or length but as the term proposes the physiological position of the system and its influence on other systems.

Presence of Tridosha at three major sites of the digestive system suggests the anatomical importance of the alimentary tract with respect to their functionality and influence on digestion. Kapha has dominant presence at the stomach (called Amashaya), Pitta at the small intestine (called Grahani), and Vata at the colon (called Pakvashaya). Interestingly, these are the major sites in where the opaquest population of diverse human microbiome is more active than anywhere else in the body. The bacterial cells harbored within the human gastrointestinal tract (GIT) outnumber the host's cells by a factor of ten and the genes encoded by the bacteria resident within the GIT outnumber their host's genes by more than 100 times.[7] The diversity and number of the colony of gut microbes are remarkably different at these three sites where Tridosha are playing their specific role in complex metabolic conversions.

The gut microbiota plays a vital part in harvesting, storing, and expending energy obtained from the diet. The absorption of fat, simple carbohydrates, and proteins begins in the duodenum and is completed in the jejunum. The distal part of the small intestine is mainly involved in the absorption of bile acids and vitamin $B_{12}$, while the colon is responsible for the absorption of water, electrolytes, and short chain fatty acids produced by bacterial fermentation.[8] Overall, the colon receives only 15% of ingested carbohydrates and 5–33% of proteins.[8] Microbiota taxonomic complexity and bacterial load increases gradually from the stomach ($10^1$–$10^3$ CFU(colony-forming unit)/ml) to the jejunum ($10^4$–$10^7$ CFU/ml) to feces ($10^{11}$–$10^{12}$ CFU/ml),[8] which mainly consists of aero-intolerant prokaryotes. In the small intestine, the transport time is quick, and the existence of digestive enzymes and bile makes the environment inhospitable to microbial life. There, the resident microbiota displays less species diversity but greater intersubject variability compared to the mouth or colon.[9] The gut microbiota of the small intestine is dominated by Streptococci, Bifidobacterium, Enterococci, and Lactobacilli which effectively develop metabolic pathways positioned on the rapid uptake and alteration of simple carbohydrates[9] Studies involving obesity and the gut microbiota emphasis the disparity of small intestine bacterial efficiency in carbohydrates and fatty acid oxidation, with the subsequent cholecystokinin-mediated feedback on the satiety reflex,[10] whereas the presence of *Lactococcus sp.* in this part of the intestine has been associated with the lipid and carbohydrate metabolisms.[11]

Fascinatingly, Ayurveda has described the role of Tridosha at various stages of the conversion of food in the digestive system that resonate with this description. The physiology of digestion can be stated using three stages known as Avastha paka,[12] wherein successive changes in the chemical and mechanical nature of food or medicine, for example, are well documented.

Kapha Dosha, which is present in the stomach, is rich in volume and density and converts the Madhura-taste-dominant food (which according to Ayurveda texts belongs to the food classes carbohydrates and proteins) and is known as Madhura Vipaka Awsatha (sweet taste phase in digestion).

## 11.4 "Vishishte Paka Vipaka" (Sus/40/10 Dalhan Tika)

This Sanskrit verse means that this exclusive intended transformation is called Vipaka. The Sanskrit term "paka" means transformation and "vi" is a prefix meaning exclusive. At this stage, primitive juice is obtained from food and is directed to the subsequent part of the digestive tract. The small intestine is the seat for Pitta Dosha and metabolic fire (Agni) where Madhura-taste-dominant Aahara Rasa undergoes conversion by Pitta resulting in Amla Paka Avastha (sour-taste-dominant phase of digestion). This results in reducing the overall volume of food by the remaining conversion of carbohydrates. The third stage of digestion in the colon (Pakvashaya) is Vata dominant where the general absorption of micronutrients takes place. Ayurveda signifies this stage of digestion as Katu Vipaka, where the Mala (solid waste) is separated from the required nutrients and the stools are formed. Simultaneously, at these important sites the essence of consumed food is extracted as Aahara Rasa which circulates through blood to form and nourish existing tissues all over the body. A step ahead, Ayurveda believes that food does not only nourish the physical components of the human body, but it is also capable of nourishing the emotions and has a huge impact on mental health. Along with the important physiological event of formation and circulation of Aahara Rasa, an important event of formation of physiological Tridosha takes place in parallel. Existing Kapha Dosha is nourished, as well as new Kapha Dosha being produced in the stomach, Pitta Dosha in the small intestine, and Vata Dosha in the colon.

A clear difference has been noted between Vipaka and Avastha Paka, although Charaka gives both numerical similarities.[13] Vipaka is the final transformation of food, whereas Avastha paka is the initial phase. Vipaka commences only after the Avastha paka has ceased.

The holistic mechanism of gut microbiota coincides, to some extent, with the doctrines of Ayurveda in the context of pharmacodynamics and pharmacokinetics.

Vipaka is commonly referred to as a post-digestive irreversible process. It is closely associated with the biotransformation of drugs/food caused by microbiota. These microbiomes themselves are sources of Agni which reside in gastrointestinal tract and are responsible for the metabolism of drugs. Gut microflora, as a whole, reveals certain specificity in the ultimate production of SCFAs (short chain fatty acids) and other nutrients, depending on the quantity and nature of the diet and medicines. Similarly, the Madhura, Amla, and Katu Vipaka of drugs (food/medicine) have been denoted to possess a qualitative degree (Taratama Bhava) depending on the nature of the drug consumed which manifests in the *Karma* (action) of the drug.

The intestinal microbiota may play an important role in mediating the metabolism and enhancement of the bioactivity of many herbs such as ginseng.[13] Gut microbiota surely play a role in decreasing as well as increasing drug activity.[14]

## 11.5 Concept of Ama with Respect to Dysbiosis

Ayurveda explains that most diseases are caused by an accumulation of Ama or errors in the biological transformation of food. Ama literally means "uncooked food," but it can be understood from a scientific perspective as endogenous toxins resulting from imbalanced or incomplete digestion. Ama can be seen as a result of reduced Agni, or digestive power. Agni has a number of different meanings and not only relates to digestive enzymes but also to the metabolic process in the different tissues or dhatus of the body. Ama is initially formed in the digestive tract, but at a later stage of disease it can escape into the tissues leading to tissue disruption and chronic inflammatory disease.

It has been suggested that compromised mucosal integrity, such as a disruption in the tight junctions, leads to dysbiosis, resulting in the formation of Ama[3] Ama is also produced at other levels of the physiology, including the cellular level. Excessive formation of free radicals contributes to the formation of Ama. A variety of free radicals and reactive oxygen species (ROS) are produced during cellular metabolism. Excessive amounts of these reactive molecules can cause damage, starting the disease process. The ability to control their concentrations may be helpful for the prevention and treatment of many disorders.

Antioxidants "scavenge" free radicals and ROS and purify them. Antioxidants can be lipid- or water-soluble; some are produced in the body and others can be obtained from food or dietary supplements. Vitamins, enzymes, and herbal mixtures are a range of natural antioxidants. Powerful antioxidants are present in the bioflavonoids found in a concentrated form in some antiaging herbs described in Ayurveda. The class of this property-bearing food, herb, or practice is termed Rasayana. The use of these Rasayana may induce a neutralizing effect in the excessive free radical activity that contributes to Ama formation.

It is interesting to interpret the meaning of Ama in terms of recent findings. Remarkable progress has been made in understanding the mechanisms of leaky gut syndrome in celiac patients. In celiac disease, the tight junctions that hold the cells of the gut wall together become loose, and as a result, undigested food and harmful substances "leak" through the gut wall and into the bloodstream, causing inflammation. The exact mechanism of this process involves a product of gluten called gliadin, which interacts with receptors on the surface of the cells in the small intestine, causing the production of zonulin. Zonulin then causes the proteins, which bind tight junctions, to relax and allow unwanted substances to enter the bloodstream. In celiac patients, this process is exaggerated and can ultimately result in a harmful autoimmune reaction. A disruption in the gut microbiome has been associated with problems in the gut barrier. It is suggested that gut dysbiosis may cause the release of zonulin but the exact mechanisms are complex and still under investigation.

## 11.6 Virudhha (Incompatible Food): A Common Causative Factor for Gut Dysbiosis and Inflammatory Disorders

A new science branch called topography, which exclusively studies the effect of various food combinations on health, is emerging. Topography reveals combinations of basic categories of food and their effects on the body. A similar unique theory in Ayurveda is called Virudhhanna. Incompatibility is a unique concept in Ayurveda. Anything edible such as medicine or food that provokes Doshas, displaces them from their normal biorhythm, and is not eliminated out of body is called Viruddha.[15] Virudhha's certain types of combinations hinder the metabolism of tissue, which inhibits the process of formation of tissue and has the opposite property to the tissue. Food, which is wrong in combination, has undergone wrong processing, been consumed in an incorrect quantity, with food of opposite qualities, consumed at an incorrect time of day and in the wrong season can become Virudhha. As well as numerous minor to serious systemic illnesses, insanity is mentioned as an obvious result of consuming Viruddha Aahara. Application of this theory for prediction and prevention is important. This theory provides a strong foundation to study the recent diet and culinary trends and their incompatibility. The combination of some prohibited combinations of diet is responsible for inflammatory reactions during digestion, forming the faulty Aahara Rasa and Ama. Virudhha Aahara has adverse gut-modulating actions and disrupts the gut flora permanently causing various disorders of the sense organs and immune system (see Table 11.1).[15]

**Table 11.1** Virudhha Aahara Classical list from Charka Samhita

**A Few Examples of Incompatible Food Items**

- **Fruits + milk** (as in milkshake deserts, ice creams, fruit followed by drinking milk or vice versa)
- **Fish + milk** either by combining or eating separately followed by each other
- **Curd heated** and used as an ingredient
- **Milk + salt** combined in recipes
- **Milk/milk products + meat** at the same time
- **Radish + milk** combined
- **Milk + melons** together
- **Buttermilk heated** and consumed or used in dishes.
- **Ghee + honey** combined in equal weight
- **Too hot + too cold food** together is an example of Virudhhanna as described in Ayurveda
- **Stale, too fermented, too sour, dry food**

**Examples of Today's Trendy Incompatible Food That May not Be Mentioned in Ayurveda**

- Almost all **cocktails**, which use wild imagination in mixing different property-bearing juices and alcohol
- **Citrus fruit flavored** milkshakes and ice creams
- Use of **milk, curd, cream, and buttermilk** in marinating or preparing curry and gravy
- **Extreme hot and cold things together** in a dish are a hit nowadays, like fried hot ice cream, hot brownie with cold ice cream
- **Fruit salad served with custard made from milk.**, Fruit-flavored rabdi (condensed milk desert), esp. a custard apple thick milk dessert (rabdi), is highly allergic due to its mucus-increasing property
- Many **unusually flavored alcoholic beverages**, such as coffee cream liquor and white chocolate, and cocktails, mocktails, and smoothies containing veggies + milk + cream + yogurt together, etc.
- **Sweets, desserts, and recipes that have honey** as an ingredient and need to be cooked or heated
- Eating **curd, rice, and pickle** together daily at night
- **Khichadi (cereal rice) and milk** together
- **Preserved salty (MSG)** synthetic oxidants, preservatives, and artificial taste enhancers

# 11.7 Prakriti (Body Constitution): Personalized Spectrum of Human Microbiome

Epigenetics is an interesting branch of science which explores environmental imprints on the genetic profile of the human body. The Ayurveda school of thought matches many of the revelations in epigenetics and can be looked upon as an ancient science of epigenetics. Ayurveda recognizes that each individual has his or her own unique psychophysiological constitution, which is affected by diet, digestion, lifestyle, stress management, and environmental factors. These are the precise nutrigenomic mechanics of how food can affect gene expression.[7]

Several studies have established the relationship between the Ayurvedic Prakriti of a person and the characteristic pattern of microbiome. Scholars found that three main Prakriti types, Vata, Pitta, and Kapha, can be addressed on the basis of an exclusive microbiome composition. The population studied was from the same region and had similar dietary habits. The main bacteria of all the subjects were from the phyla Bacteroidetes and Firmicutes. There were distinct differences between the Vata, Pitta, and Kapha groups in less common bacteria. The extreme Pitta individuals, for example, had more butyrate-producing microbes which might help protect them from inflammatory diseases. The extreme Kapha women had larger amounts of a type of bacteria called Prevotella copri, which has been associated with patients who have rheumatoid arthritis and insulin resistance. A more recent paper analyzes how the concept of Prakriti can be used as a stratification of the gut microbiome.

## 11.8 Stress and Mental Health and Ayurveda Psychobiotics

Ayurveda respects the interdependent relation of gut and brain. Worry, fear, and stress are addressed as manas bhava (mental parameters) which have influence on hunger and appetite and cause indigestion and metabolic errors. Stressors can abnormally activate adrenal glands to release cortisol, which goes into the bloodstream and affects both the gut and the gut bacteria. Cortisol can increase intestinal permeability, as seen in a leaky gut. The chemical changes in stress-related conditions can hamper the gut immune system

Ayurveda uses a wide variety of approaches to improve the mind or manas and to improve the effects of stress on gut microbiome and generated disorders. Apoptogenic herbs are scientifically accepted as a safe and effective way to manage various gut- and brain-related psychological conditions.[7]

Ayurveda has long explained that disturbances in our mental state, which are usually associated with a Vata imbalance, can be traced to problems in the nervous system and the gut. It recommends specific herbs such as Ashwagandha and Brahmi, which may interact with the microbiome. It also has a long tradition of using natural probiotics such as lassi. Modern research on the microbiome validates this concept, showing that depression and anxiety may be linked to a disrupted microbiome and may be improved through the use of probiotics.

One brain-imaging study showed that women react differently to stimuli depending on the type of bacteria they have in their gut. The same researchers had previously shown that diet could affect the brain. They gave subjects either psychobiotics (a probiotic mixture that is used for mental health) or a placebo. They then showed the subjects images of frightened faces while measuring brain activity. The subjects taking the placebo showed a normal stress response with specific areas of the brain responsible for emotions being activated. Subjects receiving the psychobiotics showed a reduced stress response in these same areas of the brain

## 11.9 Dincharya, Rutucharya, and Biorhythm of Gut Microbiome

Ayurveda theories of preserving health clearly identify daily and seasonal rhythms. Ayurveda clearly states the active period of Vata, Pitta, and Kapha at specific times of a 24-hour cycle. Early morning to late morning (6 am to 10 am) Kapha is active, Pitta Dosha is in its best active state from 10 am until the afternoon, and then Vata takes over from 2 pm to 6 pm. A further cycle is another Kapha-dominating period from 6 pm to 10 pm, Pitta from 10 pm to 2 am, and finally Vata from 2 am to 6 am. All daily activities like sleeping, eating, excreting, exercise, rest, etc. are in accordance with these Dosha naturally, which is called the biological rhythm. If these importance activities are irregular and untimely, the related Dosha is at risk of impacting overall metabolism. Gut health is at major risk as all these important daily activities are interdependent on digestion. Ayurveda uses this Dincharya as a potent mode to rectify the circadian rhythm-related metabolic errors and Dincharya has a significant role in managing gut health.[15]

Each season is represented by either one Dosha or a combination of Doshas. Late autumn and winter are cold and dry and link to the Vata Dosha. Summer is hot and naturally corresponds to the Pitta Dosha. Spring is cold and wet and resembles the Kapha Dosha. The daily routine is called Dincharya and the seasonal routine is called Rutucharya. Following Rutucharya is a scientific guideline theory which takes care of Agni, calorie needs, Dosha balance, and altered internal environment. Modern medicine also identifies the need for the circadian clock. From bacteria to humans, almost all forms of life have an internal "biological clock." Manual alterations or wrong lifestyles, like in shift workers, for instance, can lead to a higher incidence of cancer, cardiovascular disease, digestive disorders, and obesity, as well as psychiatric and neurodegenerative diseases.

Gut bacteria too has its own biological rhythms. One interesting study created jet lag in mice by forcing these normally nocturnal animals to stay awake during the day. When the researchers transferred the gut bacteria from jet-lagged mice into germ-free mice, the recipient mice developed both obesity and glucose intolerance. Food habits, diet etiquettes, food combinations, and mental state while eating food affect the composition of the microbiome Gut microbiome are active and work on the daily as well as the seasonal rhythmic pattern. The relationship between the circadian rhythms and gut microbiota appears to be bidirectional and may have important influences on health.

Ayurvedic seasonal practices (Rutucharya) of specific diets at specific times may relate to the seasonal rhythms of the microbiome. The summer season naturally decreases the Agni and a person is expected to eat easy to digest/low calorie food. Pitta-increasing food, i.e., hot, dry food is contraindicated. Early spring is Kapha vitiation season where individuals can manifest various allergies. Ayurveda recommends Kapha-pacifying food in this season. Six tastes and their impact on each Dosha are a scientific approach to maintain gut mucosa and microbiome harmony. Diet according to Dincharya and Rutucharya can be an innovative approach to study the role of the seasons in

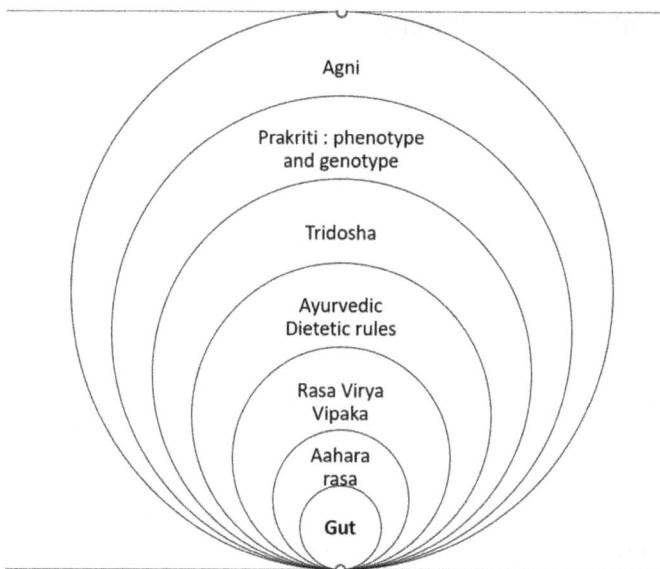

**Figure 11.1** *Reliant perspectives in Ayurveda dietetics and gut health.*

altering the nature of the gut microbiome and how an Ayurvedic regime can help restore it (see Figure 11.1).

## 11.10 Loopholes of Conventional Probiotics

The last few decades have witnessed unparalleled progress in the application of probiotics for promoting general gut health as well as their inception as biotherapeutics to alleviate certain clinical disorders related to dysbiosis. On one hand, numerous studies have substantiated the health-restoring potential for a restricted group of microbial species. On the other hand, the marketed extrapolation of a similar probiotic label to a large number of partially characterized microbial formulations seems biased. Individuals of neonatal age and/or those with some clinical conditions including malignancies, leaky gut, diabetes mellitus, and post-organ transplant rehabilitation likely fail to reap the benefits of these probiotics. Certain probiotic strains might overcome the weak immunity in these vulnerable groups and turn into opportunistic pathogens provoking life-threatening pneumonia, endocarditis, and sepsis. Moreover, the unregulated and rampant use of probiotics potentially carries the risk of plasmid-mediated antibiotic resistance transfer to the gut infectious pathogens. Through interference with commensal microflora, they can result in opportunistic performances in the host due to bacteremia and fungemia. Since substantial numbers of consumers use probiotic products worldwide, assurance of the safety of these products is necessary.[16]

## 11.11 Concept of Ayurvedic Nutraceuticals for Gut Health

Nutraceutical is a term consisting of "nutrition" and "pharmaceutics." The term is functional to products that are isolated from herbal products, dietary supplements (nutrients), specific diets, and processed foods such as cereals, soups, and beverages that other than nutrition are also used as medicine. A nutraceutical product may be defined as a substance which has physiological benefit or provides protection against chronic disease. Nutraceuticals may be indicated to expand health, delay the aging process, prevent chronic diseases, increase life expectancy, or support the metabolism. Nutraceuticals have established substantial attention due to potential nutritional, safety, and therapeutic effects. Herbal nutraceuticals and their impact on noncommunicable health conditions related to oxidative stress including allergies, and cardiovascular, cancer, diabetes, eye and immune disorders, and Alzheimer's and Parkinson's diseases, as well as obesity, is promising.

Interestingly, the whole concept of health and wellness in Ayurveda is to seek the goodness out of daily diet and the daily life regime. Nutraceuticals for the management of health conditions are the soul of Ayurveda medicine. Gut mucosa is considered the largest available effective medium for various therapies and medicines. Ayurveda preparations are combinations of herbs, cooking spices, and a few animal-derived products like cow milk, cow ghee, honey, etc. which are classified as "food."

Efficacy of the particular food, herb, or Herbo mineral combination is decided by their properties and their Rasa, Virya, and Vipaka. The chemical composition and their pharmaceutical action are explained on the basis of physical properties like heavy, light, cold, hot, rough, smooth, sticky, etc. Twenty such properties define the expression of the substance on cellular physiology when it is metabolized in the body. Six tastes and their sole or in combination presence decide the pharmacological effect of that particular substance after it undergoes the complex process of chemical conversion during digestion and other metabolic activities. Considering all these attributes of various food classes, herbs, cooking spices, and animal products, Ayurveda pharmacology groups them in their pharmacological actions on gut mucosa and other systems. This is a unique classification in Ayurveda science where a particular section of herbs or diet signifies their metabolic expression. The site of activity of these groups is gut mucosa.

## 11.12 Ayurvedic Pharmacologic Notions for Modulation of Gut Mucosa (see Figure 11.2)

### 11.12.1 Deepana: Pharmacological Expression of Nutraceuticals for Enhancing Gut Microbiome Activity

The term Deepana is elaborated by the word "Deepa," which means "kindling the fire." The diet or medicine or process which stimulates digestion is called "Deepana."[17] The Deepana process inspires digestion at a key level or even

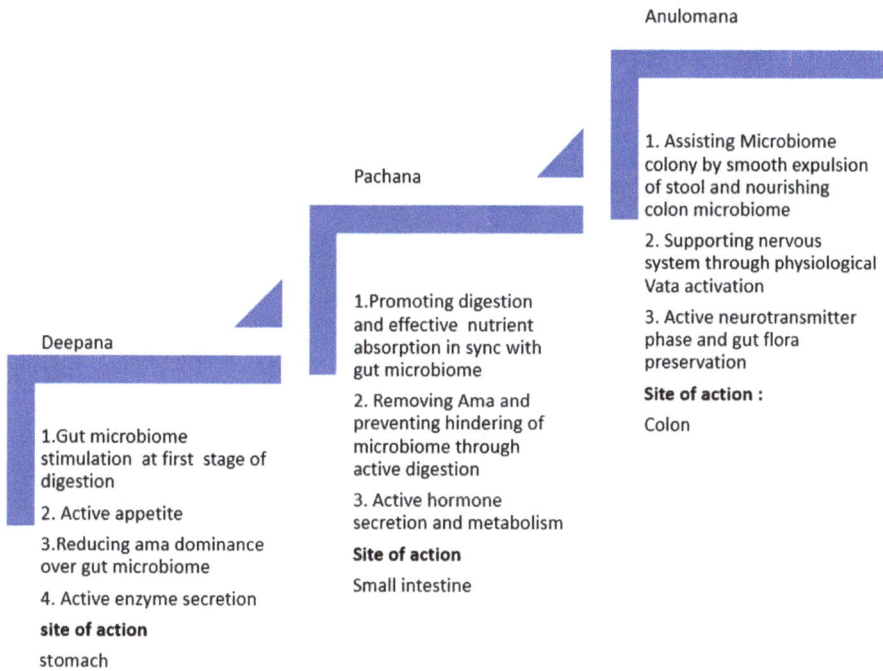

**Figure 11.2** *Ayurvedic gastrointestinal class of nutraceuticals: Impact on gut health.*

before the consumption of food itself. The processes of digestion and metabolism are an important component of health. Qualitative or quantitative impairment of Agni is the fundamental cause of all diseases.[18] Deepana action aims to preserve the equilibrium of Agni and the gut itself. The Deepana effect can be studied in terms of factors stimulating digestion. The digestive hormones like gastrin, secretin, and cholecystokinin may increase by consumption of Deepana food. More specifically, the hormones ghrelin and leptin seem to play an important role in producing the Deepana effect.

Ghrelin is an orexigenic hormone secreted in stomach mucosa. The concentration of ghrelin in plasma rises before food intake. It falls after the ingestion of food. It also activates a group of neurons in the hypothalamus called AgRP (agoutirelated peptide) neurons. Asprosin is another orexigenic hormone that activates AgRP directly. In animal studies, it is observed that AgRP neurons are activated when there is a deficiency in calories and become less active when fed. When the AgRP neurons were activated through chemical or light stimulus, they started to eat intensely in already-fed animals. So, these neurons are considered hunger-promoting neurons.[19]

Leptin is an anorexigenic hormone secreted by adipose tissue. Its main function is to maintain adequate fat storage in the body. A fall in the leptin level stimulates hunger.[19] Thus, these two hunger-promoting hormones can have a role in Deepana action.

A wide range of food items and medicines have a Deepana effect. The best form of food to kindle digestion is unctuous foods like fats/oils (Sneha).[20]

The medicines with Deepana action have a predominance of the fire element.[21] Deepana action through tastes (Rasa) is significant and tastes like salt (Lavana), bitter (Tikta), and spicy (Katu) taste have a Deepana effect. Food or herbs having properties like hot (Ushna) show a Deepana effect. Some examples of herbs with a Deepana effect are Anethum sowa (Shatapushpa), Tinospora cordifolia (Guduchi), Azadirachta indica (Nimba), Santalum album (Chandana), Prunus cerasoides (Padmaka), Piper longum (Pippali),[20] Piper nigrum (Maricha), Zingiber officinale (Shunthi), Aegle marmelos (Bilwa/wood apple), Clerodendrum phlomidis (Agnimantha), Cyperus rotundus (Musta), Terminalia chebula (Haritaki), etc.

Food and beverages such as hot/lukewarm drinking water,[22] coconut water,[22] cow's milk,[22] breast milk,[22] buttermilk, alcohol, honey, rock salt, asafoetida, etc. are supposed to be gut health promoters by keeping the digestive fire active. Not only edibles but daily regimens like timely baths[23] and appropriate exercise are also admired for enhancing appetite.

The abovementioned Deepana foods and herbs are nutraceuticals with a broad-spectrum therapeutic role in treating various psychosomatic diseases.

## 11.12.2 Pachana: Pharmacological Expression of Nutraceuticals to Enhance Nutrient Absorption through Effective Digestion

The word "Pachana" factually means digestion, cooking, boiling. In therapies, it denotes digestion or promoting digestion. It is envisioned to remove undigested food/toxins (Ama) from the body and is a prerequisite before purificatory therapies. It is prescribed for the pacification of Dosha. Food and medicines with a Pachana effect may work on the primary and secondary metabolism at organic and cellular levels. The primary metabolic and biochemical process is believed to be accelerated due to Pachana food and herbs

In experimental studies, the food conversion ratio is used to assess the Pachana activity of medicines objectively. It is calculated as the food consumed in gram percentage (gm%) by dividing fecal matter in gm% passed on the same day. Improved metabolism leads to an increase in the nutritional part (sarabhaga) and a subsequent decrease in waste products (kittabhaga). So, Pachana can result in higher food conversion ratio.

Pachana activity is intended to promoting the nutrients bioavailability in digestion. This particular target depends upon the gut microbiome and the Pachana herbs through symbiosis can increase the activity of the gut microbiome.

This process does not increase or stimulate digestive capacity at the primary level.[24] Pachana occurs at the sites of accumulation of metabolic toxins or undigested food products. Pachana herbs are especially used for psychosomatic health conditions to reduce metabolic toxins (Ama) and improve the gut brain axis by effective metabolism of hormones, enzymes, and neurotransmitters.

## 11.12.3 Anulomana: Therapeutic Rejuvenation of the Colon Microbiome

Anulomana is a term which means the kind or gentle physiological expulsion through the nearest outlet. Anulomana, according to Ayurvedic texts, is an effective path to gut health. It is a proven fact that dysbiosis or a decreased number of the gut microbiome can cause irregular bowel habits with hard dry stools. Improper expulsion of stools is considered as a major blockage in mahastrotasa and is closely related to Vata Dosha diseases. This blockage results in Ama circulation and impacts both physical as well as mental health. Anulomana herbs loosen the stools, promote active peristalsis for expulsion, and favor the microbiota with proper excretion. Herbs like Ajamoda (Ptychotis ajowan), Jeeraka (Cuminum cyminum), Balharitaki (Terminalia chebula), Yashtimadhu (Glycyrrhiza glabra), and rock salt are effective on colon mucosa to promote gut health. The efficacy of these herbs as mild laxatives is well established.

The colon is used as an effective site for therapeutic enema (basti) in Ayurveda therapies as it escapes the complex two stages of digestion and can act directly on gut microbiome as well as highly receptive mucosa for efficient absorption of drug molecules. Vata is supposed to be the prime-involving Dosha in all neurological disorders. Anulomana can be a potent practice to preserve the gut flora. All Anulomana foods or medicines are Vata pacifying and gentle in nature. The herbs are treated with a healthy form of fat such as sesame oil, castor oil, cow ghee, etc. which ensures the prebiotics results on gut microbiome. Probiotic basti can be a solution to many psychosomatic health conditions to correct the dysbiosis at the level of the large intestine.

## 11.13 Prebiotic Activity of Single or Polyherbal Ayurvedic Herbs

The prebiotic potential of remedial herbs and their capacity to modulate the gut microbiota in a specific manner to improve colonic epithelium function, reduce inflammation, and protect from opportunistic infection is a hope for therapeutic science in many noncommunicable diseases. The herbal medicines regularly used for gastrointestinal health and disease in Ayurvedic medicine, as well as other traditional systems of medicine, such as Yashtimadhu/ Licorice (*Glycyrrhiza glabra*), the polyherbal combination Triphala (*Embelica officinalis*, *Terminalia bellerica*, and *Terminalia chebula*), and Chitraka (*Plumbago officinalis*) are proving their gut protective ability along with gut microbiome preservation and a therapeutic role in improving chronic health conditions

Triphala exerts entero-protective effects and promotes health of the gut epithelium and villi through improved barrier function and nutrient absorption.[2] Licorice root is used as a demulcent, a mild laxative, and is anti-inflammatory. Chitraka is supposed to be a digestive stimulant and improve absorption of nutrients in the gut.

## 11.14 Ayurvedic Nutraceuticals and Their Role in Gut Modulation

Ayurveda considers food as medicine. Every day, every meal we eat influences the great microbial organ inside which is gut microbiome. Almost nothing influences gut bacteria as much as the food we eat. Prebiotics, probiotics, and nutraceuticals are the most powerful tool at our disposal if we want to support our good gut bacteria.

Among all other food classes described in Ayurveda cooking, spices have a significant place and role in gut health. The interest in the potential of spices is extraordinary due to the chemical compounds such as phenylpropanoids, terpenes, flavonoids, and anthocyanins. A few spices display prebiotic-like activity by encouraging the growth of beneficial bacteria and resisting the growth of pathogenic bacteria, suggesting their potential role in the regulation of intestinal microbiota and the enhancement of gastrointestinal health.[25]

An interesting study for observing their efficacy on gut health was conducted. Seven culinary spices including black pepper, cayenne pepper, cinnamon, ginger, Mediterranean oregano, rosemary, and turmeric were extracted with boiling water. Major chemical ingredients were categorized by reversed-phase high-performance liquid chromatography (RP-HPLC-DAD) technique and antioxidant dimensions were assessed by measuring calorimetrically the extent to scavenge ABTS (2, 2′-azino-bis (3-ethylbenzothiazoline-6-sulfonic acid) radical cations. Effects of spice extracts on the viability of 88 anaerobic and facultative isolates from intestinal microbiota were examined by using Brucella agar plates containing serial dilutions of extracts. A total of 14 phenolic compounds, a piperine, cinnamic acid, and cinnamaldehyde were identified and quantitated. Spice extracts displayed a high antioxidant nature that correlated with the total amount of major chemicals. All spice extracts, with the exception of turmeric, enhanced the growth of *Bifidobacterium* spp. and *Lactobacillus* spp. All spices exhibited inhibitory activity against selected Ruminococcin species. Cinnamon, oregano, and rosemary were active against selected Fusobacterium strains and cinnamon, rosemary, and turmeric were active against selected *Clostridium* spp. Some spices displayed prebiotic-like action by helping the growth of beneficial bacteria and overpowering the growth of pathogenic bacteria, signifying their possible role in the regulation of intestinal microbiota and the enhancement of gastrointestinal health.

Recent research shows that both ginger and a herbal preparation called Triphala can have beneficial effects on the microbiome. Triphala is a combination of fruits, *Embelica officinalis* (Amalaki), *Terminalia bellerica* (Bibhitaki), and *Terminalia chebula* (Haritaki). It is an important constituent of Ayurvedic gastrointestinal and rejuvenation treatment programs, particularly to help improve stool excretion. Studies have found that Triphala has different possible clinical applications which attend to Agni correction and a reduction in Pitta activities, hyperacidity, and constipation. Triphala is widely used for its biological properties such as anti-inflammatory, immunomodulatory, antibacterial, antimutagenic, apoptogenic, hypoglycemic, antineoplastic, chemoprotective and radioprotective, and antioxidant activities. The polyphenols in Triphala modulate the human gut microbiome and thereby promote the growth of beneficial Bifidobacterium and Lactobacillus while inhibiting the growth of undesirable gut microbes.[3]

Cooking spices are known for their numerous medicinal values. Ayurveda medicines, medicinal foods, and supplements characteristically have numerical spice combinations. The combinations can be looked upon as a synergism of ingredients.

A few examples of these are as follows.

**Trikatu** is a combination of three bitter spices—dry ginger, black pepper, and Piper longum. Tri means three and Katu means pungent taste. All three express a strong pungent taste. They are quickly absorbed in digestive mucosa due to their light nature according to Ayurveda. They manifest a hot property during and after digestion. All three spices have specific anatomical adaptivity. Dry ginger to the small intestine and colon digestive system, black pepper to the nervine, immune, and hormonal system, and long pepper to the respiratory system.

The action of this combination is Agni specific. Trikatu works on respiratory conditions by working on gut health.

**Trimada** is an equal portion powder of Chitraka root (leadwort or doctor bush) (*Plumbago zeylanica*), Musta root (nutgrass/*Cyperus rotundas*, and Vidanga (false pepper/*Embelica ribes*).

Trimada is traditionally used to increase the functioning of the digestive system and metabolism. Along with this, it also assists in the reduction of cholesterol as well as reduces stomach aches and chest pains. The synergy of the three potent herbs supports the maintenance of a healthy gut flora. Chitraka root (leadwort) increases the digestive fire (Agni) and improves the cellular metabolism. Nutgrass (Musta) is cold in nature and has the unique quality of pacifying Pitta present in the small intestine. It has a pleasant smell and is a calming herb with a prebiotic nature. Vidanga (false pepper) is a famous flatus-relieving herb. Vidanga is used in traditional remedies and food from ancient times because of its anti-parasitic properties. This herb is used to treat various intestinal worms. It relieves stomachache and increases appetite. All these gut-specific activities ensure gut microbiome restoration.

**Trijata** is an equal portion of three aromatic herbs cinnamon (*Cinnamomum verum*), cardamon (*Elettaria cardamomum*), and bay leaf (*Laurus nobilis*) powder. All three have their own distinguishing woody aroma. The herbs exhibit a pungent astringent sweet taste at the level of initial digestion and reflect a hot property. Trijata is used in Kapha disorders. Cinnamon decreases Vata and Kapha and promotes digestion and cures dyspepsia through promoting digestive enzymes and prebiotic assistance. Cardamon (Ela) is a warming spice, contributing a sweet and pungent taste. Cardamom is considered an excellent digestive, especially beneficial in reducing bloating and gas. It is excellent for balancing Kapha, particularly in the stomach and the lungs. The seeds are often chewed to refresh the breath and promote oral mucosa hygiene. Bay leaves (Talisa) are aromatic leaves and used as a spice in cooking. In Ayurveda, bay leaves are used as a medicine to treat various health ailments. Cinnamon leaves and bark have aromatic, astringent, stimulant, and carminative qualities and are used in rheumatoid arthritis, pain in the abdomen diarrhea, nausea, and vomiting. Trijata is one of the numerous ingredients in the excellent well-known antiaging immunity-boosting supplement Chyavanprasha, used for its catalyst nature.[7]

**Chaturbij** is a mixture of Methika/fenugreek seeds, garden cress seeds/Ahaliv (*Lepidium sativum*), black cumin/Krishn Jeeraka (*Carum bulbocastanum*), and Ajwayan/Yavani (*Carum copticum*). Fenugreek seeds (Methika) are bitter, with hot and dry properties. Fenugreek has benefits for lowering blood sugar levels, boosting testosterone, and increasing milk production in breastfeeding mothers. Fenugreek may also reduce cholesterol levels, lower inflammation, and help with appetite control. It is supposed to be a bitter tonic and reduces Kapha Dosha and can increase physiological Pitta. Garden cress seeds/ Chandrasura (*Lepidium sativum*) are a tiny nutrient powerhouse. According to Ayurveda, Chandrasura seeds have beneficial effects on female reproductive functions, as they support hormonal balances through various stages like puberty, pregnancy, and lactation. Garden cress seeds are prebiotic and favor gut microbiome. Carom seeds are a digestive stimulant, anti-diarrheal, bind stool, digest Ama/toxins, reduce mucus, reduce Vata Dosha, are intoxicating, and induce sleep. They relieve pain in the abdomen due to indigestion and black cumin seeds are an estrogen stimulant, an appetizer, and enhance menstruation and lactation. This combination is used in gut modulation in many hormonal disorders in females.[7]

**Chaturushna** is the combination of the four hot spices of Trikatu: dry ginger, black pepper, long pepper (*Piper longum*), and Pippali root (*Piper longum* root). Chatur means four and Ushna means hot. The hot property of this group is targeted towards Vata and Kapha Dosha balance.

The fourth addition to the already discussed Trikatu is *Piper longum* root. The fruits of the plant *Piper longum* are known as Pippali, and the roots as Pippali Moola. Both are used for medicinal purpose in Ayurveda. The roots are anti-inflammatory, analgesic, carminative, laxative, and expectorant. Due to their hot potency, the roots are used in Agni imbalances and excessive Kapha inside the body.

**Panchkola** is a combination of five potent spices and herbs: Pippali/long pepper fruit (*Piper longum*), Pippali root/long pepper root, Chavya (*Piper cubeba*), Chitraka/leadwort (*Plumbago zeylanica*), and Shunthi/dried ginger (*Zingiber officinale*). Chavya (*Piper cubeba* L.) fruit is an important species used in Ayurvedic medicine for different types of pain such as rheumatism, chills, flu, colds, muscular aches, and fever. It is also very effective in multiple digestive track disorders. Panchkola is indicated in many conditions causing anorexia. It improves hunger, relieves bloating, and favors digestion. It specifically targets Vata and Kapha and keeps Pitta balanced. Panchkola churnam (powder) is planned for long-term intake to maintain the metabolic fire and as an adjuvant to a balanced diet. Efficacy of this simple combination in dysbiosis and metabolic diseases like diabetes, obesity, colitis, rheumatoid arthritis, renal disorders, and piles fissures, etc. is time-tested by Ayurveda physicians. Panchkola powder, according to Ayurveda, should be consumed mixed with buttermilk as the probiotic existence with these digestive herbs favors the gut microbiome

**Shadushna** is a combination of equal proportions of six hot spice powders. The formula consists of Pippali (long pepper fruit), *Piper longum* root (long pepper root), Chavya (*Piper cubeba*), Chitraka (leadwort/*Plumbago zeylanica*), Shunthi (dried ginger/*Zingiber officinale*), and black pepper. This spice mix has properties like the Panchkola. The mixture of these gut-friendly herbs is indicated in severely diminished Agni or increased Kapha in the digestive system. Increased abnormal Kapha symptoms match with the dysbiosis or abnormal growth of unfavorable bacteria in the gut. The combination may correct the dysbiosis with its hot properties and enzymatic stimulation for gut immunity.

**Ashtvarga** is called **Hingawshatka powder** and is one of the most widely used combinations by Ayurveda practitioners for the correction of gut health in digestive system diseases, psychological conditions, joint disorders, obesity, and chronic inflammatory conditions.

Ashtvarga is a combination of eight spices Shunthi (dry ginger), Maricha (black pepper), Pippali (long pepper), Ajamoda (carom seeds), Saindhava (rock salt), Jeeraka (cumin), Krishn Jeeraka (black cumin), and Shuddha Hingu (asafoetida). It is mainly used for problems related to indigestion (gas, constipation, loose motions, hiccups). It helps increase the absorption of nutrients and reduce cramps and bloating. It's great for loss of appetite, low metabolism, and obesity. It relieves breathlessness and pressure on the chest in asthma and bronchitis. Regular consumption in small quantities increases metabolic rate and corrects digestion. Interestingly, the powder is indicated a few minutes prior to the meal with ghee. The application of this mix may stimulate the digestive enzymes and favors the gut microbiome

## 11.15 Efficacy of Traditional and Ayurvedic Functional Food in Gut Health

Probiotics are not a brainchild of modern pharmacology but have existed in traditional foods for an age. Due to ignorance of a correct lifestyle, there is an increased demand for functional foods which will gain optimum nutritional balance and also provide added health benefits. For a diverse food culture consisting in a variety of fruits and vegetables, and in some unique cooking processes, every season has a potent availability of functional foods. Fermented foods are a favorable version of probiotic potential. The therapeutic solutions of probiotics available in the market are mostly in concentrated form and devoid of the synergic association of food substances like herbs, spices, vegetables, or fruit. The science behind traditional cooking is an excellent example of functional foods which are able to provide taste, balanced nutrition, prebiotic impressions, and probiotic effects all in one dish. Ayurveda dietetics are aimed at holistic gut health through the correct food items and cooking processes. The area holds tremendous opportunity in the functional food and nutraceutical market.

It is an established fact that probiotics alone have their limitations, and they are effective unidirectionally to increase the number of gut microbiome. Gut health should not be confused with only gut bacteria. The holistic approach to gut health will be receptive to gut mucosa, active appetite (Agni), and favorable gut microbiome. To maintain or modulate the gut health, Ayurvedic herbs and nutraceuticals constantly ensure the symbiosis in keeping these segments aligned. The herbs when combined with probiotics show promising results compared to the use of only probiotics. Herbs like Deepana, Pachana, and Anulomana can regulate bacterial colonization, improve micro digestion, and help nourish the gut microbiome. The ambiguities of sole probiotics use like indigestion, nausea, bacterial infections, and dysbiosis due to incorrect probiotic consumption are well prevented with Ayurvedic nutraceuticals. Traditional cuisine is a rich source of such nutraceutical probiotics and prebiotics. Cooking spices are an unexplored area in nutraceuticals which holds innumerable possibilities in modifying gut health. The scientific use of cooking spices in many traditional probiotic recipes explains their multidirectional therapeutic role.

The following are some examples of simple traditional probiotics recipes which can be used as nutraceuticals in the modulation of the microbiome through food.

### 11.15.1 Curd Treated with Herbs

The traditional method of curd-setting is very different from probiotic yogurt. Curd and yogurt exhibit different expressions on the gut microbiome. Traditional curd preparation involved boiling of milk, cooling it to room temperature, and inoculating it with a very small portion of sour milk or curd. The blend is gently but thoroughly mixed together and kept in a clean warm place until natural fermentation takes place. The liquid milk curdles to form uniform curd. Ayurveda incorporates medicinal herbs and spices in the making of the curd. A fine powder of herbs like Chitraka (*Plumbago officinalis*), black pepper (*Piper nigrum*), cumin (*Cuminum cyminum*), Haritaki (*Terminalia chebula*), etc. are mixed with the boiling milk and this treated milk is used to set as curd. In some medicinal curds a fine layer of paste of these spices or herbs is applied inside the utensil in which the curd will be set. The association of herbs enhances the original properties of the curd and inhibits the overfermentation. The medicinal attributes of specific herbs/spices enable this probiotic mixture to target the desired anatomical site in the digestive track. For example, curd treated with Deepana herbs will be active in the stomach, Pachana herbs in curd will enable the probiotic mixture to unwind its therapeutic action at the small intestine, and so on.

Curd treated with Chitraka herbs is exclusively Deepana and Pachana and is used to increase the appetite as well as digestive strength in Grahani patients (colitis), where the Agni and digestion is impaired due to dysbiosis or other digestive conditions. The treated curd is used as an adjuvant food to be taken along with Ayurvedic medicine to make it more of a nutraceutical rather than just a food item.

## 11.15.2 Takrarishta: Novel Fermentation of Buttermilk with Herbs and Spices

Takrarishta, a fermented medicament prepared by buttermilk is a classical Ayurvedic formulation mentioned in *Charaka Samhita*. There are abundant references to Takra (buttermilk) in various Ayurvedic classics to manage various health conditions through gut health modulation.[26] Takrarishta, containing Go (cow) milk-derived buttermilk (75% curd and 25% water), Amla (*Embelica officinalis*), Haritaki (*Terminalia chebula* Retz.), Maricha (*Piper nigrum* Linn.), and Ajowan (*Carum copticum* Hirem), along with minerals, namely Sauvarcala, Saindhava, Bida, Audbhida, and Samudra (rock salt and sea salts) has satisfactorily shown its antimicrobial efficacy against some dysbiosis-causing bacterial species.[27] This formulation is prescribed in gut health generated conditions like hemorrhoids, worm infestation, loss of appetite, irritable bowel syndrome, and abdominal disorders including diarrhea.

## 11.15.3 Kanji

Kanji is a naturally fermented probiotic traditional drink widely used in summer to improve diminished appetite and restore gut health Lactic acid food fermentation is a delicate process whereby microorganisms and their enzymes are used to convert fermentable sugars in the food substrate into mainly lactic acid and other limited products. Kanji is usually made from dark or black carrots (*Daucus carota*) They are a potential source of anthocyanin pigment and have high antioxidant activity. Kanji is a spontaneous lactic acid fermentation of black carrots with the addition of salt, crushed mustard, and/or red chili powder. Traditionally, this drink is used as a remedial food in indigestion, loss of appetite, and liver disorders. It is prepared and used extensively as an appetizer in the early summer season. The hepatoprotective effect of kanji and its use as a remedial food in the hot harsh summer is being studied. A research study has been conducted to explore the antioxidation and antimicrobial potential of the traditional standard drink Kanji in comparison to commercially fermented probiotic products. The overall consumption by common people of probiotic products available in the market, due to their rosy picture with respect to their therapeutic potential, has increased. The available synthetic probiotics are consumed as wellness supplements without the need for medical supervision. Many studies, on other hand, emphasized that the homemade products are much more beneficial in comparison to market products. It has been detected that probiotic content can be better in homemade Kanji. In addition, Kanji has antioxidant and antimicrobial potential which is not present in market probiotics. Market probiotics lacks nutritional synergy making them susceptible to dysbiosis if not consumed properly or stored in the correct environment. Moreover, they are contraindicated if the host is immunologically weak or already suffering the bacterial infections. The bioactive properties in traditional probiotic food need attention and more research. There is a great need to explore such products in detail to highlight the benefits of traditional homemade drinks to the general public.

Other interesting research studies comparing traditional fermented foods for their probiotic properties highlight the importance of promoting the consumption of traditionally fermented food as probiotics instead of the market products. One study in microbial isolation of the traditional foods Idali batter, Ambil (fermented finger millet flour drink), and plain sheep's milk examines for their LAB (Lactic Acid Bacillus) presence and concentration and shows positive results when compared to the standardized use of functional food for gut dysbiosis.

Homemade Idli batter is made by mixing rice flour and black lentils properly and allowing them to ferment overnight. The sample is obtained for the standard isolation of LABs. Ambil is a fermented food prepared with finger millet flour, water, salt, and buttermilk. Ragi flour was mixed with hot water and salt was added. After thorough mixing, buttermilk was added to the mixture and Ambil was prepared. The sample of prepared Ambil was subjected to the isolation of LABs. Sheep's milk was collected from a dairy and isolation for LABs done. A total of six different isolates were isolated from the Indian fermented food and dairy products. When evaluated, these isolates exhibited similar characteristics of microscopic and biochemical features to the LABs. However, further molecular identification is essential for its species confirmation. These isolates also displayed probiotic properties when evaluated for their pH and salt tolerance. JNEC/ID/01 exhibited maximum pH as well as salt tolerance as compared to the commercial *Lactobacillus* strain, indicating its further utilization in nutraceutical formulations. The concluding results were positive.

## 11.16 Management of Dysbiosis with Nutraceuticals-based Ayurvedic Therapies

Ayurveda advocates to always preserve the Agni to avoid all kinds of health conditions. Elaborate dietetic guidelines in Ayurvedic texts throw light on many factors involved in nutrition and not just balanced food. Aahara Vidhi Vidhanam is an elaborate theory which addresses concerns regarding hygiene, purity of food, cooking processes, utensils used to cook or store the food, and the physical and mental constitution of the person eating the food. Other important parameters are season, compatibility of food combination, properties of food, etc. Dysbiosis is considered as Agni imbalance and is managed by modulation of all the factors which influence the gut and digestion and which will improve the metabolic fire. Correction of Agni through food, herbs, medicine, therapies, or other lifestyle practices such as exercise, sleep, etc. is the holistic way Ayurveda adapts to manage dysbiosis or dysbiosis-related acute or chronic health conditions.

Ayurvedic functional food, phytochemicals, and their metabolic products may inhibit pathogenic bacteria while stimulating the growth of beneficial bacteria, exerting prebiotic-like effects. Therefore, the intestinal microbiota is both a target for nutritional intervention and a factor influencing the biological activity of other food compounds acquired orally or introduced rectally. Basti or probiotic enemas have been suggested to help manage certain neurological disorders. Probiotics that are taken orally need to pass through the complex process of digestion and the small intestine, being inhospitable due to stomach acid and digestive enzymes destroys many of the valuable probiotic bacteria long before they reach the colon. A probiotic enema, however, provides an almost immediate route to the colon, where most of the gut bacteria are active in number and functions.

The Ayurvedic term for enema is basti, and basti is a much-appreciated type of panchakarma which cleanses the colon mucosa, improve microcirculation in gut mucosa, extracts impurities, and promotes health and longevity. There are multiple types of basti according to the target results. Some basti are mucosa-lubricating, which kindles the gut microbiota gently, and a few are strong and are meant to extract the Ama out of the gut. Basti are known to improve microcirculation within the large intestine, extract the hard fecal matter stuck to the colon, reduce intestinal parasites, and relieve chronic constipation. Basti can facilitate micronutrient absorption in the gut. The bastis are made up of ingredients such as sesame oil, medicated ghee, buttermilk, many different combinations of herbs, and, in special cases, bone broth. Rock salt, honey, and a few herbal ground pastes are common in all types of basti.

Honey and rock salt have a positive influence on gut microbiome and selected herbs are medicinal and many of them exhibit a prebiotic nature. Vital nutrients and herbs are absorbed through gut mucosa due to the fat-soluble nature of many vitamins. A few studies also state that sesame oil has a positive effect on colon cells, and on certain beneficial bacteria.[28]

In a more recent study, the metabolomic profile was taken after a six-day panchakarma treatment. The experimental group consisted of healthy male and female subjects whose treatment program included herbs, vegetarian diet, meditation, yoga, and massage. The results showed that 12 plasma phosphatidylcholines decreased after treatment in the experimental group as compared to the control group of 54 subjects. There were changes in metabolites across many pathways such as phospholipid biosynthesis, choline metabolism, and lipoprotein metabolism, with statistically significant changes in the plasma levels of phosphatidylcholines, sphingomyelins, and others in just six days. It is unclear whether the lipid metabolites were modulated by the gut microbiome or by the external agents such as herbs, vegetarian diet, meditation, yoga, and massage. The study of panchakarma and other Ayurvedic purification treatments is an important area of future research. It would also be useful to compare the modern use of fecal transplant treatment with all the different types of basti treatments.

## 11.17 The Future of Ayurveda Nutraceuticals in Therapeutic Gut Modulation

The health sector and its related research are witnessing a transitional moment in medicine (see Figure 11.3). New studies are emerging that will help medicinal science make better choices. The field of integrative medicine represents an important accomplishment since it combines the best of modern medicine with the best of a traditional system of natural health like Ayurveda. Integrative medicine benefits greatly from research on the microbiome because it helps us better understand the ancient practices of Ayurveda in the light of modern science.[29] Diet and lifestyle protocols are closely related to epigenetics and need the urgent attention of physicians, researchers, and pharmacists to address the benefits of good diet and the importance of Ayurvedic concepts such as Dincharya and Rutucharya, personal awareness regarding Prakriti Agni and one's own gut microbiota profile. Traditional cuisine and its nutraceutical implement can be embraced by the future scope in the revolution of food science and the global food-processing market. The organic market is touching the sky and Ayurvedic nutraceuticals for gut health may open abundant avenues for revenue. The current limitation in the management of chronic, metabolic, and noncommunicable disorders is an area where researchers, scholar students, and physicians practicing integrative medicine can contribute in terms of novel research

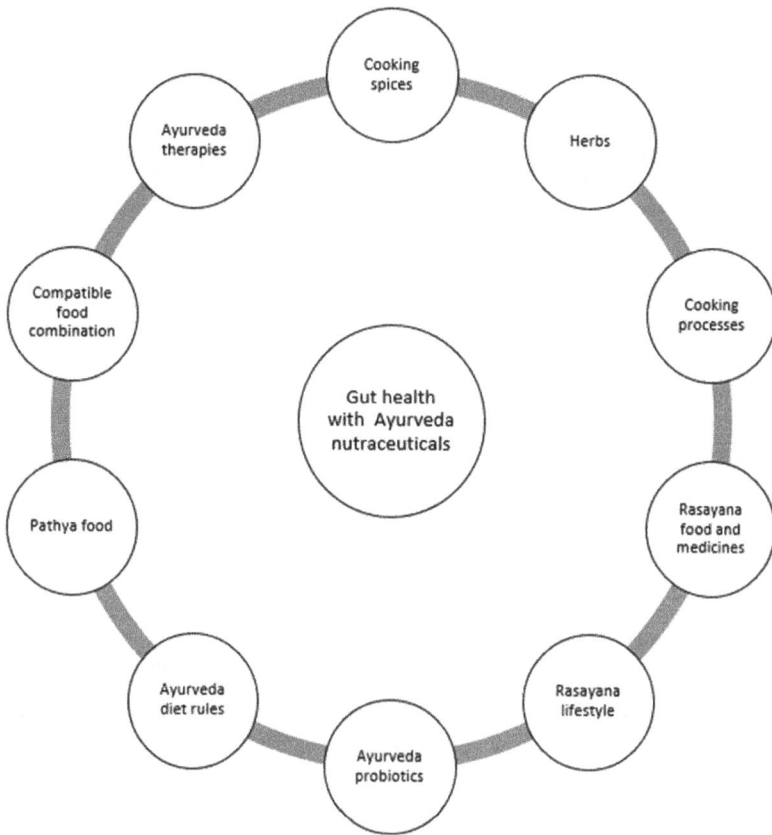

**Figure 11.3** *Holistic application of Ayurvedic nutraceuticals for gut modulation.*

ideas and products for the restoration of gut health more organically without compromising other health-related factors. Practicing as a nutritionist integrating modern nutrition and Ayurvedic wisdom with practical solutions for gut health could be a flourishing career option in the near future. Overall, Ayurvedic nutraceuticals is a broad-spectrum area of research and practice for addressing the giant market of noncommunicable diseases, including the steep surge of psychological disorders, in offering holistic noncompromising solutions through gut health modulation

# References

1. https://www.ncbi.nlm.nih.gov/pmc/articles/PMC7210818/#ref9
2. https://www.ncbi.nlm.nih.gov/pmc/articles/PMC7210818/#ref7
3. https://www.ncbi.nlm.nih.gov/pmc/articles/PMC7559905/#B13-medicina-56-00462
4. Conlon M.A., Bird A.R. The Impact of Diet and Lifestyle on Gut Microbiota and Human Health. *Nutrients.* 2015; 7(1):17–44. doi: 10.3390/nu7010017

5. Charaka Samhita Sutrasthana, 27Annapana Vidhi adhyaya, Sri Satyanarayana Shastri, Chaukhambha Bharati Academy, Varanasi, India.
6. *Food Guru: Your Guide to Eating Right*, Neemtree Publication, Pune India. Dr. Rupali Panse.
7. https://www.ncbi.nlm.nih.gov/pmc/articles/PMC4566439/
8. https://bmcmicrobiol.biomedcentral.com/articles/10.1186/s12866-018-1304-7#ref-CR2
9. https://bmcmicrobiol.biomedcentral.com/articles/10.1186/s12866-018-1304-7#ref-CR8
10. https://bmcmicrobiol.biomedcentral.com/articles/10.1186/s12866-018-1304-7#ref-CR9
11. https://www.ncbi.nlm.nih.gov/pmc/articles/PMC7210818/#ref16
12. https://www.ncbi.nlm.nih.gov/pmc/articles/PMC7210818/#ref18
13. https://www.ncbi.nlm.nih.gov/pmc/articles/PMC7210818/#ref30
14. https://www.ncbi.nlm.nih.gov/pmc/articles/PMC7210818/#ref31
15. Nutraceuticals for aging and antiaging, Publication: CRC Publication, USA, Nutritional psychiatry as basis of development of nutraceutical development for mental illness in aging population, Editors: Dr. Yashwant Pathak/Dr. Jayant Lokhande. Author: Dr. Rupali Panse.
16. https://www.tandfonline.com/doi/abs/10.1517/14740338.2014.872627; https://www.sciencedirect.com/science/article/pii/S0753332218345657
17. Sharangadhara Samhita Purvakhanda 04/01.
18. Ashtanga Hrudayam, Nidana Sthana 12/1.
19. https://www.carakasamhitaonline.com/index.php/Deepana#cite_note-6
20. Charaka Samhita, Chikitsa Sthana 15/201, Chaukhambha Bharati Academy, Author: Shri Satyanarayana Shastri.
21. Sushruta Samhita, Sutra Sthana 41/6.
22. https://www.carakasamhitaonline.com/index.php/Deepana#cite_note-Susruta-4
23. Ashtanga Hrudayam, Sutra Sthana 2/16.
24. https://www.carakasamhitaonline.com/index.php/Pachana#cite_note-Shargadara-3
25. https://www.ift.org/news-and-publications/news/2017/july/07/certain-spices-may-display-prebiotic-activity
26. Charaka Samhita, Chikitsa Sthana Chapter 14 and Chapter 15 Publication: Chaukhambha Bharati Academy, Author: Shri Satyanarayana Shastri.
27. https://www.researchgate.net/publication/228666429_In-vitro_antibacterial_activity_of_takrarishta-an_Ayurvedic_formulation
28. https://www.ncbi.nlm.nih.gov/pmc/articles/PMC7559905/#B93-medicina-56-00462
29. https://www.ncbi.nlm.nih.gov/pmc/articles/PMC7559905/#B110-medicina-56-00462

# 12

# Stress Disorder and Gut Microbiota

Triveni Shelke, Sushama Talegaonkar, and Monalisa Mishra

## Contents

## 12.1 Introduction

Stress is a common experience among the human population and can be caused by a wide variety of factors, such as work or financial pressures, relationship problems, health issues, and traumatic events. Long-term stress can have negative effects on both physical and mental health, and can lead to conditions such as depression, anxiety, and heart disease. Henceforth, it is important for individuals to find healthy ways to manage stress, such as through exercise, meditation, therapy, and social support. It is estimated that a significant proportion of the population is affected by stress and related mental health conditions (Hart & Kamm, 2002). According to the World Health Organization (WHO), an estimated 264 million people of all ages suffer from depression, and an estimated one in 13 globally develops anxiety disorders. Stress can also be a contributing factor to other mental health conditions such as post-traumatic stress disorder, obsessive-compulsive disorder, phobias, bipolar disorder, and schizophrenia.

The gut microbiota, also known as gut flora or gut microbiome, refers to the collection of microorganisms that live in the digestive tract. These microorganisms play an important role in maintaining overall health and well-being. First, the gut microbiota plays a critical role in digestion and metabolism by

DOI: 10.1201/9781003333821-12

213

breaking down food and absorbing nutrients. It also helps to protect the gut from harmful pathogens and maintain the integrity of the gut lining. Second, the gut microbiota is also thought to play a role in the development and function of the immune system. Studies have shown that a diverse and healthy gut microbiome can help to improve immune function and reduce the risk of infection and inflammation. Third, the gut microbiome has also been linked to mental health. Studies have shown that the gut microbiome can affect the production of neurotransmitters such as serotonin, which play a role in mood regulation. A healthy gut microbiome may also reduce the risk of developing conditions such as depression, anxiety, and autism (Cryan & Dinan, 2012). Finally, the gut microbiome has also been associated with various other health conditions such as obesity, type 2 diabetes, autoimmune diseases, and allergies. Overall, gut microbiota plays a crucial role in maintaining health and well-being, and a healthy gut microbiome is important for overall health (Cici, 2016).

Diet plays a crucial role in shaping the composition and diversity of the gut microbiota. Research has shown that a diet high in fruits, vegetables, whole grains, and fermented foods can promote a healthy gut microbiome, while a diet high in processed foods, sugar, and saturated fats can have a negative impact on the gut microbiome (Larroya-García et al., 2019). Fiber is an essential nutrient that helps to feed the healthy bacteria in the gut, and a diet rich in fruits, vegetables, and whole grains can provide a good source of fiber. Fermented foods like yogurt, kefir, kimchi, and sauerkraut also provide beneficial bacteria that can help to improve gut health. On the other hand, a diet high in processed foods, sugar, and saturated fats has been linked to an increase in harmful bacteria and a decrease in beneficial bacteria. This can lead to a disruption of the gut microbiome, which is associated with a number of health problems such as obesity, type 2 diabetes, and inflammatory bowel disease (Costabile et al., 2022). Additionally, recent research suggests that a Mediterranean diet, rich in fruits, vegetables, whole grains, nuts, and fish, has a positive impact on gut microbiome. This diet is associated with a lower risk of chronic diseases, such as cardiovascular disease and type 2 diabetes (Merra et al., 2022).

The chapter discusses the effects of stress on the important gut microbiota. This would enable concluding about the relation between different stress disorders and the disturbed microbiota. It would contribute significantly in the gut microbiota research with respect to anxiety and depression distress (Figure 12.1).

## 12.2  Stress and Types

Stress corresponds to the nonspecific behavioral, physical, and biochemical changes in the body that seldom has the role of a pituitary secretion called the adeno-corticotrophic hormone (ACTH). It can be a whole-body response

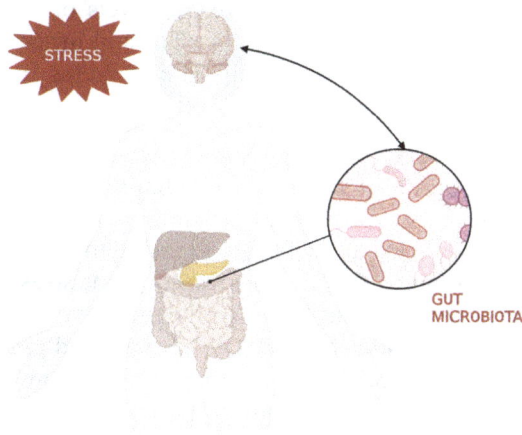

*Figure 12.1* Stress and gut microbiota correlation.

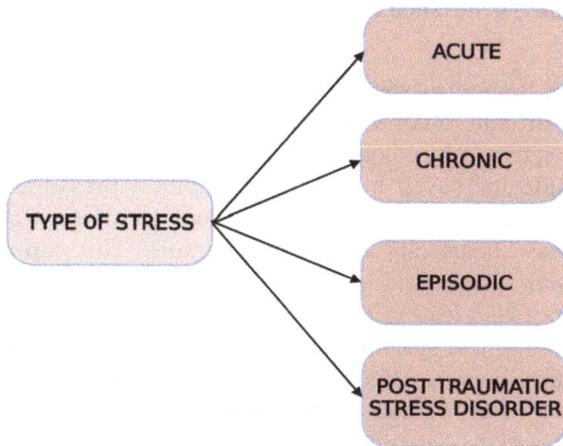

*Figure 12.2* Major types of stress.

(systemic) or a local body part specific (topical) response. Stress can be categorized into acute, acute episodic, chronic, post-traumatic stress disorder, and eustress (Figure 12.2). Acute stress is an initial response towards traumatic events. It is seldom associated with reduced cortisol levels and memory impairment. Acute stress is the most common type of stress and is typically caused by a specific event or situation, such as a job interview or public speaking engagement. This condition persists for around 28 days with symptoms like hyperarousal, intrusions, and avoiding work (Koopman et al., 1998). Tissues respond to stressful conditions when mediated by higher glucocorticoid secretions which can be manifested by the decrease in corticosteroid-binding globulins (Breuner et al., 2006). Lipid peroxidation fastens in the heart, stomach, and liver due to oxidative stress (Kovács et al., 1996). At the inflammation front, there is an increase in the levels of monocytes, neutrophils, and C-reactive protein along with IL (interleukin)-6 in the circulation (Miller et al., 2005). Cognitive behavioral therapy helps in managing acute symptoms of stress (Bryant et al., 2008).

Episodic acute stress occurs when a person experiences multiple instances of acute stress in a short period of time. This can happen when a person is dealing with a number of stressful events or situations at the same time, such as a job loss, a move to a new city, and a family illness. This can be overwhelming and can cause the person to feel a sense of constant stress, with little time to recover between events. It can have similar negative effects on the body as chronic stress, such as increased heart rate and blood pressure, weakened immune system, digestive problems, sleeping problems, anxiety and depression, musculoskeletal problems, and hormonal imbalances (Kuti et al., 2020; Lepore et al., 1997). Additionally, it could lead to a condition called Acute Stress Disorder (ASD), which is a severe emotional reaction that can happen within the first month after a traumatic event. It is characterized by symptoms such as flashbacks, avoidance behaviors, and emotional numbing (Harvey & Bryant, 2002).

Chronic stress is long-term stress that is caused by ongoing events or situations, such as a difficult job or a troubled relationship. Chronic stress can have a number of negative physiological impacts on the body (Checkley, 1996). These can include increased heart rate and blood pressure: chronic stress can cause the release of stress hormones, such as cortisol and adrenaline, which can increase heart rate and blood pressure. This can put a strain on the cardiovascular system and increase the risk of heart disease and stroke. Chronic stress can also lead to a weakened immune system: stress hormones can suppress the immune system, making it more difficult for the body to fight off infections and illnesses. Digestive problems like stress can cause changes in the digestive system, leading to symptoms such as abdominal pain, diarrhea, and constipation. Sleeping problems can interfere with the ability to fall asleep and stay asleep, leading to fatigue and insomnia (Brosschot, 2010). Chronic stress can contribute to the development of mental health conditions such as anxiety and depression (Brosschot, 2010; McEwen, 2017). It can also lead to musculoskeletal problems like muscle tension and pain, headaches, and other types of pain in the body, as well as imbalances in hormones such as insulin, which can increase the risk of diabetes and other metabolic disorders (McEwen, 2008).

Additionally, there is also post-traumatic stress disorder (PTSD) which is a type of stress that can develop after a person experiences or witnesses a traumatic event. PTSD can cause changes in the levels of stress hormones such as cortisol and adrenaline, which can lead to a number of physical symptoms, including fatigue, poor sleep, and a weakened immune system. It has been linked to an increased risk of heart disease and stroke (Barroca et al., 2022). The stress hormones released in response to traumatic events can cause changes in heart rate and blood pressure, and can also contribute to the development of plaque in the arteries. It can cause changes in breathing patterns, leading to symptoms such as shortness of breath and chest tightness and lead to an increased risk of substance abuse and addiction, as some people may use drugs or alcohol as a way to cope with their symptoms (Paulus et al., 2013).

## 12.3 Gut Microbiota

A healthy gut microbiota is important for maintaining a healthy host and is the collection of microorganisms that live in the digestive tract of humans. These microorganisms, including bacteria, viruses, and fungi, play a crucial role in maintaining the health of the host. They aid in the digestion of food, the synthesis of vitamins, and the regulation of the immune system. Imbalances in the gut microbiota, known as dysbiosis, have been linked to a variety of health conditions, including obesity, inflammatory bowel disease, and mental health disorders. (Schwiertz, 2016). The pro-inflammatory state caused by alteration of the gut microbiota balance leads to the onset of many diseases ranging from gastrointestinal and metabolic conditions to immunological and neuropsychiatric diseases (Gomaa, 2020).

There are many different types of bacteria that live in the human gut. A microarray method was developed for the detection of 40 bacterial species reported in the literature to be predominant in the human gastrointestinal tract (Gomaa, 2020). Some of the most common microbes include *Firmicutes*. This phylum includes many different types of bacteria, such as Bacillus and Clostridium. These bacteria are known to break down complex carbohydrates, such as fibers, that the host is unable to digest. *Bacteroidetes* is the other phylum which is known to break down proteins and simple sugars. *Actinobacteria* include the genus *Bifidobacterium* and *Streptococcus*, which are known for their role in maintaining the health of the gut. *Proteobacteria* include the *Escherichia coli* and *Salmonella* genus, which are known to cause infections. *Verrucomicrobia* include *Akkermansia muciniphila*, which is associated with a healthy gut and metabolic health (Wang et al., 2004) (Figure 12.3).

The autochthonous component of the intestinal microbiota is expected to provide crucial information on how to develop therapies for various gastrointestinal diseases (Ventura et al., 2009). Probiotics are live microorganisms that, when administered in adequate amounts, provide a health benefit to the host. Probiotics are used to restore or maintain the balance of the gut microbiota and can be found in food products such as yogurt and fermented foods (Schwiertz, 2016). Prebiotics are nondigestible carbohydrates that stimulate the growth or activity of beneficial microorganisms in the gut. They are usually fibers and are found in food such as artichokes, garlic, leeks, onion, and asparagus. Synbiotics are a combination of probiotics and prebiotics. They act

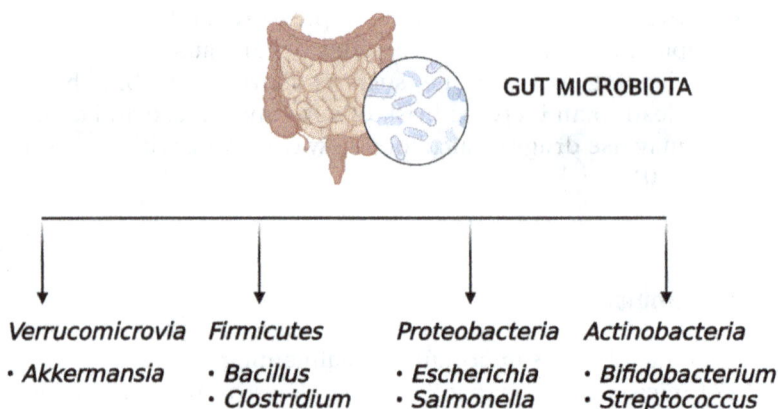

GUT MICROBIOTA

| Verrucomicrovia | Firmicutes | Proteobacteria | Actinobacteria |
| --- | --- | --- | --- |
| · Akkermansia | · Bacillus | · Escherichia | · Bifidobacterium |
| | · Clostridium | · Salmonella | · Streptococcus |

**Figure 12.3** *Common gut microbiota in humans.*

together to help the growth of beneficial bacteria and also provide the food source for those bacteria (Roberfroid, 2007). Fecal Microbiota Transplantation (FMT) is a procedure in which the feces of a healthy donor are transplanted into the colon of a patient with a gut microbiome-associated disorder. FMT has been found to be effective in treating recurrent *Clostridium difficile* infections and is also being studied as a potential treatment for other conditions such as inflammatory bowel disease (IBD), metabolic syndrome, and even autism (Cohen & Maharshak, 2017).

Low-abundant microorganisms can impact the dysbiotic signature of local microbial habitats (Cena et al., 2021). Gut dysbiosis is a condition characterized by an imbalance in the composition and/or function of the gut microbiota. This can occur as a result of a variety of factors such as poor diet, stress, antibiotics, and certain medical conditions. When gut dysbiosis occurs, the balance between beneficial and harmful bacteria is disrupted, which can lead to a wide range of health problems (Cohen & Maharshak, 2017; Kriss et al., 2018). Treatment for gut dysbiosis typically involves a combination of dietary changes, probiotics, and prebiotics, and in some cases, antibiotics or other medications may be needed. Gastrointestinal symptoms include diarrhea, constipation, bloating, and abdominal pain, immune dysfunction, such as allergies or autoimmune disease, skin conditions such as eczema or acne, fatigue, depression, or anxiety (Brüssow, 2020).

Diet composition and nutritional status are among the most critical modifiable factors of the gut microbiota ecosystem (Larroya-García et al., 2019). The types and amounts of food that we consume can have a significant impact on the gut microbiome. A diet high in processed foods and low in fruits, vegetables, and fibers can lead to gut dysbiosis, while a diet high in these foods can promote a healthy gut microbiome (De Angelis et al., 2019). Antibiotics can disrupt the balance of the gut microbiome by killing off beneficial bacteria along with harmful bacteria. This can lead to gut dysbiosis and increase the risk of infections and other health problems (Lange et al., 2016). The gut microbiome changes as we age, and the composition of the gut microbiome in older adults is different from that of younger adults. This can lead to an increased risk of certain health problems. Chronic stress can disrupt the gut microbiome by altering the gut–brain axis and the immune system. This can lead to gut dysbiosis and increase the risk of certain health problems (Kriss et al., 2018; Lange et al., 2016).

## 12.4 Gut Microbiota in Neurological Disorders

The gut microbiota has been found to play a role in the development and progression of certain neurological disorders. Research suggests that the gut–brain axis, which is the communication between the gut and the brain through the immune system, the enteric nervous system may be disrupted in these disorders (Kriss et al., 2018; Lange et al., 2016; Larroya-García et al., 2019).

Autism Spectrum Disorder (ASD) patients have a different gut microbiome compared to healthy individuals. There are indications that gut dysbiosis may contribute to the development of autism by affecting the immune system and the production of neurotransmitters. Bacterial species belonging to the *Clostridium* and *Sutterella* genus are involved in toxin production and metabolic distress is the clinical manifestation (Ding et al., 2017). Strati et al. reported that the relative abundance of the fungal genus Candida was more than double in the autistic than the neurotypical subjects (Strati et al., 2017). Fecal microbiota transplant could transform the dysbiotic gut microbiome towards a healthy one in children with autism spectrum disorders, this is called microbiota transfer therapy (Kang et al., 2019).

Studies have found that individuals with anxiety and depression have a different gut microbiome compared to healthy individuals. There are indications that gut dysbiosis may contribute to the development of these disorders by affecting the production of neurotransmitters such as serotonin. Simpson et al., stated that there is a high difference in the abundance of pro-inflammatory bacterial species like *Enterobacteriaceae* and *Desulfovibrio*, as well as the short fatty acid synthesizing bacteria *Faecalibacterium* (Simpson et al., 2021). Parkinson's disease leads to different gut microbiomes compared to healthy individuals. There are indications that gut dysbiosis may contribute to the development of Parkinson's disease by affecting the immune system and the production of dopamine (Huang & Wu, 2021; Larroya-García et al., 2019; Simpson et al., 2021). The microbes affect the neurotransmitters and hence their balance is important for neurotransmission in order to avoid neurological disorders like Parkinson's and Alzheimer's disease.

Neuropsychiatric disorders like schizophrenia and bipolar show evidence of disturbed microbiota in the gut (Mangiola, 2016). Gut microbiota alterations are widely observed in patients with schizophrenia (Samochowiec & Misiak, 2021). The gut microbiota and epigenetic mechanisms are factors that are

**Table 12.1** List of Bacteria Dominant in the Neurological Stress Disorders

| Disorder | Gut Microbiota | Reference |
|---|---|---|
| Autism Spectrum Disorder | *Clostridium, Sutterella* | (Ding et al., 2017) |
| Anxiety | *Enterobacteriaceae, Desulfovibrio, Faecalibacterium* | (Simpson et al., 2021) |
| Parkinson's | *Lactobacillus, Akkermansia, Bifidobacterium* | (Romano et al., 2021) |
| Schizophrenia | *Megasphaera, Clostridium, Klebsiella* | (Shen et al., 2018) |

currently being considered to better understand another dimension of schizophrenia (Rodrigues-Amorim et al., 2018). Glutamate synthase was more active in the guts of patients with schizophrenia and it was associated with altered gut microbiota taxonomies along with gut IgA (immunoglobulin A) levels (Xu et al., 2020). An imbalance in the microflora of the gut depletes neurotoxins as well as inflammatory mediators which leads to synaptic and neuronal damage promoting schizophrenia (Yuan et al., 2019). The relative abundance of *Succinivibrio*, *Megasphaera*, *Collinsella*, *Clostridium*, *Klebsiella*, and *Methanobrevibacter* in schizophrenia patients was significantly higher compared to health controls (Shen et al., 2018). Dietary, pro- and prebiotic interventions are potential adjuvant therapies for use in the management of mood disorders such as bipolar disorder (Gondalia et al., 2019) (Table 12.1).

## 12.5 Correlation of Stress and Microbiota

There is increasing evidence that stress can affect the composition and function of the gut microbiome, which can in turn impact various physiological processes, including immune function, nutrient metabolism, and mental health. Studies have shown that chronic stress can lead to changes in the gut microbiome, including reductions in beneficial bacteria and increases in pro-inflammatory species (Cryan & Dinan, 2012). Additionally, stress-induced changes in the gut microbiome may contribute to the development of stress-related disorders such as anxiety and depression. However, more research is needed to fully understand the relationship between stress and the gut microbiome and to determine the best ways to manipulate the microbiome to mitigate the effects of stress.

Stress can affect the gut microbiome in a number of ways, which include slowing down or speeding up the movement of food through the gut, which can affect the amount of time that bacteria have to ferment and digest food. Stress can increase the permeability of the gut lining, allowing bacteria and other toxins to enter the bloodstream. This can lead to inflammation and other immune responses. Stress can cause changes in the levels of hormones such as cortisol and adrenaline, which can affect the growth and metabolism of gut bacteria (Dinan & Cryan, 2012). Stress can decrease the number of beneficial bacteria in the gut microbiome, such as *Bifidobacterium* and

*Lactobacillus*, which can lead to an overgrowth of harmful bacteria. Stress can increase the number of pro-inflammatory bacteria in the gut microbiome, such as *Escherichia coli* and *Proteobacteria*, which can contribute to inflammation and other health problems (González Olmo et al., 2021).

Stress can have a negative impact on beneficial gut microbiota. Studies have shown that chronic stress can lead to a decrease in the number of beneficial bacteria in the gut microbiome, such as *Bifidobacterium* and *Lactobacillus*. *Bifidobacterium* and *Lactobacillus* are considered to be beneficial bacteria because they help to maintain a healthy balance of gut microbiome and have been associated with various health benefits, such as improved digestion and nutrient absorption, stronger immune function, and reduced risk of certain illnesses (Tetel et al., 2018). When the number of these beneficial bacteria decreases, it can lead to an overgrowth of harmful bacteria, which can contribute to inflammation, gut permeability, and other health problems. Stress-induced changes in the gut microbiome may also contribute to the development of stress-related disorders such as anxiety and depression (Madison & Kiecolt-Glaser, 2019).

## 12.6 Study Models for Assessing Change in Gut Microbiota

Studying stress *in vivo*, or in living organisms, is necessary as it allows for the examination of the complex interactions between the various physiological and behavioral systems that are involved in the stress response. *In vivo* studies can provide a more complete understanding of the stress response than *in vitro* studies, which only examine isolated cells or tissues. They allow for the examination of the effects of stress on the whole organism, rather than just on a single system or tissue. This is important because stress can have a wide range of effects on different parts of the body, such as the immune system, cardiovascular system, and nervous system. They allow for the examination of the effects of stress in the context of the organism's natural environment (Madison & Kiecolt-Glaser, 2019; Pearce et al., 2018). *In vivo* studies can provide information about how stress affects an organism in its natural habitat, which may not be possible to replicate in an artificial laboratory setting. They allow for the examination of the effects of stress over time. *In vivo* studies can be used to examine the long term effects of stress on an organism, which is important for understanding the development of stress-related disorders such as depression and anxiety. They allow for the examination of the potential therapeutic effects of drugs or other interventions on stress-related disorders, as it's important to evaluate the drug efficacy in the organism's natural environment (Hart & Kamm, 2002).

There are several model organisms that are commonly used to study stress in biology and physiology research, for example zebra fish are a popular model organism in stress research due to their genetic similarity to humans and their ease of use in laboratory settings. They are also transparent, which makes it easy to observe changes in physiology and behavior after stress (Steenbergen et al., 2011). The zebra fish model can be used for developing probiotics for xenobiotic detoxification and resistance against bacterial infection (Davis et al., 2016; Zhong et al., 2022). Fruit flies are widely used in genetics and neuroscience research, and have been used to study the genetic and neural mechanisms underlying stress response. The gut microbiota of *Drosophila* is linked to several physiological processes and disease development in mammals (Chiang et al., 2022; Sahu et al., 2022). *C. elegans* is a nematode worm that is commonly used as a model organism in aging and stress research. It has a simple nervous system and a short life span, making it a useful model for studying the effects of stress on aging and longevity (Hart & Kamm, 2002; Rodriguez et al., 2013). Rodents (mice and rats are widely used in stress research due to their genetic and physiological similarity to humans, as well as their availability and ease of handling in laboratory settings (Tengeler et al., 2020).

Unpredictable chronic stress in zebra fish is an adequate model to preclinical stress studies (Piato et al., 2011). (Demin et al., 2021) has shown aspects of neurogenesis, neuroprotection, and neuro-immune responses upon chronic and acute stress in zebra fish. Acute psychological stress markedly impaired spatial and cued memory in a zebra fish plus-maze test (Gaikwad et al., 2011). Acute alarm pheromone and acute caffeine produced robust anxiogenic effects in zebra fish tested in the novel tank diving test (Egan et al., 2009). High-throughput automated tracking systems make possible behavioral readouts of the stress response in zebra fish. These can be used to study behavioral genetics in the zebra fish (Clark et al., 2011). Zebra fish when treated with pentylenetetrazol showed an effect on their natural shoaling and variation in behavior that led to increased stress (Pagnussat et al., 2013). The absence of a microbiota dramatically altered locomotor and anxiety-related behavior in germ-free zebra fish larvae (Davis et al., 2016).

The *Drosophila* hematopoietic system uses developmental signals not only for hematopoiesis but also as sensors for stress and environmental changes to elicit necessary blood responses (Shim, 2015). Changes in neural plasticity are critical components of the homeostatic response to stress (Neckameyer & Nieto-Romero, 2015). Stress-inducing diets in *Drosophila* showed that female flies on a high-fat diet show increased triglyceride levels in normoxia, intermittent hypoxia, and constant hypoxia (Heinrichsen & Haddad, 2012). The associated microbes appear to display a variety of effects beneficial for the worm (Zhang et al., 2017). Stressor exposure significantly affects bacterial populations in the intestines (Bailey et al., 2011). Probiotic administration increased IgA producing cells and CD4+ cells in the lamina propria of the small intestine (Palomar et al., 2014). Male mice were more vulnerable to the anxiogenic effects of the high-fat diet stress (Bridgewater et al., 2017). Stressor exposure can disrupt the stability of the intestinal microbiota leading to increased colonization of *Citrobacter rodentium* (Bailey et al., 2010). Rifaximin treatment alleviates stress-induced local pathologies in chronically stressed mice (Kuti et al., 2020).

## 12.7 Conclusion

In conclusion, the current chapter has discussed that there is a clear link between stress disorders and the gut microbiota. Individuals with stress disorders have a distinct composition of gut microbes compared to those without stress disorders, which is linked to changes in gut permeability, inflammation, and immune function. Research also suggests that the gut microbiome may play a role in the development and maintenance of stress disorders, and that changes in the gut microbiome can affect the effectiveness of stress and anxiety treatments. However, more research is needed to fully understand the complex relationship between stress disorders and the gut microbiome, and to develop potential therapeutic interventions targeting the gut microbiome for stress disorders. Overall, the studies suggest that targeting the gut microbiome may be a viable therapeutic approach for stress disorders and could have a positive impact on mental health.

## References

Acute stress, memory, attention and cortisol. (2000). *Psychoneuroendocrinology, 25*(6), 535–549.

Bailey, M. T., Dowd, S. E., Galley, J. D., Hufnagle, A. R., Allen, R. G., & Lyte, M. (2011). Exposure to a social stressor alters the structure of the intestinal microbiota: Implications for stressor-induced immunomodulation. Brain, Behavior, and Immunity, 25(3), 397–407.

Bailey, M. T., Dowd, S. E., Parry, N. M. A., Galley, J. D., Schauer, D. B., & Lyte, M. (2010). Stressor exposure disrupts commensal microbial populations in the intestines and leads to increased colonization by *Citrobacter rodentium*. Infection and Immunity, 78(4), 1509–1519.

Barroca, I., Velosa, A., Cotovio, G., Santos, C. M., Riggi, G., Costa, R. P., Macieira, J., Machado, L. S., Simões, D. S., Pereira, P. A., Pinto, I., & Carvalho, P. S. (2022). Translation and validation of the clinician administered PTSD scale (CAPS-CA-5) for Portuguese children and adolescents. Acta Medica Portuguesa, 35(9), 652–662.

Breuner, C. W., Lynn, S. E., Julian, G. E., Cornelius, J. M., Heidinger, B. J., Love, O. P., Sprague, R. S., Wada, H., & Whitman, B. A. (2006). Plasma-binding globulins and acute stress response. Hormone and Metabolic Research = Hormon- Und Stoffwechselforschung = Hormones etMetabolisme, 38(4), 260–268.

Bridgewater, L. C., Zhang, C., Wu, Y., Hu, W., Zhang, Q., Wang, J., Li, S., & Zhao, L. (2017). Gender-based differences in host behavior and gut microbiota composition in response to high fat diet and stress in a mouse model. Scientific Reports, 7(1). https://doi.org/10.1038/s41598-017-11069-4.

Brosschot, J. F. (2010). Markers of chronic stress: Prolonged physiological activation and (un)conscious perseverative cognition. Neuroscience and Biobehavioral Reviews, 35(1), 46–50.

Brüssow, H. (2020). Problems with the concept of gut microbiota dysbiosis. Microbial Biotechnology, 13(2), 423–434.

Bryant, R. A., Mastrodomenico, J., Felmingham, K. L., Hopwood, S., Kenny, L., Kandris, E., Cahill, C., & Creamer, M. (2008). Treatment of acute stress disorder: A randomized controlled trial. *Archives of General Psychiatry, 65*(6), 659–667.

Cena, J. A. de, de Cena, J. A., Zhang, J., Deng, D., Damé-Teixeira, N., & Do, T. (2021). Low-abundant microorganisms: The human microbiome's dark matter, a scoping review. Frontiers in Cellular and Infection Microbiology, 11. https://doi.org/10.3389/fcimb.2021.689197.

Checkley, S. (1996). The neuroendocrinology of depression and chronic stress. British Medical Bulletin, 52(3), 597–617. https://doi.org/10.1093/oxfordjournals.bmb.a011570.

Chiang, M.-H., Ho, S.-M., Wu, H.-Y., Lin, Y.-C., Tsai, W.-H., Wu, T., Lai, C.-H., & Wu, C.-L. (2022). Drosophila model for studying gut microbiota in behaviors and neurodegenerative diseases. Biomedicines, 10(3), 596. https://doi.org/10.3390/biomedicines10030596.

Cici, T. (2016). Metabolic disorders and gut microbiota. Advances in Obesity, Weight Management & Control, 5(3). https://doi.org/10.15406/aowmc.2016.05.00133.

Clark, K. J., Boczek, N. J., & Ekker, S. C. (2011). Stressing zebrafish for behavioral genetics. Revneuro, 22(1), 49–62. https://doi.org/10.1515/rns.2011.007.

Cohen, N. A., & Maharshak, N. (2017). Novel indications for fecal microbial transplantation: Update and review of the literature. Digestive Diseases and Sciences, 62(5), 1131–1145.

Costabile, A., Corona, G., Sarnsamak, K., Atar-Zwillenberg, D., Yit, C., King, A. J., Vauzour, D., Barone, M., Turroni, S., Brigidi, P., & Hauge-Evans, A. C. (2022). Wholegrain fermentation affects gut microbiota composition, phenolic acid metabolism and pancreatic beta cell function in a rodent model of type 2 diabetes. Frontiers in Microbiology, 13, 1004679.

Cryan, J. F., & Dinan, T. G. (2012). Mind-altering microorganisms: The impact of the gut microbiota on brain and behaviour. Nature Reviews. Neuroscience, 13(10), 701–712.

Davis, D. J., Bryda, E. C., Gillespie, C. H., & Ericsson, A. C. (2016). Microbial modulation of behavior and stress responses in zebrafish larvae. Behavioural Brain Research, 311, 219–227.

De Angelis, M., Garruti, G., Minervini, F., Bonfrate, L., Portincasa, P., & Gobbetti, M. (2019). The food-gut human axis: The effects of diet on gut microbiota and metabolome. Current Medicinal Chemistry, 26(19), 3567–3583.

Demin, K. A., Taranov, A. S., Ilyin, N. P., Lakstygal, A. M., Volgin, A. D., de Abreu, M. S., Strekalova, T., & Kalueff, A. V. (2021). Understanding neurobehavioral effects of acute and chronic stress in zebrafish. Stress, 24(1), 1–18.

Dinan, T. G., & Cryan, J. F. (2012). Regulation of the stress response by the gut microbiota: Implications for psychoneuroendocrinology. Psychoneuroendocrinology, 37(9), 1369–1378.

Ding, H. T., Taur, Y., & Walkup, J. T. (2017). Gut microbiota and autism: Key concepts and findings. Journal of Autism and Developmental Disorders, 47(2), 480–489.

Egan, R. J., Bergner, C. L., Hart, P. C., Cachat, J. M., Canavello, P. R., Elegante, M. F., Elkhayat, S. I., Bartels, B. K., Tien, A. K., Tien, D. H., Mohnot, S., Beeson, E., Glasgow, E., Amri, H., Zukowska, Z., & Kalueff, A. V. (2009). Understanding behavioral and physiological phenotypes of stress and anxiety in zebrafish. Behavioural Brain Research, 205(1), 38–44.

Gaikwad, S., Stewart, A., Hart, P., Wong, K., Piet, V., Cachat, J., & Kalueff, A. V. (2011). Acute stress disrupts performance of zebrafish in the cued and spatial memory tests: The utility of fish models to study stress–memory interplay. Behavioural Processes, 87(2), 224–230. https://doi.org/10.1016/j.beproc.2011.04.004.

Gomaa, E. Z. (2020). Human gut microbiota/microbiome in health and diseases: A review. Antonie van Leeuwenhoek, 113(12), 2019–2040. https://doi.org/10.1007/s10482-020-01474-7.

Gondalia, S., Parkinson, L., Stough, C., & Scholey, A. (2019). Gut microbiota and bipolar disorder: A review of mechanisms and potential targets for adjunctive therapy. Psychopharmacology, 236(5), 1433–1443. https://doi.org/10.1007/s00213-019-05248-6.

González Olmo, B. M., Butler, M. J., & Barrientos, R. M. (2021). Evolution of the human diet and its impact on gut microbiota, immune responses, and brain health. Nutrients, 13(1). https://doi.org/10.3390/nu13010196.

Hart, A., & Kamm, M. A. (2002). Review article: Mechanisms of initiation and perpetuation of gut inflammation by stress. Alimentary Pharmacology and Therapeutics, 16(12), 2017–2028.

Harvey, A. G., & Bryant, R. A. (2002). Acute stress disorder: A synthesis and critique. *Psychological Bulletin*, *128*(6), 886–902. https://doi.org/10.1037/0033-2909.128.6.886.

Heinrichsen, E. T., & Haddad, G. G. (2012). Role of high-fat diet in stress response of Drosophila. PLOS ONE, 7(8), e42587. https://doi.org/10.1371/journal.pone.0042587.

Huang, F., & Wu, X. (2021). Brain neurotransmitter modulation by gut microbiota in anxiety and depression. *Frontiers in Cell and Developmental Biology*, 9. https://doi.org/10.3389/fcell.2021.649103.

Kang, D.-W., Adams, J. B., Coleman, D. M., Pollard, E. L., Maldonado, J., McDonough-Means, S., Gregory Caporaso, J., & Krajmalnik-Brown, R. (2019). Long-term benefit of microbiota transfer therapy on autism symptoms and gut microbiota. *Scientific Reports*, 9(1). https://doi.org/10.1038/s41598-019-42183-0.

Koopman, C., Hales, R., & Spiegel, D. (1998). Acute stress disorder as a predictor of post-traumatic stress symptoms. The American Journal of Psychiatry. https://doi.org/10.1176/ajp.155.5.620.

Kovács, P., Juránek, I., Stankovicová, T., & Svec, P. (1996). Lipid peroxidation during acute stress. Die Pharmazie, 51(1), 51–53.

Kriss, M., Hazleton, K. Z., Nusbacher, N. M., Martin, C. G., & Lozupone, C. A. (2018). Low diversity gut microbiota dysbiosis: Drivers, functional implications and recovery. Current Opinion in Microbiology, 44, 34–40.

Kuti, D., Winkler, Z., Horváth, K., Juhász, B., Paholcsek, M., Stágel, A., Gulyás, G., Czeglédi, L., Ferenczi, S., & Kovács, K. J. (2020). Gastrointestinal (non-systemic) antibiotic Rifaximin differentially affects chronic stress-induced changes in colon microbiome and gut permeability without effect on behavior. Brain, Behavior, and Immunity, 84, 218–228.

Lange, K., Buerger, M., Stallmach, A., & Bruns, T. (2016). Effects of antibiotics on gut microbiota. *Digestive Diseases*, *34*(3), 260–268. https://doi.org/10.1159/000443360.

Larroya-García, A., Navas-Carrillo, D., & Orenes-Piñero, E. (2019). Impact of gut microbiota on neurological diseases: Diet composition and novel treatments. Critical Reviews in Food Science and Nutrition, 59(19), 3102–3116.

Lepore, S. J., Miles, H. J., & Levy, J. S. (1997). Relation of chronic and episodic stressors to psychological distress, reactivity, and health problems. International Journal of Behavioral Medicine, 4(1), 39–59. https://doi.org/10.1207/s15327558ijbm0401_3.

Madison, A., & Kiecolt-Glaser, J. K. (2019). Stress, depression, diet, and the gut microbiota: Human–bacteria interactions at the core of psychoneuroimmunology and nutrition. *Current Opinion in Behavioral Sciences*, *28*. https://doi.org/10.1016/j.cobeha.2019.01.011.

Mangiola, F. (2016). Gut microbiota in autism and mood disorders. World Journal of Gastroenterology, 22(1), 361. https://doi.org/10.3748/wjg.v22.i1.361.

McEwen, B. S. (2008). Central effects of stress hormones in health and disease: Understanding the protective and damaging effects of stress and stress mediators. European Journal of Pharmacology, 583(2–3), 174–185. https://doi.org/10.1016/j.ejphar.2007.11.071.

McEwen, B. S. (2017). Neurobiological and systemic effects of chronic stress. Chronic Stress (Thousand Oaks, Calif.), 1. https://doi.org/10.1177/2470547017692328.

Merra, G., Noce, A., Marrone, G., Cintoni, M., Tarsitano, M. G., Capacci, A., & De Lorenzo, A. (2022). Influence of Mediterranean diet on human gut microbiota. In *Kompass Nutrition & Dietetics* (pp. 1–7). https://doi.org/10.1159/000523727.

Miller, G. E., Rohleder, N., Stetler, C., & Kirschbaum, C. (2005). Clinical depression and regulation of the inflammatory response during acute stress. Psychosomatic Medicine, 67(5), 679–687.

Neckameyer, W. S., & Nieto-Romero, A. R. (2015). Response to stress in Drosophila is mediated by gender, age and stress paradigm. Stress, 18(2), 254–266.

Pagnussat, N., Piato, A. L., Schaefer, I. C., Blank, M., Tamborski, A. R., Guerim, L. D., Bonan, C. D., Vianna, M. R. M., & Lara, D. R. (2013). One for all and all for one: The importance of shoaling on behavioral and stress responses in zebrafish. *Zebrafish*, *10*(3), 338–342.

Palomar, M. M., Galdeano, C. M., & Perdigón, G. (2014). Influence of a probiotic lactobacillus strain on the intestinal ecosystem in a stress model mouse. *Brain, Behavior, and Immunity*, 35. https://doi.org/10.1016/j.bbi.2013.08.015.

Paulus, E. J., Argo, T. R., & Egge, J. A. (2013). The impact of posttraumatic stress disorder on blood pressure and heart rate in a veteran population. *Journal of Traumatic Stress*, *26*(1), 169–172. https://doi.org/10.1002/jts.21785.

Pearce, S. C., Coia, H. G., Karl, J. P., Pantoja-Feliciano, I. G., Zachos, N. C., & Racicot, K. (2018). Intestinal in vitro and ex vivo Models to Study Host-Microbiome Interactions and Acute Stressors. *Frontiers in Physiology*, *9*. https://doi.org/10.3389/fphys.2018 .01584.

Piato, Â. L., Capiotti, K. M., Tamborski, A. R., Oses, J. P., Barcellos, L. J. G., Bogo, M. R., Lara, D. R., Vianna, M. R., & Bonan, C. D. (2011). Unpredictable chronic stress model in zebrafish (Danio rerio): Behavioral and physiological responses. Progress in Neuro-Psychopharmacology and Biological Psychiatry, 35(2), 561–567.

Roberfroid, M. (2007). Prebiotics: The concept revisited. The Journal of Nutrition, 137(3), 830S–87S.

Rodrigues-Amorim, D., Rivera-Baltanás, T., Regueiro, B., Spuch, C., de Las Heras, M. E., Vázquez-Noguerol Méndez, R., Nieto-Araujo, M., Barreiro-Villar, C., Olivares, J. M., & Agís-Balboa, R. C. (2018). The role of the gut microbiota in schizophrenia: Current and future perspectives. *The World Journal of Biological Psychiatry: The Official Journal of the World Federation of Societies of Biological Psychiatry*, *19*(8), 571–585.

Rodriguez, M., Basten Snoek, L., De Bono, M., & Kammenga, J. E. (2013). Worms under stress: C. elegans stress response and its relevance to complex human disease and aging. *Trends in Genetics*, *29*(6), 367–374. https://doi.org/10.1016/j.tig.2013.01.010.

Romano, S., Savva, G. M., Bedarf, J. R., Charles, I. G., Hildebrand, F., & Narbad, A. (2021). Meta-analysis of the Parkinson's disease gut microbiome suggests alterations linked to intestinal inflammation. *NPJ Parkinson's Disease*, *7*(1). https://doi.org/10.1038/ s41531-021-00156-z.

Sahu, S., Jaysingh, P., & Mishra, M. (2022). Drosophila melanogaster as an in vivo model for the investigation of host-microbiota interaction. In *Prebiotics, Probiotics and Nutraceuticals* (pp. 275–300). Singapore: Springer Nature Singapore.

Samochowiec, J., & Misiak, B. (2021). Gut microbiota and microbiome in schizophrenia. Current Opinion in Psychiatry, *34*(5), 503–507. https://doi.org/10.1097/yco .0000000000000733.

Schwiertz, A. (2016). *Microbiota of the Human Body: Implications in Health and Disease*. Springer.

Shen, Y., Xu, J., Li, Z., Huang, Y., Yuan, Y., Wang, J., Zhang, M., Hu, S., & Liang, Y. (2018). Analysis of gut microbiota diversity and auxiliary diagnosis as a biomarker in patients with schizophrenia: A cross-sectional study. Schizophrenia Research, 197, 470–477.

Shim, J. (2015). Drosophila blood as a model system for stress sensing mechanisms. *BMB Reports*, *48*(4), 223–228. https://doi.org/10.5483/bmbrep.2015.48.4.273.

Simpson, C. A., Diaz-Arteche, C., Eliby, D., Schwartz, O. S., Simmons, J. G., & Cowan, C. S. M. (2021). The gut microbiota in anxiety and depression – A systematic review. *Clinical Psychology Review*, *83*, 101943. https://doi.org/10.1016/j.cpr.2020.101943.

Steenbergen, P. J., Richardson, M. K., & Champagne, D. L. (2011). The use of the zebrafish model in stress research. Progress in Neuro-Psychopharmacology and Biological Psychiatry, 35(6), 1432–1451.

Strati, F., Cavalieri, D., Albanese, D., De Felice, C., Donati, C., Hayek, J., Jousson, O., Leoncini, S., Renzi, D., Calabrò, A., & De Filippo, C. (2017). New evidences on the altered gut microbiota in autism spectrum disorders. *Microbiome*, *5*(1). https://doi.org /10.1186/s40168-017-0242-1.

Tengeler, A. C., Dam, S. A., Wiesmann, M., Naaijen, J., van Bodegom, M., Belzer, C., Dederen, P. J., Verweij, V., Franke, B., Kozicz, T., Arias Vasquez, A., & Kiliaan, A. J. (2020). Gut microbiota from persons with attention-deficit/hyperactivity disorder affects the brain in mice. Microbiome, 8(1), 44.

Tetel, M. J., de Vries, G. J., Melcangi, R. C., Panzica, G., & O'Mahony, S. M. (2018). Steroids, stress and the gut microbiome-brain axis. Journal of Neuroendocrinology, 30(2). https://doi.org/10.1111/jne.12548.

Ventura, M., Turroni, F., Canchaya, C., Vaughan, E. E., O'Toole, P. W., & van Sinderen, D. (2009). Microbial diversity in the human intestine and novel insights from metagenomics. Frontiers in Bioscience, 14(9), 3214–3221.

Wang, R.-F., Beggs, M. L., Erickson, B. D., & Cerniglia, C. E. (2004). DNA microarray analysis of predominant human intestinal bacteria in fecal samples. Molecular and Cellular Probes, 18(4), 223–234.

Xu, R., Wu, B., Liang, J., He, F., Gu, W., Li, K., Luo, Y., Chen, J., Gao, Y., Wu, Z., Wang, Y., Zhou, W., & Wang, M. (2020). Altered gut microbiota and mucosal immunity in patients with schizophrenia. Brain, Behavior, and Immunity, 85, 120–127.

Yuan, X., Kang, Y., Zhuo, C., Huang, X.-F., & Song, X. (2019). The gut microbiota promotes the pathogenesis of schizophrenia via multiple pathways. *Biochemical and Biophysical Research Communications*, *512*(2), 373–380.

Zhang, F., Berg, M., Dierking, K., Félix, M.-A., Shapira, M., Samuel, B. S., & Schulenburg, H. (2017). Caenorhabditis elegans as a model for microbiome research. *Frontiers in Microbiology*, *8*. https://doi.org/10.3389/fmicb.2017.00485.

Zhong, X., Li, J., Lu, F., Zhang, J., & Guo, L. (2022). Application of zebrafish in the study of the gut microbiome. *Animal Models and Experimental Medicine*, *5*(4), 323–336. https://doi.org/10.1002/ame2.12227.

# 13

# Polyphenolic Nutraceuticals to Combat Oxidative Stress through Microbiota Modulation

Aaishwarya B. Deshmukh and Jayvadan K. Patel

## Contents

DOI: 10.1201/9781003333821-13

# 13.1 Introduction

Nutraceuticals, compounds that offer medical or health benefits, along with the prevention and/or treatment of a disease, have shown to improve conditions related to oxidative stress (1, 2). Oxidative stress is a triggering cause for many diseases, however, it does act on a second plane, creating disturbance in the balance of human colonic microbiota as the real and primary cause. In addition, involvement of dysbiosis in disease development can be thought of by linking the oxidative stress with an inflammatory progression (3). Some recent studies have shown the necessity of discovering the biomarkers that portray the health status of patients with degenerative pathologies, viz. the cardiovascular patient group (4). Human gut microbiota is one such example, and the biotransformation of the nutraceuticals can be considered as a direct indicator of the biomarker presence (e.g., butyric acid). On the basis of compelling evidence from clinical studies and practices, microbiota is the second target for nutraceutical administration (5). Moreover, a nutraceutical drug, as compared to a classical drug, normally consists of a complex of bioactive substances, the effect of which is in turn affected by human colonic biotransformations (6). One instance is the metabolic syndrome that progresses as a side effect of weight gain and/or metabolic alterations, and nutraceuticals are said to be a groundbreaking strategy to diminish chronic inflammation. The pathological developments are thoroughly associated with the disproportion of the microbiota of the human colon (7).

Polyphenols are the most significant plant secondary metabolites and are of considerable fascination because of their health-promoting actions, like antioxidant, antibacterial, anti-inflammatory, anti-adipogenic, and neuro-protective activities. But, due to their complicated structures and high-molecular-weights, the majority of dietary polyphenols remain unabsorbed through the gastrointestinal tract (GIT), causing their biotransformation into bioactive, low-molecular-weight phenolic metabolites in the large intestine by existing gut microbiota. Dietary polyphenols can modify the intestinal microbes composition and, consecutively, polyphenols are catabolized by gut microbes to release bioactive metabolites (8). Much literature data advocates that a diet rich in fruits and vegetables could diminish the incidence of many diseases, including specific cancers, majorly due to the presence of natural polyphenols. There are many polyphenols, like resveratrol, epigallocatechin gallate, and curcumin, which have been comprehensively studied, and the mainstream effects of which are attributed to their antioxidant and anti-inflammatory properties. Several mechanisms are found to be involved, viz. modulation of molecular events and signalling pathways linked with cell survival, proliferation, differentiation, migration, angiogenesis, hormonal activities, detoxification enzymes. and immune responses (9).

## 13.2 Interface between Nutraceutical/Drug and Human Microbiota

The nutraceutical pharmacodynamics varies from that of drugs, given that the molecule complex holding the bioactive potential acts multidirectionally. The pharmacological effect is unswervingly reliant on the concentration of the main component, and so, diverse technologies are engaged in potentiation of their biological action (10). Some natural nutraceutical products, viz. green tea, are also a source of xenobiotics, known for their antioxidative stress effects. A metabolomic study evidently showed the links between active molecules and variances in their sources of origin, processing methods, as well as *in vivo* uses. In addition, the xenobiotics interactions with biological fluids like saliva, Hydrochloric acid (HCl), pepsin, bile salts, etc., the biotransformations process, and metabolite arrays resoluted by the microbiota affect the ultimate therapeutic effect. The interface of the metabolomic pattern with the physiological functions is replicated in the manifestation of the outcome of health promotion (11). The encounter of the degenerative progression etiologies (obesity, diabetes, for instance) and the critical point of the connection of the dysbiosis (Figure 13.1), makes an innovative method for refining the metabolic imbalance (12).

The effect of antibiotics, which directly depends on the fermentative action of the colon, since they are metabolized at this point, intermingles with the human microbiota, suggesting the ability to categorize the metabolites after administration. Similar behavior is exerted by most products based on the phenolic compounds (nutraceuticals); thus, biological action being an

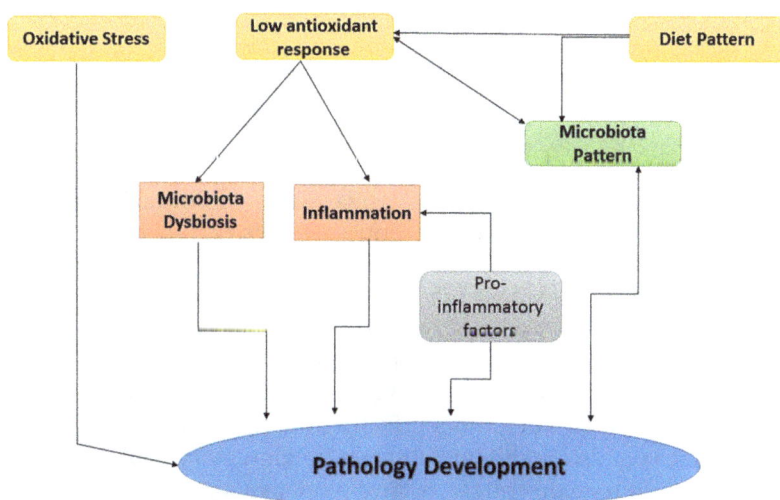

**Figure 13.1** *Diagrammatic illustration of the oxidative stress-dysbiosis-pathology progression pathway.*

manifestation of the existence of these metabolites rather than that of the biologically active molecules (13). Biotransformation in the colon regulates the modifications or reductions in the effects of many of these *in vitro* products (14). However, the extent of bioavailability is governed by the alteration in the inflammatory process, at the individual level, which, during its progression, alters the microbiota structure. The advancements in oxidative stress modify both the immune response and metabolic rate thus favoring the microbial modifications (15, 16). The *in vivo* bioavailability varies considerably from the *in vitro* study results. The therapeutic index is a valuable factor to investigate the pharmacological effect of a product and/or molecule (17); interface with the colonic microbiota being critical for articulating the therapeutic value. The *in vivo* bioavailability shown by the microbial metabolite products exercises a direct alteration on the forms of various pathogenic groups. These constituents augment the growth of the favorable strains at the expense of the residual microbial fingerprint. The clinical consequence is, thus, secondarily exercised by the plasticity of the human colonic microbial pattern. Thus, nutraceuticals interactions with microbiota encompass not just mutual interaction, but have clinical significance on human health as well (18).

In addition, the microbiota interactions are expressed in terms of the kind of biotransformation process that follows, since the microbial pattern responds and regulates the clinical effect. Moreover, absorption can be considered as a direct effect of the degree of degradation and biotransformation which in turn influences the pharmacological response. In the biotransformation process, the chief factor which is responsible for rendering end products stable and in turn enabling their transit into the blood stream is the enzymatic action. For example, the alteration of water-soluble to liposoluble state is the characteristic way of promoting the fraction of molecules absorbed in the intestinal lumen (19, 20). This development depends on individual variations and the capacity of the individual pattern to acquire those definite molecules that could confirm a reduction in the microbial risk groups for the evolution and stimulation of oxidative stress. This multifaceted course, predisposed to numerous exogenous factors and distinct genetic heritage, assists the biotransformation and absorption, as well as bioavailability, of the nutraceuticals (21). A grave opinion on many study data restates that the bioactivity of the nutraceuticals depends on the chemical structure and stability at the time of microbiota activity. A few *in vitro* vs. *in vivo* studies also expose another remarkable perception for it elucidates the physiological pathway of nutraceuticals (polyphenols) degradation during the period of microbiota's fermentative action. The nutraceuticals intermingle with human microbiota affecting the physiological balance of the body, though it may drop with age and the inflammatory proliferation which develops into a more acute phase during oxidative stress. This dire opinion defines diminished bioavailability and, lastly, dysbiosis. Microbiological modulation of the microbiota as well as the metabolomic response are influenced by the capacity to colonize *in vivo*, but, they are a restraining factor in *in vitro* study. Much research has been directed into static systems, and the dynamic response (comparable to that of the *in vivo*) is presumed to be established on the identification of certain biomarkers (e.g., butyric acid level).

## 13.3 Polyphenols

Polyphenols, plant secondary metabolites, are chemically categorized by the presence of at least one aromatic ring with one or more hydroxyl groups attached and they aid plants to endure and proliferate, and shield against microbial infections or herbivorous animals, or tempting pollinators. Polyphenols constitute a group of natural products that encompasses a wide number of different compounds, extending from simplest low-molecular-weight molecules to most complex large derived molecules (22, 23). Polyphenols (Table 13.1) can be classified into flavonoids and non-flavonoids (24). Flavonoids, the major polyphenols and widely distributed in the plant kingdom, are made up of fifteen carbon skeletons with two aromatic rings connected to a three-carbon bridge. The chief subclasses of flavonoids comprise of flavonols, flavan-3-ols, flavanones, flavones, isoflavones, anthocyanins, dihydrochalcones, and proanthocyanidins. The non-flavonoid polyphenols, phenolic acids, can be subdivided into hydroxycinnamic acids and hydroxybenzoic acids (22, 23).

They encompass a huge class of antioxidants, for instance flavonoids, phenolic acids and their derivatives, lignans, and stilbenes. The chief phenolic acids contain hydroxybenzoic acids (e.g., gallic, p-hydroxybenzoic, vanillic, and syringic acid) and hydroxy-cinnamic acids (e.g., ferulic, caffeic, p-coumaric, chlorogenic, and synapic acid); though, because of structural similarity, other polyphenols are also considered analogues of phenolic acid, like capsaicin,

**Table 13.1** Classification of Polyphenols and Their Sources

| Polyphenols | Sub-Types | Sources |
|---|---|---|
| Phenolic acids | Bonzoic acid | Benzoic acid (Blueberry) |
|  | Cinnamic acid and derivatives | Caffeic acid (Coffee) |
| Flavonoids | Flavonoids | 2-phenylchromone (Celery) |
|  | Flavonones | Flavonones (Grape fruit) |
|  | Isoflavones | Soy isoflavone (Soybean) |
|  | Chalcones | Chalcones (Phloretin) |
|  | Flavanols | 3-flavanol (Cocoa) |
|  | Flavonols | Quercetin (Tea) |
|  | Flavanonols | Flavanonols (Orange) |
|  | Anthocyanins | Petunidin chloride (Eggplant) |
| Polyphenolic amide | Capsaicinoids | Capsaicin (Chili) |
|  | Avenanthramides | Avenanthramide (Oat) |
| Non-flavonoids | Stilbenes | Resveratrol (Grape) |
|  | Lignans | Phyllanthin (Sesame) |

rosmarinic acid, gingerol, and gossypol. A key source of gallic acid is tea, while coffee, lettuce, carrots, berries, sweet potatoes, prunes, peaches, apples, tomatoes, and grapes are some of the rich sources of hydroxy-cinnamic acids. As far as most abundant diet polyphenol is concerned, flavonoids are considered at the top, and are further classified into flavones, flavonols, flavan-3-ols, flavanones, isoflavones, and anthocyanins. These flavonoids consists of the basic phenylbenzopyrone skeleton with two aromatic rings. In addition, flavonoids can exist both in free and conjugated form in nature. Food sources like onions, cherries, apples, broccoli, cabbage, tomatoes, berries, tea, red wine, cumin, and buckwheat are rich in flavonoids. Citrus fruits, grapes, and the medicinal herbs of Rutaceae, Rosaceae, and Leguminosae are rich in flavanones; flavanols like catechin, epicatechin, epigallocatechin, epicatechin gallate, and epigallocatechin gallate (EGCG), are present in medicinal herbs and diet plants like tea, apples, berries, cocoa, and catechu. The chief sources of flavones like luteolin, apigenin, and tangeritin are leaves, rinds, barks, and pollens; isoflavones include daidzein, genistein, and glycitein, found in soybeans and other legumes. Anthocyanidines, which are a characteristically colored group of flavonoids, are found in flowers and red, blue, or purple fruits (25). Since polyphenols are widely distributed, they have been investigated enourmously for the prevention and treatment of several pathological conditions, including cancer, neurodegenerative disorders, metabolic and cardiovascular diseases, and strokes.

## 13.4 The Biological Significance of Dietary Polyphenols

The total dietary intake of polyphenol is as high as 1 g per day for each adult, i.e., ten times higher than the intake of vitamin C, and 100 times higher than that of vitamin E and carotenoids (26). Studies have shown that most of the dietary polyphenol intake remains unabsorbed in the small intestine, accumulates in the large intestine, and is broadly metabolized by the gut microbiota (27). Thus, intestinal microbiota have a significant function in the biotransformation and metabolism of the original polyphenolic structures into metabolites with low-molecular-weight and readily absorbable property, contributing to host health benefits. Conversely, limited knowledge prevails concerning the potential mechanism among dietary polyphenols, gut microbes, and host health. Polyphenols impact the composition of host gut microbiota, which in turn affect the host's metabolism. Consecutively, intestinal microbiota can break down polyphenols into low-molecular-weight bioactive phenolic metabolites to modify the regulatory metabolism linkage.

Remarkable attention has been applied by food researchers, nutritionists, and consumers in these recent years. Apart from defensive actions of polyphenols against pathogens and atmospheric agents, they have also been shown to exhibit antimicrobial and antioxidant properties, thus protecting plant tissues from the noxious effects of reactive oxygen species (28). Many *in vitro* and *in vivo* studies have revealed health-promoting effects of polyphenols by various mechanisms that include antioxidant, anti-inflammatory, antibacterial, anti-adipogenic, and neuro-protective actions.

## 13.4.1 Antioxidant Properties

The efficacy of phenolic compounds in the attenuation of oxidative process is hypothetically associated with their reactive species scavenging activity, by the vitue of presence of the hydroxyl group on the benzene ring, which makes it possible for polyphenols to transfer H-atoms from the active Hydroxyl (OH) group of the polyphenol to the free radical (29), permitting them to circuitously trigger antioxidant responses and produce nontoxic levels of intermediates, explicitly the electrophilic forms of hydroquinone and quinone (30). Conversely, polyphenols constrain the formation of or deactivation of free radical active species and precursors, hence decreasing the oxidation rate and eventually subduing the production of free radicals. Polyphenols donate an electron to the free radical, as a result neutralizing the radical, and rendering themselves to convert to a stable (less reactive) radical, and consequently stopping the reaction (31). A study has shown that treatment of hepatoblastoma cell line (HepG2) cells with (-)-epigallocatechin-3-gallate from green tea led to stimulation of nuclear translocation of nuclear factor erythroid 2-related factor 2 (Nrf2), which alters the gene of expression of antioxidant in the cell (32). In yet another study, resveratrol showed enhanced antioxidant defenses by augmenting the activity of endogenous antioxidant enzymes such as catalase (CAT), superoxide dismutase (SOD), glutathione peroxidase (GPx), and glutathione-S-transferase (GST) in pancreatic tissue (33).

## 13.4.2 Anti-Inflammatory Properties

Inflammation induced by oxidative stress is facilitated by the stimulation of cellular signalling processes of nuclear factor kappa B (NF-κB) activation as well as activator protein1 (AP-1) DNA binding (34). This distresses the pro-inflammatory gene expression such as interleukin-1beta (IL-1β), IL-6, tumor necrotic factor alpha (TNF-α), and inducible nitric oxide synthase (iNOS) (35). Studies in animals as well as clinical studies advocate that polyphenols have the capacity to prompt anti-inflammatory properties (36); though the exact mechanisms merit further explanations, polyphenols have certainly shown benefits in diverse disorders (37). A study by Monagas et al. (2009) demonstrated that dihydroxylated phenolic acids which were produced from dietary proanthocyanidins expressively dropped the secretion of cytokines, including TNF-α, IL-1β, and IL-6 in healthy volunteers (38). Moreover, 0.8% quercetin supplementation in male C57Bl/6J mice reduced interferon-, IL-1α, and IL-4 (39). In another study, treatment with 10 mg/kg of quercetin likewise diminished the plasma nitrate plus nitrite (NOx) concentration and TNF-α production causing an anti-inflammatory effect in adipose tissue of obese Zucker rats (40).

### 13.4.3 Effects on Mitochondria and Healthy Aging

Mitochondrial dysfunction has been linked with aging as well as age-related disease (41, 42); a diminution in the mitochondrial function leading to loss of necessary energy production is assumed to be responsible in age-related decline. Thus, preventing mitochondrial dysfunction can serve as an operative approach to counter the undesirable effects associated with aging (43–46). Studies have shown that long-standing quotidian intake of polyphenols improved age-related cardiac effects like inflammation and cell apoptosis, in turn conserving the heart morphology (47). Furthermore, grape pomace polyphenol was recommended as prospective therapy due to its action on modulation of the transient receptor potential canonical 3 and nuclear factor of activated T cells c3 (TRPC3-NFATc3) signalling which further showed to regulate ventricular cardiac fibroblasts and myocardial fibrosis (48). Phenolic metabolite mixtures formed by the fermentation of fruits and vegetables with bacteria *Lactobacillus rhamnosus* and *L. casei* were studied in the invertebrate animal model *C. elegans*. It was observed that in nematodes, the phenolic metabolite mixture and the metabolite protocatechuic acid stimulated molecular and cellular aspects of mitochondrial function, which was beneficial for optimal health, as a result leading to healthy aging (49). To be precise, protocatechuic acid having antioxidant properties showed positive effects on mitochondrial function and energy production (50). New indication also suggests that other phenolic acid representing polyphenol metabolites like gallic, vanillic, and syringic acids stimulate longevity pathways in *C. elegans* (51). Subsequently, mitochondrial dysfunction has been said to contribute not only in aging but also in noncommunicable diseases, making it an key target for polyphenol. Nevertheless, for accurate estimation of polyphenol intake in clinical settings, quantification of biomarkers might be necessary. Besides, an inclusive comprehension of polyphenol biotransformation and identification of the different metabolites in the body are crucial. Numerous research has exhibited that polyphenols modify the mitochondrial metabolism, biogenesis, as well as redox status (52); though titrating the doses employed in *in vivo* studies to clinical studies is the main challenge. Nonetheless, polyphenols and their metabolites have good prospects to impact human health.

### 13.4.4 Neuroprotection

Recent studies recommend that polyphenols exercise their neuroprotective effect by induction of survival mechanisms, the same as that during caloric restriction and physical activity, with activation of longevity signals and action outside the ambit of antioxidant properties which includes sirtuins and mitochondrial biogenesis (53–55). In a study by Sun et al. (2021), it has been demonstrated that xanthohumol, a flavonoid present in hops, improved memory and attenuated deposition of $\beta$-amyloid in the hippocampus of amyloid precursor protein/presenilin 1 (APP/PS1) mice by regulating the rapamycin/microtubule-associated protein 1 light chain 3 II (mTOR/LC3II) signalling pathways (55).

## 13.5 Polyphenic Compounds as Nutraceuticals

Grape has a high flavonoid content, which renders protection against cardio-vascular progression (56), by virtue of its antioxidant and anti-inflammatory effects, providing cardio- and neuroprotection (57). The *in vivo* studies in animals have shown that the biological effect of the flavonoids in grapes can be associated by their interface with the colon microbiota. The same results have also been shown in *in vitro* studies, though the effect is due to chlorogenic acid presence, and the blood glucose-lowering effect is directly dependent on the amount of this compound in the beverage consumed (58). Another nutraceutical, resveratrol, present in the species of the berries of genus *Vaccinium* (59), as well as in grapes, combats oxidative stress by exerting antioxidant and anti-inflammatory effects on the cyclooxygenase-1 enzyme. Stilbenes, through antioxidant protection, have be shown to exert antitumour effects (60). A study has shown recently that resveratrol undergoes degradation to dihydroresveratrol by the microbial constituent of the microbiota (61), which leads to a limitation or possible effect different from the parent compound. Besides this occurrence, a step in the biotransformation process is common for polyphenolic components, which in turn control the response to oxidative stress.

Curcumin, the main ingredient in turmeric (*Curcuma longa*) exhibits antioxidant activity combined with a strong anti-inflammatory effect. Curcumin, with its ability to cross the blood-brain barrier and exertion of neuroprotective activity in neurodegenerative pathologies, has garnered much attention (62). The antioxidant effect, expressed as a defense against oxidative stress, is observed *in vivo* as the oxidation of the lipid component (63). The direct use has shown reduced bioavailability; though curcumin is dynamic on the human microbiota (64), where it exercises striking antimicrobial action, as seen against *Staphylococcus aureus*, *Salmonella* spp., and some *Candida* species (65, 66). Moreover, the *in vitro* effect of the curcumin on the HepG2 cancer cells has been found to be modest; the curcumin administered directly has shown to affect the cell's morphophysiological facet without breaking down the cellular progression (67). The mechanism of curcumin has also be shown to depend on the effect of modulation on the microbiota in cardiovascular patients (68), which established (*in vitro* simulation) alterations of the microbial pattern and a balance of the metabolic activity (69).

## 13.6 Polyphenol and Gut Microbiota Interaction

The absorption of polyphenol is very low (70), with about 90% of these compounds stuck at the colon, where they are metabolized by means of an array of enzymes, such as esterase, glucosidase, demethylation, dihydroxylation, and decarboxylation activities of bacteria (71), subsequently getting converted to smaller metabolites like phenolic acids and short chain-fatty acids, more or less most of which gets absorbed through the intestinal mucosa. Fascinatingly, the microbial bioconversion ability of each person impacts the ultimate metabolite produced and eventually influences the bioavailability. Undeniably, due to the fact that all individuals have a peculiar and unique signature of intestinal microbiota, such as to make an equivalence with a fingerprint, human intestinal microbiota composition can modify the influence of polyphenol on host health (71, 72). Alternatively, polyphenols and their metabolites also influence the ecology-modulating microbiota of the intestine. By this logic, numerous phenolic compounds have been recognized to be prospective antimicrobial agents with both bacteriostatic or bactericidal action. Additionally, they can also inhibit infection-causing bacteria within intestinal and urinary tract cells, proposing that a few phenolic compounds can be explored as antimicrobial agents against human infection (71). Notwithstanding these positive effects, it is imperative not to overlook the fact that unwarranted amounts of polyphenols might hinder the development of beneficial microbiota in the colon, which is said to be accountable for the bioconversion of polyphenols, and as a consequence indirectly impede their own bioavailability. Subsequently, dietary supplementation may exhibit a non-desirable influence on human health in the place of supporting it (72).

Residing in a host gut with shared sympathetics, microbiota is the natural occupant of the GIT (73), where, it executes a well-maintained alignment and equilibrium within the host homeostasis (74). The dysbiosis of gut microbiota has been found responsible for host vulnerability leading to a huge range of communicable and noncommunicable diseases (73). The gut ecosystem is a crucial participant in preserving host health by not only delivering several nutrients but also modifying energy balance besides immune responses (74). Furthermore, polyphenols improve homeostasis of intestinal microbiota and exert beneficial effects on host health by defensive actions against pathogenic invasion as well as risk of obesity, type 2 diabetes, inflammatory bowel disease, cancer, and cardiovascular, liver, and central nervous system disorders (75). Polyphenols found in red wine have been shown to control the gut microbiota profile in patients with metabolic syndrome by augmenting *Bifidobacterium*, *Lactobacillus*, and butyrate-producing bacteria, such as *Faecalibacterium prausnitzii* and *Roseburia*, in feces (76). A study by Ray and Mukherjee (2021) (77) examined the outcome of dietary polyphenol and their association with intestinal microbial ecology, biological activities, and human well-being and disease.

*Vigna radiate* (mung bean) is one of the most vital edible legume crops (78), rich in protein, carbohydrates, vitamins, and minerals (79). Mung bean seed coat is a major byproduct of the mung bean industry. It is rich in polyphenols and dietary fiber but is usually discarded, although its health benefits have now been revealed. Studies show that mung bean seed coat water extract exerts anti-inflammatory effects in LPS(lipopolysaccharide)-induced inflammation in RAW264.7 cells, acute liver injury mice (80), and 3T3-L1 adipocytes

(81). Additionally, antioxidant activity of ethanolic extract has been observed *in vivo* as well as *in vitro* studies (82–84). Bound polyphenols from mung bean seed coat have also been shown to exert an inhibitory effect against α-amylase and α-glucosidase thereby lowering glycemic markers in diabetic db/db and KK-Ay mice (83–85). A new study in high-fat diet-induced obese mice showed decreased fasting blood glucose, fat accumulation, and serum lipid levels; modifying the gut microbiota, particularly Akkermansia, by mung bean seed coat polysaccharides was observed (86).

Disparities in the production and eradication of reactive oxygen species (ROS) leads to oxidative stress, that modifies intracellular signallings and inflammatory status (87). The bioactive compounds having the capacity to decrease intracellular ROS levels can alleviate oxidative stress and the progression of insulin resistance and inflammation. In a study by Jang et al. (2014), it has been demonstrated that mung bean seed coat extract improved superoxide dismutase, catalase, and glutathione peroxidase activity in db/db mice by the virtue of its antioxidative activity (83). In yet another study by Saeting and Chandarajoti et al. (88), it was shown that mung bean water extract improved the percentage of cellular glucose uptake in insulin-resistant HepG2 cells (83, 84). Many phenolic compounds, like agrimonolide, desmethylagrimonolide, quercetin, luteolin, luteolin-7-O-glucoside, kaempferol, and apigenin, have shown glucose-lowering effects (89). Flavonoids have been shown to correlate between antioxidative and anti-inflammatory effects in a study by Chanput et al., (2016) (90).

The GIT is inhabited by numerous microbiota, phyla majorly being *Firmicutes, Bacteroidetes, Proteobacteria*, etc. (91), however, precise microbiota composition may differ in conditions like diarrhea and antibiotic therapy and/or nutritional interventions (92). Diet, by influencing the gut microbiota, changes the implication of well-being favorably or detrimentally. The chief bacteria in the gut system is Prevotella, that uptakes diet rich in carbohydrates, whereas *Bacteroides* is accountable for uptake of animal protein and saturated fat-rich diet (93–94). Limited bacteria, specially *Flavonifractor plautii, Slackia equolifaciens*, and *Slackia isoflavoniconvertens*, are involved in the metabolism of several polyphenols (95). The mechanism of polyphenol in alteration of gut microbiota necessities rectification and exhibits its function through a direct or indirect way. They are implicated in activation as well as suppression of bacterial growth; suppressed bacterial growth is considered as a bacteriostatic or bactericidal effect of polyphenols that averts the active pathogenic bacteria development. Hence, it is crucial to consider the level and characteristic features of these compounds. The indirect effect of polyphenol metabolites cause the expansion of one group of bacteria by stimulating the growth of another group of bacteria (96, 97). The impact of polyphenol intake on the copiousness and multiplicity of gut microbiota has been associated with a range of substrate inclinations and metabolic capabilities of the gut microbial community (98). Polyphenol have also been shown to affect the *Firmicutes/*

*Bacteroidetes* (F/B) ratio via overpowering particular bacterial species (99). In a randomized, double-blind, placebo-controlled human trial, oral consumption of epigallocatechin-3-gallate and resveratrol for 12 weeks in obese individuals at 282 and 80mg/day, respectively, positively attenuated fecal richness of *Bacteroidetes* and *Faecalibacterium prausnitzii* (100). In another study, rats treated with quercetin at 30mg/kg/day attenauted gut microbiota impairment elicited by a high-fat diet by sinking the F/B ratio and lessening the profusion of obese-related bacteria like that of *Erysipelotrichaceae, Bacillus*, and *Eubacterium cylindroides* (101).

Polyphenol extracts/nutraceuticals or food has also been shown to alter the gut microbiota composition. A study by Chen et al. (2018) showed that the canine treated with green tea polyphenol extracts for a period of 18 weeks repressed the levels of *Bacteroidetes* and *Fusobacteria* in addition to improvement in the abundance of *Firmicutes* (102). In a study it was demonstrated that when the mice fed with dietary anthocyanins at 5% and 10% freeze-dried black raspberry powder were challenged with azoxymethane/DSS (dextran sodium sulfate) for a period of 12 weeks, stimulation in the fecal profusion of beneficial bacteria like *Faecalibacterium prausnitzii, Lactobacillus*, and *Eubacterium rectale*, in addition to deterioration in number of pathogens, like *Desulfovibrio* spp. and *Enterococcus* spp., was observed (103). A current study has disclosed that treatment with wild blueberry polyphenolic extract and blueberries isolated fraction in a high-fat sucrose diet, amplified the development of polyphenol-degrading bacteria, specifically *Adlercreutzia equolifaciens* in obese mice, signifying that adding these microbes in polyphenol metabolism could be intricated in alleviation of metabolic disorders related to obesity and diabetes by employing bioactive molecules (104). By and large, the polyphenol structure, optimizing doses, and microbe strain might influence polyphenol action on bacterial growth and metabolism. Polyphenol may upsurge the supplements of helpful bacteria, for example, *Bifidobacterium* and *Lactobacillus* responsible for safeguarding gut barrier function, along with *Faecalibacterium prausnitzii* which is implicated in anti-inflammatry effect by suppressing stimulation of nuclear factor kappa B (NF-κB), as well as *Roseburia* spp, which are producers of butyric acid (105). A study has also proved that gram-positive bacteria are susceptible to polyphenols contrary to gram-negative bacteria; these deviations may be because of the dissimilarity in the cell wall composition of these types of bacteria (106).

## 13.6.1 *In Vivo* Modulation of Dietary Polyphenols on Gut Microbiota of Humans

Clinical studies have established the regulatory effects of polyphenols on human intestinal microbiota. Studies have shown upsurged levels of *Bifidobacterium* and *Lactobacillus*, two intestinal protective agents in the human gut following supplementation with polyphenols such as anthocyanins and flavonoids, the results being consistent with the findings in *in vitro* and *in vivo* animal studies (107, 108). A study by Vendrame et al. (2011) demonstrated a rise in the numbers of *Bifidobacteria* and lactic acid bacteria in healthy volunteers when treated with blueberries which are rich in anthocyanins (109). Dry fruit, viz. almond and almond skin, are profoundly high in a variety of flavonoids, like catechin, flavonol, and flavanone glycosides, and a study has shown a rise in the number of *Bifidobacteria* and *Lactobacillus* in feces in almond and/or almond skin-supplemented diet (110); Moreno-Indias et al. have also revealed that polyphenols present in red wine can intensify the number of *Bifidobacteria* and *Lactobacillus* (111). Moreover, a polyphenol-rich diet can control the quotient of *Firmicutes* to *Bacteroides* in the human body. A study has also demonstrated that daily ingestion of cranberries, which are rich in proanthocyanidins, can diminish the abundance of *Firmicutes* in the body and escalate the abundance of *Bacteroides* (112); nevertheless, polyphenols of tea were used by Yuan et al. to arbitrate in healthy individuals and found dissimilar results. The diet that interfered with tea polyphenols caused a rise in the quantity of *Firmicutes* in feces, a drop in the number of *Bacteroides*, and an rise in the ratio of *Firmicutes* to *Bacteroides* (113). Queipo-Ortu et al. instituted that the collective effect of alcohol and polyphenols might augment the number of *Enterococcus*, *Prevotella*, *Bacteroides*, *Bifidobacterium*, *Bacteroides uniformis*, *Eggerthella lenta*, and *Blautia coccoides–Eubacterium*, but did not affect the levels of *Lactobacillus* (114).

## 13.6.2 Effects of Polyphenols on Gut Microbiota

Recently, novel approaches have been developed for manipulating the microbiota; like fecal transplantation, phage therapy, use of pre/probiotics, as well as adoption of an appropriate diet (115). Moreover, the significance of research on microbiota lies in the conceivable association between its composition and the brain, via the signal mediator metabolite formed by these bacteria. For instance, butyrate (a short chain-fatty acid, SCFA), formed during the fermentation of fiber, can energize and lift mitochondria improving brain health. Likewise, dietary polyphenols have been revealed to interact with the gut microbial communities, viz. *Lactobacilli* and *Bifidobacteria*, improving butyrate production to diminish colitis and avert colitis-associated colorectal cancer, and equivalently declining the existence of pathogenic microbes (116). Lately, a study has revealed that microbiota discharges metabolites like hydrogen sulfide ($H_2S$) and nitric acid ($HNO_3$) along with SCFAs, which sequentially interferes in mitochondrial respiratory chain and adenosine triphosphate (ATP) production, affecting gene expression of inflammatory cytokines (117). The feature of human microbiota and the dynamics of mitochondria may be re-modified and influenced by diet and/or metabolites to reinstate the equilibrium of the system (Figure 13.2). Polyphenol influence has also been ascribed to the anti-inflammatory metabolites which are produced by the gut microbiota and responsible for a reduction in the symptoms of inflammatory bowel diseases. Thus, these beneficial facets are a synergy between the impact of

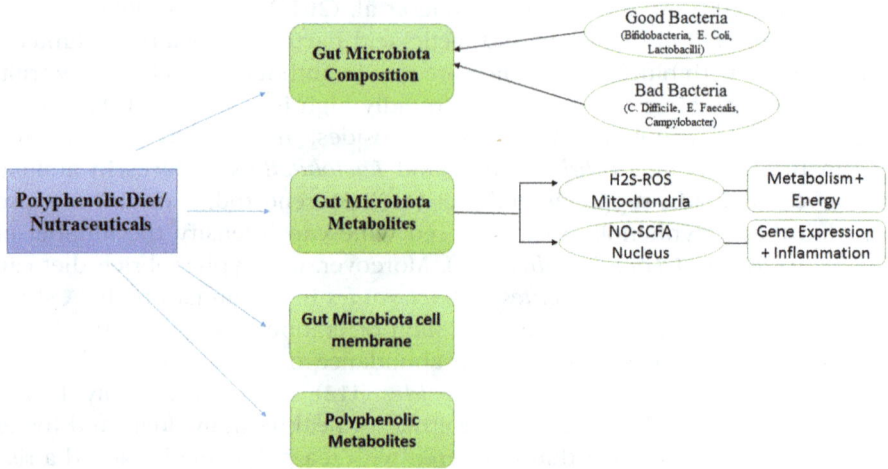

**Figure 13.2** *The effect of a polyphenol-rich diet/nutraceutical on the host via the metabolites produced by the microbiota.*

their metabolites on the augmentation of beneficial microbial range while attenuating the opportunistic pathogenic microbes through mechanisms related to oxidative stress reduction (118–121).

## 13.7 Polyphenols: A Natural Source of Antioxidants

### 13.7.1 Oxidative Stress and Antioxidant Supplementation

Antioxidants are substances that decrease the severity of oxygen species either via formation of a less active radical or quenching the free radicals chain reaction on biomolecules such as proteins, lipids, carbohydrates, or DNA (122). There are a few antioxidants that can interrelate with other antioxidants rejuvenating their original properties; the mechanism known as the "antioxidant network." The antioxidants are endogenous or exogenously obtained as a diet or a dietary supplement. There are a few dietary supplements/nutraceuticals that augment endogenous antioxidant activity without having any effect on the neutralization process of free radicals (123). Endogenous antioxidants preserve optimum cellular functions and accordingly systemic health. But, under some circumstances they are insufficient, requiring extra antioxidants to uphold optimum cellular functions (124). Humans have highly multifaceted antioxidant systems (enzymatic and nonenzymatic) working synergistically and together to defend the cells and organ systems of the body against damage from free radicals like SOD, CAT, and GPx. Nonenzymatic antioxidants do exist which exert an antioxidant effect by acting as enzymatic cofactors and flavonoids (a specific group of polyphenols) that include vitamin A (retinol) (122), vitamin E (tocopherol) (125), vitamin C (ascorbic acid), thiol antioxidants (glutathione, thioredoxin, and lipoic acid), melatonin, carotenoids, and micronutrients (iron, copper, zinc, selenium, manganese) (126). Amongst nonenzymatic antioxidants, polyphenols have been acknowledged by many researchers in the last few years seeing their valuable effects in the alleviation of many chronic diseases (127, 128). Over 8000 phenolic structures are presently recognized, over 4000 being flavonoids (129–131).

## 13.7.2 Oxidative Stress and Lipid Peroxidation

Free radicals are the chemical species comprising one or more unpaired electrons, which incorporate many O-, C-, N-, or S-centred radicals. Amongst them, the O-centred radicals like superoxide radical and the highly reactive hydroxyl radical are most predominant in the biological systems (132). A r hydrogen peroxide, is also one of the commonest ROS. The term "oxidative stress" was originally mentioned in 1970, subsequent to Harman's free radical theory of aging (1956) (133), stating the oxidative encounter of erythrocytes with hydrogen peroxide (134). After more than a decade, in 1985, the term "oxidative stress" was given definition, as an imbalance between oxidants and antioxidants (135), concentrating on the oxidative damage of cells, tissues, and organs (136). Ever since, this notion has advanced considerably, and a redefinition of oxidative stress has been given, as a dysfunction of cellular redox signalling and redox control (137, 138). Recently, a dissimilarity between oxidative eustress and oxidative distress has been given, which says, oxidative eustress as a physiological situation vital for redox signalling, and oxidative distress, on the other hand, is a supraphysiological state that causes biomolecule impairment (139). Up to now, numerous publications have verified and established the relationship between oxidative stress with several human diseases, including cardiometabolic disease. Certainly, now, it is virtually impossible to find a human disease not associated with the oxidative stress. Conventional concept defines the oxidative stress as an overall imbalance between the ROS and the cellular antioxidants. This disparity transpires due to a disproportionate production of ROS, and/or an insufficient concentration/activity of the cellular antioxidants (nonenzymatic or enzymatic) (140).

## 13.7.3 Polyphenols and Their Antioxidant Properties

Dietary polyphenols have been shown to exhibit an antioxidant effect in many studies since they are one of the most important groups of natural antioxidants and anti-inflammatory agents found in the human diet, comprising of fruits, vegetables, grains, essential oils, and their derived foods and beverages, and even nutraceuticals (141). Polyphenols have been established to avert lipid oxidation of poly unsaturated fatty acids (PUFAs), evading organoleptic and sensory deterioration, formation of toxic substances, and, especially, reserving the bioactive and functional properties of omega-3 PUFAs of marine origin due to their antioxidant actions (142, 143). Furthermore, studies have shown that a polyphenol and omega-3 PUFAs combination communally impacted their pharmacological contours and bioavailability as polyphenols inhibit omega-3 PUFAs oxidation, supporting their intestinal uptake though conserving their bioactivity (144, 145); and omega-3 PUFAs consecutively impacted the metabolism and bioaccessibility of polyphenols (146, 147). Furthermore, on conjugation as lipophenols, they exhibit the following prospective benefits: upsurged lipophilicity, cell penetration, bioavailability of explicit polar phenolic drugs, rendering suitable solubility of hydrophobic drugs to grow into tissue/tumor-specific, limiting auto-oxidation of the conjugate PUFAs, and covering their hydroxyl polar functions and therefore by decreasing their biotransformation or the speed of oxidative degradation, amplifying antioxidant properties (148). The omega-3 PUFAs and polyphenol combinations in food are not only beneficial for holding their bioactive value and bioavailability but also for elimination or limiting the damaging prospective effects of high PUFAs intake regarding oxidation. A recent genome-wide association study (GWAS) (149) has demonstrated that both polyphenols (predominantly resveratrol and flavonoids) and omega-3 PUFAs possibly control the genes associated with immune responses and disease pathways, in addition to numerous individual effects on gene expression.

Polyphenols have the capacity to scavenge lipid peroxyl radicals (150), which are a fundamental part of oxidative stress theory (151). A first epidemiological study signifying a counter link between flavonoid intake and mortality from coronary heart disease (CHD) was published in 1993 (152). Polyphenols exhibit great *in vitro* antioxidant capacity, which made an assumption that the *in vitro* antioxidant capacity of all food or plant extracts is a direct determinant of their valuable effects on human health. Succeeding this notion, *in vitro* antioxidant capacities of numerous foods and beverages estimated with Oxygen Radical Absorbance Capacity assay were published (153). In addition, a number of other methods for example trolox equivalent antioxidant capacity, 2,2-diphenyl-1-picrylhydrazyl, and ferric reducing antioxidant power assay were also established (154–156). Eventually, rising scientific indications explicated numerous complex mechanisms of absorption, distribution, metabolism, and excretion (ADME) of polyphenols as a molecular basis of low bioavailability displayed by them. It was further found that the *in vivo* antioxidant activity of polyphenols comprised considerably higher complex mechanisms than the free radical scavenging effects; these molecular mechanisms that were indirectly associated with the antioxidant enzymes were also intricated in their health-supporting properties (157).

## 13.7.4 Antioxidant Effects of Polyphenol-Molecular Mechanism

With the advancement in understanding of oxidative stress and revelation of the complex metabolic processes of polyphenols, the perception that polyphenols facilitate a health-promoting effect only by scavenging free radicals *in vivo* has been nullified. Certainly, it has been clear that polyphenol metabolites do not scavenge significant quantities of free radicals *in vivo* and that α-tocopherol is the crucial composite terminating the lipid peroxidation chain reaction. Therefore, briefing the cutting-edge scientific confirmations from both fields, the foremost mechanism by which polyphenols back the cellular antioxidant defense mechanism has been projected lately (158); viz. post consumption, minor concentrations of metabolized polyphenols reach the cells, and some of them, like hydroxytyrosol, catechin, epicatechin, and delphinidin, as well as carnosic acid, are oxidized by free radicals, in free radical-scavenging reactions. An imperative aim of the oxidized polyphenol is a cytosolic protein, Keap1 (Kelch-like ECH associated protein 1), which controls the action of transcription factor Nrf2 (nuclear factor, erythroid 2-related factor 2). There are a few polyphenol, like resveratrol and curcumin, which have the capacity to bind with Keap1 directly, without being oxidized. The regulatory function of Keap1 in turn is to assist in ubiquitination of Nrf2, resulting in its proteasomal degradation. Post binding a polyphenolic compound, Keap1 is incapacitated and the half-life of Nrf2 is prolonged, which leads to migration of Nrf2 to the nucleus, binding to the antioxidant response element (electrophile response element), and recruitment of gene transcription involved in the antioxidant defense, as well as detoxification. Further to Nrf2, many transcription factors, like c-Maf, c-Jun, c-Fos, Fra1, Bach1, Nrf1 or c-Myc, have also been found to be involved in the antioxidant response element-mediated transcription in multifaceted interactions. Furthermore, protein kinases, like that of protein kinase C or phosphoinositide-3-kinase, have been demonstrated in the phosphorylation of Nrf2, which is, again, a dire step for its nuclear translocation. Contemporary studies have shown that polyphenol metabolites have an impending effect in the modulation of kinases' activities and thus can be suggestive of multilevel regulation of Nrf2-mediated transcription.

A surfeit of cellular functions of nutritional polyphenols has been demonstrated, apart from the Keap1/Nrf2/antioxidant response element pathway, that is indirectly connected with the enzymatic antioxidant, but, however, is still precisely associated with the elusive regulation of cellular redox balance defense. Many studies have demonstrated polyphenol effects on cellular progressions involved in chronic inflammation, endothelial dysfunction, impaired insulin signalling, adipose tissue remodeling, or mitochondrial dysfunction of cardiometabolic disorders (159–162). Rising scientific evidence indicates molecular mechanisms of health benefits exerted by polyphenols to include their binding to specific proteins, and consequent effects on cell signalling pathways. For example, in silico docking analyses have exposed that curcumin has the capacity to bind to kinases like Transforming growth factor (TGF)-β-activated kinase 1 (mitogen-activated protein kinase kinase kinase 7), 3-phosphoinositide-dependent protein kinase 1, serine/threonine kinase (AKT) 1, and AKT2, all of which are responsible for redox-sensitive pro-inflammatory transcription factor NF-κB regulation. Undeniably, NF-κB is recognized as a significant intermediary of inflammation, a common fundamental pathology involved in cardiometabolic diseases and many other pathogenesis. Consequently, a pre-exposure to curcumin (1 μM) in human umbilical vein endothelial cells preceding TNF-α stimulation, decreases activation of NF-κB. Autonomously, curcumin has also been found to reduce monocyte adhesion as well as transendothelial migration and modify expression of genes of antioxidant defense, metabolism, cell signalling, focal adhesion, intercellular junction, and cytoskeleton organization (163), which is overall relevant to an better endothelial function. Likewise, pre-exposure of human umbilical vein endothelial cells to physiologically appropriate concentrations of plasma anthocyanins' metabolites (including their gut microbiota metabolites) has also been shown to decline the TNF-α-induced monocyte cell adhesion. Studies related to gene expression analysis have validated gene modulation involved in cell adhesion, leucocyte transendothelial migration, regulation of actin cytoskeleton, or NF-κB signalling.

Succeeding bioinformatic analysis in addition to in silico docking confirmed that anthocyanins' metabolite binds to many cell-signalling proteins, such as dual specificity mitogen-activated protein kinase kinase 2 as well as NF-κB inhibitor kinase alpha, and possibly controls their activity. The in silico docking studies with the help of western blot analysis established diminished mitogen-activated protein kinase and p65 unit of NF-κB phosphorylation, relevant to the modulation of upstream kinases, and decreased leucocyte transendothelial migration and inflammation (164). Furthermore, flavanol colonic metabolites have been shown to stimulate endothelial nitric oxide synthase in human endothelial cells by AKT and Adenosine monophosphate (AMP)-activated protein kinase signalling and surge in intracellular nitric oxide, which in turn has a crucial role in endothelial function regulation (165). In recent times, an integrated systems' biology approach has been employed to explicate the multi-target and multilayer cellular actions of circulating epicatechin metabolites on endothelial cells, demonstrating gene modulation, and microRNA expressions modifications and DNA methylation. In silico docking study revealed constructive binding of epicatechin metabolites to p38 mitogen-activated protein kinase, which has regulatory control on many transcription factors like nuclear factor-κB (NF-κB), cAMP-response element binding (CREB1), Cellular myelocytomatosis oncogene (c-Myc), c-Jun, Signal transducer and activator of transcription 3 (STAT3) or Specificity protein 1 (SP1) (166).

An important consideration that ought to be discussed regarding the contribution of nutritional polyphenols to the cellular antioxidant defense is that they are present at low cellular concentrations, hence, they might not scavenge substantial volumes of free radicals, but instead, modify and control transcription of genes which are involved in antioxidant defense and detoxification. Conversely, polyphenols at high concentration may prompt toxicity; these deliberations are incorporated in the theory of hormesis (167), which applies to nutritional polyphenols as well (168). Prospective toxicities of polyphenols at high doses should always be deliberated, since over-the-counter supplements are extensively available. The safety and toxicity (169) of polyphenol nutraceuticals/food becomes even more significant due to inter-individual variability in response.

## 13.8 Summary

There are abundant indications in the literature to highlight the potential benefits of dietary polyphenols on host health through gut microbiota interactions and modulations. Many studies have validated the association of dietary polyphenols and gut microbiota with potential mechanisms, viz. alteration of composition of gut microbiota, gut microbiota metabolites production, biotransformation, metabolism of dietary polyphenols, etc. Though, profound understanding of these mechanisms is required, particularly in view of the metabolic pathways which might sanction novel therapeutic targets in the future. Besides, polyphenolic compounds have a natural antioxidant property that augments the nutritional value of food by impeding oxidative degradation and alleviating oxidative stress. Polyphenols have been broadly studied for their beneficial effects in oxidative stress-related pathologies. Certainly, bioavailability of nutritional polyphenols is low and hardened by complex mechanisms of absorption, distribution, metabolism, and excretion. However, interplay between polyphenols and modulation of gut microbiota in turn regulates and controls a plethora of cellular processes including, but not limited to, modification of transcription of genes involved in antioxidant defense.

## References

1. Catinean A, Neag MA, Muntean DM, Bocsan IC, Buzoianu AD. An overview on the interplay between nutraceuticals and gut microbiota. *PeerJ* 2018; 6: e4465.
2. Santini A, Cammarata SM, Capone G, Ianaro A, Tenore GC, Pani L, Novellino E. Nutraceuticals: Opening the debate for a regulatory framework. *Br J Clin Pharmacol* 2018; 84(4): 659–672.
3. Buttó LF, Haller D. Dysbiosis in intestinal inflammation: Cause or consequence. *Int J Med Microbiol* 2016; 306(5): 302–309.
4. Hon KW, Abu N, Ab Mutalib NS, Jamal R. Exosomes as potential biomarkers and targeted therapy in colorectal cancer: A mini-review. *Front Pharmacol* 2017; 28: 583.
5. Swanson HI. Drug metabolism by the host and gut microbiota: A partnership or rivalry? *Drug Metab Dispos* 2015; 43(10): 1499–1504.
6. Marín L, Miguélez EM, Villar CJ, Lombó F. Bioavailability of dietary polyphenols and gut microbiota metabolism: Antimicrobial properties. *BioMed Res Int* 2015; 2015: 905215.
7. Rani V, Deep G, Singh RK, Palle K, Yadav UC. Oxidative stress and metabolic disorders: Pathogenesis and therapeutic strategies. *Life Sci* 2016; 148: 183–193.
8. Wang X, Qi Y, Zheng H. Dietary polyphenol, gut microbiota, and health benefits. *Antioxidants (Basel)* 2022; 11(6): 1212.
9. Briguglio G, Costa C, Pollicino M, Giambò F, catania S, Fenga C. Polyphenols in cancer prevention: New insights (review). *Int J Funct Nutr* 2020; 1(2): 9.
10. Vamanu E. Antioxidant properties of mushroom mycelia obtained by batch cultivation and tocopherol content affected by extraction procedures. *BioMed Res Int* 2014; 2014: 974804.
11. Fujimura Y, Kurihara K, Ida M, et al. Metabolomics-driven nutraceutical evaluation of diverse green tea cultivars. *PLOS ONE* 2011; 6(8): e23426.
12. Rajani C, Jia W. Disruptions in gut microbial-host co-metabolism and the development of metabolic disorders. *Clin Sci (Lond)* 2018; 132(7): 791–811.

13. Klaassen CD, Cui JY. Review: Mechanisms of how the intestinal microbiota alters the effects of drugs and bile acids. *Drug Metab Dispos* 2015; 43(10): 1505–1521.
14. Vamanu E, Gatea F, Sârbu I. *In vitro* ecological response of the human gut microbiome to bioactive extracts from edible wild mushrooms. *Molecules* 2018; 23(9): 2128.
15. Morgan ET, Dempsey JL, Mimche SM, et al. Physiological regulation of drug metabolism and transport: Pregnancy, microbiome, inflammation, infection, and fasting. *Drug Metab Dispos* 2018; 46(5): 503–513.
16. Xu X, Jia X, Mo L, Liu C, Zheng L, Yuan Q, Zhou X. Intestinal microbiota: A potential target for the treatment of postmenopausal osteoporosis. *Bone Res* 2017; 5: 17046.
17. Lin D, Xiao M, Zhao J, et al. An overview of plant phenolic compounds and their importance in human nutrition and management of type 2 diabetes. *Molecules* 2016; 21(10): 1374.
18. Laparra JM, Sanz Y. Interactions of gut microbiota with functional food components and nutraceuticals. *Pharmacol Res* 2010; 61(3): 219–225.
19. Banks WA. Characteristics of compounds that cross the blood-brain barrier. *BMC Neurol* 2009; 9; S3.
20. Marín L, Miguélez EM, Villar CJ, Lombó F. Bioavailability of dietary polyphenols and gut microbiota metabolism: Antimicrobial properties. *BioMed Res Int* 2015; 2015: 905215.
21. Santini A, Novellino E. Nutraceuticals in hypercholesterolaemia: An overview. *Br J Pharmacol* 2017; 174(11): 1450–1463.
22. Crozier A, Jaganath IB, Clifford MN. Dietary phenolics: Chemistry, bioavailability and effects on health. *Nat Prod Rep* 2009; 26(8): 1001–1043.
23. Tsao R. Chemistry and biochemistry of dietary polyphenols. *Nutrients* 2010; 2(12): 1231–1246.
24. SanchezTapia M, Tovar AR, Torres N. Diet as regulator of gut microbiota and its role in health and disease. *Arch Med Res* 2019; 50(5): 259–268.
25. Fenga C, Costa C, Caruso E et al. Current evidence on the protective effect of dietary polyphenols on breast cancer. *Farmacia* 2016; 64: 1–12.
26. Scalbert A, Johnson IT, Saltmarsh M. Saltmarsh M. Polyphenols: Antioxidants and beyond. *Am J Clin Nutr* 2005; 81(1): 215S–217S.
27. Ma G, Chen Y. Polyphenol supplementation benefits human health via gut microbiota: A systematic review via meta-analysis. *J Funct Foods* 2020; 66: 103829.
28. Šamec D, Karalija E, Šola I, Vujčić Bok V, Salopek-Sondi B. The role of polyphenols in abiotic stress response: The influence of molecular structure. *Plants(Basel)* 2021; 10(1): 118.
29. Papuc C, Goran GV, Predescu CN, Nicorescu V, Stefan G. Plant polyphenols as antioxidant and antibacterial agents for shelf-life extension of meat and meat products: Classification, structures, sources, and action mechanisms. *Compr Rev Food Sci Food Saf* 2017; 16(6): 1243–1268.
30. Wu X, Li M, Xiao Z, et al. Dietary polyphenols for managing cancers: What have we ignored? *Trends Food Sci Technol* 2020; 101: 150–164.
31. Tsao R. Chemistry and biochemistry of dietary Polyphenols. *Nutrients* 2010; 2(12): 1231–1246.
32. Mi Y, Zhang W, Tian H, et al. EGCG evokes Nrf2 nuclear translocation and dampens PTP1B expression to ameliorate metabolic misalignment under insulin resistance condition. *Food Funct* 2018; 9(3): 1510–1523.
33. Palsamy P, Subramanian S. Modulatory effects of resveratrol on attenuating the key enzymes activities of carbohydrate metabolism in streptozotocin–nicotinamide-induced diabetic rats. *Chem Biol Interact* 2009; 179(2–3): 356–362.
34. Liu T, Zhang L, Joo D, Sun S-C. NF-κB signaling in inflammation. *Signal Transduct Target Ther* 2017; 2: 17023.
35. Opal SM, DePalo VA. Anti-inflammatory cytokines. *Chest* 2000; 117(4): 1162–1172.

36. Zhang H, Tsao R. Dietary polyphenols, oxidative stress and antioxidant and anti-inflammatory effects. *Curr Opin Food Sci* 2016; 8: 33–42.
37. Li H, Christman LM, Li R, Gu L. Synergic interactions between polyphenols and gut microbiota in mitigating inflammatory bowel diseases. *Food Funct* 2020; 11(6): 4878–4891.
38. Monagas M, Khan N, Andrés-Lacueva C, Urpí-Sardá M, Vázquez-Agell M, Lamuela-Raventós RM, Estruch R. Dihydroxylated phenolic acids derived from microbial metabolism reduce lipopolysaccharide-stimulated cytokine secretion by human peripheral blood mononuclear cells. *Br J Nutr* 2009; 102(2): 201–206.
39. Stewart LK, Soileau JL, Ribnicky D, et al. Quercetin transiently increases energy expenditure but persistently decreases circulating markers of inflammation in C57BL/6J mice fed a high-fat diet. *Metabolism* 2008; 57(7): S39–S46.
40. Rivera L, Morón R, Sánchez M, Zarzuelo A, Galisteo M. Quercetin ameliorates metabolic syndrome and improves the inflammatory status in obese Zucker rats. *Obesity (Silver Spring)* 2008; 16(9): 2081–2087.
41. Stockburger C, Eckert S, Eckert GP, Friedland K, Muller WE. Mitochondrial function, dynamics, and permeability transition: A complex love triangle as a possible target for the treatment of brain aging and Alzheimer's disease. *J Alzheimers Dis* 2018; 64(s1): S455–S467.
42. Friedland-Leuner K, Stockburger C, Denzer I, Eckert GP, Muller WE. Mitochondrial dysfunction: Cause and consequence of Alzheimer's disease. *Prog Mol Biol Transl Sci* 2014; 127: 183–210.
43. Cenini G, Lloret A, Cascella R. Oxidative stress in neurodegenerative diseases: From a mitochondrial point of view. *Oxid Med Cell Longev* 2019; 2019: 2105607.
44. Muller WE, Eckert A, Kurz C, Eckert GP, Leuner K. Mitochondrial dysfunction: Common final pathway in brain aging and Alzheimer's disease–therapeutic aspects. *Mol Neurobiol* 2010; 41(2–3): 159–171.
45. Madreiter-Sokolowski CT, Sokolowski AA, Waldeck-Weiermair M, Malli R, Graier WF. Targeting mitochondria to counteract age-related cellular dysfunction. *Genes (Basel)* 2018; 9(3): 165.
46. Lejri I, Agapouda A, Grimm A, Eckert A. Mitochondria- and oxidative stress-targeting substances in cognitive decline-related disorders: From molecular mechanisms to clinical evidence. *Oxid Med Cell Longev* 2019; 2019: 9695412.
47. Chacar S, Hajal J, Saliba Y, et al. Long-term intake of phenolic compounds attenuates age-related cardiac remodeling. *Aging Cell* 2019; 18(2): e12894.
48. Saliba Y, Jebara V, Hajal J, et al. Transient receptor potential canonical 3 and nuclear factor of activated T cells C3 signaling pathway critically regulates myocardial fibrosis. *Antioxid Redox Signal* 2019; 30(16): 1851–1879.
49. Dilberger B, Passon M, Asseburg H, et al. Polyphenols and metabolites enhance survival in rodents and nematodes—impact of mitochondria. *Nutrients* 2019; 11(8): 1886.
50. Semaming Y, Sripetchwandee J, Sa-Nguanmoo P, Pintana H, Pannangpetch P, Chattipakorn N, Chattipakorn SC. Protocatechuic acid protects brain mitochondrial function in streptozotocin-induced diabetic rats. *Appl Physiol Nutr Metab* 2015; 40(10): 1078–1081.
51. Dilberger B, Weppler S, Eckert G. Impact of phenolic acids on the energy metabolism and longevity in C. elegans. *bioRxiv* 2020. https://doi.org/10.1101/2020.06.23.166314.
52. Di Giacomo M, Zara V, Bergamo P, Ferramosca A. Crosstalk between mitochondrial metabolism and oxidoreductive homeostasis: A new perspective for understanding the effects of bioactive dietary compounds. *Nutr Res Rev* 2019; 33(1): 90–101.
53. Franco R, Navarro G, Martinez-Pinilla E. Antioxidant defense mechanisms in erythrocytes and in the central nervous system. *Antioxidants (Basel, Switzerland)* 2019; 8(2): 46.

54. Jayasena T, Poljak A, Smythe G, Braidy N, Münch G, Sachdev P. The role of polyphenols in the modulation of sirtuins and other pathways involved in Alzheimer's disease. *Ageing Res Rev* 2013; 12(4): 867–883.
55. Sun X-L, Zhang J-B, Guo Y-X, et al. Xanthohumol ameliorates memory impairment and reduces the deposition of β-amyloid in APP/PS1 mice via regulating the mTOR/LC3II and Bax/Bcl-2 signalling pathways. *J Pharm Pharmacol* 2021; 73(9): 1230–1239.
56. Caleja C, Ribeiro A, Barreiro MF, Ferreira ICFR. Phenolic compounds as nutraceuticals or functional food ingredients. *Curr Pharm Des* 2017; 23(19): 2787–2806.
57. Georgiev V, Ananga A, Tsolova V. Recent advances and uses of grape flavonoids as nutraceuticals. *Nutrients* 2014; 6(1): 391–415.
58. Bidel S, Tuomilehto J. The emerging health benefits of coffee with an emphasis on type 2 diabetes and cardiovascular disease. *Eur Endocrinol* 2013; 9(2): 99–106.
59. Nasri H, Baradaran A, Shirzad H, Rafieian-Kopaei M. New concepts in nutraceuticals as alternative for pharmaceuticals. *Int J Prev Med* 2014; 5(12): 1487–1499.
60. Rimando AM, Wilhelmina K, Magee JB, Dewey J, Ballington JR. Resveratrol, pterostilbene, and piceatannol in vaccinium berries. *J Agric Food Chem* 2004; 52(15): 4713–4719.
61. Kawabata K, Yoshioka Y, Terao J. Role of intestinal microbiota in the bioavailability and physiological functions of dietary polyphenols. *Molecules* 2019; 24(2): 370.
62. Andrew R, Izzo AA. Principles of pharmacological research of nutraceuticals. *Br J Pharmacol* 2017; 174(11): 1177–1194.
63. Mythri RB, Srinivas Bharath MM. Curcumin: A potential neuroprotective agent in Parkinson's disease. *Curr Pharm Des* 2012; 18(1): 91–99.
64. Abdel-Lateef E, Mahmoud F, Hammam O, et al. Bioactive chemical constituents of Curcuma longa L. rhizomes extract inhibit the growth of human hepatoma cell line (HepG2). *Acta Pharm* 2016; 66(3): 387–398.
65. Singh G, Kapoor IPS, Singh P, de Heluani CS, de Lampasona MP, Catalan CAN. Comparative study of chemical composition and antioxidant activity of fresh and dry rhizomes of turmeric (Curcuma longa Linn.). *Food Chem Toxicol* 2010; 48(4): 1026–1031.
66. Pandit RS, Gaikwad SC, Agarkar GA, Gade AK, Rai M. Curcumin nanoparticles: Physico-chemical fabrication and its *in vitro* efficacy against human pathogens. *3 Biotech* 2015; 5(6): 991–997.
67. Shoji M, Nakagawa K, Watanabe A, et al. Comparison of the effects of curcumin and curcumin glucuronide in human hepatocellular carcinoma HepG2 cells. *Food Chem* 2014; 151: 126–132.
68. Vamanu E, Sarbu I. Impact of Curcuma longa consumption on the gut microbiota composition of cardiovascular patients in proceedings of the conference, 12th world congress on polyphenols applications, Bonn, 2018.
69. Nelson KM, Dahlin JL, Bisson J, Graham J, Pauli GF, Walters MA. The essential medicinal chemistry of curcumin. *J Med Chem* 2017; 60(5): 1620–1637.
70. Tuohy KM, Conterno L, Gasperotti M, Viola R. UP-regulating the human intestinal microbiome using whole plant foods, polyphenols, and/or fiber. *J Agric Food Chem* 2012; 60(36): 8776–8782.
71. Selma MV, Espin JC, Tomas-Barberan FA. Interaction between phenolics and gut microbiota: Role in human health. *J Agric Food Chem* 2009; 57(15): 6485–6501.
72. Duda-Chodak A. The inhibitory effect of polyphenols on human gut microbiota. *J Physiol Pharmacol* 2012; 63(5): 497–503.
73. Lazar V, Ditu L-M, Pircalabioru GG, Picu A, Petcu L, Cucu N, Chifiriuc MC. Gut microbiota, host organism, and diet trialogue in diabetes and obesity. *Front Nutr* 2019; 6: 21.
74. Takiishi T, Fenero CIM, Câmara NOS. Intestinal barrier and gut microbiota: Shaping our immune responses throughout life. *Tissue Barriers* 2017; 5(4): e1373208.

75. Tsai Y-L, Lin T-L, Chang C-J, Wu T-R, Lai W-F, Lu C-C, Lai H-C. Probiotics, prebiotics and amelioration of diseases. *J Biomed Sci* 2019; 26(1): 3.
76. Moreno-Indias I, Sánchez-Alcoholado L, Pérez-Martínez P, Andrés-Lacueva C, Cardona F, Tinahones FJ, Queipo-Ortuño MI. Red wine polyphenols modulate fecal microbiota and reduce markers of the metabolic syndrome in obese patients. *Food Funct* 2016; 7: 1775–1787.
77. Ray SK, Mukherjee S. Evolving interplay between dietary polyphenols and gut microbiota—An emerging importance in healthcare. *Front Nutr* 2021; 8: 634944.
78. Hou D, Yousaf L, Xue Y, et al. Mung bean (Vigna radiata L.): Bioactive polyphenols, polysaccharides, peptides, and health benefits. *Nutrients* 2019; 11(6): 1238.
79. Nair RM, Yang R-Y, Easdown WJ, Thavarajah D, Thavarajah P, Hughes JD, Keatinge J. Biofortification of mungbean (Vigna radiata) as a whole food to enhance human health. *J Sci Food Agric* 2013; 93(8): 1805–1813.
80. Sae-Tan S, Kumrungsee T, Yanaka N. Mungbean seed coat water extract inhibits inflammation in LPS-induced acute liver injury mice and LPS-stimulated RAW246.7 macrophages via the inhibition of TAK1/IκBα/NF-κB. *J Food Sci Technol* 2020; 57(7): 2659–2668.
81. Buathong N, Chandarajoti K, Sae-tan S. Anti-inflammatory potential of mung bean seed coat water extract in lipopolysaccharide- induced 3T3-L1 adipocytes. *J Agric Nat Resour* 2021; 55: 777–786.
82. Cao D, Li H, Yi JY, et al. Antioxidant properties of the mung bean flavonoids on alleviating heat stress. *PLOS ONE* 2011; 6(6): e21071.
83. Jang Y-H, Kang M-J, Choe E-O, Shin M, Kim J-I. Mung bean coat ameliorates hyperglycemia and the antioxidant status in type 2 diabetic db/db mice. *Food Sci Biotechnol* 2014; 23(1): 247–252.
84. Yao Y, Chen F, Wang M, Wang J, Ren G. Antidiabetic activity of mung bean extracts in diabetic KK-ay mice. *J Agric Food Chem* 2008; 56(19): 8869–8873.
85. Zheng Y, Liu S, Xie J, et al. Antioxidant, α-amylase and α-glucosidase inhibitory activities of bound polyphenols extracted from mung bean skin dietary fiber. *LWT Food Sci Technol* 2020; 132(17): 109943.
86. Hou D, Zhao Q, Yousaf L, Xue Y, Shen Q. Beneficial effects of mung bean seed coat on the prevention of high-fat diet-induced obesity and the modulation of gut microbiota in mice. *Eur J Nutr* 2021; 60(4): 2029–2045.
87. Dong K, Ni H, Wu M, Tang Z, Halim M, Shi D. ROS-mediated glucose metabolic reprogram induces insulin resistance in type 2 diabetes. *Biochem Biophys Res Commun* 2016; 476(4): 204–211.
88. Saeting O, Chandarajoti K, Phongphisutthinan A, Hongsprabhas P, Sae Tan S. Water extract of mungbean (Vigna radiata L.) inhibits protein tyrosine Phosphatase-1B in insulin-resistant HepG2 cells. *Molecules* 2021; 26(5): 1452.
89. Huang Q, Chen L, Teng H, Song H, Wu X, Xu M. Phenolic compounds ameliorate the glucose uptake in HepG2 cells' insulin resistance via activating AMPK: Anti-diabetic effect of phenolic compounds in HepG2 cells. *J Funct Foods* 2015; 19: 487–494.
90. Chanput W, Krueyos N, Ritthiruangdej P. Anti-oxidative assays as markers for anti-inflammatory activity of flavonoids. *Int Immunopharmacol* 2016; 40: 170–175.
91. Dueñas M, Cueva C, Muñoz-González I, et al. Studies on modulation of gut microbiota by wine polyphenols: From isolated cultures to omic approaches. *Antioxidants (Basel)* 2015; 4(1): 1–21.
92. Etxeberria U, Fernández-Quintela A, Milagro FI, Aguirre L, Martínez JA, Portillo MP. Impact of polyphenols and polyphenol-rich dietary sources on gut microbiota composition. *J Agric Food Chem* 2013; 61(40): 9517–9533.
93. Moco S, Martin FPJ, Rezzi S. Metabolomics view on gut microbiome modulation by polyphenol-rich foods. *J Proteome Res* 2012; 11(10): 4781–4790.
94. Scalbert A, Johnson IT, Saltmarsh M. Polyphenols: Antioxidants and beyond. *Am J Clin Nutr* 2005; 81(1): 215S–217S.

95. Tomás-Barberán FA, Selma MV, Espín JC. Interactions of gut microbiota with dietary polyphenols and consequences to human health. *Curr Opin Clin Nutr Metab Care* 2016; 19(6): 471–476.
96. Selma MV, Espín JC, Tomás-Barberán FA. Interaction between phenolics and gut microbiota: Role in human health. *J Agric Food Chem* 2009; 57(15): 6485–6501.
97. Mahowald MA, Rey FE, Seedorf H, et al. Characterizing a model human gut microbiota composed of members of its two dominant bacterial phyla. *Proc Natl Acad Sci U S A* 2009; 106(14): 5859–5864.
98. Ozdal T, Sela DA, Xiao J, Boyacioglu D, Chen F, Capanoglu E. The reciprocal interactions between polyphenols and gut microbiota and effects on bioaccessibility. *Nutrients* 2016; 8(2): 78.
99. Most J, Penders J, Lucchesi M, Goossens GH, Blaak EE. Gut microbiota composition in relation to the metabolic response to 12-week combined polyphenol supplementation in overweight men and women. *Eur J Clin Nutr* 2017; 71(9): 1040–1045.
100. Etxeberria U, Arias N, Boqué N, Macarulla MT, Portillo MP, Martínez JA, Milagro FI. Reshaping faecal gut microbiota composition by the intake of trans-resveratrol and quercetin in high-fat sucrose diet-fed rats. *J Nutr Biochem* 2015; 26(6): 651–660.
101. Li Y, Rahman SU, Huang Y, et al. Green tea polyphenols decrease weight gain, ameliorate alteration of gut microbiota, and mitigate intestinal inflammation in canines with highfat- diet-induced obesity. *J Nutr Biochem* 2020; 78: 108324.
102. Chen L, Jiang B, Zhong C, et al. Chemoprevention of colorectal cancer by black raspberry anthocyanins involved the modulation of gut microbiota and SFRP2 demethylation. *Carcinogenesis* 2018; 39(3): 471–481.
103. Rodríguez-Daza MC, Daoust L, Boutkrabt L, et al. Wild blueberry proanthocyanidins shape distinct gut microbiota profile and influence glucose homeostasis and intestinal phenotypes in high-fat high- sucrose fed mice. *Sci Rep* 2020; 10(1): 2217.
104. Moreno-Indias I, Sánchez-Alcoholado L, Pérez-Martínez P, et al. Red wine polyphenols modulate fecal microbiota and reduce markers of the metabolic syndrome in obese patients. *Food Funct* 2016; 7(4): 1775–1787.
105. Cardona F, Andrés-Lacueva C, Tulipani S, Tinahones FJ, Queipo-Ortuño MI. Benefits of polyphenols on gut microbiota and implications in human health. *J Nutr Biochem* 2013; 24(8): 1415–1422.
106. Miller DJ, Fort PE. Heat shock proteins regulatory role in neurodevelopment. *Front Neurosci* 2018; 12: 821.
107. Molan A-L, Liu Z, Plimmer G. Evaluation of the effect of blackcurrant products on gut microbiota and on markers of risk for colon cancer in humans. *Phytother Res* 2014; 28(3): 416–422.
108. Tzounis X, Rodriguez-Mateos A, Vulevic J, Gibson GR, Kwik-Uribe C, Spencer JP. Prebiotic evaluation of cocoa-derived flavanols in healthy humans by using a randomized, controlled, double-blind, crossover intervention study. *Am J Clin Nutr* 2011; 93(1): 62–72.
109. Vendrame S, Guglielmetti S, Riso P, Arioli S, Klimis-Zacas D, Porrini M. Six-week consumption of a wild blueberry powder drink increases bifidobacteria in the human gut. *J Agric Food Chem* 2011; 59(24): 12815–12820.
110. Liu Z, Lin X, Huang G, Zhang W, Rao P, Ni L. Prebiotic effects of almonds and almond skins on intestinal microbiota in healthy adult humans. *Anaerobe* 2014; 26: 1–6.
111. Moreno-Indias I, Sánchez-Alcoholado L, Pérez-Martínez P, Andrés-Lacueva C, Cardona F, Tinahones FJ, Queipo-Ortuño MI. Red wine polyphenols modulate fecal microbiota and reduce markers of the metabolic syndrome in obese patients. *Food Funct* 2016; 7: 1775–1787.
112. Rodríguez-Morató J, Matthan NR, Liu J, de la Torre R, Chen C-YO. Cranberries attenuate animal-based diet-induced changes in microbiota composition and functionality: A randomized crossover controlled feeding trial. *J Nutr Biochem* 2018; 62: 76–86.

113. Yuan X, Long Y, Ji Z, et al. Green tea liquid consumption alters the human intestinal and oral microbiome. *Mol Nutr Food Res* 2018; 62(12): e1800178.
114. Queipo-Ortuño MI, Boto-Ordóñez M, Murri M, et al. Influence of red wine polyphenols and ethanol on the gut microbiota ecology and biochemical biomarkers. *Am J Clin Nutr* 2012; 95(6): 1323–1334.
115. Frezza PD, Edeas M, Paule A. Microbiota and phage therapy: Future challenges in medicine. *Med Sci (Basel)* 2018; 6(4): 86.
116. Zhao Y, Jiang Q. Roles of the polyphenol-gut microbiota interaction in alleviating colitis and preventing colitis-associated colorectal cancer. *Adv Nutr* 2021; 12(2): 546–565.
117. Saint-Georges-Chaumet Y, Edeas M, Carbonetti N. Microbiota–mitochondria intertalk: Consequence for microbiota–host interaction. *Pathog Dis* 2016; 74(1): ftv096.
118. Chakraborty MS, Mukherjee C. Study of dietary polyphenols from natural herbal sources for providing protection against human degenerative disorders. *Biocatal Agr Biotechnol* 2021; 33: 101956.
119. Friedman JM. Leptin and the endocrine control of energy balance. *Nat Metab* 2019; 1(8): 754–764.
120. Aragones G, Ardid-Ruiz A, Ibars M, Suarez M, Blade C. Modulation of leptin resistance by food compounds. *Mol Nutr Food Res* 2016; 60(8): 1789–1803.
121. Ibars M, Ardid-Ruiz A, Suarez M, Muguerza B, Blade C, Aragones G. Proanthocyanidins potentiate hypothalamic leptin/stat3 signalling and POMC gene expression in rats with diet-induced obesity. *Int J Obes (Lond)* 2017; 41(1): 129–136.
122. Finaud J, Lac G, Filaire E. Oxidative stress: Relationship with exercise and training. *Sports Med* 2006; 36(4): 327–358.
123. McLeay Y, Stannard S, Houltham S, Starck C. Dietary thiols in exercise: Oxidative stress defence, exercise performance, and adaptation. *J Int Soc Sports Nutr* 2017; 14(1): 1–8.
124. Rousseau I, Margaritis AS. Does physical exercise modify antioxidant requirements? *Nutr Res Rev* 2008; 21(1): 3–12.
125. Sacheck JM, Blumberg JB. Role of vitamin E and oxidative stress in exercise. *Nutrition* 2001; 17(10): 809–814.
126. Kurutas EB. The importance of antioxidants which play the role in cellular response against oxidative/nitrosative stress: Current state. *Nutr J* 2015; 15(71): 1–22.
127. Milner JA. Reducing the risk of cancer. In: Goldberg I, editor. *Functional Foods: Designer Foods, Pharmafoods, Nutraceuticals.* New York: Chapman & Hall, 1994; 39–70.
128. Duthie GG, Brown KM. Reducing the risk of cardiovascular disease. In: Goldberg I, editor. *Functional Foods: Designer Foods, Pharmafoods, Nutraceuticals.* New York: Chapman & Hall, 1994; 19–38.
129. Harborne JB, Williams CA. Advances in flavonoid research since 1992. *Phytochemistry* 2000; 55(6): 481–504.
130. Bravo L. Polyphenols: Chemistry, dietary sources, metabolism, and nutritional significance. *Nutr Rev* 1998; 56(11): 317–333.
131. Cheynier V. Polyphenols in foods are more complex than often thought. *Am J Clin Nutr* 2005; 81: 223S–29S.
132. Kehrer JP, Klotz LO. Free radicals and related reactive species as mediators of tissue injury and disease: Implications for health. *Crit Rev Toxicol* 2015; 45(9): 765–798.
133. Harman D. Aging: A theory based on free radical and radiation chemistry. *J Gerontol* 1956; 11(3): 298–300.
134. Paniker NV, Srivastava SK, Beutler E. Glutathione metabolismof the red cells: Effect of glutathione reductase deficiency on the stimulation of hexose monophosphate shunt under oxidative stress. *Biochim Biophys Acta* 1970; 215(3): 456–460.
135. Sies H. Oxidative stress: Introductory remarks. In: Sies H, editor. *Oxidative Stress.* London: Academic Press, Elsevier Ltd, 1985; 1–8.

136. Sies H, Cadenas E. Oxidative stress: Damage to intact cells and organs. *Philos Trans R Soc Lond B Biol Sci* 1985; 311(1152): 617–631.
137. Jones DP. Redefining oxidative stress. *Antioxid Redox Signal* 2006; 8(9–10): 1865–1879.
138. Jones DP. Radical-free biology of oxidative stress. *Am J Physiol Cell Physiol* 2008; 295(4): C849–C868.
139. Sies H. Oxidative stress: Eustress and distress in redox homeostasis. In: Fink G, editor. *Stress: Physiology, Biochemistry, and Pathology.* London: Academic Press, Elsevier Ltd, 2019; 153–163.
140. Birben E, Sahiner UM, Sackesen C, Erzurum S, Kalayci O. Oxidative stress and antioxidant defense. *World Allergy Organ J* 2012; 5(1): 9–19.
141. Zhang H, Tsao R. Dietary polyphenols, oxidative stress and antioxidant and anti-inflammatory effects. *Curr Opin Food Sci* 2016; 8: 33–42.
142. Mei J, Ma X, Xie J. Review on natural preservatives for extending fish shelf life. *Foods* 2019; 8(10): 490.
143. Pezeshk S, Ojagh SM, Alishahi A. Effect of plant antioxidant and antimicrobial compounds on the shelf-life of seafood—a review. *Czech J Food Sci* 2016; 33(3): 195–203.
144. Dasilva G, Boller M, Medina I, Storch J. Relative levels of dietary EPA and DHA impact gastric oxidation and essential fatty acid uptake. *J Nutr Biochem* 2018; 55: 68–75.
145. Maestre R, Douglass JD, Kodukula S, Medina I, Storch J. Alterations in the intestinal assimilation of oxidized pufas are ameliorated by a polyphenol-rich grape seed extract in an *in vitro* model and caco-2 cells. *J Nutr* 2013; 143(3): 295–301.
146. Molinar-Toribio E, Ramos-Romero S, Fuguet E et al. Influence of Omega-3 PUFAs on the metabolism of proanthocyanidins in rats. *Food Res Int* 2017; 97: 133–140.
147. Gu C, Suleria HAR, Dunshea FR, Howell K. Dietary lipids influence bioaccessibility of polyphenols from black carrots and affect microbial diversity under simulated gastrointestinal digestion. *Antioxidants (Basel)* 2020; 9(8): 762.
148. Crauste C, Rosell M, Durand T, Vercauteren J. Omega-3 polyunsaturated Lipophenols, how and why? *Biochimie* 2016; 120: 62–74.
149. Warburton A, Vasieva O, Quinn P, Stewart JP, Quinn JP. Statistical analysis of human microarray data shows that dietary intervention with n–3 fatty acids, flavonoids and resveratrol enriches for immune response and disease pathways. *Br J Nutr* 2018; 119(3): 239–249.
150. Erben-Russ M, Bors W, Saran M. Reactions of linoleic acid peroxyl radicals with phenolic antioxidants: A pulse radiolysis study. *Int J Radiat Biol Relat Stud Phys Chem Med* 1987; 52(3): 393–412.
151. Siti HN, Kamisah Y, Kamsiah J. The role of oxidative stress, antioxidants and vascular inflammation in cardiovascular disease (a review). *Vascul Pharmacol* 2015; 71: 40–56.
152. Hertog MG, Feskens EJ, Hollman PC, Katan MB, Kromhout D. Dietary antioxidant flavonoids and risk of coronary heart disease: The Zutphen elderly study. *Lancet* 1993; 342(8878): 1007–1011.
153. U.S. Department of Agriculture, Agricultural Research Service. USDA database for the oxygen radical absorbance capacity (ORAC) of selected foods. Release 2, 2010.
154. Prior RL, Hoang H, Gu L, et al. Assays for hydrophilic and lipophilic antioxidant capacity (oxygen radical absorbance capacity (ORAC(FL))) of plasma and other biological and food samples. *J Agric Food Chem* 2003; 51(11): 3273–3279.
155. Gillespie KM, Chae JM, Ainsworth EA. Rapid measurement of total antioxidant capacity in plants. *Nat Protoc* 2007; 2(4): 867–870.
156. Litescu SC, Eremia S, Radu GL. Methods for the determination of antioxidant capacity in food and raw materials. *Adv Exp Med Biol* 2010; 698: 241–249.
157. Cunningham E. What has happened to the ORAC database? *J Acad Nutr Diet* 2013; 113(5): 740.
158. Forman HJ, Davies KJ, Ursini F. How do nutritional antioxidants really work: Nucleophilic tone and para-hormesis versus free radical scavenging *in vivo*. *Free Radic Biol Med* 2014; 66: 24–35.

159. Krga I, Milenkovic D, Morand C, Monfoulet LE. An update on the role of nutrigenomic modulations in mediating the cardiovascular protective effect of fruit polyphenols. *Food Funct* 2016; 7(9): 3656–3676.
160. Kim HS, Quon MJ, Kim JA. New insights into the mechanisms of polyphenols beyond antioxidant properties; lessons from the green tea polyphenol, epigallocatechin 3-gallate. *Redox Biol* 2014; 2: 187–195.
161. Goszcz K, Duthie GG, Stewart D, Leslie SJ, Megson IL. Bioactive polyphenols and cardiovascular disease: Chemical antagonists, pharmacological agents or xenobioticsthat drive an adaptive response? *Br J Pharmacol* 2017; 174(11): 1209–1225.
162. Kerimi A, Williamson G. At the interface of antioxidant signalling and cellular function: Key polyphenol effects. *Mol Nutr Food Res* 2016; 60(8): 1770–1788.
163. Monfoulet LE, Mercier S, Bayle D, Tamaian R, Barber-Chamoux N, Morand C, Milenkovic D. Curcumin modulates endothelial permeability and monocyte transendothelial migration by affecting endothelial cell dynamics. *Free Radic Biol Med* 2017; 112: 109–120.
164. Krga I, Tamaian R, Mercier S, et al. Anthocyanins and their gut metabolites attenuate monocyte adhesion and transendothelial migration through nutrigenomic mechanisms regulating endothelial cell permeability. *Free Radic Biol Med* 2018; 124: 364–379.
165. Álvarez-Cilleros D, Ramos S, Goya L, Martín MÁ. Colonic metabolites from flavanols stimulate nitric oxide production in human endothelial cells and protect against oxidative stress-induced toxicity and endothelial dysfunction. *Food Chem Toxicol* 2018; 115: 88–97.
166. Milenkovic D, Berghe WV, Morand C, et al. A systems biology network analysis of nutri(epi)genomic changes in endothelial cells exposed to epicatechin metabolites. *Sci Rep* 2018; 8(1): 15487.
167. Rattan S. Aging, health, hormesis and future lines of investigation. *Aging Sci* 2014; 2: 1000e111.
168. Son TG, Camandola S, Mattson MP. Hormetic dietary phytochemicals. *NeuroMolecular Med* 2008; 10(4): 236–246.
169. Yates AA, Erdman JW Jr, Shao A, Dolan LC, Griffiths JC. Bioactive nutrients – Time for tolerable upper intake levels to address safety. *Regul Toxicol Pharmacol* 2017; 84: 94–101.

# 14

# The Role of Functional Foods and Nutraceuticals in Gastrointestinal Health

Dan DuBourdieu, Jamil Talukder, Ajay Srivastava,
Rajiv Lall, and Ramesh C. Gupta

## Contents

DOI: 10.1201/9781003333821-14

# 14.1 Introduction

The gastrointestinal (GI) system has a pivotal physiological role in the absorption of essential nutrients and metabolites from the GI tract (GIT). Alongside the essential nutrients, microbes and their toxins and other harmful substances are also absorbed from the GIT. The GI system appears to suffer from a variety of diseases and syndromes, such as gastritis, intestinal mucositis, chronic inflammatory bowel diseases (IBD) including Crohn's disease (CD) and ulcerative colitis (UC), peptic ulcers, dysbiosis, chronic enteropathy, celiac disease, leaky gut syndrome, cancer, etc. Damage to the GI system can also be caused by: (1) nonsteroidal anti-inflammatory drugs (NSAIDS) overdosage, (2) chemotherapy, (3) metabolic disorders, and (4) radiation exposure (Banerjee and Gupta, 2019; Gupta et al., 2019; Glassner et al., 2020).

The GI microbiome (consisting of bacteria, viruses, protozoa, fungi, and archaea) plays an immense role in promoting GI health and in the prevention and treatment of diseases. Alterations in the GI microbiome can lead to inflammatory and immunomodulatory diseases not only in the GIT (Belkaid and Hand, 2014; Halfvarson, 2017; Glassner et al., 2020), but also in other organs/systems and pathways (cardiovascular, central nervous, hepatic, renal, endocrine, immune, etc.) (Noverr and Huffnagle, 2004; Clapp et al., 2017; Lee et al., 2020; Golovinskaia and Wang, 2022). Altered microbiota-gut–brain axis can lead to mental diseases (Mayer et al., 2014; Clapp et al., 2017; Butler et al., 2019; Cryan et al., 2019), gut-liver axis can lead to hepatic diseases (Tripathi et al., 2018), and gut-kidney axis can lead to renal diseases (Chen et al., 2019). Prevention and therapeutic interventions of these diseases can be achieved through microbiome-based strategies involving selected diets, functional foods, prebiotics, probiotics, postbiotics, and nutraceuticals (Voreades et al., 2014; Liu et al., 2015; Kim et al., 2016; Uranga et al., 2016; Clapp et al., 2017; Fritsch et al., 2022).

Phytoconstituents present in functional foods and nutraceuticals can exert their biological effects by serving as substrates for biochemical reactions, cofactors for enzymatic reactions, enzyme modulators, enhancement of absorption, and stability of essential nutrients and nutraceuticals. They can also scavenge and eliminate toxic compounds from the GIT and serve as selective growth factors and substrates for beneficial bacteria, as well as inhibitors of deleterious intestinal bacteria (Keerthana et al., 2019; Gupta et al., 2021).

Most nutraceuticals are unstable, poorly soluble, and absorbed in the GIT, thereby limiting their bioavailability (Kang et al., 2009; Jhanwar and Gupta, 2014; Pandit et al., 2019). Some of these issues can be resolved using stabilizers, emulsifiers, bioenhancers, nanoparticles, and other new technologies (Keservani et al., 2010; Kesarwani et al., 2013; Jain and Patil, 2015; Das et al., 2016; Yurdakok-Dikmen et al., 2018; Srivastava et al., 2019).

Insult to the GIT by diseases and toxicants can be monitored by employing a variety of biomarkers, such as the presence of occult blood in feces, evaluation of the GI content and blood/serum, histopathological examination, and prediction of effects on GI absorption and contractility using *in vitro/ex vivo* systems (Banerjee and Gupta, 2019; Dinesh et al., 2022). The use of many biomarkers can aid us in the evaluation of therapeutic efficacy and safety of functional foods and nutraceuticals in GI diseases.

This chapter describes the role of functional foods and nutraceuticals in the prevention and therapeutic interventions of GI diseases, with a specific focus on TurmiZn in leaky gut syndrome.

## 14.2 Biomarkers of Foods, Nutraceuticals and GI Health and Disease

### 14.2.1 Foods and Nutraceuticals

Many functional foods and nutraceuticals with antioxidative, anti-inflammatory, fatty acid, prebiotic, probiotic, synbiotic, and immunomodulating properties have been discovered that ameliorate the signs of GI diseases (Banerjee and Gupta, 2019; Talukder, 2019). An appropriate food is an integral part of normal body functions as well as for the digestive system that helps in the absorption of nutrients, prevention of nutritional deficiencies and malnutrition, repair of damaged intestinal epithelium, restoration of normal luminal bacterial populations, promotion of normal GI motility, and maintenance of normal immune functions (Zoran, 2003). Recently, Banerjee and Gupta (2019) and Gupta et al. (2019) described a number of biomarkers for safety and toxicity of foods and nutraceuticals in general and GI health and disease in particular.

In the food and nutraceutical industries, biomarkers play pivotal roles in the identification and quantification of chemical ingredients, pharmacokinetics and toxicokinetics, food-herb-drug interactions, safety and toxicity evaluations, and decision-making policies (Gupta et al., 2019).

These compounds can be identified and quantitated in the food ingredients/ nutraceuticals and in body fluids and tissues, and they often serve as biomarkers of food/nutraceutical intake. For example, plasma levels of alkylresorcinol C17 and alkylresorcinol C19 serve as good biomarkers of whole grain wheat and rye intake; β-alanine for beef; eicosapentaenoic acid (EPA) and 3-carboxy-4-methyl-5-propyl-2-furanpropanoic acid (CMPF) for fish; linoleic acid for seeds, nuts, vegetable oil, etc. (Gupta et al., 2019). Some biomarkers are specific, while others are neither specific nor validated. These biomarkers can not only aid in identifying the food or nutraceutical consumed but also in pharmacokinetics and toxicokinetics, phytotherapy, and interaction in polypharmacy.

Some plant-based nutraceuticals have toxic principle(s), mentioned in parentheses: St. John's wort (hypericin), goldenseal (hydrastine), ginkgo biloba (ginkgotoxins), kava (flavokawain B), ephedra (ephedrine), pennyroyal oil (ketone pulegone), *Aristolochia* (aristolochic acid), bitter melon (momordins and vicine), lychee (hypoglycin A), comfrey (pyrrolizidine alkaloid), green tea (epigallocatechin-3-gallate), and many others (Gupta et al., 2018, 2019). Detection of these phytotoxic compounds or their metabolite(s) in the body tissues or fluids often serves as a biomarker of exposure, and the level of exposure can serve as a biomarker of effect. Thus, with the aid of validated biomarkers, the food and nutraceutical industries will have greater confidence in high-quality foods and nutraceuticals (Gupta et al., 2019).

## 14.2.2 GI Health and Disease

A number of biomarkers for GI damage have been tested to investigate their usefulness in tracking adverse events. Some of these biomarkers are listed in Table 14.1.

Some other fecal biomarkers of GI damage include lysozyme, leukocyte esterase, elastase, myeloperoxidase, TNF-α, IL-β, IL-4, IL-10, alpha-1 antitrypsin, alpha-2-macroglobulin, and M2-pyruvate kinase (Banerjee and Gupta, 2019).

Currently, in the area of GI biomarker research, scientists are trying to understand GI metabolomics and develop and validate novel metabolome-based biomarkers. GI tissue metabolomic profiles provide an information-rich matrix that can lead to the identification of metabolites such as lipids and organic acids, as well as amino acids that may impact overall GI metabolism.

## 14.3 Foods and Functional Foods

Food usually consists of protein, carbohydrate, fat, and other nutrients which are used in the body of an organism to provide energy and growth, and to maintain vital processes. Functional food consists of ingredients that provide health benefits beyond nutritional values. These have gained recognition for promoting good health and well-being and are also known as nutraceuticals. Nutraceuticals prevent nutrient deficiencies, promote proper growth and development, and protect organisms against disease(s). The concept of "Functional Food" was coined in Japan in the 1980s (Katan, 2004) based on "foods for specified health use" (FOSHU). A second definition of functional foods was developed by Functional Food Science in Europe (FUFOSE): functional food is a food with certain beneficial effects on one or more target functions in the body beyond the basic nutritional effects to improved health state and well-being or reduction of risk of diseases. It is consumed as a part of a normal diet and is not used in the form of a pill or capsule or any other form of dietary supplement. However, the agencies of the Japanese government started approving foods with proven benefits to provide better health to the overall population (Lang, 2007). Furthermore, a functional food can have a component in which a health-promoting component has been added or

**Table 14.1** Biomarkers for GI Damage.

| Blood Biomarkers | Brief Description | Applications |
|---|---|---|
| Citrulline | An intermediate metabolic amino acid produced mainly by enterocytes of the small intestine | A promising biomarker of mucosal mass and absorptive enterocyte mass, atrophy of Celiac disease, and a safety biomarker of small intestinal injury |
| Diamine oxidase (DAO) | An enzyme that catabolizes substrates such as histamine and diamines | Biomarker of small intestine lesions and mucositis |
| CD64 | A high-affinity Fragment crystalizable receptor I (FcRI) receptor for IgG, serves as a ligand for acute phase reactants, C-reactive protein (CRP) and amyloid P | A biomarker of GI inflammation (e.g., IBD) and injury |
| Gastrins | Gastrins are a family of sequence-related carboxyamidated peptides produced by the endocrine G cells of the gastric antrum and duodenum in response to various GI stimuli | Indicative of duodenal ulcers, mucosal damage, chronic lymphocytic-plasmacytic enteritis, bacterial infections, tumors, etc. |
| C-reactive protein (CRP) | CRP is a hepatic protein produced in response to acute and chronic inflammatory conditions | An indirect biomarker of GI inflammation. Also a good biomarker of bacterial and viral infections, autoimmune disorders, malignancy, and tissue necrosis |
| Matrix metalloproteinases (MMPs) | MMPs are zinc-dependent endopeptidases | Often used as tissue-specific biomarkers of chemotherapy-induced gut-injury |
| Pepsinogen I and II | These are precursors of pepsin and are produced by the gastric mucosa and released into the gastric lumen and peripheral circulation | Used as biomarkers of severe inflammation of gastric mucosa and its progression toward atrophic gastritis |
| **Fecal Biomarkers** | | |
| Calprotectin | Calprotectin is a calcium-binding protein (36.5-kDa nonglycosylated protein) found in abundance in neutrophils. Lower concentrations are also found in monocytes and reactive macrophages. The release of calprotectin is most likely a consequence of cell disruption and death | Calprotectin reflects the flux of leukocytes into the intestinal lumen. A very good biomarker of GI inflammation |
| Lactoferrin | Lactoferrin, an iron-binding glycoprotein, is secreted by most mucosal membranes and is a major component of the secondary granules of polymorphonuclear neutrophils (PMNs) | Lactoferrin in feces is an indicator of intestinal inflammation |

(*Continued*)

**Table 14.1 (Continued)** Biomarkers for GI Damage.

| Blood Biomarkers | Brief Description | Applications |
|---|---|---|
| Polymorphonuclear neutrophil elastase (PMN-e) | PMN-e is a neutral proteinase normally stored in the azurophil granules of PMNs | Used as an indicator of GI inflammation |
| Bile acids | The fecal bile acids are a complex mixture of metabolites of bile acids produced by intestinal microorganisms | Increases in bile acids are indicators of malabsorption, which can cause diarrhea |
| Fatty acid-binding proteins: I-FABP and L-FABP | There are two fatty acid-binding proteins (FABPs): intestinal FABP (I-FABP) and liver FABP (L-FABP). Both are very small proteins and are released from GI enterocytes into the blood after cellular damage | These are good biomarkers of cellular damage |
| MicroRNAs (miRNAs) | miRNAs are small, endogenous noncoding RNAs that act as posttranscriptional regulators of gene expression | Fecal miRNA assay is being developed as a screening tool for human colon cancer, active ulcerative colitis, and GI toxicity |
| Fecal S100A12 | Fecal S100A12 is similar to calprotectin, and it activates NF-κB signal transduction and enhances cytokine release | Fecal S100A12 is a sensitive and specific biomarker for IBD |

from which a component for specific health reasons has been removed, or a component has been modified by technological or chemical means to provide a specific health benefit, or in which the bioavailability of a component has been modified, or a combination of any of them.

Conventional functional foods include fruits, vegetables, nuts, seeds, legumes, whole grains, seafood, herbs, spices, beverages, and fermented foods. The functional foods can originate from either a plant or animal. In addition, there are some modified functional foods such as fortified milk alternatives (e.g., almond, rice, coconut, and cashew milk), fortified dairy products (e.g., vitamin D-added milk and yogurt), fortified grains (e.g., bread and pasta), fortified cereals and granola, fortified eggs (containing egg yolk antibodies IgYs), and fortified juices. Based on their activities, functional foods can be grouped as: (1) dietary fiber, (2) phytochemicals, (3) cholesterol reduction, (4) vitamins and minerals fortification, and (5) probiotics, prebiotics, and synbiotics (Roberfroid, 2000).

## 14.3.1 Benefits of Functional Foods

Functional foods or fortified foods usually contain higher amounts of nutrients, including vitamins, minerals, healthy fats, and fiber. They correlate with various health benefits including the prevention of nutrient deficiencies. For instance, rates of iron deficient-associated anemia were reduced to half in Jordan by the introduction of iron-fortified wheat flour (Dwyer et al., 2015). Fortification is being used to prevent some deficiencies, e.g., iodized salt to prevent goiter. Functional foods also contain antioxidants which neutralize harmful free radicals in the body. Thus, they can prevent cell damage and certain chronic conditions, including heart disease, cancer, and diabetes (Pham-Huy et al., 2008). Functional foods are rich in fiber, which leads to slower digestion and helps in controlling blood sugar levels. They may also help prevent different digestive disorders, such as constipation, hemorrhoids, acid reflux, diverticulitis, and ulcers (Anderson et al., 2009).

Functional foods also perform important roles in prenatal and postnatal growth and development since they contain micronutrients such as iron, zinc, calcium, vitamins, and omega-3 fatty acids. To achieve proper growth and development in infants, essential micronutrients are required (Morrison and Regnault, 2016). Greenberg et al. (2011) described that folic acid (vitamin $B_9$) is an essential nutrient that is required for DNA replication and as a substrate for many enzymatic reactions, amino acid synthesis, and vitamin metabolism. The MRC (Medical Research Council) Vitamin Study Research Group recommended folic acid supplementation before and after pregnancy for all women (1991). It is noted that folic acid may prevent pregnancy-related complications and neural tube defects which can affect the brain and spinal cord development. Defects may be decreased by 50–70% (Greenberg et al., 2011).

## 14.3.2 Functional Foods Help Gut Microbiome

The gut microbiome (GM) of the human GIT contains about 100 trillion microorganisms (Bresalier and Chapkin, 2020), including bacteria, fungi, viruses, protists, and archaea (Quigley, 2017). The intestinal tract is the largest microecosystem in the human body. There are more than 2000 known living species in the human GIT, which collectively contain more than 100 times the genomic DNA of humans (Thursby and Juge, 2017). The gut microbiota plays an important role in the regulation of metabolism and host energy, as well as in the development and maintenance of host immune function. This microbiota also synthesizes nutrients and essential vitamins (Wallace, 2020), which in turn influence normal host physiology.

Perhaps the best-known group of functional foods for gut health are probiotics, which maintain or improve gut health via several mechanisms. They occupy the gut mucosal lining to make a barrier against the colonization of pathogenic bacteria, inhibit the growth of pathogens, and enhance the gut immune response by contact and cross talk with the host via the GIT mucosa.

The unhealthy gut experiences digestive issues like bloating, gas, diarrhea, and food allergies which may lead to anxiety, depression, chronic fatigue, fibromyalgia, mood swings, irritability, skin problems like eczema and rosacea, frequent illnesses, autoimmune disease, hormonal imbalances, poor memory and concentration including attention deficit disorder or attention deficit hyper-activity disorder (Mayer et al., 2014; Clapp et al., 2017; Butler et al., 2019; Cryan et al., 2019). Eighty % of immune system functions depend on gut health. To achieve a healthy gut, bone broth and fermented foods may play important roles, as bone broth contains collagen and amino acids and is easy to digest. Collagen supports healthy connective tissue and joints, and supports skin, hair, and nails. In addition, collagen helps gut healing and supports intercellular junctions such as the tight junction of the GIT lining. Thus, collagen may help greatly with the symptoms of leaky gut syndrome, irritable bowel syndrome (IBS), acid reflux, Crohn's disease (CD), and ulcerative colitis (UC). Bone broth contains amino acids that are required to synthesize collagen in the body. Fermented foods contain probiotics to stabilize the gut microbiome, prebiot-ics to nourish the beneficial bacteria, and enzymes to aid in the breakdown of food for better absorption. Many fermented foods also contain prebiotics to nourish the beneficial bacteria, the probiotics of the gut. Sauerkraut is one of the fermented foods that boost the immune system and deliver probiotics including *Lactobacilli* that make for a healthy gut (Zabat et al., 2018).

### 14.3.3 Functional Foods, Gut Microbiome, and Gut–Brain Axis

Functional foods that originate from plants possess many phytochemicals including polyphenols, carotenoids, phytosterols, lignans, alkaloids, gluco-sinolates, and terpenes. Phytochemicals act as antioxidants, promote redox homeostasis, and act as anti-inflammatory agents that may positively regulate the gut microbiome (GM). Phytochemicals modulate the GM by producing short-chain fatty acids, inhibiting pathogens, and stimulating beneficial bacte-ria (Wang et al., 2022). Therefore, phytochemicals improve gut microbial diver-sity and abundance to support a healthy gut. Furthermore, Mukonowenzou et al. (2021) demonstrated that phytochemicals have important roles in Paneth cells for the maturation of enterocytes.

Recent studies show that gut microbiota produces metabolites including some neurotransmitters such as glutamate, GABA (gamma-aminobutyric acid), sero-tonin, and dopamine which modulate brain functions (Cryan et al., 2019; Chen et al., 2021). In addition, modification of the GM helps to combat neurodegen-eration (Sasmita, 2019).

Figure 14.1 shows that gut microbiota can either produce neurotransmitter precursors, catalyze the synthesis of neurotransmitters through dietary metab-olism, or some combination thereof. Some bacterial taxa may signal through their metabolites to promote the synthesis and release of neurotransmitters by enteroendocrine cells (e.g., metabolites produced by spore-forming bacte-ria serve as signaling molecules to regulate the biosynthesis of serotonin by increasing the expression of its rate-limiting gene TPH1 in enterochromaffin cells). Neurotransmitters synthesized by bacteria and enteroendocrine cells can enter the blood circulation and be transported to other parts of the body.

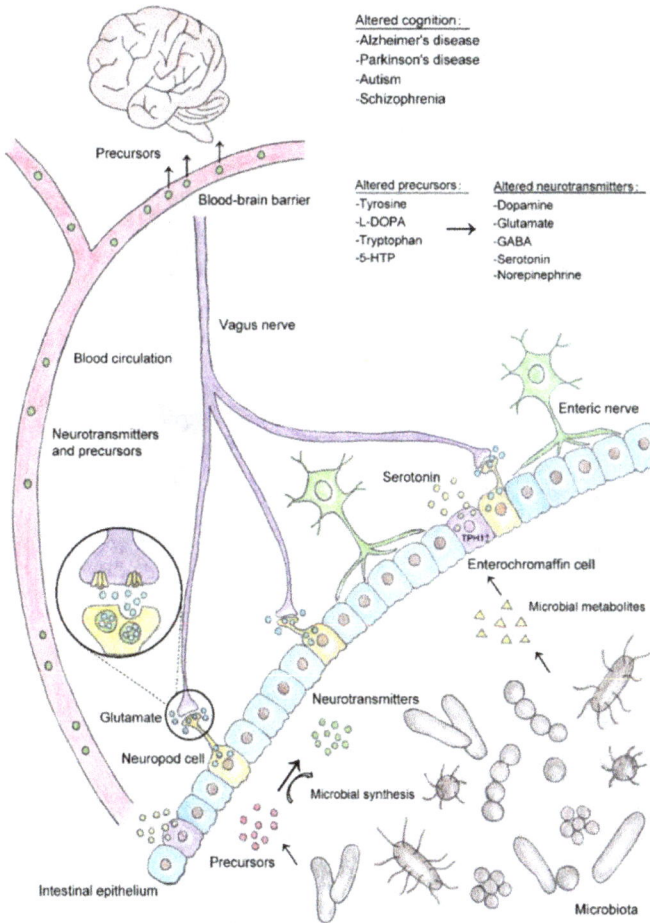

**Figure 14.1** *Gut microbial-mediated neurotransmitter synthesis and its impacts on cognition. (Courtesy, Chen et al., 2021).*

Some neurotransmitter precursors can cross the blood–brain barrier (BBB) and participate in the synthesis cycle of neurotransmitters in the brain. In addition, neuropod cells located in the intestinal epithelium synthesize and release neurotransmitters such as glutamate, which can transmit sensory signals to the brain within milliseconds through the vagus nerve. Gut microbiota-modulated changes in neurotransmitter/precursor synthesis may lead to alterations in brain function and influence cognition in neurological diseases such as Alzheimer's disease, Parkinson's disease, autism, and schizophrenia (Figure 14.2).

Bad mood, increasing age, drugs, dietary changes, and circadian rhythms can disrupt gut microbiota homeostasis. When gut dysbiosis occurs, beneficial bacteria in the gut are transformed into pathogenic bacteria, producing a large

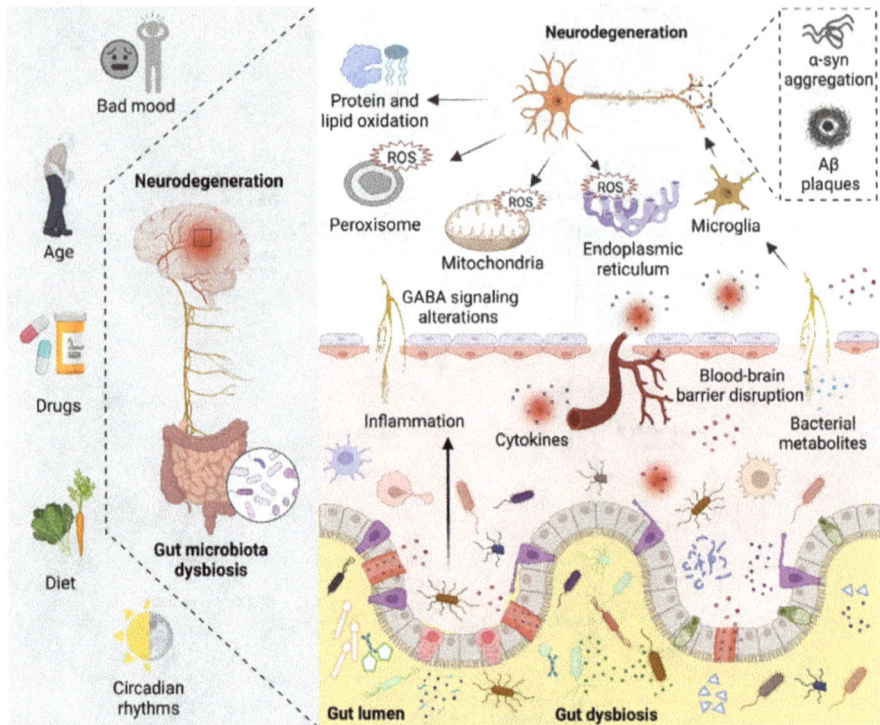

**Figure 14.2** *The role of the gut microbiota in neurodegeneration is depicted schematically. (Courtesy, Wang et al., 2022). Note: Abbreviations: 5-HTP, 5-hydroxytryptophan; l-DOPA, l-3,4-dihydroxy-phenylalanine; GABA, gamma-aminobutyric acid.*

number of harmful metabolites and proinflammatory molecules, resulting in increased BBB permeability and peripheral inflammatory responses, thereby aggravating oxidative stress in the brain. Increased levels of reactive oxygen species (ROS) in neuronal mitochondria, endoplasmic reticulum, and peroxisomes, increased protein and lipid oxidation, and accumulation of neurotoxic proteins lead to neurodegeneration (Wang et al., 2022).

## 14.3.4 Gut and Iron Transport Tocopheryl Polyethylene Glycol Succinate (ITPGS)

Tocopheryl polyethylene glycol succinate (TPGS) is being used as an efficient source of natural vitamin E, both for therapeutic and nutritional purposes. Vitamin E-TPGS (a water-soluble derivative of vitamin E) is a nonionic surfactant used as a solubilizer, absorption enhancer, emulsifier, and antioxidant. On the other hand, ovotransferrin (IT) is an iron-binding glycoprotein from the transferrin family, found in avian egg white. It has various functions including iron adsorption (Giansanti et al., 2012), immunomodulatory (Hirota et al., 1995), antioxidant activity (Kim et al., 2012), Superoxide dismutase (SOD)-like superoxide anion scavenging activity (Ibrahim et al., 2007), and antimicrobial effects (Wang et al., 2021). IT deprives pathogenic bacteria of iron, thereby acting as an antimicrobial agent (Giansanti et al., 2012). Biotechnological applications of IT, IT-related peptides, and some other natural molecules include stimulation of immunity, antimicrobial activities, iron transport, and homeostasis in various health disorders (Giansanti et al., 2012). In addition, Huang et al. (2010) revealed the oxygen radical absorbance capacity of peptides from IT and their interaction with phytochemicals. In essence, ITPGS is a novel formulation that consists of two molecules IT and TPGS (Srivastava et al., 2019). By having α-tocopherol and IT, ITPGS (Figure 14.3) appears to be a unique formulation that exerts a wide range of biological and pharmacological activities.

Chen et al. (2011) reported that berberine chloride (BBR) is a substrate of P-glycoprotein (P-gp), and that it plays an important role in the absorption of BBR (Pan et al. (2002). Srivastava et al. (2019) hypothesized that ITPGS would be a better bioenhancer than TPGS, because with potentially less pathogenic bacteria present, less energy is required by enterocytes and the gut to fight pathogens.

The cytoplasmic esterases hydrolyze ITPGS to liberate free α-tocopherol that localizes in the cell membranes and quenches free radicals and protects the membrane from lipid peroxidation and damage (Yan et al., 2007; Traber and Atkinson, 2007; Jiang, 2014). Srivastava et al. (2019) described that ITPGS works as a free radical scavenger and antioxidant in stressed cells to promote a healthy environment although both TPGS and IT molecules have shown antioxidant properties via different mechanisms.

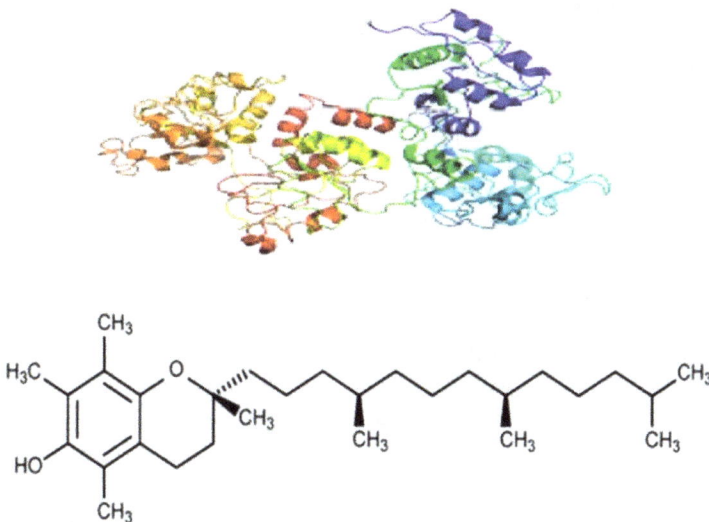

**Figure 14.3** *Structural formula of ITPGS (IT.TPGS).*

Different factors such as diet, disease, infection, medications, toxicants, aging, etc. can cause dysbiosis. In addition, many microorganisms can induce inflammation in the GIT where dysbiosis takes place. A dysbiosis of GIT is usually observed in inflammatory bowel disease (IBD) which may be associated with the systemic immune system (Noverr and Huffnagle, 2004). Talukder et al. (2014) demonstrated that an iron-binding protein (lactoferrin) ameliorates $PGE_2$ mediated inhibition of glucose absorption in enterocytes via the $Ca^{2+}$- and cAMP-signaling pathways. They concluded that iron-binding protein molecules such as Lf or IT appear to play an important role in significantly reducing inflammation of the intestine and restoring the absorption of nutrients. Thus, ITPGS would work as an inflammatory regulator or balancer to maintain normal gut health.

An ample number of studies revealed that the iron-binding protein exhibits antimicrobial properties (Farnaud and Evans, 2003; Talukder et al., 2018; Talukder, 2019). Furthermore, it has been shown that *Pseudomonas* spp., *Escherichia coli*, and *Streptococcus mutans* are the most sensitive and *Proteus* spp. and *Klebsiella* spp. are the most resistant to the antibacterial action of IT (Valenti et al., 1982). Pathogenic bacteria require more iron than nonpathogenic bacteria for their replication, growth, and development.

Direct oral administration of iron may produce an excessive amount of unabsorbed iron in the gut. This would provide enough iron to the environment of pathogenic bacteria for their growth and replication which may lead to a decreased number of beneficial bacteria (probiotics), finally culminating in dysbiosis (Yilmaz and Li, 2018). Interestingly, IT molecules chelate iron from pathogenic bacteria (Gram positive and Gram negative) where it acts as an antimicrobial agent. In contrast, IT molecules do not kill nonpathogenic bacteria while concurrently enhancing the replication and growth of probiotic bacteria (*Lactobacillus* and *Bifidobacteria*). Taken together, ITPGS promotes a healthy gut environment for normal microbial growth and allows for nutrients to be more readily absorbed. This is due to a reduction of a pathogenic bacterial population that would compete for nutrients in the intestine.

## 14.4 Leaky Gut Syndrome

The gastrointestinal tract (GIT) plays a major role in the health of both humans and animals. This is because the GIT has major functions for transportation, digestion, and absorption of food and water. The GIT is also the site of 70–80% of the immune cells of the body (Wiertsema et al., 2021). As the GIT is where many pathogens are normally encountered first in the body, nature put a lot of the immune cells there along with the barrier mucosal tract that keeps microbiota and noxious compounds in the lumen. However, various environmental and pathological factors can impair the integrity of the intestinal barrier by impinging on the mucosal lining and causing inflammation and various diseases. With changes in microbiota (Rizzetto et al., 2018; Chelakkot et al., 2018) or activation of the immune system in the GI tract, inflammatory diseases can occur (Odenwald and Turner, 2017). Inflammation and intestinal permeability changes are known to play a role in various GI problems such as celiac disease (Caio et al., 2019), Crohn's disease (Cushing and Higgins, 2021), and irritable bowel syndrome (Gecse et al., 2012). These inflammatory bowel diseases result in enhanced production of proinflammatory cytokines found in mucosal tissues. Cytokines are a diverse set of proteins made by immune and nonimmune cells and they play a role in regulating immunity by acting as key signaling molecules. Proinflammatory cytokines, including interleukins (IL-1β, IL-6, and IL-10), get released and help promote the inflammatory reactions that damage the intestinal epithelial (Liu et al., 2019) and can lead to systemic low-grade inflammation labeled with the controversial term, "leaky gut."

While the diseases are real, the question about what role increased intestinal permeability or a leaky gut plays in these diseases that can also affect the rest of the body or at a systemic level (Arrieta et al., 2006; Fasano and Shea-Donohue, 2005) is still being elucidated. On the face of this, it would make sense that a leaky gut that has increased permeability might allow bacteria and toxins or other noxious compounds to enter the bloodstream through intestinal tight junctions and cause numerous problems. Leaky gut and altered intestinal permeability issues are thought by some to be associated with certain diseases and conditions such as lupus (Pan et al., 2021), type 1 diabetes (Carratu et al., 1999; Kuitunen et al., 2002; Sapone et al., 2006; Zhou et al., 2020), multiple sclerosis (Parodi and Kerlero de Rosbo, 2021), chronic fatigue syndrome (Maes et al., 2007; Lupo et al., 2021), fibromyalgia (Erdrich et al., 2020), rheumatoid arthritis (Matei et al., 2021), allergies (Assa et al., 2014; Stefka et al., 2014; Zuccotti et al., 2015), asthma (Farshchi et al., 2017), acne (Bowe and Logan, 2011), obesity (Gasmi et al., 2021), heat stress (Koch et al., 2019; Lian et al., 2020), and other conditions such as autism (Al-Ayadhi et al., 2021).

In a normally functioning intestine, the intracellular junctions between epithelial cells are considered to be "tight," as they fuse together and reduce the ability of large molecules and water to pass between cells. However, sometimes the tight junctions get compromised for any number of reasons, such as chemotherapy (Chelakkot et al., 2018), aspirin (Oshima et al., 2008), alcohol (Hou et al., 2022), or pathogens (Paradis et al., 2021), and allow more than normal permeability of large molecules and other various substances. Testing of leaky gut in individuals can be done by drinking and then measuring for levels of indigestible sugars such as mannitol or lactulose in the urine. Other tests measure zonulin in serum, although they may be unreliable (Vojdani et al., 2017). Figure 14.4 details how stressors are thought to cross the intestinal tract barrier at the gap junctions between epithelial cells and cause health consequences.

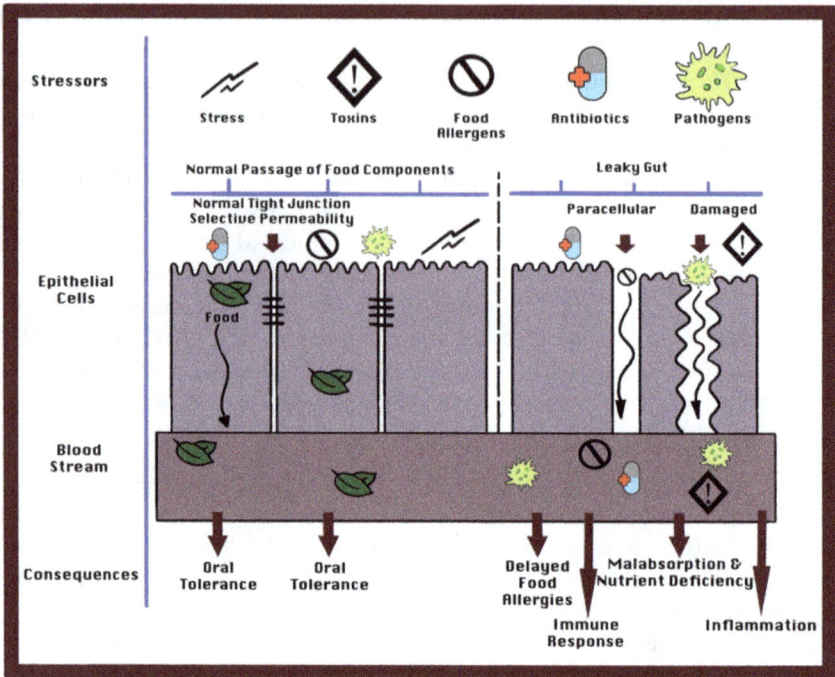

***Figure 14.4*** *Normal and leaky gut absorbance.*

Let's explore a hypothetical situation. Suppose a patient walks into a traditional or alternative-type medical clinic and starts complaining of various GI symptoms including abdominal pain, bloating, indigestion, diarrhea, or constipation. Then suppose they also complain about fatigue, headaches, confusion, difficulty concentrating, mood swings, nervousness, poor memory, anxiety, irritability, and confusion. Then suppose they complain about skin issues like rashes, acne, or eczema and go on to complain about joint pain, muscle pain, asthma, bladder infections, or vaginal infections. If you are the practitioner trying to sort all these problems out, then you have your work cut out for you as some or all of these symptoms can be attributed to altered (typically increased) intestinal permeability or the controversial concept called leaky gut syndrome. "Traditional" medical professionals will tend to talk about leaky gut to explain hyperpermeability of the intestines while "alternative" medical professionals expand on this and talk about leaky gut syndrome as an underlying cause of whole-body symptoms. Leaky gut syndrome is really a "catchall" term, based on a relative increase of intestinal permeability to cause numerous body symptoms. Leaky gut might not be a condition but rather a symptom. Leaky gut is not a specifically recognized medical diagnosis or condition at this time. Part of that may be due to a lack of recognized testing to produce reliable results. However, the term is used in alternative medicine with the understanding that while it might not be specifically recognized in medical schools, it does not mean it's not there. Whether it's a cause or a symptom or a condition, this increased intestinal permeability does lead to health problems in the rest of the body.

## 14.4.1 What Wisdom a Patient Wants to Know Regarding Leaky Gut Symptoms

Patients want to know what wisdom is needed to fix their leaky gut symptoms. The place to start is the removal of whatever stresses are causing it in the first place. While that may be difficult to figure out, it may be related to diet such as high-fat food, food allergies, or GI pathogens. A number of nutrients, minerals, probiotics, and nutraceuticals have been used over time to help patients maintain their normal GI functions and help repair the damage that occurred in the GI tract. Getting good sleep, exercising, and managing stress also is part of the wisdom. Apart from removing stresses, changing foods, and adding probiotics, a patient with leaky gut symptoms should consider certain vitamins, amino acids, micronutrients, minerals, and nutraceuticals that are known to help maintain intestinal integrity (Farré et al., 2020).

# 14.5 Effects of Nutrients and Nutraceuticals on Intestinal Integrity

## 14.5.1 Vitamins

Vitamin A and vitamin D play a role in regulating GI homeostasis. These vitamins regulate the expression of proteins on tight junction interfaces of intestinal epithelial cells and are important for barrier function in the GIT (Cantorna et al., 2019). Deficiencies of these vitamins adversely affect microbial diversity in the GIT in animals and humans (Ooi et al., 2013; Lv et al., 2016) and can lead to pathogenic increases. Supplementing vitamin A-deficient children has helped improve the intestinal barrier as tested by the mannitol/lactulose test methodology (Thurnham et al., 2000). Studies of supplementation with vitamin D showed improvement in GI permeability while reducing (C-reactive protein) CRP markers of inflammation in patients with IBD (Raftery et al., 2015). As such, it is likely that vitamin supplementation helps out different components of the mucosal barrier.

## 14.5.2 Minerals

Certain minerals also have beneficial effects on diseases associated with leaky gut syndrome. Not having enough zinc disrupts the epithelial barrier function via disassembling tight junction proteins (Zhong and Zhou, 2019). It has been shown (Giacomo et al., 2001) that zinc supplementation can help resolve permeability alterations in patients with Crohn's disease. Supplementing with zinc can also help improve intestinal permeability in children with acute shigellosis (Alam et al., 1994) and in experimental malnutrition (Rodriguez et al.,

1996). There are other benefits to using zinc for inflammatory bowel diseases (Solomons et al., 1977; Sturniolo et al., 1980; Hendricks and Walker, 1988) as there can be zinc deficiency with IBD.

## 14.5.3 Amino Acids

There are certain amino acids that play an important role in intestinal barrier integrity. Among these amino acids is glutamine. Glutamine is considered to be a conditionally essential amino acid as its consumption will increase during times of stress such as trauma, sepsis, and post-surgery. Glutamine has a number of functions in the body including protein synthesis and nitrogen donation, and it helps attenuate renal oxidative damage (Tsai et al., 2012). Another important role is serving as a precursor to adenosine triphosphate (ATP) that is used, in turn, for energy in biological reactions. Many fast-growing cells such as intestinal cells and immune system cells use glutamine as their predominant source of energy (Newsholme et al., 1985; Alpers, 2000). If glutamine is not present, alterations in tight junctions can occur that lead to increased permeability (Li and Neu, 2009). Some inflammatory gut diseases are known to improve with glutamine use. A strategy to involve the use of glutamine to reduce intestinal permeability from stress factors and to help maintain the intestinal barrier makes sense (Foitzik et al., 1997; Yoshida et al., 1998; Rao and Samak, 2012). Glutamine also can affect the production of cytokines by reducing proinflammatory ones such as IL-6 and IL-8 and by increasing anti-inflammatory IL-10 levels in T and B lymphocytes as well as epithelial cells (Coeffier et al., 2003). It has also been shown (Akobeng et al., 2016; Zhou et al., 2019) that patients with IBS with diarrhea or Crohn's disease can safely improve their condition when oral dietary glutamine is given. The human gut has little capacity to synthesize glutamine. As such, the gut relies on the supply of glutamine from the diet and other sources under physiologic and pathophysiologic conditions. It would appear that glutamine supplementation can help with barrier function and mucosal integrity of the gut by serving as an essential nutrient for gut mucosal epithelial cell growth. It is believed that glutamine can activate epidermal growth factor receptors which leads to the stabilization of tight junctions and actomyosin between cells. This involves mechanisms of various kinase enzymes such as Protein kinase C (PKC) and Mitogen-activated protein kinase (MAPK) (Rao and Samak, 2012).

Another amino acid that shows potential benefit in humans in normalizing gut issues is arginine. Arginine is considered a semi-essential amino acid that is a substrate for certain enzymes such as nitric oxide synthases. Nitric oxide (NO) is necessary for the maintenance of a normal epithelial barrier in the intestine (Alican and Kubes, 1996). While glutamine supplementation has more reported human clinical evidence for efficacy, oral supplementation of arginine in animal trials has shown some improvement of jejunum morphology following heat stress-induced intestinal damage (Xia et al., 2019). It has also shown improvement in intestinal immune function (Qiao et al., 2005), a reduction of the colonic paracellular permeability (Coburn et al., 2012; Xia et al., 2019), reduced intestinal paracellular permeability of a molecule of 400 Da, and bacterial translocation (Viana et al., 2010). With these promising animal studies, it is clear that more arginine research should be carried out in humans with leaky gut issues.

## 14.5.4 Short-Chain Fatty Acids

There are a number of dietary fibers that get converted into short-chain fatty acids by the host's microbiota and into beneficial beta-glucans that help reduce intestinal permeability (Mall et al., 2018). The short-chain fatty acids such as acetate, propionate, and butyrate play a role as energy substrates for the GIT. For example, butyrate is an important energy substrate for colonocytes (Marsman and McBurney, 1995). Supplementation of butyrate has shown some promise in patients with IBS (Banasiewicz et al., 2013) as it helps increase certain beneficial microflora (Verhoog et al., 2019). However, it is not clear whether the indiscriminate use of butyrate supplementation is wise. Butyrate can actually be detrimental to barrier function in circumstances when inflammatory mediators TNF-$\alpha$ and IFN-$\gamma$ occur (Vancamelbeke et al., 2019). More research is required to clarify when to use butyrate supplementation.

## 14.5.5 Botanicals

There are a number of plants and botanical extracts that have been used to help normalize leaky gut issues. Combinations of these various extracts can be found in any number of commercial products. Among these is the root from *Glycyrrhiza glabra* which contains licorice (Murray, 2020). This traditional medicine root has been used for thousands of years for coughs, infections, stomach pains, heartburn, inflammation (Yang et al., 2017), and other issues. The chemical form of licorice that typically is used is deglycyrrhizinated licorice (DGL) in which glycyrrhizin has been removed to help reduce the side effects of licorice. Glycyrrhizin can cause elevations in blood pressure whereas the DGL form appears to reduce those issues.

Another commercial ingredient used in leaky gut products is arabinogalactan. Arabinogalactan is a starch like compound from larch trees that has been used as a prebiotic fiber that can favorably affect microbial balance in the GI tract. Arabinogalactan may also have a direct effect on the immune system by acting on the gut-associated lymphoid tissues (Dion et al., 2016). As such, this may help explain its use for improving cold symptoms. It also helps stimulate butyrate production needed for intestinal mucosal integrity and short-chain fatty acids, and decreases ammonia in the GIT (Kelly, 1999).

Extracts from the root of marshmallow (*Althaea officinalis*) have been used for centuries to treat cough issues. However, it is now also in products intended for leaky gut syndrome as it is believed that it can provide a protective film on inflamed mucosa (Bonaterra et al., 2020) and help reduce inflammation (Deters et al., 2010).

The slippery elm tree (*Ulmus rubra*) has been used in healing for centuries for various conditions such as sore throat and IBS (Hawrelak and Myers, 2010). This is because the bark of slippery elm contains mucilage and therefore it coats and soothes the throat, stomach, and intestines. As slippery elm contains antioxidants (Langmead et al., 2002) that help relieve inflammatory bowel conditions, it is found in a number of commercial leaky gut treatment products.

*Aloe vera* (*Aloe barbadensis* Miller) is a plant that contains various vitamins, minerals, enzymes, sugars, lignin, saponins, amino acid, and salicylic acid. It has been used for centuries for cosmetics, treating skin wounds, and other dermal issues. It has also been used in commercial products for treating leaky gut as there is some evidence (Le Phan et al., 2021) that oral use improved age-related leaky guts issues in mice.

## 14.6 TurmiZn and Leaky Gut

One common factor in many GI health issues is inflammation. While there are a number of nutraceuticals that are known to help with inflammation as discussed here, curcumin and its metabolite tetrahydrocurcumin have received considerable attention for their anti-inflammatory capabilities (Peng et al., 2021). Both curcumin and tetrahydrocurcumin have excellent antioxidative capabilities (Jakubczyk et al., 2020). Curcumin is used for arthritis, metabolic syndrome, hyperlipemia, anxiety, and muscle soreness (Hewlings and Kalman, 2017). This is important as oxidative stress is an underlying factor for many health conditions and inflammation. However, curcumin and tetrahydrocurcumin have poor bioavailability as they are not very water-soluble. Among the efforts to increase the bioavailability of curcumin is to chelate it to metals. Zinc is one metal that has shown promise in increasing the solubility and bioavailability of curcumin or tetrahydrocurcumin. The use of zinc to bond both curcumin and tetrahydrocurcumin simultaneously has resulted in chelation complexes termed "TurmiZn" (DuBourdieu et al., 2021). These chelation complexes can take into account the capabilities of curcumin, tetrahydrocurcumin, and zinc simultaneously (Figure 14.5).

Heat is one of the stresses that can cause leaky gut in humans and animals. Elevated heat as little as 45°C can stimulate a thermoregulatory mechanism in the body that shifts splanchnic blood flow to peripheral blood flow. This can result in hypoxia in the GI tract and lead to disruption of the intestinal barrier. Tight junctions and adherens junctions are affected, and this leads to the disruption between intestinal cells. This disruption then provokes reactive oxygen species and hampered antioxidant defenses (King et al., 2015) while leading to inflammation and increased passage of toxins and pathogens into the blood and the symptoms of leaky gut syndrome.

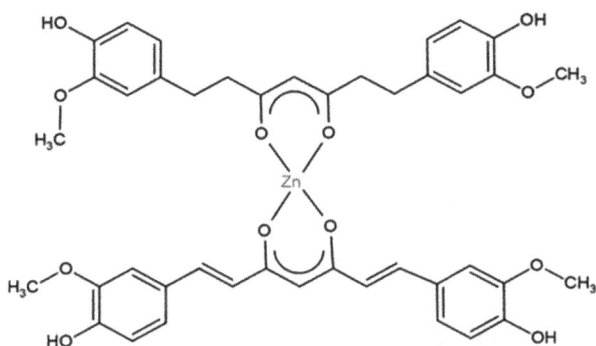

**Figure 14.5** *Molecular model of a chelation complex of TurmiZn.*

Heat in animals such as cows can cause milk production to decrease (Fontoura et al., 2022), which then can become an economic issue besides being a health issue and an increasing effect of global warming. Models of heat stress in rodents have been used to study the effects of oral rehydration solutions and GI inflammation (Miyamoto et al., 2021) and other aspects such as gene expression that drive heat stress effects (Kotlarz et al., 2022). Significant morphological changes in the intestine will occur in rats after being exposed to 45°C for 25 minutes (Giblot Ducray et al., 2016).

TurmiZn was tested in an animal model of leaky gut syndrome induced by heat stress (Kachhadiya, 2022). Rats from both sexes were fed TurmiZn at 25mg/kg in test groups (N = 10/group) for 15 days. Laparotomy was performed and both the renal arteries were ligated, and then the small intestine at the ileocecal valve was ligated. An 18-gauge catheter was inserted 1–2cm distal to the pyloric sphincter, a syringe containing 5ml of FITC-Dextran 4000 MW (200mg/kg) in isotonic saline was connected to the catheter, and the small intestine was gently filled with the solution. The insertion site of the catheter was ligated to avoid leakage of the solution. After suturing the abdominal site, the animal was subjected to heat stress in a preheated climatic chamber at 4 °C for 25 minutes at a relative humidity of 55%. The animals had access to food and water during and after heating. Four hours after the heat stress experiments, rats were anesthetized and euthanized by rapid decapitation. Blood was collected from each rat to obtain serum for measurements of pro-and anti-inflammatory immune responses. Measurements of interleukins in serum were compared in all groups and controls. Samples of small intestines from each rat were used for morphological analysis. Loss of structural integrity in intercellular junctions was measured using a 4-kDa FITC-Dextran molecule oral gavage (Lambert et al., 2002) to check intestinal barrier functions compared in all groups and the control animals.

The results showed heat stress-induced changes in intestinal permeability as evidenced by widening morphology between intestinal gap junctions, subsequent FITC-Dextran increases into serum from the GI tract, increases in inflammatory interleukins in serum, and increases in oxidative stress parameters. The use of TurmiZn helped prevent these heat stress changes from occurring. As seen in Figure 14.6 morphology of intestinal jejunum, the gap junctions in the control animals are close together but get wider when heat stress occurs. TurmiZn helps prevent this widening.

FITC-Dextran uptake from the intestines into serum under these heat stress conditions (Figure 14.7) indicates that TurmiZn helped reduce uptake to close to normal levels in control animals.

Heat stress induces the release of various inflammatory interleukins. TurmiZn helps prevent the release of IL-1β, IL-10 (Figures 14.8 and 14.9), and others during heat stress induction of leaky gut.

Oxidative stress also occurs when heat induces a leaky gut to produce ROS that can cause cellular damage. TurmiZn helps prevent various oxidative stress parameters such as malondialdehyde release (Figure 14.10).

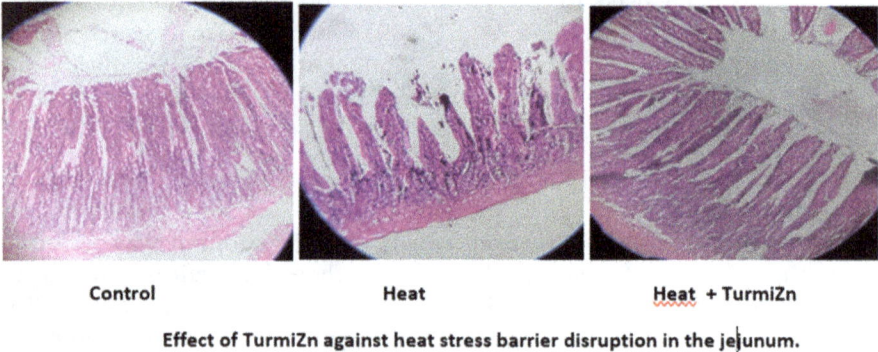

|       Control       |        Heat        |    Heat + TurmiZn    |

Effect of TurmiZn against heat stress barrier disruption in the jejunum.

*Figure 14.6* *Jejunum morphology in heat stress.*

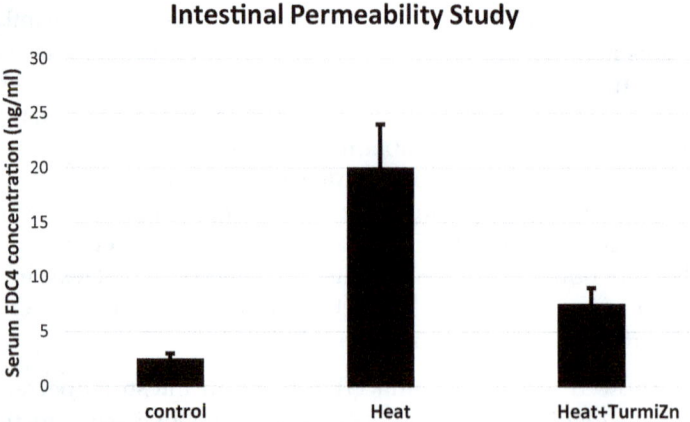

**Intestinal Permeability Study**

*Figure 14.7* *FITC-Dextran uptake in rats.*

## IL-10 in heat stress leaky gut model

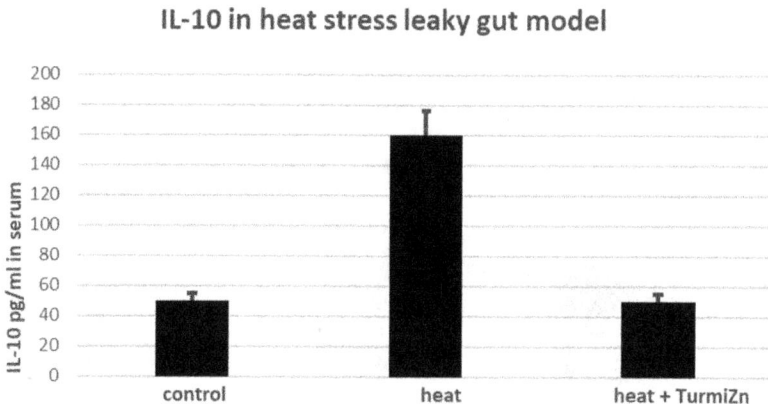

*Figure 14.8* IL-10 release in heat stress-induced leaky gut.

## IL-1 Beta in heat stress leaky gut model

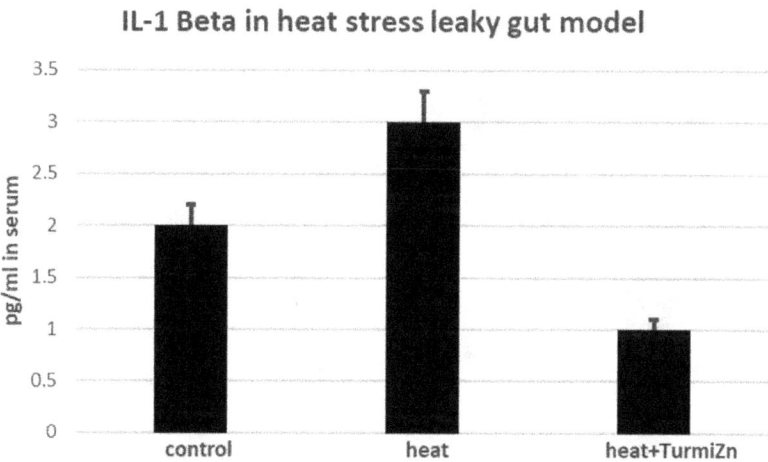

*Figure 14.9* IL-1β release in heat stress-induced leaky gut.

The data of this study is consistent with TurmiZn acting as an antioxidant to reduce reactive oxygen species that can damage cells and also reduce the inflammatory response caused by heat stress-induced leaky gut (Figure 14.11).

From this study of heat stress-induced leaky gut, TurmiZn was able to reduce proinflammatory cytokine production, reduce oxidative stress, and reduce intestinal barrier disruption. These results are consistent with the ability of TurmiZn to provide the beneficial effects of curcumin, tetrahydrocurcumin, and zinc in the GI tract. This data suggests that TurmiZn can be added to the list of effective nutraceuticals that have been used to improve GI function. While more research is required, the example of TurmiZn as a chelation complex that improves the benefits of curcumin is a step in the right direction for patients that want to reduce or prevent leaky gut issues.

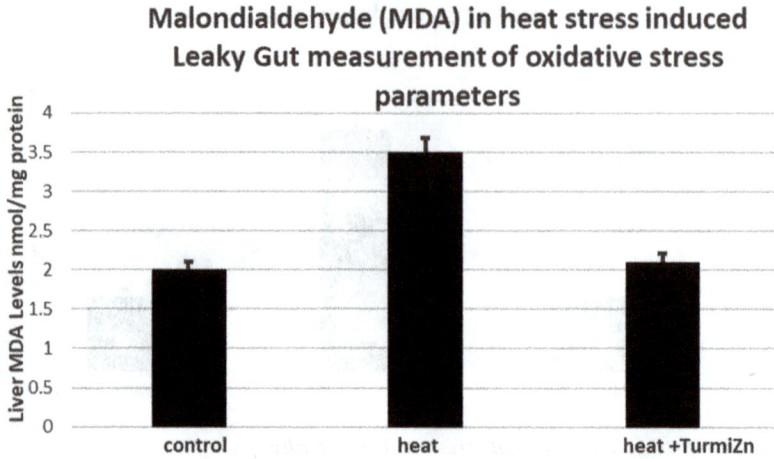

**Figure 14.10** *Oxidative stress parameter MDA in heat stress-induced leaky gut.*

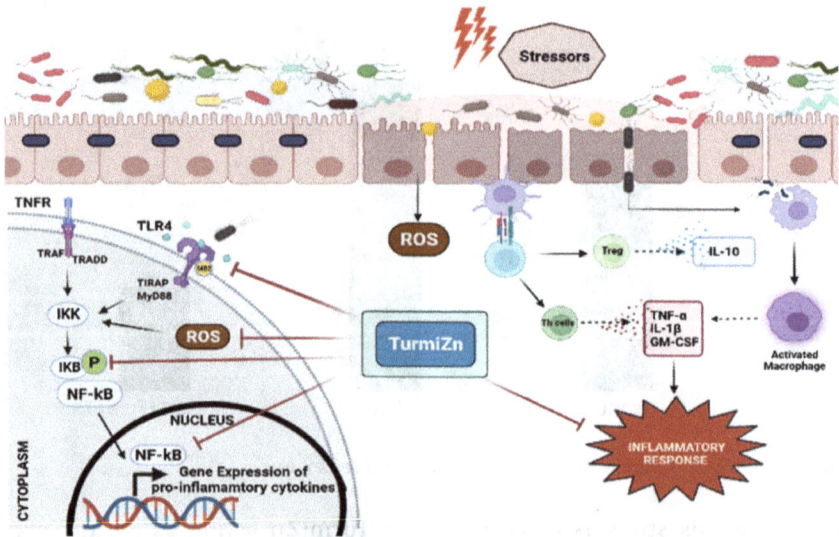

**Figure 14.11** *TurmiZn model of reducing the effects of leaky gut.*

## 14.7 Conclusion and Future Perspective

The GI tract is one part of the gateway to overall health. Functional foods and nutraceuticals are another part of this gateway. A number of the functional foods and nutraceuticals discussed here are examples of having antioxidant or immune-modulating capabilities necessary for improved health, but they suffer from bio-availability issues. The improvement of the bioavailability of nutraceuticals and functional foods is one area that future research will be keying in on. Increased bioavailability of any nutraceutical or functional food would lead to using less of any particular ingredient to achieve the same biological effect that a higher amount of a less bioavailable active would require. TurmiZn is an example of the kind of nutraceutical that would fall into this category. By complexing the more soluble tetrahydrocurcumin to curcumin via zinc chelation, increases in solubility occur over just curcumin while also allowing the health benefits of the other components to occur in one complex. This allows for better bioavailability and better efficacy to achieve improvements in leaky gut conditions. The use of TPGS as a soluble version of vitamin E allows for increased bioavailability and efficacy, especially in conjunction with ovotransferrin. The kinds of novel nutraceuticals such as TurmiZn and ITPGS that increase bioavailability and efficacy over their parent compounds will be the future of functional foods. Placing these kinds of innovative nutraceuticals into foods will turn normal foods into functional foods and allow the GI tract to optimize the health of the individual.

## Acknowledgment

The authors would like to thank Ms Robin B. Doss for her technical assistance in preparation of this chapter.

## References

Alam, A.N., Sarker, S.A., Wahed, M.A., Khatun, M., Rahaman, M.M. (1994) Enteric protein loss and intestinal permeability changes in children during acute shigellosis and after recovery: Effect of zinc supplementation. *Gut* 35(12): 1707–1711.

Anderson, J.W., Baird, P., Davis, R.H. Jr., Ferreri, S., Knudtson, M., et al. (2009) Health benefits of dietary fiber. *Nutr. Rev.* 67(4): 188–205.

Arrieta, M.C., Bistritz, L., Meddings, J.B. (2006) Alterations in intestinal permeability. *Gut* 55(10): 1512–1520.

Assa, A., Vong, L., Pinnell, L.J., Avitzur, N., Johnson-Henry, K.C., Sherman, P.M. (2014) Vitamin D deficiency promotes epithelial barrier dysfunction and intestinal inflammation. *J. Infect. Dis.* 210(8): 1296–1305.

Akobeng, A.K., Elawad, M., Gordon, M. (2016) Glutamine for induction of remission in Crohn's disease. *Cochrane Database Syst. Rev.* 2: CD007348. doi: 10.1002/14651858. CD007348.pub2.

Alican, I., Kubes, P. (1996) A critical role for nitric oxide in intestinal barrier function and dysfunction. *Am. J. Physiol.* 270(2 Pt 1): G225–G237.

Alpers, D.H. (2000) Is glutamine a unique fuel for small intestinal cells? *Curr. Opin. Gastroenterol.* 16(2): 155.

Al-Ayadhi, L., Zayed, N., Bhat, R.S., Moubayed, N.M.S., Al-Muammar, M.N., El-Ansary, A. (2021) The use of biomarkers associated with leaky gut as a diagnostic tool for early intervention in autism spectrum disorder: A systematic review. *Gut Pathog.* 13(1): 54. doi: 10.1186/s13099-021-00448-y.

Banasiewicz, T., Krokowicz, Ł., Stojcev, Z., Kaczmarek, B.F., Kaczmarek, E., et al. (2013) Microencapsulated sodium butyrate reduces the frequency of abdominal pain in patients with irritable bowel syndrome. *Colorectal Dis.* 15(2): 204–209.

Banerjee, A., Gupta, R.C. (2019) Gastrointestinal toxicity biomarkers. In Gupta, R.C. (Ed.), *Biomarkers in Toxicology*, 2nd edn. Academic Press/Elsevier, Amsterdam, pp. 277–285.

Belkaid, Y., Hand, T. (2014) Role of the microbiota in immunity and inflammation. *Cell* 157(1): 121–141.

Bonaterra, G.A., Bronischewski, K., Hunold, P., Schwarzbach, H., Heinrich, E.U., et al. (2020) Anti-inflammatory and antioxidative effects of Phytohustil® and root extract of *Althaea officinalis* L. on macrophages *in vitro. Front. Pharmacol.* 11: 290. doi: 10.3389/fphar.2020.00290.

Bowe, W.P., Logan, A.C. (2011) Acne vulgaris, probiotics and the gut-brain-skin axis - Back to the future? *Gut Pathog.* 3(1): 1. doi: 10.1186/1757-4749-3-1.

Bresalier, R.S., Chapkin, R.S. (2020) Human microbiome in health and disease: The good, the bad, and the bugly. *Dig. Dis. Sci.* 65(3): 671–673.

Butler, M.I., Mörkl, S., Sandhu, K.V., Cryan, J.F., Dinan, T.G. (2019) The gut microbiome and mental health: What should we tell our patients?: Le microbiote Intestinal et la Santé Mentale: Que Devrions-Nous dire à nos Patients? *Can. J. Psychiatry* 64(11): 747–760.

Cantorna, M.T., Snyder, L., Arora, J. (2019) Vitamin A and vitamin D regulate the microbial complexity, barrier function, and the mucosal immune responses to ensure intestinal homeostasis. *Crit. Rev. Biochem. Mol. Biol.* 54(2): 184–192.

Caio, G., Volta, U., Sapone, A., Leffler, D.A., De Giorgio, R., et al. (2019) Celiac disease: A comprehensive current review. *BMC Med.* 17(1): 142. doi: 10.1186/s12916-019-1380-z.

Carratu, R., Secondulfo, M., de Magistris, L., Iafusco, D., Urio, A, et al. (1999) Altered intestinal permeability to mannitol in diabetes mellitus type I. *J. Pediatr. Gastroenterol. Nutr.* 28: 264–269.

Chelakkot, C., Ghim, J., Ryu, S.H. (2018) Mechanisms regulating intestinal barrier integrity and its pathological implications. *Exp. Mol. Med.* 50(8): 1–9.

Chen, W., Miao, Y.-Q., Fan, D.-J., Yang, S.-S., Lin, X., et al. (2011) Bioavailability study of berberine and the enhancing effects of TPGS on intestinal absorption in rats. *AAPS PharmSciTech* 12(2): 705–711.

Chen, Y.-Y., Chen, D.-Q., Chen, L., Liu, J.-R., Vaziri, N.D., et al. (2019) Microbiome-metabolome reveals the contribution of gut-kidney axis on kidney diseases. *J. Transl. Med.* 17(1): 5.

Chen, Y., Xu, J., Chen, Y. (2021) Regulation of neurotransmitters by the gut microbiota and effects on cognition in neurological disorders. *Nutrients* 13(6): 2099. doi: 10.3390/nu13062099.

Clapp, M., Aurora, N., Herrera, L., Bhatia, M., Wilen, E., Wakefield, S. (2017) Gut microbiota's effect on mental health: The gut-brain axis. *Clin. Pract.* 7(987): 131–136.

Coburn, L.A., Gong, X., Singh, K., Asim, M., Scull, B.P., et al. (2012) L-arginine supplementation improves responses to injury and inflammation in dextran sulfate sodium colitis. *PLOS ONE* 7(3): e33546. doi: 10.1371/journal.pone.0033546.

Coeffier, M., Marion, R., Ducrotte, P., Dechelotte, P. (2003) Modulating effect of glutamine on IL-1beta-induced cytokine production by human gut. *Clin. Nutr.* 22(4): 407–413.

Cushing, K., Higgins, P.D.R. (2021) Management of Crohn's disease: A review. *JAMA* 325(1): 69–80.

Cryan, J.F., O'Riordan, K.J., Cowan, C.S.M., Sandhu, K.V., Bastiaanssen, T.F.S., et al. (2019) The microbiota-gut-brain axis. *Physiol. Rev.* 99(4): 1877–2013.

Cryan, J.F., O'Riordan, K.J., Sandhu, K., Peterson, V., Dinan, T.G. (2020) The gut microbiome in neurological disorders. *Lancet Neurol.* 19(2): 179–194.

Das, R., Biswas, S., Banerjee, E.R. (2016) Nutraceutical-prophylactic and therapeutic role of functional food in health. *J. Nutr. Food Sci.* 6(4): 4. doi: 10.4172/2155-9600.1000527.

Deters, A., Zippel, J., Hellenbrand, N., Pappai, D., Possemeyer, C., Hensel, A. (2010) Aqueous extracts and polysaccharides from Marshmallow roots (*Althea officinalis* L.): Cellular internalisation and stimulation of cell physiology of human epithelial cells *in vitro. J. Ethnopharmacol.* 127(1): 62–69.

Dinesh, N., Slovak, J.E., Kogan, C., Kopper, J.J. (2022) Preliminary evaluation of serum zonulin in canine chronic enteropathies. *J. Small Anim. Pract.* 2022: 1–7.

Dion, C., Chappuis, E., Ripoll, C. (2016) Does Larch arabinogalactan enhance immune function? A review of mechanistic and clinical trials. *Nutr. Metab. (Lond.)* 13: 28. doi: 10.1186/s12986-016-0086-x.

DuBourdieu, D., Prasad, S., Lall, R. (2021) Curcuminoid–metal complexes for oxidative stress. In Gupta, R.C., Lall, R., Srivastava, A. (Eds.), *Nutraceuticals: Efficacy, Safety, and Toxicity*, 2nd edn. Academic Press/Elsevier, Amsterdam, pp. 571–584.

Dwyer, J.T., Wiemer, K.L., Dary, O., Keen, C.L., King, J.C., et al. (2015) Fortification and health: Challenges and opportunities. *Adv. Nutr.* 6(1): 124–131.

Erdrich, S., Hawrelak, J.A., Myers, S.P., Harnett, J.E. (2020) Determining the association between fibromyalgia, the gut microbiome and its biomarkers: A systematic review. *BMC Musculoskelet. Disord.* 21(1): 181. doi: 10.1186/s12891-020-03201-9.

Farnaud, S., Evans, R.W. (2003) Lactoferrin-A multifunctional protein with antimicrobial properties. *Mol. Immunol.* 40(7): 395–405.

Farré, R., Fiorani, M., Abdu Rahiman, S., Matteoli, G. (2020) Intestinal permeability, inflammation and the role of nutrients. *Nutrients* 12(4): 1185. doi: 10.3390/nu12041185.

Farshchi, M.K., Azad, F.J., Salari, R., Mirsadraee, M., Anushiravani, M.A. (2017) A Viewpoint on the leaky gut syndrome to treat allergic asthma: A novel opinion. *J. Evid. Based Complem. Altern. Med.* 22(3): 378–380.

Fasano, A., Shea-Donohue, T. (2005) Mechanisms of disease: The role of intestinal barrier, function in the pathogenesis of gastrointestinal autoimmune diseases. *Nat. Clin. Pract. Gastroenterol. Hepatol.* 2(9): 416–422.

Foitzik, T., Stufler, M., Hotz, H.G., Klinnert, J., Wagner, J., et al. (1997) Glutamine stabilizes intestinal permeability and reduces pancreatic infection in acute experimental pancreatitis. *J. Gastrointest. Surg.* 1(1): 40–46.

Fontoura, A.B.P., Javaid, A., Sáinz de la Maza-Escolà, V., Fubini, S.L., Grilli, E., et al. (2022) Heat stress develops with increased total-tract gut permeability, and dietary organic acid and pure botanical supplementation partly restores lactation performance in Holstein dairy cows. *J. Dairy Sci.* 105(9): 7842–7860.

Fritsch, D.A., Jackson, M.I., Wernimont, S.M., Feld, G.K., MacLeay, J.M., et al. (2022) Microbiome function underpins the efficacy of a fiber-supplemented dietary intervention in dogs with chronic large bowel diarrhea. *BMC Vet. Res.* 18(1): 245. doi: 10.1186/s12917-022-03315-3.

Gasmi, A., Mujawdiya, P.K., Pivina, L., Doşa, A., Semenova, Y., et al. (2021) Relationship between gut microbiota, gut hyperpermeability and obesity. *Curr. Med. Chem.* 28(4): 827–839.

Gecse, K., Róka, R., Séra, T., Rosztóczy, A., Annaházi, A., et al. (2012) Leaky gut in patients with diarrhea-predominant irritable bowel syndrome and inactive ulcerative colitis. *Digestion* 85(1): 40–46.

Sturniolo, G.C., Di Leo, V., Ferronato, A., D'Odorico, A., D'Incà, R. (2001) Zinc supplementation tightens "leaky gut" in Crohn's disease. *Inflammatory Bowel Dis.* 7(2): 94–98.

Giansanti, F., Leboffe, L., Pitari, G., Ippoliti, R., Antonini, G. (2012) Physiological roles of ovotransferrin. *Biochim. Biophys. Acta* 1820(3): 218–225.

Giblot Ducray, H.A., Globa, L., Pustovyy, O., Reeves, S., Robinson, L., et al. (2016) Mitigation of heat stress-related complications by a yeast fermentate product. *J. Therm. Biol.* 60: 26–32.

Glassner, K.L., Abraham, B.P., Quigley, E.M.M. (2020) The microbiome and inflammatory bowel disease. *J. Allerg. Clin. Immunol.* 145(1): 16–27.

Golovinskaia, O., Wang, C.-K. (2022) Nutraceuticals in digestive therapy. Nutr funct foods boost digest Metab Imm health 2022: 477–500.

Greenberg, J.A., Bell, S.J., Guan, Y., Yu, Y.H. (2011) Folic acid supplementation and pregnancy: More than just neural tube defect prevention. *Rev. Obstet. Gynecol.* 4(2): 52–59.

Gupta, R.C., Srivastava, A., Lall, R. (2018) Toxicity potential of nutraceuticals. In Nicolotti, O. (Ed.), *Computational Toxicology-Methods and Protocols*. Springer Nature, New York, pp. 367–394.

Gupta, R.C., Srivastava, A., Sinha, A., Lall, R. (2019) Biomarkers of foods and nutraceuticals: Applications in efficacy, safety and toxicity. In Gupta, R.C., Srivastava, A., Lall, R. (Eds.), *Nutraceuticals in Veterinary Medicine*. Springer Nature, Cham, Switzerland, pp. 693–710.

Gupta, R.C., Doss, R.B., Banerjee, A., Lall, R., Srivastava, A., Sinha, A. (2021) Nutraceuticals in gastrointestinal disorders. In Gupta, R.C., Lall, R., Srivastava, A. (Eds.), *Nutraceuticals: Efficacy, Safety, and Toxicity*, 2nd edn. Academic Press/Elsevier, Amsterdam, pp. 141–155.

Halfvarson, J. (2017) Dynamics of the human gut microbiome in inflammatory bowel disease. *Nat. Microbiol.* 2017: 13.

Hawrelak, J.A., Myers, S.P. (2010) Effects of two natural medicine formulations on irritable bowel syndrome symptoms: A pilot study. *J. Alternati. Complem. Med.* 16(10). doi: 10.1089/acm.2009.0090.

Hendricks, K.M., Walker, A.W. (1988) Zinc deficiency in inflammatory bowel disease. *Nutr. Rev.* 46(12): 401–408.

Hewlings, S.J., Kalman, D.S. (2017) Curcumin: A review of its effects on human health. *Foods* 6(10): 92. doi: 10.3390/foods6100092.

Hirota, Y., Yang, M.P., Araki, S., Yoshihara, K., Furusawa, S., et al. (1995) Enhancing effects of chicken egg white derivatives on the phagocytic response in the dog. *J. Vet. Med. Sci.* 57(5): 825–829.

Hou, Z., Ding, Q., Li, Y., Zhao, Z., Yan, F., et al. (2022) Intestinal epithelial β klotho is a critical protective factor in alcohol-induced intestinal barrier dysfunction and liver injury. *eBio. Med.* 82: 10418. doi: 10.1016/j.ebiom.2022.104181.

Huang, W.Y., Majumder, K., Wu, J. (2010) Oxygen radical absorbance capacity of peptides from egg white protein ovotransferrin and their interaction with phytochemicals. *Food Chem.* 123(3): 635–641.

Ibrahim, H.R., Hoq, M.I., Aoki, T. (2007) Ovotransferrin possess SOD-like superoxide anion scavenging activity that is promoted by copper and manganese binding. *Int. J. Biol. Macromol.* 41(5): 631–640.

Jain, G., Patil, U.K. (2015) Strategies for enhancement of bioavailability of medicinal agents with natural products. *Int. J. Pharm. Sci. Res.* 6: 5315–5324.

Jakubczyk, K., Drużga, A., Katarzyna, J., Skonieczna-Żydecka, K. (2020) Antioxidant potential of curcumin-A meta-analysis of randomized clinical trials. *Antioxidants (Basel)* 9(11): 1092. doi: 10.3390/antiox9111092.

Jhanwar, B., Gupta, S. (2014) Biopotentiating using herbs: Novel technique for poor bioavailable drugs. *Int. J. PharmTech Res.* 6: 443–454.

Jiang, Q. (2014) Natural forms of vitamin E: Metabolism, antioxidant, and anti-inflammatory activities and their role in disease prevention and therapy. *Free Radic. Biol. Med.* 72: 76–90.

Kachhadiya, H.P. (2022) Pharmacological evaluation of Turmizn in leaky gut syndrome. Master's Thesis. Department of Pharmacology, Institute of Pharmacy, Nirma University, Gujarat, India. May 2022.

Kang, M.J., Cho, J.Y., Shim, B.H., Kim, D.K., Lee, J. (2009) Bioavailability enhancing activities of natural compounds from medicinal plants. *J Pant Res.* 3: 1204–1211.

Katan, M.B. (2004) Health claims for functional foods. *BMJ* 328(7433): 180. doi: 10.1136/bmj.328.7433.180.

Keerthana, M., Jemimah, G., Reddy, T.S., Bonagiri, Y., Gupta, A.V.S., et al. (2019) Nutraceuticals for prevention of various disease conditions. Indo. *Am. J. Pharmaceut. Sci.* 6(11): 14421–14427.

Kelly, G.S. (1999) Larch arabinogalactan: Clinical relevance of a novel immune-enhancing polysaccharide. *Altern. Med. Rev.* 4(2): 96–103.

Keservani, R.K., Kesharwani, R.K., Vyas, N., Jain, S., et al. (2010) Nutraceutical and functional food as a future food. A review. *Der Pharm. Lttre* 2: 106–116.

Kesarwani, K., Gupta, R., Mukerjee, A. (2013) Bioavailability enhancers of herbal origin: An overview. *Asian Pac. J. Trop. Biomed.* 3(4): 253–266.

Kim, J., Moon, S.H., Ahn, D.U., Paik, H.D., Park, E. (2012) Antioxidant effects of ovotransferrin and its hydrolysates. *Poult. Sci.* 91(11): 2747–2754.

Kim, B., Hong, V.M., Yang, J., Hyun, H., Im, J.J., et al. (2016) A review of fermented foods with beneficial effects on brain and cognitive function. *Prev. Nutr. Food Sci.* 21(4): 297.

King, M.A., Clanton, T.L., Laitano, O. (2015) Hyperthermia, dehydration and osmotic stress: Unconventional sources of exercise-induced reactive oxygen species. *Am. J. Physiol. Regul. Integr. Comp. Physiol.* 310: 105–114.

Koch, F., Thom, U., Albrecht, E., Kuehn, C. (2019) Heat stress directly impairs gut integrity and recruits distinct immune cell populations into the bovine intestine. *PNAS* 116(21): 10333–10338.

Kotlarz, K., Mielczarek, M., Wang, Y., Dou, J., Suchocki, T., Szyda, J. (2022) Identification of functional features underlying heat stress response in Sprague–Dawley rats using mixed linear models. *Sci. Rep.* 12(1): 7671. doi: 10.1038/s41598-022-11701-y.

Kuitunen, M., Saukkonen, T., Ilonen, J., Akerblom, H.K., Savilahti, E. (2002) Intestinal permeability to mannitol and lactulose in children with type 1 diabetes with the HLA-DQB1*02 allele. *Autoimmunity* 35(5): 365–368.

Lambert, G.P., Gisolfi, C.V., Berg, D.J., Moseley, L., Oberly, L.W., Kregel, K.C. (2002) Molecular biology of thermoregulation selected contribution: Hyperthermia-induced intestinal permeability and the role of oxidative and nitrosative stress. *J. Appl. Physiol. (1985)* 92(4): 1750–1761.

Lang, T. (2007) Functional foods. *BMJ* 334(7602): 1015–1016.

Langmead, L., Dawson, C., Hawkins, C., Banna, N., Loo, S., Rampton, D.S. (2002) Antioxidant effects of herbal therapies used by patients with inflammatory bowel disease: An *in vitro* study. *Aliment. Pharmacol. Ther.* 16(2): 197–205.

Le Phan, T.H., Park, S.Y., Jung, H.J., Kim, M.W., Cho, E., et al. (2021) The role of processed *Aloe vera* gel in intestinal tight junction: An *in vivo* and *in vitro* study. *Int. J. Mol. Sci.* 22(12): 6515. doi: 10.3390/ijms22126515.

Lee, G., You, H.J., Bajaj, J.S., Joo, S.K., Yu, J., et al. (2020) Distinct signatures of gut microbiome and metabolites associated with significant fibrosis in non-obese NAFLD. *Nat. Commun.* 11(1): 4982. doi: 10.1038/s41467-020-18754-5.

Li, N., Lewis, P., Samuelson, D., Liboni, K., Neu, J. (2004) Glutamine regulates Caco-2 cell tight junction proteins. *Am. J. Physiol. Gastrointest. Liver Physiol.* 287(3): G726–G733.

Li, N., Neu, J. (2009) Glutamine deprivation alters intestinal tight junctions via a PI3-K/Akt mediated pathway in Caco-2 cells. *J. Nutr.* 139(4): 710–714.

Lian, P., Braber, S., Garssen, J., Wichers, H.J., Folkerts, G., et al. (2020) Beyond heat stress: Intestinal integrity disruption and mechanism-based intervention strategies. *Nutrients* 12(3): 734. doi: 10.3390/nu12030734.

Liu, X., Cao, S., Zhang, X. (2015) Modulation of gut microbiota-brain axis by probiotics, prebiotics, and diet. *J. Agr. Food Chem.* 63(36): 7885–7895.

Liu, F., Lee, S.A., Riordan, S.M., Zhang, L., Zhu, L. (2019) Effects of anti-cytokine antibodies on gut barrier function. *Mediators Inflamm.* 2019: 7028253. doi: 10.1155/2019/7028253.

Lupo, G.F.D., Rocchetti, G., Lucini, L., Lorusso, L., Manara, E., et al. (2021) Potential role of microbiome in chronic fatigue syndrome/myalgic encephalomyelits (CFS/ME). *Sci. Rep.* 11(1): 7043. doi: 10.1038/s41598-021-86425-6.

Lv, Z., Wang, Y., Yang, T., Zhan, X., Li, Z., et al. (2016) Vitamin A deficiency impacts the structural segregation of gut microbiota in children with persistent diarrhea. *J. Clin. Biochem. Nutr.* 59(2): 113–121.

Mall, J.P.M., Casado-Bedmar, M., Winberg, M.E., Brummer, R.J., Schoultz, I., Keita, Å.V. (2018) A β-glucan-based dietary fiber reduces mast cell-induced hyper permeability in ileum from patients with Crohn's disease and control subjects. *Inflam. Bowel Dis.* 24(1): 166–178.

Maes, M., Coucke, F., Leunis, J.C. (2007) Normalization of the increased translocation of endotoxin from Gram negative enterobacteria (leaky gut) is accompanied by a remission of chronic fatigue syndrome. *Neuro Endocrinol. Lett.* 28(6): 739–744.

Maes, M., Leunis, J.C. (2008) Normalization of leaky gut in chronic fatigue syndrome (CFS) is accompanied by a clinical improvement: Effects of age, duration of illness and the translocation of LPS from gram-negative bacteria. *Neuro Endocrinol. Lett.* 29(6): 902–910.

Marsman, K.E., McBurney, M.I. (1995) Dietary fiber increases oxidative metabolism in colonocytes but not in distal small intestinal enterocytes isolated from rats. *J. Nutr.* 125(2): 273–282.

Matei, D., Menon, M., Alber, D.G., Klein, N., Blair, P.A., et al. (2021) Intestinal barrier dysfunction plays an integral role in arthritis pathology and can be targeted to ameliorate disease. *Med.* 2: 7. doi: 10.1016/j.medj.2021.04.013.

Mayer, E.A., Padua, D., Tillisch, K. (2014) Altered brain-gut axis in autism: Comorbidity or causative mechanisms? *BioEssays* 36(10): 933–939.

Miyamoto, K., Suzuki, K., Ohtaki, H., Nakamura, M., Yamaga, H., et al. (2021) A novel mouse model of heatstroke accounting temperature and relative humidity. *J. Intensive Care* 9(1): 35. doi: 10.1186/s40560-021-00546-8.

Morrison, J.L., Regnault, T.R. (2016) Nutrition in pregnancy: Optimizing maternal diet and fetal adaptations to altered nutrient supply. *Nutrients* 8(6): 342. doi: 10.3390/nu8060342.

Mukonowenzou, N.C., Adeshina, K.A., Donaldson, J., Ibrahim, K.G., Usman, D., Erlwanger, K.H. (2021) Medicinal plants, phytochemicals, and their impacts on the maturation of the gastrointestinal tract. *Front. Physiol.* 12: 684464. doi: 10.3389/fphys.2021.684464.

Murray, M.T. (2020) *Glycyrrhiza glabra* (licorice). *Textbook Nat. Med.* 2020: 641–647.e3. doi: 10.1016/B978-0-323-43044-9.00085-6.

Newsholme, E.A., Crabtree, B., Ardawi, M.S. (1985) Glutamine metabolism in lymphocytes: Its biochemical, physiological and clinical importance. *Q. J. Exp. Physiol.* 70(4): 473–489.

Noverr, R.P., Huffnagle, G.B. (2004) Does the microbiota regulate immune responses outside the gut? *Trends Microbiol.* 12(12): 562–568.

Odenwald, M.A., Turner, J.R. (2017) The intestinal epithelial barrier: A therapeutic target? *Nat. Rev. Gastroenterol. Hepatol.* 14(1): 9–21.

Ooi, J.H., Li, Y., Rogers, C.J., Cantorna, M.T. (2013) Vitamin D regulates the gut microbiome and protects mice from dextran sodium sulfate-induced colitis. *J. Nutr.* 143(10): 1679–1686.

Oshima, T., Miwa, H., Joh, T. (2008) Aspirin induces gastric epithelial barrier dysfunction by activating p38 MAPK via claudin-7. *Am. J. Physiol. Cell Physiol.* 295(3): C800–C806.

Pan, G.Y., Wang, G.J., Liu, X.D., Fawcett, J.P., Xie, Y.-Y. (2002) The involvement of P-glycoprotein in berberine absorption. *Pharmacol. Toxicol.* 91(4): 193–197.

Pan, Q., Guo, F., Huang, Y., Li, A., Chen, S., et al. (2021) Gut microbiota dysbiosis in systemic lupus erythematosus: Novel insights into mechanisms and promising therapeutic strategies. *Front. Immunol.*. doi: 10.3389/fimmu.2021.799788.

Pandit, A.P., Joshi, S.R., Dalal, P.S., Patole, V.C. (2019) Curcumin as a permeability enhancer enhanced the antihyperlipidemic activity of dietary green tea extract. *BMC Complement. Altern. Med.* 2019: 19.

Paradis, T., Bègue, H., Basmaciyan, L., Dalle, F., Bon, F. (2021) Tight junctions as a key for pathogens invasion in intestinal epithelial cells. *Int. J. Mol. Sci.* 22(5): 2506. doi: 10.3390/ijms22052506.

Parodi, B., Kerlero de Rosbo, N. (2021) The gut-brain axis in multiple sclerosis: Is its dysfunction a pathological trigger or a consequence of the disease? *Front. Immunol.* 12: 718220. doi: 10.3389/fimmu.2021.718220.

Peng, Y., Ao, M., Dong, B., Jiang, Y., Yu, L., et al. (2021) Anti-inflammatory effects of cur-cumin in the inflammatory diseases: Status, limitations and countermeasures. *Drug Des. Devel. Ther.* 15: 4503–4525.

Pham-Huy, L.A., He, H., Pham-Huy, C. (2008) Free radicals, antioxidants in disease and health. *Int. J. Biomed. Sci.* 4(2): 89–96.

Prevention of neural tube defects: Results of the medical research council vitamin study. MRC Vitamin Study Research Group, No authors listed (1991). *Lancet* 338(8760): 131–137.

Qiao, S.F., Lu, T.J., Sun, J.B., Li, F. (2005) Alterations of intestinal immune function and regulatory effects of L-arginine in experimental severe acute pancreatitis rats. *World J. Gastroenterol.* 11(39): 6216–6218.

Quigley, E.M. (2017) Gut microbiome as a clinical tool in gastrointestinal disease manage-ment: Are we there yet? *Nat. Rev. Gastroenterol. Hepatol.* 14(5): 315–320.

Raftery, T., Martineau, A.R., Greiller, C.L., Ghosh, S., McNamara, D., et al. (2015) Effects of vitamin D supplementation on intestinal permeability, cathelicidin and disease mark-ers in Crohn's disease: Results from a randomized double-blind placebo-controlled study. *U. Eur. Gastroenterol. J.* 3(3): 294–302.

Ramaa, C.S., Shirode, A.R., Mundala, A.S., Kadam, V.J. (2006) Nutraceuticals- an emerg-ing era in the treatment and prevention of cardiovascular diseases. *Curr. Pharm. Biotechnol.* 7(1): 15–23.

Rao, R.K., Samak, G. (2012) Role of glutamine in protection of intestinal epithelial tight junctions. *J. Epithel Biol. Pharmacol.* 5: 47–54.

Rizzetto, L., Fava, F., Tuohy, K.M., Selmi, C. (2018) Connecting the immune system, systemic chronic inflammation and the gut microbiome: The role of sex. *J. Autoimmun.* 92: 12–34.

Roberfroid, M.B. (2000) *Functional Foods Concept to Product*, 1st edn. Gibson, G.R., William, C.M. (Eds.), Woodhead Publishing, Abington, Cambridge, pp. 9–25.

Rodriguez, P., Darmon, N., Chappuis, P., Candalh, C., Blaton, M.A., et al. (1996) Intestinal paracellular permeability during malnutrition in guinea pigs: Effect of high dietary zinc. *Gut* 39(3): 416–422.

Sasmita, A.O. (2019) Modification of the gut microbiome to combat neurodegeneration. *Rev. Neurosci.* 30(8): 795–805.

Sapone, A., de Magistris, L., Pietzak, M., Clemente, M.G., Tripathi, A., et al. (2006) Zonulin upregulation is associated with increased gut permeability in subjects with type 1 diabetes and their relatives. *Diabetes* 55(5): 1443–1449.

Stefka, A.T., Feehley, T., Tripathi, P., Qiu, J., McCoy, K., et al. (2014) Commensal bacte-ria protect against food allergen sensitization. *Proc. Natl Acad. Sci. (USA)* 111(36): 13145–13150.

Surjushe, A., Vasani, R., Saple, D.G. (2008) *Aloe vera*: A short review. *Indian J. Dermatol.* 53(4): 163–166.

Solomons, N.W., Rosenberg, I.H., Sandstaed, H.H., Vo-Khactu, K.P. (1977) Zinc deficiency in Crohn's disease. *Digestion* 16(1–2): 8795.

Sturniolo, G.C., Molokhia, M.M., Shields, R., Turnberg, L.A. (1980) Zinc absorption in Crohn's disease. *Gut* 21(5): 387–391.

Srivastava, A., Lall, R., Talukder, J., DuBourdieu, D., Gupta, R.C. (2019) Iron transport tocopheryl polyethylene glycol succinate in animal health and diseases. *Molecules* 24(23): 4289. doi: 10.3390/molecules24234289.

Talukder, J.R., Griffin, A., Jaima, A., Boyd, B., Wright, J. (2014) Lactoferrin ameliorates pros-taglandin $E_2$-mediated inhibition of $Na^+$-glucose cotransport in enterocytes. *Can. J. Physiol. Pharmacol.* 92(1): 9–20.

Talukder, J., Srivastava, A., Ray, A., Lall, R. (2018) Treatment of infectious endometritis with a novel protein, VPI-O22 in cows. *FASEB J.* doi: 10.1096/fasebj.2018.32.1_supplement .882.12.

Talukder, J. (2019) Nutraceuticals in gastrointestinal conditions. In Gupta, R.C., Srivastava, A., Lall, R. (Eds.), *Nutraceuticals in Veterinary Medicine*. Springer Nature, Cham, Switzerland, pp. 467–479.

The European Parliament and the Council of the European Union. (2006). Regulation no 1924/2006 of the European Parliament and of the council on nutrition and health claims made on foods. *Official Journal of the European Union*. 404: 9–25.

Thurnham, D.I., Northrop-Clewes, C.A., McCullough, F.S., Das, B.S., Lunn, P.G. (2000) Innate immunity, gut integrity, and vitamin A in Gambian and Indian infants. *J. Infect. Dis.* 182(suppl. 1): S23–S28.

Thursby, E., Juge, N. (2017) Introduction to the human gut microbiota. *Biochem. J.* 474(11): 1823–1836.

Traber, M.G., Atkinson, J. (2007) Vitamin E, antioxidant and nothing more. *Free Radic. Biol. Med.* 43(1): 4–15.

Tripathi, A., Debelius, J., Brenner, D.A., Karin, M., Loomba, R., et al. (2018) The gut-liver axis and the intersection with the microbiome. *Nat. Rev. Gastroenterol. Hepatol.* 15(7): 397–411.

Tsai, P.H., Liu, J.J., Yeh, C.L., Chiu, W.C., Yeh, S.L. (2012) Effects of glutamine supplementation on oxidative stress-related gene expression and antioxidant properties in rats with streptozotocin-induced type 2 diabetes. *Br. J. Nutr.* 107(8): 1112–1118.

Uranga, J.A., López-Miranda, V., Lombó, F., Abalo, R. (2016) Food, nutrients and nutraceuticals affecting the course of inflammatory bowel disease. *Pharmacol. Rep.* 68(4): 816–826.

Valenti, P., Antonini, G., Fanelli, M.R., Orsi, N., Antonini, E. (1982) Antibacterial activity of matrix-bound ovotransferrin. *Antimicrob. Agents Chemother.* 21(5): 840–841.

Wallace, R.K. (2020) The microbiome in health and disease from the perspective of modern medicine and Ayurveda. *Medicina (Kaunas)* 56(9): 462. doi: 10.3390/medicina56090462.

Wang, X., Zihao, W., Changhu, X. (2021) The past and future of ovotransferrin: Physicochemical properties, assembly and applications. *Trends Food Sci. Technol.* 116: 47–62.

Wang, Y., Zhang, Z., Li, B., He, B., Li, L., et al. (2022) New insights into the gut microbiota in neurodegenerative diseases from the perspective of redox homeostasis. *Antioxidants (Basel)* 11(11): 2287. doi: 10.3390/antiox11112287.

Vancamelbeke, M., Laeremans, T., Vanhove, W., Arnauts, K., Ramalho, A.S., et al. (2019) Butyrate does not protect against inflammation-induced loss of epithelial barrier function and cytokine production in primary cell monolayers from patients with ulcerative colitis. *J. Crohns Colitis* 13(10): 1351–1361.

Viana, M.L., Santos, R.G., Generoso, S.V., Arantes, R.M., Correia, M.I., Cardoso, V.N. (2010) Pretreatment with arginine preserves intestinal barrier integrity and reduces bacterial translocation in mice. *Nutrition* 26(2): 218–223.

Verhoog, S., Taneri, P.E., Roa Díaz, Z.M., Marques-Vidal, P., Troup, J.P., et al. (2019) Dietary factors and modulation of bacteria strains of *Akkermansia muciniphila* and *Faecalibacterium prausnitzii*: A systematic review. *Nutrients* 11(7): 1565. doi: 10.3390/nu11071565.

Vojdani, A., Vojdani, E., Kharrazian, D. (2017) Fluctuation of zonulin levels in blood vs stability of antibodies. *World J. Gastroenterol.* 23(31): 5669–5679.

Voreades, N., Kozil, A., Weir, T.L. (2014) Diet and the development of the human intestinal microbiome. *Front. Microbiol.* 5: 594.

Wiertsema, S.P., van Bergenhenegouwen, J., Garssen, J., Knippels, L.M.J. (2021) The interplay between the gut microbiome and the immune system in the context of infectious diseases throughout life and the role of nutrition in optimizing treatment strategies. *Nutrients* 13(3): 886. doi: 10.3390/nu13030886.

Xia, Z., Huang, L., Yin, P., Liu, F., Liu, Y., et al. (2019) L-arginine alleviates heat stress-induced intestinal epithelial barrier damage by promoting expression of tight junction proteins via the AMPK pathway. *Mol. Biol. Rep.* 2019. doi: 10.1007/s11033-019-05090-1.

Yan, A., Bussche, A.V.D., Kane, A.B., Hurt, R.H. (2007) Tocopheryl polyethylene glycol succinate as a safe, antioxidant surfactant for processing carbon nanotubes and fullerenes. *Carbon* 24(13): 2463–2470.

Yang, R., Yuan, B.C., Ma, Y.S., Zhou, S., Liu, Y. (2017) The anti-inflammatory activity of licorice, a widely used Chinese herb. *Pharm. Biol.* 55(1): 5–18.

Yilmaz, B., Li, H. (2018) Gut microbiota and iron: The crucial actors in health and disease. *Pharmaceuticals (Basel)* 11(4): 98. doi: 10.3390/ph11040098.

Yoshida, S., Matsui, M., Shirouzu, Y., Fujita, H., Yamana, H., Shirouzu, K. (1998) Effects of glutamine supplements and radiochemotherapy on systemic immune and gut barrier function in patients with advanced esophageal cancer. *Ann. Surg.* 227(4): 485–491.

Yurdakok-Dikmen, B., Turgut, Y., Filazi, A. (2018) Herbal bioenhancers in veterinary phytomedicine. *Front. Vet. Sci.* 2018: 5.

Zabat, M.A., Sano, W.H., Wurster, J.I., Cabral, D.J., Belenky, P. (2018) Microbial community analysis of Sauerkraut fermentation reveals a stable and rapidly established community. *Foods* 7(5): 77. doi: 10.3390/foods7050077.

Zhou, Q., Verne, M.L., Fields, J.Z., Lefante, J.J., Basra, S., et al. (2019) Randomized placebo-controlled trial of dietary glutamine supplements for post infectious irritable bowel syndrome. *Gut* 68(6): 996–1002.

Zhou, H., Sun, L., Zhang, S., Zhao, X., Gang, X., Wang, G. (2020) Evaluating the causal role of gut microbiota in Type 1 diabetes and its possible pathogenic mechanisms. *Front. Endocrinol.* 2020. doi: 10.3389/fendo.2020.00125.

Zhong, W., Zhou, Z. (2019) Sealing the leaky gut represents a beneficial mechanism of zinc intervention for alcoholic liver disease. In Watson, R.R., Preedy, R.R. (Eds.), *Dietary Interventions in Gastrointestinal Diseases*. Academic Press, San Diego, pp. 91–106.

Zoran, D. (2003) Nutritional management of gastrointestinal disease. *Clin. Tech. Small Anim. Pract.* 18(4): 211–217.

Zuccotti, G., Meneghin, F., Aceti, A., Barone, G., Callegari, M.L., et al. (2015) Probiotics for prevention of atopic diseases in infants: Systematic review and meta-analysis. *Allergy* 70(11): 1356–1371.

# 15

# Traditional Therapy of Prebiotics and Probiotics as Treatment for Anxiety and Stress

Jesna John and Yashwant Pathak

## Contents

N obel Prize winner Eli Metchnikoff was studying why some members of the Bulgarian population around the late 1800s and early 1900s were living so much longer than others. He focused on Bulgarians who were living past 100. He came to realize that the villagers were drinking fermented yogurt daily. The drink contained *Lactobacillus bulgaricus*, a probiotic which seemed to be responsible for their life span. Metchnikoff believed the colon was a stock of waste matter that only harmed the human. He realized the way to defeat the bacteria that accumulate in the colon is through the ingestion of probiotics in the form of yogurt. Metchnikoff also recommended probiotics to delay senility, but other medical professionals never accepted that proposal.

Probiotics are found naturally in the body. Probiotics are live bacteria that are found in the gut. They are ingested through foods such as yogurt and passed on from the mother to the child during childbearing. The function of probiotics, according to the Cleveland Clinic, is to maintain a healthy balance. During an infection, bad bacteria enter the body and disrupt the balance of good bacteria and bad bacteria. Probiotics work to restore the ratio of good bacteria to bad bacteria. The exact mechanism of how probiotics work isn't known exactly but there are several theories. One theory is that probiotics change the composition of the bacteria in the gut and help return the gut to its normal condition.[1] Another theory is that probiotics affect the intestinal mucosa. Studies have found that some probiotics treat diarrhea by stimulation of lactase activity. The method in which probiotics treat infections vary depending on the type of bacteria, the route of the administered probiotic, and how frequently it is taken.

The development of the microbiome can be seen *in vitro*. It is formed through transmission of the placenta and amniotic fluid. One week into their birth, the microbiome develops drastically. The bacteria in the gut colonize very rapidly during this time period. If the microbiome doesn't develop properly in this time period it is associated with conditions such as cardiovascular disease, sepsis, and atopic disease.[2] Researchers came to find that whether an infant is breastfed or given formula can impact the development of their microbiome. Researchers concluded that the undigestible sugars found in breast milk act as a foundation allowing for the growth of bacteria.[3] The cause behind the transition of an infant-like microbiome to an adult microbiome is the quitting of breast feeding. The relation between diet and microbiome starts from infancy and continues well into adulthood.

Probiotics have been shown to be effective in treating antibacterial-associated diarrhea.[4] A yeast probiotic was shown to significantly reduce the frequency of diarrhea and shorten its duration. Although this study showed the potential of this yeast being used as treatment against diarrhea, more studies need to be conducted to see if it can be used as the sole treatment. Studies have also showed the use of probiotics in the treatment of yeast infections and common colds, but it is uncommon for probiotics to be prescribed as treatment for these conditions.

The mechanism of action for probiotics is still being studied. A study published in *Annals of Nutrition and Metabolism* explored several theories behind how probiotics behave in the body. One way the study established that probiotics can be helpful in fighting off harmful pathogens and bacteria in the body is by strengthening the epithelial barrier. The intestinal barrier acts as one of the main defense systems against the environment of the organism. The intestinal barrier contains a mucus layer and antimicrobial peptides and it secretes immunoglobin. There are a few proposed ways that probiotics help promote the integrity of the barrier. A few studies say that the probiotic *Lactobacilli* regulates genes that are responsible for encoding for proteins that are embedded into the barrier. Another study says that the probiotic *Escherichia coli* helps prevent disrupting the barrier and helps in repairing the barrier. Probiotics are also known to release metabolites such as arganine, glutamine, and fatty acids, which protect the gut barrier.

There are varieties of probiotics on the market that are available for purchase by the consumer. A quick Google search of "probiotic" yields dozens of pages of different probiotics to purchase. These range from digestive probiotics to women's probiotics to healthy hair probiotics. This raises the question of just how probiotics are seen as beneficial. One of the major benefits of taking probiotics is that they can help in the prevention of disease, according to a study published in the *Brazilian Archives of Biology and Technology*.[5] Probiotics do so by competing with pathogens for the few receptors that are necessary for the growth of such pathogens. A probiotic, *Lactobacillus*, is reported to reduce the occurrence and severity of diarrhea. Other probiotics can trigger immune responses which prevent pathogens from harming the gut. Probiotics are also used to treat irritable bowel syndrome, necrotizing enterocolitis, atopy, Crohn's disease, and ulcerative colitis. A study published in *Environmental Health* found that the frequency of sick days in participants who took the probiotic *L. reuteri* was much less than the participants who took the placebo.[6] This same probiotic was also shown to reduce levels of streptococcus bacteria in young adults.[7] As previously stated, probiotics can also reduce the incidence of antibiotic-related diarrhea. Probiotics have also been tested to be proven helpful for constipation in older adults. Although it seems as if probiotics always are beneficial, there may be the chance that probiotics can't treat the problems the seller claims they can. For example, there are many probiotics on the market that are targeted towards treating UTIs. However, according to the National Institute of Health, their review of studies that investigate a correlation between probiotics and UTI treatment have revealed that there is no evidence of probiotics playing a beneficial role in the treatment of UTIs. This chapter will seek to investigate if there are incidents of whether probiotics can be beneficial in treating anxiety and stress, just as they can be used to treat a multitude of conditions.

Unknown to many, there is a difference between prebiotics and probiotics. As discussed earlier, probiotics are a type of live bacteria that can be found in certain foods or supplements. Prebiotics are found in carbs and the stomach is unable to digest them. The bacteria in the gut eat this undigestible substance. Prebiotics are typically found in foods that are rich in fiber which can include beans, oats, berries, garlic, onions, and more. When the bacteria in the gut consume the fiber, they convert it into an acid called butyrate. This acid is important because it provides cells in the colon with most of their energy.[8] A study published in the *American Society of Microbiology* also found that when participants are not given a diet rich in prebiotics, the body isn't able to produce adequate amounts of butyrate which can be harmful to the colon.[9] There are numerous studies that have shown that prebiotics can be beneficial in treating conditions such as IBS (irritable bowel syndrome) and high blood sugar. This study found that prebiotics reduces the activity of Crohn's disease. Prebiotics are beneficial in maintaining homeostasis of the microbiome.[10] Many researchers believe that prebiotics can be helpful in treating inflammatory bowel disease if a specific regime can be established for patients.

There are many examples of prebiotics and probiotics being used in a traditional, holistic manner. For example, garlic is a significant herb that used to be used as a drug in prehistoric times due to its ability to treat conditions. It is used in traditional medicine to fight diseases and conditions like cancer, diabetes, cardiovascular diseases, snakebites, respiratory disorders, and more. Garlic contains fructans which act as prebiotics. Numerous studies have shown that the presence of garlic helps bacteria grow in the gut.[11]

Many people have heard of the gut–brain connection. But can what one eats truly affect one's mental health? Everyone has had feelings of "butterflies" in their stomach or nervous situations causing inability to eat. That is because these emotions can cause a response in the gastrointestinal system. Similar to the brain being able to control movement, the brain can control the actions of the stomach. For example, even by thinking about eating, the stomach can start releasing digestive acids. Just as a troubled mind can cause a troubled gut, if the gut is experiencing distress, it can also send signals to the brain. The gut and emotions are closely intertwined. There are several manners in which the gut communicates with the brain. The typical pathways it uses to do so include the neural, endocrine, and immune pathways. Substances that are released by the gut can be transported through blood to the brain. An inflammatory response in the intestinal system sends signals to the brain. When the GI tract is inflamed, it causes a stress response from the microbiome which includes the release of neurotransmitters and cytokines. The elevated levels of cytokines in the body cause the blood-brain barrier to be more permeable. This allows the released neurotransmitters to easily gain access to the brain which can cause anxiety, depression, and memory loss.[12] There are certain cytokines that stimulate the hypothalamic pituitary adrenal axis, HPA. The stimulation of the HPA eventually leads to the release of cortisol which is a stress hormone. This is important because hyperactivity of the HPA is one of the major indicators of depression and anxiety. A study found that, in rats, when the stimulus that causes HPA hyperactivity is removed, it reverses their abnormal behaviors. Evidently, the gut plays a significant role in the mental status of humans. This leads to the question of if probiotics, which are ingested, play a role in mental health. Probiotics play a role in preventing dysfunction caused by stress. When rats were given probiotics, it led to decreased levels of corticosterone. This means that probiotics suppress the HPA axis.[13] This suggests that probiotics may be able to regulate the response of the HPA in stressful situations. If the hyperactivity of the HPA can be regulated, it can help reduce feelings such as stress and anxiety.

An individual can experience stress from a multitude of sources. Reasons for people's stress in today's day and age usually include work, education, financial concerns, happiness in life, and burnout. Stress is not only bad for mental health, it also has effects on the well-being of the body. Stress can include likelihood of disease, hypertension, cardiovascular diseases, and digestive system diseases.[14,15]

Stress doesn't always mean something negative. Sometimes stress will keep the body alert to avoid danger. The body's fight-or-flight reaction is helpful in reacting to stress. There can be potential negative side effects of stress including but not limited to anxiety, depression, and panic attacks. Therefore, it is essential that researchers continue to research ways anxiety can be treated, and prebiotics and probiotics may be an answer.

A study published in LWW journals sought to explore if stress can be alleviated by probiotic supplements. The study conducted a systematic review of several experiments to determine whether probiotic supplements make a difference in symptoms of stress. It was found that there is a lot of potential in probiotics for relieving stress and preventing stress.[16] Another study sought to specifically see if probiotics can be used in the treatment of stress in cancer patients. The patients were given the Hamilton Anxiety Scale to determine levels of stress throughout the study. The study found that there was no statistical difference in levels of depression and anxiety between cancer patients that received probiotics and those that didn't.[17]

Another experiment conducted at the University of Missouri showed that common probiotics can reduce stress levels, as seen in zebra fish. In this study, zebra fish received doses of *Lactobacillus plantarum*, which is commonly found in probiotic supplements such as yogurt. In both the placebo and experimental group, the scientist introduced stressors such as reducing water levels. Zebra fish are known to be a model fish and are frequently used in drug screenings so there may be many parallels between how humans and zebra fish handle probiotics in relation to stress. The stressors that were introduced to the fish have been tested and proven to create tension in the fish. The scientists then analyzed the gene pathways of the fish and came to realize that zebra fish who were given the prebiotics had a reduction in the metabolic pathways that are linked to stress. The bacteria in the gut that grew thanks to the probiotics changed the gene expression of pathways that are responsible for stress. Previous studies also showed that fish who are experiencing stress are frequently found at the bottom of their tanks. However, the fish that were given probiotics spent more time at the top of their tanks, which is another indication of them experiencing less stress.[18]

Overall, there are a handful of studies available on the treatment of stress with prebiotics and probiotics. However, many of these studies are done in animals or haven't investigated different kinds of stress. The research that is available now shows a lot of promise in using prebiotics and probiotics to homeopathically treat stress. More research needs to be conducted to see if specific treatment plans can help alleviate a variety of stresses.

# References

1. *Int J Antimicrob Agents* 2012;40(4):288–296.
2. Barrett F, Kerr C, Murphy K, et al. The individual-specific and diverse nature of the preterm infant microbiota. *Arch Dis Child-Fetal* 2013;98(4):F334–F340.
3. Gritz EC, Bhandari V. The human neonatal gut microbiome: A brief review. *Front Pediatr* 2015;3: 3–18
4. McFarland LV, Surawicz CM, Greenberg RN, et al. Prevention of b-lactam-associated diarrhea by *Saccharomyces boulardii* compared with placebo. *Am J Gastroenterol* 1995;90(3):439–448.
5. Hemaiswarya S, Raja R, Ravikumar R, Carvalho IS. Mechanism of action of probiotics. *Braz Arch Biol Technol* 2013;56(1):113–119. doi: 10.1590/s1516-89132013000100015.
6. Tubelius P, Stan V, Zachrisson A. Increasing work-place healthiness with the probiotic Lactobacillus reuteri: A randomised, double-blind placebo-controlled study. *Environ Health* 2005;4:25. doi: 10.1186/1476-069X-4-25.

7. Caglar E, Cildir SK, Ergeneli S, Sandalli N, Twetman S. Salivary mutans strepto-cocci and lactobacilli levels after ingestion of the probiotic bacterium Lactobacillus reuteri ATCC 55730 by straws or tablets. *Acta Odontol Scand* 2006;64(5):314. doi: 10.1080/00016350600801709.

8. Bourassa MW, Alim I, Bultman SJ, Ratan RR. Butyrate, neuroepigenetics and the gut microbiome: Can a high fiber diet improve brain health? *Neurosci Lett* 2016;625:56–63. doi: 10.1016/j.neulet.2016.02.009.

9. Baxter NT, Schmidt AW, Venkataraman A, et al. Dynamics of human gut microbiota and short-chain fatty acids in response to dietary interventions with three ferment-able fibers. *mBio* 2019;10(1). doi: 10.1128/mbio.02566-18.

10. Markowiak P, Śliżewska K. Effects of probiotics, prebiotics, and Synbiotics on human health. *Nutrients* 2017;9(9):1021. doi: 10.3390/nu9091021.

11. El-Saber Batiha G, Magdy Beshbishy A, Wasef G, et al. Chemical constituents and pharmacological activities of garlic (Allium sativum L.): A review. *Nutrients* 2020;12(3):872.

12. Gądek-Michalska A, Tadeusz J, Rachwalska P, Bugajski J. Cytokines, prostaglan-dins and nitric oxide in the regulation of stress-response systems. *Pharmacol Rep* 2013;65(6):1655–1662.

13. Ait-Belgnaoui A, Durand H, Cartier C, et al. Prevention of gut leakiness by a probiotic treatment leads to attenuated HPA response to an acute psychological stress in rats. *Psychoneuroendocrinology* 2012;37(11):1885–1895.

14. Steptoe A, Kivimäki M, Lowe G, Rumley A, Hamer M. Blood pressure and fibrino-gen responses to mental stress as predictors of incident hypertension over an 8-year period. *Ann Behav Med* 2016;50(6):898–906.

15. Murray CD, Flynn J, Ratcliffe L, et al. Effect of acute physical and psychological stress on gut autonomic innervation in irritable bowel syndrome. *Gastroenterology* 2004;127(6):1695–703.

16. Zhang N, Liao X, Zhang Y, Li M, Wang W, Zhai S. Probiotic supplements for reliev-ing stress in healthy participants: A protocol for systematic review and meta-anal-ysis of randomized controlled trials. *Medicine* 2019;98(20):e15416. doi: 10.1097/MD.0000000000015416.

17. Ye, Z, Zhang Y, Du M, et al. The correlation between probiotics and anxiety and depression levels in cancer patients: A retrospective cohort study. *Front Psychiatry* 2022;13:830081.

18. Davis D, Doerr H, Grzelak A, et al. Lactobacillus plantarum attenuates anxiety-related behavior and protects against stress-induced dysbiosis in adult zebrafish. *Sci Rep* 2016;6:33726. doi: 10.1038/srep33726.

# 16

# Oral Beta-Lactamase Therapies Designed for the Prevention of Antibiotic-Induced Disruption of the Gut Microbiome

Sabrina Strelow, Sarvadaman Pathak, and Yashwant V. Pathak

## Contents

## 16.1 Introduction

The human gut is one of the most densely populated microbial ecosystems, with a vast majority of the microbes unable to be cultivated in the laboratory [1]. Until recently the collection of microbes that compose the human gut, "the microbiome," was inert and impacted very little by the foods, toxins, and medications that are orally introduced to the body [2]. It was believed to be relatively stable, homeostatic, and possess the ability to bounce back to normal composition after minor insults [2]. New technologies such as bioinformatics and high-throughput DNA sequencing created a revolution in our knowledge of the gut microbiome crumbling the old notion that endogenous microbes are of little physiologic importance [2]. It has now been established that the gut microbiome is a complex, evolving environment with a central role in human metabolism, nutrition, physiology, and immune function [3]. During development the primitive microbiome matures from a relatively sterile environment in infants to the adult composition by acquiring taxonomic

DOI: 10.1201/9781003333821-16

diversity and microbial complexity [2]. This transformation both parallels and contributes to the development of normal host physiology and thus perturbations could have drastic consequences on normal development and physiologic processes [2]. Imbalances in the composition of the gut microbiome have been linked to localized gastrointestinal conditions such as irritable bowel syndrome (IBS) and inflammatory bowel disease (IBD) as well as systemic manifestations of disease processes including obesity and type 2 diabetes [3].

Much of the decades of work done regarding the effects of antibiotics on indigenous microflora has been done on isolated culture strains in the laboratory [4]. As a result, much of the current understanding has been about narrow subsets of organisms in isolation from the remaining community of gut microbiota [4]. Recently, study has shifted to more of a broad ecological perspective to understand how they impact the homeostasis of the gut microenvironment in terms of its taxonomic composition and the emergence of drug resistance [4]. The importance of considering the system is exemplified by the drug Ciprofloxacin, which has very little activity against cultured anaerobic bacteria but has a profound influence on the composition of a mostly anaerobic organism-composed gut microbiota [5]. In general, antibiotics have been found to alter the genomic, taxonomic, and functional capacity of the gut microbiota regardless of their administration route [4]. They serve to reduce overall bacterial diversity while expanding membership of specific taxa in a rapid and sometimes persistent manner [4]. The consequence of these antibiotic disturbances can range from minor pathologies such as self-limited diarrhea to more severe life-threatening pathogenic infections [6]. One of the first described ecological consequences of antibiotics on the gut was loss of resistance to colonization in mice treated with streptomycin [7]. Loss of "competitive exclusion" due to decreased microbiome density enhanced the susceptibility of streptomycin-treated mice to be colonized with a secondary *Salmonella enteritidis* infection [7]. Broad spectrum oral antibiotic use, particularly beta-lactam antibiotics, is one of the leading risk factors for disease associated with such pathogens as *Salmonella typhimurium* and *Clostridium difficile* which is consistent with a metabolic disruption in the beneficial anaerobes and decreased taxonomic diversity in the gut microbiome after their administration [8].

Beta-lactam antibiotics include many natural or semisynthetic drugs developed and marketed beginning in the 1930s after the introduction of penicillin [9]. They currently constitute about 65% of the antibiotic market and are the most prescribed antibiotic group in both inpatient and ambulatory settings [9]. They are used for both prophylaxis and empiric therapy in cases of acute otitis media, Group A strep pharyngitis, pneumonia, bloodstream infections, intraabdominal infections, and urinary tract infections [10]. This class of drugs includes the penicillins, cephalosporins, carbapenems, and monobactams which all share a lactam ring [9]. This ring can irriversibly bind to and inactivate the enzyme DD-transpeptidase, a penicillin-binding protein that catalyzes cross-linking of peptidoglycan in bacteria cell walls [11].

The inhibition of cell wall remodeling during replication and growth is the mechanism by which beta-lactam anitbiotics exert their bacteriocidal effect that is perceived as a major advantage in severe infections [11]. Not only are they well tolerarated, efficacious, and carry minimal toxicity but they are also recommended by many national and international treatment guidelines which makes them so widely prescribed [12].

A myriad of natural enzymes called beta-lactamases are produced by a variety of bacteria, particularly gram-negative species [13]. They work to hydrolyze the lactam chemical ring structure, thus inactivating the beta-lactam antibiotic [13]. The secretion of beta-lactamases by pathogenic bacteria constitutes a powerful primary mechanism of resistance to beta-lactam antibiotics [13]. With their significant prescription rates and extensive therapeutic use, resistance to beta-lactams is a rapidly growing public health challenge [14]. When antibiotics are improperly chosen, used too frequently, or in too small of a dose there is selection and survival of resistant bacteria strains [14]. Selection pressures from drug administration promote the evolution of pathogens through the horizontal transfer of antimicrobial resistance genes among bacteria in such a densely populated ecosystem as the human gut microbiota [1]. To combat the emerging resistance and the negative consequences of gut microbiome disruption the active antimicrobial agent must be degraded in or removed from the gastrointestinal tract before it can cause dysfunction but without altering the therapeutic efficacy of the drug [9]. Thus beta-lactamase enzymes are not only a problem but also could be harvested to be a potential protective solution [15].

## 16.2 Normal Composition of Gut Bacteria

The microbiota of the gut is a collection of microganisms, particularly bacteria, archaea, and eukaryota, that inhabit all parts of the gastrointestinal tract (GI), establishing a symbiotic relationship with the host [16]. These microorganisms have a vital role in maintence of health by aiding digestion, synthesizing vitamins, and maintaining epithelial integrity, and alongside the immune system preventing the colonization of pathogens [16]. The sheer numbers of bacteria in the human gastrointestinal tract outnumber the amount of host cells by ten times [3]. The international Metagenomics of the Human Intestinal Tract (Meta-HIT) project derived a gene catalogue of the human gut microbiome, identifying more than 3.3 million different bacteria genes which is 150 times greater than the compostion of the human genome [17]. The overall microbiome of the gut is composed primarily of strict anaerobes within two dominant phyla, Bacteroides and Firmcutes, composing 90% of the microorgamnisms [18]. Other subdominant phyla categories include Actinobacteria, Verrucomicrobia, Proteobacteria, and Fusobacteria [18].

The indigenous microbiota begins to establish itself from birth and evolves as the host develops [1]. By the age of 3, the diverse makeup and functional capacity of the human gut microbiome resembles that of the adult form [16]. The compostion of the intestinal microbiota is fairly stable at the phylum level despite the abundance of factors that can influence it's makeup [3]. Originally, suggestions were made about the presence of a "core microbiota" that was an organism-level composition found to be conserved between all humans [19]. It was confirmed that between most individuals the Bacteroidetes and Firmicutes are largely conserved despite minor variation in their relative proportions to each other [18]. This proportion variability in humans is largely attributable to differences in physical activity levels as well dietary exposure to toxins, food additives, and antibiotics [18]. Host and environmental selective factors both shape the composition of the gut microbiota [20]. A sequencing study of the gut microbiomes of 1,135 Dutch participants showed that 18.7% of the variation in interindividual microbial concentration could be linked to a variety of exogenous and intrinsic factors including diseases, drugs, smoking, and dietary differences [20]. However, at the interindividual level there is considerably greater variation due to functional redundancy in the roles that gut bacterial species carry out within the host [3]. There is more observable similiarity in the repertoire of microbial genes that are present rather than the toxonomic compositon suggesting more of a functional rather than organism-level way to define the core microbiota [19].

By location in the gastrointestinal tract, the microbiota density and composition are stratified along a gradient, reflective of chemical, nutritional, and immuno-logic influences [21]. The small intestine, for example, creates an environment only suitable for rapidly growing faculatative anaerobes due to their ability to tolerate high levels of bile acids, oxygen, and antimicrobials [21]. Additonally, a short transit time through this protion of the GI tract is another selction pressure that requires that bacteria have the abilty to adhere to tissue or mucus for continued colonization [21]. In contrast, the conditions of the colon allow for more dense and diverse microbial communities than any other body habitus [21]. Anaerobic bacteria that thrive on the complex carbohydrates that are unable to be digested in the small intestine are abundant here and further protected by the increased amounts of mucus present in this region [21].

## 16.3 Antibiotic Use and Its Role in Causing Dysbiosis

The human microbiota is constantly exposed to various modern lifestyle stressors, including the consumption of chlorinated water, food additives, contaminants, pesticicides, and antibiotics [18]. Overall, the microbiome is an extremely plastic entity, allowing it to adapt to mild fluctuations and be reconfigured in response to the aforementioned lifestyle stressors [22]. However, the homeostatic equilibirum can be permanently disrupted by continuous exposure or repeated insults [19]. This chronic alteration of gut microbial composition is known as dysbiosis [19]. The degree of disruption depends on not only the strength and duration of the perturbing factor but also on the stability of an individual's microbiota, assuming there is some individual variation [22]. Dysbiosis can shift the microbiome from an environment of mutualistic harmony to one that has potential deleterious effects on the host, allowing for various pathologic conditions and the selection of more virulent organisms [22]. During severe pertubations such as treatment with antibiotics, the environment becomes one of low taxonomic diversity [23]. Eventually some species have the ability to recover and resemble the pretreatment state while other sare depleted to undetectable levels or allowed to grow unchecked, causing prolonged dysbiosis [23].

Antibiotics are a unique class of drugs having not only an effect on the individual to which they are directly given but also on the community through control of infection spread and evolving antibiotic resistance [24]. The gut microbiota is a human reservoir for antibiotic resistance and with each additional antibiotic exposure has increased potential for aquisition and propagation of novel resisistance genes [25]. The cost of antibiotic use due to resistance has become evident as some of the most clinically important infections are no longer able to be treated with what were once considered to be the most effective drugs [24]. However, the cost of antibiotics on an indidividual's own health due to the collateral damage they inflict on a previously healthy human's microbiome is just coming to light [24]. The degree to which the gut microbiota changes after an antibiotic use depends not only on the chemical nature of the antibiotic, but also the route of administration, duration, dose, and the level of resistance that develops [26].

Several classes of antibiotics are used readily for medical management of bacterial infections and have been shown to improve clinical outcomes, although many are overprescribed or improperly prescribed [27]. Their worldwide consumption rates have increased 46% between 2000 and 2018 creating great concern for increasing levels of antimicrobial resistance [27]. In 2021 alone, the Center for Disease Control and Prevention (CDC) reports 211.1 million prescriptions for oral antibiotics in the United States, the equivalent of 636 prescriptions per 1,000 persons [28]. As many as 30% of the oral antibiotics prescribed in the United States are estimated to be unneccessary across all types of medical conditions [29]. In high-income contries such as the United States, these prescription rates have remained relatively stable but they are increasing rapidly in developing and low-income regions of North Africa, the Middle East, and South Asia [27]. Broad-spectrum penicillin usage rates were found to be stable for the duration of the 2000 to 2018 study period with highest use identified in high-income countries [27]. Carbapenem cosumption was also found to be highest among high-income countries but with an increasing usage rate instead of a stable one [27]. Conversely, the consumption of third-generation cephalosporins was low in high-income areas but usage increased drastically in the Middle East, North Africas and South Asia [27].

While there have been reports of many different types of antibiotics creating microbial shifts in the gut microenvironment, beta-lactam antibiotics are one of the most well studied and important covariates that influence its composition [26]. During an explorative intervention study, it has been demonstrated the intravenous beta-lactam therapy with a combination of cefazolin, ampicillin, and sulbactam exerts changes in both the active and total bacterial taxa [30]. During beta-lactam administration there has been an observed initial reduction in gram-negative organisms by the sixth day after the start of intervention and an overall collapse of microbiome diversity by the eleventh day [31]. Bacteria that thrive and bloom during or after antibiotic intervention are organisms that display improved colonization and survival mechanisms [30]. Active Firmicutes including *Enterococcus durans* and naturally antibiotic-resistant Bacteroidetes were shown to expand dramatically after a course of beta-lactams [30]. Maximum imbalance in the gut microbiota occurs around the fourteenth day of antibiotic intervention [31].

Successful use of antibiotics relies on integrated knowledge of their pharmacodynamic (PD) and pharmacokinetic (PK) properties. The pattern of a drugs antimicrobial killing can be time dependent, concentration dependent, or a hybrid of both patterns [32]. Beta-lactams, for example, have a time-dependent killing mechanism [33]. The minimum inhibitory concentration (MIC) defines a level of susceptibility or resistance of a bacterial strain to a specific antibiotic by completely preventing visible *in vitro* growth [14]. It is regarded to have the greatest importance in optimizing therapy and must be used alongside PK parameters such as volume of distribution, elimination half-life, clearance, and maximal concentration that describe the fate of the drug once inside this organism [14]. The duration of exposure is the percentage of the dosing interval that remains above the MIC of the pathogen [33]. To maximize the duration of exposure the dose can be increased, the dosing interval can be shortened, or the infusion time can be prolonged [33]. At such effective concentrations, antibiotic use is not pathogen specific for the intended target and instead produces co-lateral effects on the gut microbiota [26].

## 16.4 Beta-Lactam Antibiotics

Beta-lactam antibiotics are so named because they share a highly reactive 3-carbon and 1-nitrogen four-membered lactam ring [9]. They are categorized into subclasses including penicilins, cepaholsporins, monobactams, and carbapenems based on the chemical structure that is joined to the ring [34]. Each subclass has developed from a need to increase the spectrum of the drug activity to encompass additional bacterial species or to combat certain resistance mechanisms [12]. The basic structure of penicillins contains a thiazolidine ring attached to the lactam ring, creating a 6-aminopenicilling acid nucleus that is essential for its pharmacologic action and antibacterial properties [34]. Penicillins are active against mostly gram-positive organisms, some gram-negative cocci, and non-beta-lactamase-producing anaerobes [34]. They are extremely susceptible to hydrolysis by beta-lactamases and have no activity against gram-negative rods [34]. Penicillins have a short half-life requiring repeated parenteral dosing in severe systemic infection [9]. They do not readily penetrate the cerebral spinal fluid in the absence of inflammation, but do achieve therapeutic levels in pleural, pericadial, peritoneal, synovial fluid, and urine [9]. Extended-spectrum penicillins such as the aminopenicillins retain the antibacterial spectrum previously mentioned for penicillin but have improved activity against gram-negative rods [34]. Cephalosporins, in contrast, contain an 7-aminocephalosporanic acid nucleus and are divided into five generations based on a numerically broadening spectrum of antimicrobial activity [9]. In contrast to the previously mention subclasses, monobactams have a linked sulfonic acid group instead of a fused ring system [35]. They have a spectrum of activity that is uniquely limited to aerobic gram-negative bacteria [34]. Finally, the carbapenems have a beta-lactam ring fused to a 5-membered ring similar to that of penicillin with a carbon atom instead of a sulfur atom at postion one and a double bond between carbons two and three [35]. They possess a broad spectrum of activity against both gram-negative and gram-positive bacteria and are increasingly used to treat infections caused by multidrug-resistant pathogens [35].

Peptidoglycan is a vital stability component of bacterial cell walls that is relatively well conserved among both gram-positive and gram-negative bacteria [9]. Gram-positve bacteria have a much thicker wall structure with upwards of ten layers while gram-negative walls only have one–two layers of peptidoglycan [9]. It is composed of glycan chains of N-acetylglucosamin and N-acetylmuramic disacharide subunits which are linked to higly conserved tetrapeptide and pentapeptides [9]. The target of the beta-lactam class of anitbitoics is bacterial DD-peptidases that catalzye the final step in peptidoglycan biosynthesis [36]. Once the transpeptidase is acylated by the beta-lactam antibiotic, the terminal transpeptidation process is interrupted and the bacteria undergoes a loss of viability and lysis [9]. The percentage of time that the drug serum concentration of a beta-lactam antibiotic exceeds its MIC, is a PD-PK parameter that closely correlates with its antibacterial efficacy [32]. Since beta lactams have a time-dependent effect, continuous drug infusions may have an advantage of traditional bolus dosing methods [9]. It is also observed that faster growing bacteria are killed more rapidly by this class of antibiotics while dormant bacteria are phenotypically tolerant and have drastically reduced lysis rates [37].

The primary mechanism of resistance to this class of antibiotics is achieved by bacterial production of beta-lactamase enzymes that have evolved from a DD-peptidase ancestory and are capable of catalyzing hydrolysis of the beta-lactam ring [36]. However, the resistance mechanism to beta-lactam antibotics seems to be multifactorial and pathogen dependent, driven by other additional mechanism such as efflux pumps, permeability modifications, and mutations in penicillin-binding proteins [38]. Enzymes to degrade penicillin were originally descovered in *E. coli* but can be produced by many gram-negative organisms as well as some gram-positive ones [39]. Treponema pallidum and Group A streptococci are two of the few bacterial species that do not produces these inactivating enzymes [40]. Beta-lactamases can be classified by a molecular classification scheme with classes A, C, and D all utilizing serine for beta-lactam hydrolysis and class B which is a metalloenzyme that needs divalent zinc ions to complete hydrolysis of the ring [12]. Some of the most concerning culprits of antibiotic resistance to beta-lactams are *Streptococcus pneumononiaoe* and gram-negative bacteria such as *Pseudomonas aeruginosa* [9]. Extended spectrum beta-lactamases (ESBLs) are bacteria-produced enzymes that are of growing concern because they are able to hydrolyze more stable antibiotics including extended spectrum third- and fourth-generation cephalosporins [41].

Original beta-lactamase inhibitors such as clavulanic acid, sulbactam, and tazobactam resemble beta-lactam molecules but do not have potent antibacterial properties, they instead protect hydrolyzable penicillin from inactivation by beta-lactamase enzymes [34]. Inhibition of beta-lactames through the use of small molecule inhibitors is a method of overcoming class-specific resistance by preventing hydrolysis and inactivation of the antibiotic while simultaneously restoring potency against gram-negative organisms [42]. The inhibitors are available in fixed combinations with specific penicillins and cephalosporins, extending the spectrum of the anitbitoics [34]. Their efficacy is greatest against class A beta-lactamases that are plasmid encoded versus class C enzymes that are chromosomally encoded [34]. Thus, they have excellent activity against those produced by staphylocci, *Salmonella*, *Shigella*, *E. coli*, *H. influenzae*, *N. gonorrhoae*, and *K. pneumoniae* that produce class A beta-lactamases and poor activity against *S. marcescens*, *P. aeruginosa*, *Enterobacter* sp., and *Citrobacter* sp. that produce class C [34]. An exception to the general rule is their ability to inhibit the beta-lactamases produced by *B. fragilis* and *M. catarrrhalis* which are chromosomally encoded [34]. The newer beta-lactamase inhibitors have broader profile of inhibition agaisnst class C beta-lactamases and include avibactam, vaborbactam, and relebactam [42]. Unfortunately they still have no action against class B metallo-beta-lactamases and a lack of oral bioavailibity, making them less useful clinically [42].

## 16.5 Consequences of Antibiotic Use on Microbiome Function

The bacteria of the gut microbiome initially respond to antibiotic therapy by activating protective mechanisms to attenuate the antimicrobial drug effects while also altering overall metabolic status [31]. Early life antibiotic exposure leads to lifelong phenotype variations such a predisposition to obesity [43]. Throughout the life span there are profound insult-associated changes in the capacity to metabolize and transport hormones, cholesterol, bile acids, and vitamins [31]. The repertoire of antibiotic-induced changes in the gut microbiota disturbs the regulation of anaerobiosis and aerobiosis due to altered oxygen availability [43]. This closely relates to the epithelial metabolism of the gut utilization of micronutrients such as copper and vitamin E and macronutrients including amino acids [43]. Administration of beta-lactams has a negative effect on production of key metabolites involved in major cellular functions such as acetyl phosphate and acetyl-CoA [30]. It has also been demonstrated in mice that microbiota disturbances secondary to antibiotic administration alter both serotonin and bile acid levels in the colon, resulting in delayed gastrointestinal motility [44].

The undisturbed intestinal microbiota offers a protective barrier against invasive pathogen colonization due to limited nutrients and high microbial densities. [45]. Conversely, dysbiosis leaves it vulnerable to pathogenic colonization due to alterations in mucosal carbohydrate availability [8]. Under normal circumstances, *Clostridium difficile* is not a significant component of the human colonic microflora, but the altered nutrient conditions favor expansion of the species [46]. *C. difficile* is a gram-positive, spore-forming anaerobe that is highly resistant to beta-lactam antibiotics due to production of a beta-lactamase [47]. This resistance allows the pathogen to replicate unchecked in the gut and causes severe diarrheal disease in antibiotic-treated patients [47]. This problem plagues almost half a million individuals in the United States alone every year and is responsible for 29,000 yearly deaths [48]. It has become increasingly difficult to treat due to the high resistance *C. difficile* exhibits for a wide array of antibiotics, allowing it ultimately to result in pseudomembranous colitis, intestinal rupture, and death [47].

## 16.6 Oral Beta-Lactamases as an Emerging Solution

Since beta-lactam antibiotics exert a time-dependent effect on bacteria, finding a strategy to minimize the time they can affect gut microbiome while still preserving their therapeutic efficacy is a problem of great clinical importance [9]. A viable strategy is to prophylactically eliminate biologically active antimicrobials that are excreted into the gastrointestinal tract before they can disrupt the composition of the intestinal flora [15]. To solve this problem of antibiotic-mediated dysbiosis, beta-lactamases were harnessed as therapeutics [15]. These enzymes function to destroy the antibiotics in the proximal portion of the intestine before they can pass to and disturb the microbiota of the colon [15].

P1A is a beta-lactamase that was originally isolated from *Bacillus licheniformis* [49]. Both P1A and its derivative SYN-004 have been designed to be orally delivered in concert with intravenous beta-lactam administration [49]. SYN-004 (ribaxamase) has a broader degradation profile and hydrolyzes both cephalosporins and penicillins [49]. These two subclasses are not only the most widely used intravenous (IV) antibiotics but also are excreted in high concentrations into the upper GI tract via the bile [49]. Ribaxamase has an enteric coating that protects it from degradation by stomach acid and mediates release at a pH of greater than 5.5 at the site of antibiotic biliary excretion in the upper small intestine [50].

In pigs, the combination of ceftriaxone, a third-generation cephalosporin, and ribaxamase showed no significant posttreatment changes in the composition of the gut microbiota or increased frequency of antibiotic-resistant genes from pretreatment levels [51]. In phase 2b clinical studies, orally administered SYN-004 has been shown to degrade IV-administered ceftriaxone, thus decreasing the concentration of the drug in the intestinal fluid [15]. It was also shown that ribaxamase protected the diversity of the human gut microbiome and significantly reduced incidence of secondary *C. difficile* infection [15]. A major limitation is that many beta-lactams are administered orally, not systemically, and ribaxamase is not appropriate for co-administration with oral antibiotics [52]. Beta-lactam antibiotics including amoxicillin are absorbed in the proximal small intestine [53]. Since the ribaxamase release is also in the proximal small intestine, it degrades the antibiotic in the GI tract prior to its systemic absorption [52]. Concurrent oral administration of both ribaxamase and amoxicillin to canines resulted in no detectable antibiotic levels in the blood, confirming the degradation mechanism [52].

To expand the utility of ribaxamase to oral beta-lactam antibiotics, delayed release formulation SYN-007 was developed [52]. It is dual-coated with enteric coated-pellets packed into an enteric-coated capsule, to prevent its release in the upper portion of the small intestine [50]. This design allows it to pass to its target in the distal small bowel beyond the point where antibiotic absorption takes place, and instead be released upon encountering a pH greater than seven in the ileum, allowing the active enzyme to degrade the antibiotic before it reaches the bacteria of the colon [52]. Its efficacy was evaluated in dogs by collecting metagenomic and resistome analyses of fecal DNA before and after exposure to oral amoxicillin therapy as well as serum antibiotic levels during the 5-day study period [54]. In canine models, it was shown that SYN-007 protected the gut microbiome from oral amoxicillin-mediated dysbiosis without significantly altering the antibiotics systemic absorption and efficacy [52]. Animals that receive only amoxicillin showed loss of microbial diversity and the emergence of antibiotic-resistance genes [52]. Amoxicillin exposure showed increased populations of Proteobacteria, Furmiculates, and Fusobacteria phyla which were reduced when SYN-007 was added to the regimen [15]. The pathogenic transfer of antibiotic resistance was also mitigated in the cohort of animals receiving amoxicillin + SYN-007 [52]. Broadening the microbiome protection to include oral antibiotics greatly expands the clinical functionality or oral beta-lactamase therapy [54].

## 16.7 Conclusion

It has been established that antibiotics, while therapeutically important, are simultaneously detrimental to the homeostasis of the human gut microbiome. The dysbiosis they cause makes way for a variety of metabolic disturbances and colonization by pathogenic bacteria including *C. difficile*, states with negative impact on the health of the host. The disturbed environment additionally promotes the spread of antibiotic-resistance genes that has a negative impact on the community.

As we have developed a better understanding of the mechanisms leading to the antibiotic-induced dysbiosis, the magnitude of biochemical activities that are perturbed, and the resulting vulnerability to pathogens we have recognized a need to protect the homeostatic balance of the gut microbiome from the harmful costs of beta-lactam antibiotic use. It has led to development of complementary and alternative strategies to maintain human health such as administration of oral beta-lactamases to remove biologically active antimicrobials from the gastrointestinal tract before they can cause destruction. Microbiota protectors, such as ribaxamase, have the potential to impact the way antibiotics are prescribed in the future, enhance clinical outcomes for patients, and save many healthcare dollars. As demonstrated in proof-of-concept studies in both humans and dogs, these microbiota protectors are the first solution to attenuating antibiotic-mediated dysbiosis and curbing the problem of emerging bacterial resistance to beta-lactam antibiotics.

## 16.8 Future Trends

Amoxicillin and amoxicillin plus beta-lactamase inhibitor, clavulanate, is the most prescribed oral antimicrobial with more than 70 million prescriptions yearly in the United States alone [15].

Amoxicillin + clavulanate is routinely used to treat resistant infections caused by beta-lactamase-producing pathogens [55]. However, administration of the combination drug incurs more side effects than amoxicillin alone, including severe antibiotic-associated diarrhea due to disruption of the gut microbiome [55]. Amoxicillin exposure additionally results in emergence of plasmid-encoded class A beta-lactamase genes in the microbiome, perpetuating the spread of antimicrobial resistance [56]. Ribaxamase is notably sensitive to beta-lactamase inhibitors *in vitro* but could protect the gut microbiome in dogs treated with amoxicillin/clavulanate [54].

These paradoxical observations may be due to sufficiently high beta-lactamase concentrations in the gastrointestinal tract to overcome the inhibition with clavulanate [54]. Due to high prescription rates, protection of the gut microbiome from antibiotics combined beta-lactamase inhibitors remains an unmet need that warrants further investigation.

## References

1. J. Penders, E. Stobberingh, P. Savelkoul and P. Wolffs, "The human microbiome as a reservoir of antimicrobial resistance," *Front Mirobiol*, 4, p. 87, 2013.
2. M. Blaser, "The microbiome revolution," *J Clin Invest*, 124(10), pp. 4162–4165, 2014.

3. M. J. Bull and N. T. Plummer, "Part 1: The human gut microbiome in health and disease," *Integr Med (Encinitas)*, 13(6), pp. 17–22, 2014.
4. S. R. Modi, J. J. Collins and D. A. Relman, "Antibiotics and the gut microbiota," *J Clin Invest*, 124(10), pp. 4212–4218, 2014.
5. L. Dethlefsen, S. Huse, M. Sogin and D. Relman, "The pervasive effects of an antibiotic on the human gut microbiota, as revealed by deep 16S rRNA sequencing," *PLOS Biol*, 6(11), p. e280, 2008.
6. L. Beaurgerie and J.-C. Petit, "Microbial-gut interactions in health and disease: Antibiotic-associated diarrhoea," *Best Pract Res Clin Castroenterol*, 18(2), pp. 337–352, 2004.
7. M. Bohnhoff and P. Miller, "Enhanced susceptibility to salmonella infection in streptomycin-treated mice get access arrow," *J Infect Dis*, 111(2), pp. 117–127, 1962.
8. K. Ng, J. Ferreyra, S. Higginbottom, J. Lynch, P. Kashyao, S. Gopinath and N. Naidu, "Microbiota-liberated host sugars facilitate post-antibiotic expansion of enteric pathogens," *Nature*, 502(7469), pp. 96–99, 2013.
9. N. Pandey and M. Cascella, *Beta lactam antibiotics*. Treasure Island (FL): StatPearls [Internet], 2022.
10. K. Holten and E. Onusko, "Appropriate prescribing of oral beta-lactam antibiotics," *Am Fam Phys*, 62(3), pp. 611–620, 2001.
11. D. W. Yip and V. Gerriets, *Penicillin*. Treasure Island (FL): StatPearls [Internet], 2022.
12. K. Bush and P. Bradford, "β-lactams and β-lactamase inhibitors: An overview," *Cold Spring Harb Perspect Med*, 6(8), 2016. https://www.ncbi.nlm.nih.gov/pmc/articles/PMC4968164/
13. A. Andremont, J. Cervesi, P.-A. Bandinelli, F. Vitry and J. de Gunzburg, "Spare and repair the gut microbiota from antibiotic-induced dysbiosis: State-of-the-art," *Drug Discov Today*, 26(9), pp. 2159–2163, 2021.
14. B. Kowalska-Krochmal and R. Dudek-Wicher, "The minimum inhibitory concentration of antibiotics: Methods, interpretation, clinical relevance," *Pathogens*, 10(2), p. 165, 2021.
15. S. Connelly, B. Fanelli, N. Hasan, R. Colwell and M. Kaleko, "Low dose oral beta-lactamase protects the gut microbiome from oral beta-lactam-mediated damage in dogs," *AIMS Public Health*, 6(4), pp. 477–487, 2019.
16. S. M. Jandhyala, R. Talukdar, C. Subramanyam, H. Vuyyuru, M. Sasikala and D. N. Reddy, "Role of the normal gut microbiota," *World J Gastroenterol*, 21(29), pp. 8787–8803, 2015.
17. J. Qin, R. Li, J. Raes, M. Arumugam, K. Burgdorf, C. Manichanh and T. Nielsen, "A human gut microbial gene catalog established by metagenomic sequencing," *Nature*, 464(7285), pp. 59–65, 2013.
18. F. Magne, M. Gotteland, L. Gauthier, A. Zazueta, S. Pesoa, P. Navarrete and R. Balamurugan, "The Firmicutes/Bacteroidetes Ratio: A relevant marker of gut dysbiosis in obese patients?" *Nutrients*, 12(5), p. 1474, 2020.
19. E. Thursby and N. Juge, "Introduction to the human gut mucrobiota," *Biochem J*, 474(11), pp. 1823–1836, 2017.
20. A. Zhernakova, A. Kurlshikov, M. Bonder, E. Tigchelaar, M. Schirmer, T. Vatanen and Z. Mujagic, "Population-based metagenomics analysis reveals markers for gut microbiome composition and diversity," *Science*, 352(6285), pp. 565–569, 2016.
21. G. Donaldson, S. Lee and S. Mazmanian, "Gut biogeopgraphy of the bacterial microbiota," *Nat Rev Microbiol*, 14(1), pp. 20–32, 2016.
22. M. Candela, E. Biagi, S. Maccaferri, S. Turroni and P. Brigidi, "Intestinal microbiota is a plastic factor responding to environmental changes," *Trends Microbiol*, 20(8), pp. 385–391, 2012.
23. L. Dethlefsen and D. Relman, "Incomplete recovery and individualized responses of the human distal gut microbiota to repeated antibiotic perturbation," *Proc Natl Acad Sci U S A*, 108, pp. 4554–4561, 2011.

24. M. Blaser, "Antibiotic use and its consequences for the normal microbiome," *Science*, 352(6285), pp. 544–545, 2016.
25. M. Francino, "Antibiotics and the human gut microbiome: Dysbioses and accumulation of resistances," *Front Microbiol*, 6, p. 1543, 2016.
26. M. Ferrer, C. Mendez-Garcia, D. Rojo, C. Barbas and A. Moya, "Antibiotic use and microbiome function," *Biochem Pharmacol*, 134, pp. 114–126, 2016.
27. A. J. Browne, M. G. Chipeta, G. Haines-Woodhouse, E. Kumaran, B. Hamadani and S. Zaraa, "Global antibiotic consumption and usage in humans, 2000–18: A spatial modelling study," *Lancet Planet Health*, 5(12), pp. 893–904, 2021.
28. Centers for Disease Control and Prevention, "Outpatient antibiotic prescriptions — United States, 2021," Cent, 4 Oct 2022 [Online]. Available: https://www.cdc.gov/antibiotic-use/data/report-2021.html. [Accessed 27 Dec 2022].
29. K. Fleming-Dutra, A. Hersch and D. Shapiro, "Prevalence of inappropriate antibiotic prescriptions among US ambulatory care visits, 2010–2011," *JAMA*, 315(17), pp. 1864–1873, 2016.
30. M. Ferrer, V. Santos, S. Ott and A. Moya, "Gut microbiota disturbance during antibiotic therapy: A multi-omic approach," *Gut Microbes*, 5(1), pp. 64–70, 2014.
31. A. Perez-Cobas, M. Gosalbes, A. Friedrichs, H. Knecht, A. Artacho, K. Eismann and W. Otto, "Gut microbiota disturbance during antibiotic therapy: A multi-omic approach," *Gut*, 62(11), pp. 1591–1601, 2013.
32. M. D. Reed, "Optimal antibiotic dosing: The pharmacokinetic-pharmacodynamic interface," *Postgrad Med*, 108(7), pp. 17–24, 2000.
33. R. Moehring and C. Sarubbi, "Prolonged infusions of beta-lactam antibiotics," UpToDate, 23 Jun 2021 [Online]. Available: https://www.uptodate.com/contents/prolonged-infusions-of-beta-lactam-antibiotics#:~:text=Beta%2Dlactam%20antibiotics%20demonstrate%20a,more%20effectively%20than%20short%20infusions. [Accessed 8 Jan 2023].
34. B. Katzung and T. Vanderah, *Basic & Clinical Pharmacology*. New York: McGraw Hill, 2021.
35. T. Palzkill, "Metallo-β-lactamase structure and function," *Ann N Y Acad Sci*, 1277, pp. 91–104, 2013.
36. R. Pratt, "β-lactamases: Why and how," *J Med Chem*, 59(18), pp. 8207–8220, 2016.
37. A. Lee, S. Wang, H. Merideth, B. Zhuang, Z. Dai and L. You, "Robust, linear correlations between growth rates and β-lactam–mediated lysis rates," *PNAS*, 115(16), pp. 4069–4074, 2018.
38. C. Tooke, P. Hinchliffe, E. Bragginton, C. Colenso, V. Hirvonen, Y. Tekebayashi and J. Spencer, "β-lactamases and β-lactamase inhibitors in the 21st century," *J Mol Biol*, 431(18), pp. 3472–3500, 2019.
39. E. Abraham and E. Chain, "An enzyme from bacteria able to destroy penicillin. 1940," *Rev Infect Dis*, 10(4), pp. 677–678, 1988.
40. V. Schaar, I. Uddback, T. Nordstrom and K. Riesbeck, "Group A streptococci are protected from amoxicillin-mediated killing by vesicles containing β-lactamase derived from Haemophilus influenzae," *J Antimicrob Chemother*, 69(1), pp. 117–120, 2014.
41. S. Ghafourian, H. Sadeghifard, S. Soheili and Z. Sekawi, "Extended spectrum beta-lactamases: Definition, classification and epidemiology," *Curr Issues Mol Biol*, 17(1), pp. 11–22, 2015.
42. K. Bush and P. Bradford, "Interplay between β-lactamases and new β-lactamase inhibitors," *Nat Rev Microbiol*, 17(5), pp. 295–306, 2019.
43. C. Mu and W. Zu, "Antibiotic effects on gut microbiota, metabolism, and beyond," *Appl Microbiol Biotechnol*, 103(23–24), pp. 9277–9285, 2019.
44. X. Ge, C. Ding, W. Zhao, L. Xu, H. Tian, J. Gong and M. Zhu, "Antibiotics-induced depletion of mice microbiota induces changes in host serotonin biosynthesis and intestinal motility," *J Transl Med*, 15(13), 2017.

45. B. Stecher, S. Chaffron, R. Kappeli, S. Hapfelmeier, S. Freedrich, T. Weber and J. Kirundi, "Like will to like: Abundances of closely related species can predict susceptibility to intestinal colonization by pathogenic and commensal bacteria," *PLOS Pathog*, 6(1), 2010. https://journals.plos.org/plospathogens/article?id=10.1371/journal .ppat.1000711

46. K. Wilson, "The microecology of Clostridium difficile," *Clin Infect Dis*, 16, pp. S214–S218, 1993.

47. B. Sandhu, A. Edwards, S. Anderson, E. Woods and S. McBride, "Regulation and anaerobic function of the Clostridioides difficile β-lactamase," *Antimicrob Agents Chemother*, 64(1), pp. e01496–19, 2020.

48. F. Lessa, Y. Mu, W. Bamberg, Z. Beldavs, G. Dumyati, J. Dunn and M. Farley, "Burden of Clostridium difficile infection in the United States," *N Engl J Med*, 372(9), pp. 825–834, 2015.

49. M. Kaleko, J. A. Bristol, S. Hubert, T. Parsley, G. Widmer, S. Tzipori and P. Subramanian, "Development of SYN-004, an oral beta-lactamase treatment to protect the gut microbiome from antibiotic-mediated damage and prevent Clostridium difficile infection," *Anaerobe*, 41, pp. 58–67, 2016.

50. A. Bristol, S. H. F. Hubert and H. Baer, "Formulation development of SYN-004 (ribaxamase) oral solid dosage form, a β-lactamase to prevent intravenous antibiotic-associated dysbiosis of the colon," *Int J Pharm*, 534(1–2), pp. 25–34, 2017.

51. S. Connelly, J. Bristol, S. Hubert, P. Subramanian, N. Hasan, R. Colwell and M. Kaleko, "SYN-004 (ribaxamase), an oral beta-lactamase, mitigates antibiotic-mediated dysbiosis in a porcine gut microbiome model," *J Appl Microbiol*, 123(1), pp. 66–79, 2017.

52. S. Connelly, B. Fanelli, N. Hasan, R. Colwell and M. Kaleko, "Oral beta-lactamase protects the canine gut microbiome from oral amoxicillin-mediated damage," *Microorganisms*, 7(5), p. 150, 2019.

53. W. Barr, E. Zola, E. Candler, S. Hwang, A. Tendolkar, R. Shamburek and B. Parker, "Differential absorption of amoxicillin from the human small and large intestine," *Clin Pharmacol Ther*, 56(3), pp. 279–285, 1994.

54. S. Connelly, B. Fanelli, N. Hasan, R. Colwell and M. Kaleko, "SYN-007, an orally administered beta-lactamase enzyme, protects the gut microbiome from oral amoxicillin/clavulanate without adversely affecting antibiotic systemic absorption in dogs," *Microorganisms*, 8(2), p. 152, 2020.

55. J. Kuehn, Z. Ismael, P. Long, C. Barker and M. Sharland, "Reported rates of diarrhea following oral penicillin therapy in pediatric clinical trials," *J Pediatr Pharmacol Ther*, 20(2), pp. 90–104, 2015.

56. P. Bradford, "Extended-spectrum β-lactamases in the 21st century: Characterization, epidemiology, and detection of this important resistance threat," *Clin Microbiol Rev*, 14(4), pp. 933–951, 2001.

# 17

# Gut Microbiota with Functional Food Components and Nutraceuticals

Vivek Patel, Dhara Patel, and Jayvadan Patel

## Contents

## 17.1 Introduction

The term "microbiota" applies to the entire population of microorganisms in a given location (1). The largest population of microorganisms is the microbiota of the human gut, which is comprised of approximately 100 trillion microorganisms (most of them bacteria, but also fungi, viruses and archaea) (2–7). The collection of genes found in intestinal microorganisms forms a genetic repertoire that is one level above the human genome. (8). The microbiota offers a great deal of help to the host with a variety of physiological functions such as strengthening gut integrity or intestinal epithelium (9), harvesting energy (10), protecting against pathogens (11) and regulating host immunity (12). The human gut microbiota is complex, lively and unique to each individual and influenced by various factors such as diet, age, antibiotic intake, xenobiotics, early life microbiota exposure, changes in hygiene practices, pollution and socioeconomic status (13).

DOI: 10.1201/9781003333821-17

Of these factors, the diet is considered a major driver for changes in gut bacterial diversity that may affect its functional relationships with the host (14). Studies have shown that several diseases, such as inflammatory bowel disease (IBD), cancer, cardio-metabolic diseases, obesity and diabetes, are associated with an imbalance of the bacterial composition of the gut, which is referred to as a symbiosis (15, 16). Dietary interventions may be effective in restoring the gut to a healthier state. Overall, a balanced gut microbiota composition confers benefits to the host, while microbial imbalances are linked with metabolic and immune mediated disorders (17).

Instead of taking drugs, like non-steroidal anti-inflammatory drugs (NSAIDs) that, in some cases, could possibly do more harm than good, the use of dietary intervention with functional foods provides a window of opportunity for gut health and the treatment of gastrointestinal diseases (18, 19). Diet plays a key role in the provision of adequate nutrients to meet the basic nutritional necessities for maintenance and growth, while giving the consumer a feeling of satisfaction and well-being. In addition, some food components provide beneficial effects beyond basic nutrition, leading to the concept of functional foods and nutraceuticals (20). Functional foods and nutraceuticals offer an opportunity to improve human health, reduce health care expenses and support economic development in rural communities. Some functional food components influence the growth and/or metabolic activity of the gut microbiota and, thereby, its composition and functions (21). Therefore, the intestinal microbiota is both a target for nutritional intervention to improve health and a factor influencing the biological activity of other food compounds acquired orally. This chapter emphasizes the reciprocal interaction between the gut microbiota and functional food components and nutraceuticals and the significance of these interactions on human health.

## 17.2 Gut Microbial Ecology

The human gastrointestinal (GI) tract is a complex system and the largest internal organ of the body. The human GI starts from the oral cavity, continues through the stomach and intestine and finally ends at the anus. It also acts as a barrier against pathogens and the intestinal lumen. The community of microorganisms existing in the human GI tract consists of nearly a thousand commensal and symbiotic microbial species. These include bacteria, viruses (including bacteriophages), archaea, and unicellular eukaryotes, etc., They are collectively known as "Gut Microbiota". In recent years, research involving the human microbiota has increased and shown that it produces metabolites that play a key role in the host's immune system through a complex series of chemical interactions and signaling pathways (22–24). The distribution of different strains or species of bacteria within the gut determines the metabolic profile of the microbiota, which could have potential physiological effects on health (25). The intestinal microbiota develops after birth; some factors, such as the mode of birth, infant nutrition, antibiotic use, diet and age determine its colonization rate (Figure 17.1).

In general, *bifidobacterium* populations are dominant in the first months of life, especially in breastfed infants (up to 90% of the total fecal bacteria) due to the bifidogenic effect of breast milk, while a more-diverse microbiota is found in formula-fed infants, weaning children and adults (27). Eating habits, food consumption and lifestyle have health impacts. The composition of this bacterial ecosystem is dynamic and susceptible to changes driven by dietary factors and diverse disease conditions (28, 29). As a result, some gut diseases result from an imbalance of intestinal microbiota and are related to diet; therefore, diet has implications on gut health (30, 31). The human gut has the following functions: (a) it breaks food down into nutrients, (b) it facilitates the absorption of nutrients into the blood through the intestinal walls and (c) it prevents foreign and toxic molecules from entering the bloodstream (32, 33). Gut malfunction, therefore, has a direct negative impact on human health. Research studies have shown that several diseases (inflammatory bowel disease, cancer, cardio-metabolic diseases, obesity and diabetes) are associated with an imbalance of the bacterial composition of the gut, which is referred to as dysbiosis (34, 35) (Figure 17.2). Overall, a balanced gut microbiota composition confers benefits to the host, while microbial imbalances are linked with metabolic and immune mediated disorders.

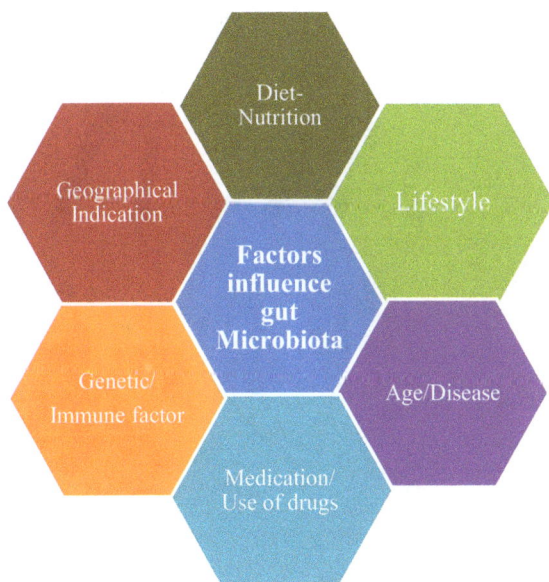

*Figure 17.1* Factors that affect gut microbiota

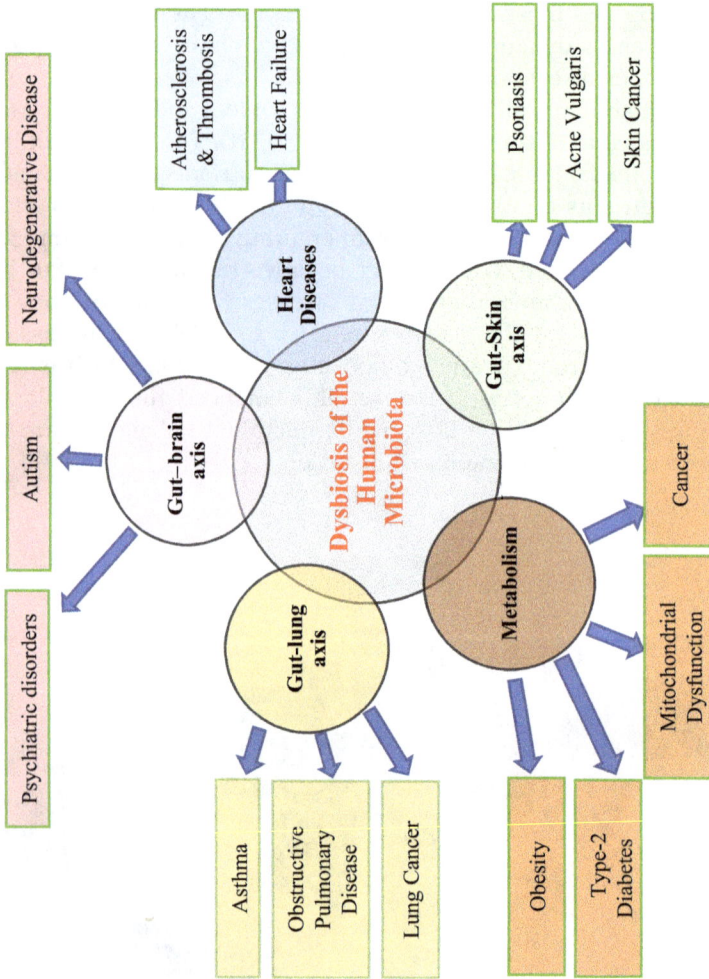

*Figure 17.2  Human microbial dysbiosis in human disease*

## 17.3 Functional Foods and Nutraceuticals

The phrase "Let food be the medicine and medicine be the food," coined by Hippocrates over 2500 years ago is getting a lot of interest today as food scientists and consumers realize the many health benefits of certain foods (36). Functional foods and nutraceuticals are two new terms used to describe health-promoting foods or their extracted components. Although the concept of functional foods has been frequently discussed in research studies, there is no internationally recognized definition of this term (37). Also, despite efforts to establish regulations, there is no scientific consensus to discriminate between functional foods, nutraceuticals and dietary supplements. It is more appropriate to describe nutraceuticals as healthful products that are formulated and taken in the form of dosage. On the other hand, functional foods are products that are consumed as foods and not in dosage form (38). Functional foods are classified as traditional or staple foods that support vital nutritional levels and have potentially positive effects on host health, including the reduction of disease by optimizing the immune system's ability to avoid and control infections by pathogens, as well as pathologies that cause functional modifications in the host. Functional foods, as defined by Health Canada, are products that look like traditional foods but are proven to offer some physiological benefits. The combination of foods with some herbal medicines forms the basis for most outstanding traditional functional foods (39).

Functional foods include the following:

- Foods enhanced with biologically active substances (for example, probiotics)
- Derived food compounds added to conventional foods (for example, prebiotics)
- Normal foods containing inherent biologically active substances (for example, dietary fiber, dietary polyphenol, phytochemical)

Some of the main types of functional foods, besides conventional fermented ones, include nutraceuticals, probiotics, prebiotics and synbiotics (which are a mixture of probiotics and prebiotics) (Figure 17.3).

Nutraceutical terminology was first introduced by Dr. Stephen L. DeFelice in 1989 and acted as a link between nutrition and the pharmaceutical field. After 1994, when the place of dietary supplements in maintaining people's health was recognized, the term "nutraceuticals" was extended to comprise dietary supplements category, too (40, 41). On the other hand, Health Canada states nutraceuticals as "a product prepared from foods, but sold in the form of pills or powder or in other medicinal forms, not usually associated with foods" which play an important role in modifying and/or maintaining physiological functions or offering protection against chronic diseases. Nutraceuticals are found in a mosaic of products emerging from (a) the food industry, (b)

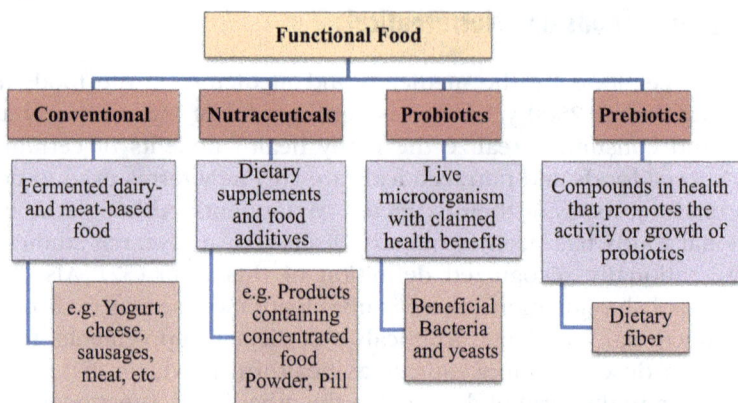

**Figure 17.3** *Classification of functional foods*

the herbal and dietary supplement market, (c) the pharmaceutical industry and (d) newly merged pharmaceuticals/agribusiness/nutrition conglomerates. They may range from isolated nutrients, herbal products, dietary supplements and diets to genetically engineered "designer" foods and processed products such as cereals, soups and beverages (42–44).

Nutraceuticals can be categorized as potential nutraceuticals and established nutraceuticals. Some potential nutraceuticals could become established only after efficient clinical data on their health and medical benefits are obtained. It should be noted that most nutraceutical products are still part of the "potential class" (45–48).

Functional foods and nutraceuticals affect biological responses in the body, promoting health benefits in some important areas like cancer prevention, cardiovascular health, gastrointestinal health, neurodegenerative diseases, cognition and cardiometabolic syndrome (Figure 17.4).

Functional foods are known to alter physiological mechanisms at the gastrointestinal tract (GIT) level by increasing biochemical parameters and improving neuronal functions (49). Dietary components with biological effects are vulnerable to being metabolized by intestinal bacteria during the gastrointestinal passage, prior to being absorbed. The colon has the highest bacterial load and establishes an active site of metabolism rather than a simple excretion route. The metabolic activity of the gut microbiota on bioactive food components can alter the host's exposure to these components and their potential health effects. Additionally, some functional food components influence the growth and/or metabolic activity of the gut microbiota and, thereby, its composition and functions. Some of the main types of functional foods, besides fermented conventional ones, include prebiotics, probiotics, dietary fibers, nutraceuticals and synbiotics (which are a mixture of probiotics and prebiotics).

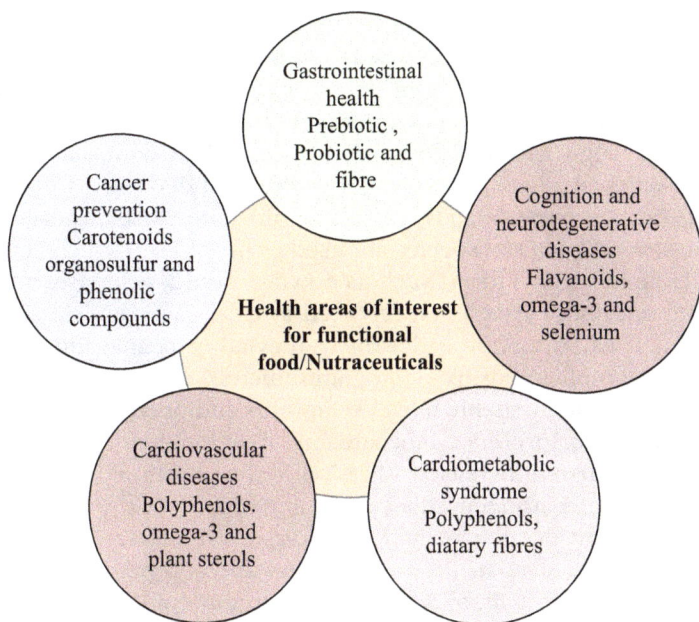

**Figure 17.4** *Health areas of interest for functional food/nutraceuticals*

## 17.3.1 Probiotics and Gut Microbiota

The history of probiotics dates back as far as the initial intake of fermented milks, over 2000 years ago. The scientific attention in this area was enhanced by the work of Metchinkoff (1907) to transmute the toxic flora of the large intestine into a host-friendly colony of *Bacillus bulgaricus*. A probiotic can be defined as a live microbial feed supplement, which when administered in sufficient amounts beneficially affects the host by improving its intestinal microbial balance. The definition of probiotics according to the Food and Agriculture Organization/World Health Organization is "Live microorganisms which when administered in adequate amounts confer a health benefit on the host" (50, 51). Probiotic microorganisms are generally lactic acid bacteria (LAB), which are included under the "Generally Recognized As Safe (GRAS)" category by the US Food and Drug Administration (FDA) (52). Presently, the food industry has seen significant growth and progress in developing functional foods, mainly by using probiotic bacteria as ingredients in the formulation of its products and as food additives. LAB belong to the phylum *Firmicutes*, class Bacilli, and order *Lactobacillales*, which includes over 50 genera placed in six families, (comprising *Lactobacillus, Levilactobacillus, Lacticaseibacillus, Limosilactobacillus, Lactococcus, Pediococcus, Enterococcus, Leuconostoc, Oenococcus, Streptococcus, Tetragenococcus, Aerococcus, Carnobacterium, Weissella, Alloiococcus, Symbiobacterium* and *Vagococcus*) and more than 300 species (52). Currently, the food industry has been significant growth in developing functional foods/nutraceuticals, mainly by applying probiotic bacteria. Two main sources of LAB isolation have emerged; they are classified according to the source: one from dairy products and the other from non-dairy products. Sour buttermilk, unfermented goat milk drinks, sour milk, ice cream and yogurt as isolate sources included in dairy-based products. Within non-dairy products, two categories are included, fermented and non-fermented, both groups include cereals, fruits, vegetables, meats and fish. Nowadays, several bacterial species are used as probiotics, which are commercially available in various forms such as powder, liquid, gel, paste and capsule etc. Specific probiotics have been reported to treat gastrointestinal (GI) complications such as suppressing diarrhea, alleviating lactose intolerance and postoperative complications, providing anti-microbial and anti-colorectal cancer activities, reducing irritable bowel symptoms and preventing inflammatory bowel disease. Major probiotic mechanisms of action comprise enhancement of the epithelial barrier, increased adhesion to the intestinal mucosa and associated inhibition of pathogen adhesion, competitive exclusion of pathogenic microorganisms, production of anti-microorganism substances and modulation of the immune system. Probiotic agents are non-pathogenic, non-toxic and resistant to gastric acid, and they adhere to gut epithelial tissues producing antibacterial substances (52). Examples of some commercially available probiotics are given in Table 17.1.

## 17.3.2 Prebiotics and Gut Microbiota

The prebiotics concept was introduced for the first time in 1995 by Glenn Gibson and Marcel Roberfroid (54). Prebiotics are nondigestible food ingredients, mostly oligosaccharides, which beneficially affect the host by stimulating the growth, activity or both of specific intestinal bacteria. In order to be classified as a prebiotic, the following criteria must be fulfilled: (1) resistance to gastric acidity and mammalian enzymes; (2) susceptibility to fermentation by gut microbiota; and (3) ability to stimulate the growth and/or activity of beneficial intestinal bacteria. The possible beneficial effects of prebiotics include the control of intestinal transit time and bowel habits and a reduction in the risk of atherosclerosis, osteoporosis, obesity, type-2 diabetes, cancer, infections and allergies, although their effectiveness in humans is still controversial (55). The biological effects of prebiotics mainly depend on their influence on the composition of gut microbiota and derived metabolites; although some roles could be due to their own structure and direct action (e.g. inhibition of pathogen adhesion by homology with bacterial receptors).

Carbohydrates are the main source of short chain fatty acids (SCFAs) – acetate, propionate and butyrate. Due to the action of SCFAs, the composition and diversity of microbiota can be changed in a positive way. The metabolites decrease intestinal pH, suppress the growth of intestinal pathogens and influence intestinal motility. Prebiotics naturally exist in various dietary food

**Table 17.1** Examples of Some Commercially Available Probiotics (53)

| Brand Name | Strain | Clinical Application |
|---|---|---|
| Dicoflor | *Lactobacillus rhamnosus GG* | • Treatment and prevention of antibiotics-associated diarrhea and infectious diarrhea<br>• Management of irritated bowel syndrome<br>• Synergistic eradication of *H. Pylori* |
| Enterogermina | *Bacillus clausii* | • For treatment of diarrhea and restoration of gut health |
| Enterolactis | *Lactobacillus casei* | • Indicated for restoring the intestinal flora affected by dietary imbalances and antibiotic therapies |
| Nutriflor | *Lactobacillus acidophilus DDS-1*<br>*Lactobacillus bulgaricus DDS-14*<br>*Bifidobacterium bifidum*<br>*Lactobacillus rhamnosus* | • Indicated in cases of reduced or compromised intestinal flora and as probiotic support during or after antibiotic therapy<br>• It can be useful in vaginitis, urinary infections, skin irritation and respiratory problems |
| Probactiol Duo | *Saccharomyces boulardii*<br>*Lactobacillus acidophilus NCFM*<br>*Lactobacillus paracasei Lpc-37*<br>*Bifidobacterium lactis Bi-07*<br>*Bifidobacterium lactis Bi-04* | • Support natural bowel movement and natural resistance |
| VSL#3 | *Streptococcus thermophilus*<br>*Bifidobacterium breve*<br>*Bifidobacterium longum*<br>*Bifidobacterium infantis*<br>*Lactobacillus acidophilus*<br>*Lactobacillus plantarum*<br>*Lactobacillus paracasei*<br>*Lactobacillus delbrueckii* subsp. *bulgaricus* | • It is used to treat irritable bowel syndrome (symptoms include abdominal pain, cramping, bloating and diarrhea or constipation) and ulcerative colitis |
| Yakult | *Lactobacillus casei shirota* | • Helps prevent constipation<br>• Reduces the chances of upper respiratory tract infections<br>• Reduces anxiety and stress<br>• Improve heart health |
| Aciforce | *Lactococcus lactis*<br>*Lactobacillus acidophilus*<br>*Enterococcus faecium*<br>*Bifidobacterium bifidum* | • It is used to treat irritable bowel syndrome (symptoms include abdominal pain, cramping, bloating and diarrhea or constipation) and ulcerative colitis |
| Baciluc | *Lactobacillus acidophilus*<br>*Lactobacillus rhamnosus* | • Treating diarrhea caused by antibiotics |
| Proflora | *Lactobacillus acidophilus*<br>*Lactobacillus delbrueckii* subsp. *bulgaricus*<br>*Streptococcus thermophilus*<br>*Bifidobacterium* | • It is necessary during and after antibiotic treatment to restore intestinal flora and prevent diarrhea induced by the antibiotic effect; Proflora Daily strains had shown in studies a superiority in the reduction of abdominal pain, flatulence, bloating and belching associated with IBS when taken daily |

products including asparagus, sugar beet, garlic, chicory, onion, Jerusalem artichoke, wheat, honey, banana, barley, tomato, rye, soybean, human and cow's milk, peas, beans, etc., and recently, seaweeds and microalgae. Because of their lower concentration in foods, they are manufactured on an industrial scale. Some of the prebiotics are produced by using lactose, sucrose and starch as raw material. Fructo-oligosaccharides (FOS), galacto-oligosaccharides (GOS), xylo-oligosaccharides (XOS), lactulose, non-digestible carbohydrates inulin, cellulose, resistant starches, hemicelluloses and pectins are the most used prebiotics in current medical practice, as shown in Table 17.2 (56). The key effects of prebiotics include modulation of gut microbiota composition

**Table 17.2** Types of Prebiotic Oligosaccharides, Health Benefits, Responsible Microorganisms and References

| Prebiotic Oligosaccharides | Benefit to Host | Proposed Responsible Microorganism | References |
|---|---|---|---|
| HMO (human milk oligosaccharides) | Anti-inflammatory effect, regulation of permeability of host cells, protection from diarrhea, necrotizing enterocolitis and respiratory tract infections, diabetes, prevents binding of pathogens like *campylobacter jejuni* and rotavirus to host cell | *Bifidobacterium longum* subsp. *Infantis* *Bacteroides* | (55–58) |
| FOS | Anti-inflammatory effect, improved IBS symptoms, lower blood glucose level, anti-cancer, diarrhea treatment, reduces atopic dermatitis | *Bifidobacteria* *Faecalibacterim Prausnitzii Bacteroidetes* | (59–61) |
| Inulin | Improved bowel function, increased bifidobacterial population, lower serum lipopolysaccharides level, immunomodulatory action, increased mineral absorption, cardiovascular effects, anti-cancer | *Bifidobacteria* *Bacteroidetes* | (62–66) |
| GOS | Immunomodulatory action, pathogen adherence inhibition, improved IBS symptoms, reduces atopic dermatitis | *Bifidobacteria* *Lactobacilli* | (67, 68) |
| MOS | Lower IBS symptoms, increased expression of proinflammatory mediators, lower proinflammatory cytokines, prevent binding of pathogens to host cell | *Lactobacilli* | (69, 70) |
| XOS | Immunomodulatory action, increased plasma HDL concentration, anti-inflammatory effect, reduction in triglycerides, lower dose requirement for clinical efficacy, anti-cancer | *Bifidobacteria* *Lactobacilli* | (71–73) |

and production of energy metabolism, increasing mineral absorption function and improvement of the intestinal barrier function.

### 17.3.3 Dietary Fiber and Gut Microbiota

Dietary fiber is the food material, more precisely the plant material, that is not hydrolyzed by enzymes secreted by the digestive tract, but digested by the microflora in the gut. Dietary fibers mostly include non-starch polysaccharides such as cellulose, hemicellulose, gums and pectin, lignin, resistant dextrin and resistant starches. Chemically dietary fiber means carbohydrate polymers with a degree of polymerization not lower than 3, which are neither digested nor absorbed in the small intestine (74–78). Dietary fibers may be divided into two forms based on their water solubility:

1. Insoluble dietary fiber (IDF): includes celluloses, some hemicelluloses and lignins which are fermented to a limited extent in the colon.
2. Soluble dietary fiber (SDF): includes β-glucans, pectins, gums, mucilages and hemicelluloses which are fermented in the colon.

IDF and SDF compounds are collectively known as non-starch polysaccharides (NSP). The soluble components of dietary fiber by the benefit of their bulking and viscosity producing capabilities, delay the gastric emptying of the stomach. This affects the rate of digestion and the uptake of nutrients and creates a feeling of satiety. Soluble fiber has been shown to selectively lower serum LDL cholesterol and improve glucose tolerance. It also enhances insulin receptor binding and improves glycemic response. In the colon, dietary fiber increases fecal bulking due to increased water retention, increased transit time and increased fecal bacterial mass caused by soluble fiber fermentation. The fiber also promotes the growth of *Bifidobacteria* in the gut (especially FOS). Persons consuming generous amounts of dietary fiber, compared to those who have minimal fiber intake, have a lower risk of coronary heart disorder, stroke, diabetes, obesity and certain GI disorders. Research reveals that certain soluble fibers enhance immunity in humans. Some potential negative effects of dietary fiber include reduced absorption of vitamins, minerals, proteins and calories. It is recommended that dietary fiber intake for adults generally fall in the range of 20 to 35 g/day. Several case histories have reported that consumption of excessive amounts of dietary fiber causes diarrhea (78, 79). Table 17.3 lists different types of dietary fibers, and their food sources and health benefits.

### 17.3.4 Polyunsaturated Fatty Acids (PUFA) and Gut Microbiota

PUFAs are also called "essential fatty acids" as they are vital to the functioning of the body and are introduced externally by the diet. PUFAs have two subdivisions: Omega-3-(n-3) fatty acids and Omega-6-(n-6) fatty acids. The main omega-3-fatty acids are α-linolenic acid (ALA), eicosapentanoic acid

**Table 17.3** Types of Dietary Fibers, Sources, Health Benefits and References

| Category | Examples | Food Source | Health Benefits | References |
|---|---|---|---|---|
| Insoluble dietary fibers | Cellulose | Beans, brown rice, flour, nuts, vegetables | Fecal bulking, SCFA production, enhance immune function | (79–81) |
| | Hemicellulose | | | (77, 81, 82) |
| | Fructans | | | (80, 81) |
| Soluble dietary fibers | Pectin | Fruits, vegetables | Slow glucose absorption and binding of bile acids, modulate microbial composition | (79, 81, 82) |
| | B-glucan | Algae, cereal grains (e.g., barley or oats), mushrooms, other marine plants | Prebiotic, SCFA production, slow glucose absorption and binding of bile acids, modulate microbial composition | (79, 82) |
| | Oligofructose | Commercially available from chemical degradation by endoglycosidase enzymes; naturally in banana, asparagus, chicory root, dandelion greens, garlics, artichokes, leeks, Onion, wheat, barley, rye | Prebiotic, decrease plasma LPS in diabetics | (81, 82) |
| | Inulin | Leeks, asparagus, onions, wheat, garlic, chicory, oats, soybeans, bananas, agave, Jerusalem artichoke | SCFA production, reduce body weight, blood cholesterol and blood glucose concentration, decrease plasma LPS in diabetics | (79, 81, 82) |
| | Fructooligosaccharides | Transfructosylation of sucrose; naturally in artichoke, asparagus, banana, chicory, garlic, onion | | (79, 81) |
| | Galactooligosaccharides | Synthesized by glycosylation of lactose; used in beverages, confectionery products, fermented and flavored milks, infant formula, meal replacers | Prebiotic, promote gastrointestinal health due to fermentability, change composition and/or activity of the gastrointestinal microbiota | (79, 80, 82) |
| | Resistance starches | Bananas, beans, lentils, peas, whole grains | | (77–79) |
| | Maltodextrin | Synthesized from highly processed corn, potato, rice, or wheat; potential application as fat replacer in butter and margarines, dairy products; low-fat salad dressings, mayonnaise, spreads, and used in nonallergenic infant formula, rehydration/recovery/ energy drinks | | (81, 82) |
| | Guar gum | Made from the endosperm of the plant *Cyamopsis tetragonolobus*; used in bakery, cereal, dairy products, meat products | | (79–82) |
| | Arabinooligosaccharides | Bars, cereals, dairy products, isotonic beverages, sports drink | Prebiotic, SCFA production | (81, 82) |
| | Xylooligosaccharides | Bamboo shoots, bars, cereals, dairy products, fruits, honey, isotonic beverages, sports drinks, vegetables | Prebiotic, SCFA production | (81, 82) |

(EPA) and docosahexanoic acid (DHA). ALA is the precursor of EPA and DHA. EPA and DHA are generally found in fatty fishes such as mackerels, salmon, herring, trout, bluefin tuna and fish oil. Major sources of ALA are generally flaxseed, soybeans, canola, some nuts (eg. walnuts) and red/black currant seeds. Omega-6-PUFAs mainly consist of linoleic acid (LA), λ- linolenic acid (GLA) and arachidonic acid (ARA). LA occurs mainly in vegetable oils e.g. corn, sunflower, soya bean and safflower. ARA is found in animal products such as meat, poultry and eggs. Omega-3-PUFAs can improve intestinal immunity. Omega-3-PUFAs could reduce intestinal epithelial cell damage caused by LPS, sodium dextran sulfate or hydrogen peroxide and increase intracellular mitochondrial activity and cell membrane integrity. Stress exposure increases intestinal dysfunction and decreases intestinal immunity. Chronic stress causes a series of anomalies in the intestine, including decreased fecal water content, increased production of pro-inflammatory cytokines (TNF-α, Il-1β, IFN-γ and IL-6) and abnormal changes in the microbiota composition (particularly *Bifidobacterium*, *Lactobacillus* and *Roseburia* and *Prevotella* spp.). Omega-3-PUFAs have been shown to effectively counteract these adverse effects. Emerging research evidence shows the benefits of omega-3-oils in other areas of health including pre-mature infant health, asthma, bipolar and depressive disorders, dysmenorrhea and diabetes. Omega-3 fatty acids have been shown to be advantageous at various stages of life. Infant formulas nowadays contain DHA along with ARA, which closely mimic breast milk. The FDA recommends a maximum of 3 g/day intake of EPA and DHA omega-3 fatty acids, with no more than 2 g per day from a dietary supplement (83–85).

## 17.3.5 Phytochemicals and Gut Microbiota

Phytochemicals are defined as bioactive non-nutrient plant compounds present in fruits, vegetables, grains and other plant foods, whose digestion has been linked to a reduction in the risk of major chronic diseases. The different compounds included in the group can be classified according to common structural features, including phenolics, carotenoids, alkaloids and nitrogen containing and organosulfur compounds (86). Phenolics, flavonoids and phytoestrogens have raised particular interest because of their potential effects as antioxidants (87), anti-estrogenics (88), anti-inflammatories and immunomodulatories (89–93), cardioprotectives (88) and anticarcinogenics (94). Only 5–10% of phytochemicals are absorbed in the small intestine, while the remaining 90–95% are transformed by the resident colonic microbiota. Phytochemicals contribute to the maintenance of human GI health largely via modulation of the gut microbial balance with simulation inhibition of pathogens and the simulation of beneficial bacteria. The bioavailability and effects of polyphenols significantly depend on their transformation by specific components of the gut microbiota via esterase, glucosidase, demethylation, dehydroxylation and decarboxylation activities (95). Many dietary polyphenols are glycosides that are transformed into aglycones through commensal bacterial glycohydrolases, thereby altering their bioavailability and affecting positively or negatively their activities and/or functional effects on the mammalian tissues (96, 97). Polyphenols are generally present in plant foods as a bound form, most often conjugated as glycosides, and most of them are metabolized by gut microbiota resulting in the formation of aglycones (98, 99). The microbiota metabolites of polyphenols are well absorbed in the intestine, and their entero-hepatic circulation confirms that the residence time in plasma for the metabolites is extended compared to that of their parent compounds, and finally are excreted via urine. The gut microbiota has been demonstrated to be essential for the production of active isoflavone metabolites with estrogen-like activity; additionally, the metabolites produced show different anti-inflammatory properties (89). Similarly, the flavonoid quercetin produced by gut microbial enzymes exerts a higher effect in the down-regulation of the inflammatory responses than the glycosylated form present in vegetables (quercetin or 3-rhamnosylquercetin) (90). This effect is exerted by inhibiting cytokine and inducible nitric oxide synthase expression through inhibition of the NF-kappaB pathway both in vitro and in vivo (90). In contrast, the ellagitanin punicalagin that is the most potent antioxidant found in pomegranate juice is extensively metabolized to hydroxy-6Hdibenzopyran-6-one derivatives, which did not indicate significant antioxidant activity compared to punicalagin (91). Phytochemicals and their derived products can also affect the intestinal ecology as a significant part of them are not fully absorbed and are metabolized in the liver, excreted through the bile as glucuronides and accumulated in the ileal and colorectal lumen (92). For example, the intake of flavonol-rich foods has been shown to alter the composition of the gut microbiota, exerting prebiotic-like effects (93). Unabsorbed dietary phenolics and their metabolites have been shown to exert antimicrobial or bacteriostatic activities (94). These metabolites selectively inhibit pathogen growth and stimulate the growth of commensal bacteria, including also some known probiotics (93, 94), thus influencing the microbiota composition. Plant phenolic compounds from olives (94), tea (93), wine (94) and berries (95, 96) have established antimicrobial properties. Tea phenolics have been shown to inhibit the growth of *Bacteroides* spp., *Clostridium* spp. (*C. perfringens* and *C. difficile*), *Escherichia coli* and *Salmonella typhimurium* (96). The level of inhibition was related to the chemical structure of the compound and bacterial species. In this sense, caffeic acid generally exerted a more significant inhibitory effect on pathogen growth than epicatechin, catechin, 3-Omethylgallic acid and gallic acid. Another in vitro study showed that (+)-catechin increased the counts of *Clostridium coccoides-Eubacterium rectale* group and *Escherichia coli*, but inhibited those of *Clostridium histolyticum* (90). The effects of (−)-epicatechin were less pronounced, increasing the growth of *Clostridium coccoides-Eubacterium rectale* group (98). Interestingly, the growth of beneficial bacteria (*Bifidobacterium* spp. and *Lactobacillus* spp.) was relatively unaffected or favored (97, 99). Resveratrol, a potent antioxidant found in wine, favored the increase of *Bifidobacterium* and *Lactobacillus* counts (100) and abolished the expression of virulence factors of Proteus mirabilis to invade

**Table 17.4** Examples of Phytochemicals, Source and Health Benefits (112)

| Phytochemicals | Source | Benefits |
|---|---|---|
| Carotenoids<br>Alpha-carotene<br>Beta-carotene<br>Lutein<br>Lycopene | Carrots, fruits, vegetable<br>Green vegetables<br>Tomato products (ketchup,<br>sauces) | Neutralize free radicals, which may cause<br>damage to cells<br>Reduce the risk of macular degeneration<br>Reduce the risk of prostate cancer |
| Phenolics<br>Anthocyanidins<br>Catechins<br>Flavanones<br>Flavones<br>Lignans<br>Tannins (proanthocyanidins) | Fruits<br>Tea<br>Citrus<br>Fruits/vegetables<br>Flax, rye, vegetables<br>Cranberries, cranberry products,<br>cocoa, chocolate | Neutralize free radicals<br>Reduce risk of cancer<br>Prevention of cancer, renal failure<br>Improve urinary tract health<br>Reduce risk of cardiovascular disease |
| Plant sterols<br>Stanol ester | Corn, soy, wheat, wood oils | Lower blood cholesterol levels by inhibiting<br>cholesterol absorption |
| Soy phytoestrogens Soy phytoestrogens &<br>Isoflavones:<br>Daidzein, Genistein<br>Isoflavones:<br>Daidzein<br>Genistein | Soybeans and soy-based foods | Menopause symptoms, such as hot flashes<br>Protect against heart disease and some<br>cancers<br>Lower LDL and total cholesterol |

human urothelial cells (101). Anthocyanins from berries also have been evidenced to inhibit the growth of pathogenic *Staphylococcus* spp., *Salmonella* spp., *Helicobacter pylori* and *Bacillus cereus* (100, 102). Phenolics and flavonoids may also reduce the adhesion ability of *L. rhamnosus* to intestinal epithelial cells (103–107). Tea catechins have also been shown to modify the mucin content of the ileum which could modulate bacterial adhesion and colonization (108–111). Therefore, polyphenols appear to have potential to confer health benefits via modulation of the gut microecology. However, the effects of the interplay between polyphenols and specific gut microbiota functions remain largely uncharacterized. Examples of phytochemicals and their sources and health benefits are shown in Table 17.4.

## 17.3.6 Micronutrients and Microbiome

Micronutrients include organic and inorganic elements and compounds, such as minerals and vitamins, which are crucial for the maintenance of host health and are not used for energy balance (113). Such micronutrients are generally found in foods and dietary supplements and are crucial for the regulation of biosynthetic cellular reactions, for example, those involved in immune and energy function, as well as in biological processes such as growth, bone health and fluid balance. Inadequate levels of micronutrients, resulting from reduced intake and/or poor absorption, are known to lead to specific micronutrient deficiency diseases, which represent a major global health concern

(114). Micronutrient deficiencies can also worsen infections and non-communicable chronic diseases, such as osteoporosis, hyperthyroidism, cardiovascular disease and cancer, with a potentially dramatic impact on quality of life, morbidity and mortality. For example, in children, vitamin D deficiency may contribute to unbalanced immune responses as adults, resulting in a higher incidence and progression of autoimmune diseases (115). Minerals, particularly zinc, play a critical role in B and T-cell-dependent immune activities (116). Moreover, multiple studies indicate that micronutrient deficiency may contribute to the progression of some human cancers (117). Micronutrients also modulate the abundance and diversity of the gut microbiota resulting in beneficial or detrimental outcomes for the host (118–119).

The micronutrient–microbiome axis is bidirectional. On the one hand, microbes in the gut are consumers of micronutrients for their growth and functioning. The host's nutrition and micronutrient supplementation largely impacts the gut microbiota composition and functions. In particular, supplementation of vitamin A (120), vitamin C (121), vitamin $B_{12}$ (122) and vitamin D (123) contribute to changes in the composition of the gut microbiota by promoting colonization of several bacterial species from the *Bifidobacterium*, *Lactobacillus* and *Roseburia* genera. Assessing the effect of mineral deficiency or supplementation on the gut microbiota is an emerging field (124), and it has been shown that iron (125), calcium (126), zinc (127) and magnesium (128) supplementation modulate the gut microbiota. Minerals and trace elements can alter the composition of the intestinal microbiota, gut barrier function, compartmentalized metabolic inflammation, and cellular glucose transport (129). Examples of some functional foods and drugs with identical targets available on the global market are shown in Table 17.5.

**Table 17.5** Some Functional Foods and Drugs with Identical Targets Available on Global Market (36)

| Food | Target | Drugs |
|------|--------|-------|
| Enriched with phytosterol-stanolesters | Low density lipoprotein cholesterol | Statins, Ezetimibe |
| Containing bioactive peptides | Blood pressure | Antihypertensive drugs (such as thiazide diuretics) |
| Containing melatonin | Quality of sleep | Benzodiazepines |
| Containing omega-3 fatty acids | Depression | Antidepressants |
| Containing glucan | Blood sugar values | Insulin |
| Containing prebiotics | Bowel frequency | Laxatives |
| Containing probiotics | Immune functioning Diarrhea (wet stools) | Loperamide |
| Containing extra calcium or vitamin D, or both | Bone health | Alendronate, calcitonin, Oestrogens |
| Containing protein or bioactive peptides | Obesity and type 2 diabetes | Orlistat, Rimonabant |

## 17.4 Conclusion

The gut immune system undergoes daily exposure to a plethora of antigens contained in the environment as well as in food. The gut microbiota exerts an enormous impact on the nutritional and health status of the host via modulation of the immune and metabolic functions. The microbiome provides additional enzymatic activities involved in the transformation of dietary compounds. It is evident that dietary modifiers, including the consumption of probiotics, prebiotics, dietary fibers, polyphenols and micronutrients have been demonstrated to influence gut health and the overall well-being of the host. Recent advancement in the field of gut microbiota are providing the new research platform to functional foods, nutraceuticals and probiotics development.

## References

1. Ballan R, Battistini C, Xavier-Santos D, Saad SMI. Interactions of probiotics and prebiotics with the gut microbiota. *PMBTS* 2022; 171: 265–300.
2. Bull MJ, Plummer NT. Part 1: The human gut microbiome in health and disease. *Integr Med (Encinitas)* 2014; 13(6): 17–22.
3. Rath CM, Dorrestein PC. The bacterial chemical repertoire mediates metabolic exchange within gut microbiomes. *Curr Opin Microbiol* 2012; 15(2): 147–154.
4. Thursby E, Juge N. Introduction to the human gut microbiota. Biochem J 2017; 474(11): 1823–1836.
5. Backhed F, Ley RE, Sonnenburg JL, Peterson DA, Gordon JI. Host-bacterial mutualism in the human intestine. *Science* 2005; 307(5717): 1915–1920.
6. Neish AS. Microbes in gastrointestinal health and disease. *Gastroenterology* 2009; 136(1): 65–80.
7. Gill SR, Pop M, DeBoy RT, et al. Metagenomic analysis of the human distal gut microbiome. *Science* 2006; 312(5778): 1355–1359.
8. Fan Y, Pedersen O. Gut microbiota in human metabolic health and disease. *Nat Rev Microbiol* 2021; 19(1): 55–71.
9. Ding RX, Goh WR, Wu RN, et al. Revisit gut microbiota and its impact on human health and disease. *J Food Drug Anal* 2019; 27(3): 623–631.
10. Natividad JMM, Verdu EF. Modulation of intestinal barrier by intestinal microbiota: Pathological and therapeutic implications. *Pharmacol Res* 2013; 69(1): 42–51.
11. Besten GD, van Eunen KV, Groen AK, Venema K, Reijngoud D-J, Bakker BM. The role of short-chain fatty acids in the interplay between diet, gut microbiota, and host energy metabolism. *J Lipid Res* 2013; 54(9): 2325–2340.
12. Bäumler AJ, Sperandio V. Interactions between the microbiota and pathogenic bacteria in the gut. *Nature* 2016; 535(7610): 85–93.
13. Gensollen T, Iyer SS, Kasper DL, Blumberg RS. How colonization by microbiota in early life shapes the immune system. *Science* 2016; 352(6285): 539–544.
14. Laparra JM, Sanz Y. Interactions of gut microbiota with functional food components and nutraceuticals. *Pharmacol Res* 2010; 2010(61): 219–225.
15. Nadal I, Donat E, Ribes-Koninckx C, Calabuig M, Sanz Y. Imbalance in the composition of the duodenal microbiota of children with coeliac disease. *J Med Microbiol* 2007; 56(12): 1669–1674.
16. Santacruz A, Marcos A, Wärnberg J, et al. Interplay between weight loss and gut microbiota composition in overweight adolescents. *Obesity (Silver Spring)* 2009; 17(10): 1906–1915.

17. Ley RE, Lozupone CA, Hamady M, Knight R, Gordon JI. Worlds within worlds: Evolution of the vertebrate gut microbiota. *Nat Rev Microbiol* 2008; 6(10): 776–788.
18. Gatt M, Reddy BS, MacFie J. Review article: Bacterial translocation in the critically ill - Evidence and methods of prevention. *Aliment Pharmacol Ther* 2007; 25(7): 741–757.
19. Sawicki CM, Livingston KA, Obin M, Roberts SB, Chung M, McKeown NM. Dietary fiber and the human gut microbiota: Application of evidence mapping methodology. *Nutrients* 2017; 9(2): 1–21.
20. Montalto M, D'Onofrio F, Gallo A, Cazzato A, Gasbarrini G. Intestinal microbiota and its functions. *Dig Liver Dis* 2009; 3(2): 30–34.
21. Roberfroid MB, Delzenne NM. Dietary fructans. *Annu Rev Nutr* 1998; 18: 117–143.
22. Gerritsen J, Smidt H, Rijkers GT, de Vos WM. Intestinal microbiota in human health and disease: The impact of probiotics. *Genes Nutr Genes* 2011; 6(3): 209–240.
23. Lozupone CA, Stombaugh JI, Gordon JI, Jansson JK, Knight R. Diversity, stability and resilience of the human gut microbiota. *Nature* 2012; 489(7415): 220–230.
24. Keeney KM, Yurist-Doutsch S, Arrieta M-C, Finlay BB. Effects of antibiotics on human microbiota and subsequent disease. *Annu Rev Microbiol* 2014; 68: 217–235.
25. Graf D, Cagno RD, Fak F, et al. Contribution of diet to the composition of the human gut microbiota. *Microb Ecol Health Dis* 2015; 26: 26164.
26. Turroni F, Milani C, Ventura M, Sinderen DV. The human gut microbiota during the initial stages of life: Insights from bifidobacterial. *Curr Opin Biotechnol* 2022; 73: 81–87.
27. Leeming ER, Johnson AJ, Spector DT. Roy CILe. Effect of diet on the gut microbiota: Rethinking intervention duration. *Nutrients* 2019; 11(2): 2862.
28. Xu J, Mahowald MA , Ley RE, et al. Evolution of symbiotic bacteria in the distal human intestine. *PLoS Biol* 2007; 19(7): e156.
29. Sanz Y, Sánchez E, De Palma G, Medina M, Marcos A, Nova E. Indigenous gut microbiota, probiotics, and coeliac disease. In: Overton Linda T, Ewente MR, editors. *Child Nutrition & Physiology*. New York: Nova Science Publishers, Inc.; 2008, pp. 210–224.
30. Conlon MA, Bird AR. The impact of diet and life style on gut microbiota and human health. *Nutrients* 2015; 7(1): 17–44.
31. Cencic A, Chingwaru W. The role of functional foods, nutraceuticals, and food supplements in intestinal health. *Nutrients* 2010; 2(6): 611–625.
32. Dahiya DK, Puniya M, Shandilya UK, et al. Gut microbiota modulation and its relationship with obesity using prebiotic fibers and probiotics: A review. *Front Microbiol* 2017; 8: 563.
33. Zhang Y-J, Li S, Gan R-Y, Zhou T, Xu D-P, Li H-B. Impact of gut bacteria on human health and disease. *Int J Mol Sci* 2015; 16(4): 7493–7519.
34. Biedermann L, Rogler G. The intestinal microbiota: Its role in health and disease. *Eur J Pediatr* 2015; 174(2): 151–167.
35. Balmer JM, Longman RS, Iliev ID, Sonnenberg GF, Artis D. Regulation of inflammation by microbiota interaction with the host. *Nat Immunol* 2017; 18(8): 851–860.
36. El Sohaimy SA. Functional foods and nutraceuticals-modern approach to food science. *World Appl Sci J* 2012; 20(5): 691–708.
37. Aronson JK. Defining 'nutraceuticals': Neither nutritious nor pharmaceutical. *Br J Clin Pharmacol* 2017; 83(1): 8–19.
38. Hasler, CM. Functional foods: Their role in disease prevention and health promotion. *Food Technol* 1998; 52: 63–70.
39. Health Canada. Nutraceuticals/functional foods and health claims on foods; 2002. https://www.canada.ca/en/health-canada/services/food-nutrition/food-labelling/health-claims/nutraceuticals-functional-foods-health-claims-foods-policy-paper.html.
40. Maddi VS, Aragade PD, Digge VG, Nitaliker MN. Importance of nutraceuticals in health management. *Phcog Rev* 2007; 1: 377–379.

41. Brower V. Nutraceuticals: Poised for a healthy slice of the healthcare market? *Nat Biotechnol* 1998; 16(8): 728–731.
42. Wildman REC, editor. *Handbook of Nutraceuticals and Functional Foods*. Boca Raton: CRC Press; 2001, pp. 13–30.
43. Bull E. What is nutraceutical? *Pharm J* 2000; 265: 57–58.
44. Dureja H, Kaushik D, Kumar V. Developments in nutraceuticals. *Indian J Pharmacol* 2003; 35: 363–372.
45. Pandey M, Verma RK, Saraf SA. Nutraceuticals: New era of medicine and health. *Asian J Pharm Clin Res* 2010; 3: 11–15.
46. Alisi A, Bedogni G, Baviera G, et al. Randomised clinical trial: The beneficial effects of VSL#3 in obese children with non-alcoholic steatohepatitis. *Aliment Pharmacol Ther* 2014; 39(11): 1276–1285.
47. Riva A, Togni S, Giacomelli L, et al. Effects of a curcumin-based supplementation in asymptomatic subjects with low bone density: A preliminary 24-week supplement study. *Eur Rev Med Pharmacol Sci* 2017; 21(7): 1684–1689.
48. Adrian Catinean A, Neag MA, Muntean DM, Bocsan JC, Buzoianu AD. An overview on the interplay between nutraceuticals and gut microbiota. *Peer J* 2018; 6: e4465.
49. Di Cerbo A, Morales-Medina JC, Palmieri B, et al. Functional foods in pet nutrition: Focus on dogs and cats. *Res Veter Sci* 2017; 112: 161–166.
50. Food and Agriculture Organization. *World Health Organization (FAO) Probiotics in Food: Health and Nutritional Properties and Guidelines for Evaluation*. FAO; Rome, Italy: 2006. This definition was adopted by the International Scientific Association for Probiotics and Prebiotics (ISAPP) in 2013.
51. Feord J. Lactic acid bacteria in a changing legislative environment. *Antonie Leeuwenhoek* 2012; 82(1–4): 353–360.
52. Bermudez-Brito M, Plaza-Diaz J, Munoz-Quezada S, Gomez-Llorente C, Gil A. Probiotic mechanisms of action. *Ann Nutr Metab* 2012; 61(2): 160–174.
53. Glenn G, Roberfroid M. Dietary modulation of the human colonic microbiota: Introducing the concept of prebiotics. *J Nutr* 1995; 125(6): 1401–1412.
54. Bode L. Human milk oligosaccharides: Every baby needs a sugar mama. *Glycobiology* 2012; 22(9): 1147–1156.
55. Chichlowski M, De Lartigue G, German JB, Raybould HE, Mills DA. Bifidobacteria isolated from infants and cultured on human milk oligosaccharides affect intestinal epithelial function. *J Pediatr Gastroenterol Nutrr* 2012; 55(3): 321–327.
56. Newburg DS, Walker WA. Protection of the neonate by the innate immune system of developing gut and of human milk. *Pediatr Res* 2007; 61(1): 2–8.
57. White BA, Lamed R, Bayer EA, Flint HJ. Biomass utilization by gut microbiomes. *Annu Rev Microbiol* 2014; 68: 279–296.
58. Lewis S, Burmeister S, Brazier J. Effect of the Prebiotic oligofructose on relapse of Clostridium difficile-associated diarrhea: A randomized, controlled study. *Clin Gastroenterol Hepatol* 2005; 3(5): 442–448.
59. Moro G, Arslanoglu S, Stahl B, Jelinek J, Wahn U, Boehm GA. A Mixture of prebiotic oligosaccharides reduces the incidence of atopic dermatitis during the first six months of age. *Arch Dis Child* 2006; 91(10): 814–819.
60. Paineau D, Payen F, Panserieu S, et al. The effects of regular consumption of short-chain fructo-oligosaccharides on digestive comfort of subjects with minor functional bowel disorders. *Br J Nutr* 2008; 99(2): 311–318.
61. Costabile A, Kolida S, Klinder A, et al. A double-blind, placebo-controlled, cross-over study to establish the bifidogenic effect of a very-long-chain inulin extracted from globe artichoke (Cynara Scolymus) in healthy human subjects. *Br J Nutr* 2010; 104(7): 1007–1017.
62. Dewulf EM, Cani PD, Claus SP, et al. Insight into the prebiotic concept: Lessons from an exploratory, double blind intervention study with inulin-type fructans in obese women. *Gut* 2013; 62(8): 1112–1121.

63. Fernandes R, do Rosario VA, Mocellin MC, Kuntz MGF, Trindade EBSM. Effects of inulin-type fructans, galacto-oligosaccharides and related Synbiotics on inflammatory markers in adult patients with overweight or obesity: A systematic review. *Clin Nutr* 2017; 36(5): 1197–1206.

64. Klinder A, Forster A, Caderni G, Femia AP, Pool-Zobel BL. Fecal water genotoxicity is predictive of tumor-preventive activities by inulin-like oligofructoses, probiotics (Lactobacillus rhamnosus and Bifidobacterium lactis), and their synbiotic combination. *Nutr Cancer* 2004; 49(2): 144–155.

65. Propst EL, Flickinger EA, Bauer LL, Merchen NR, Fahey GC Jr. A dose-response experiment evaluating the effects of oligofructose and inulin on nutrient digestibility, stool quality, and fecal protein catabolites in healthy adult dogs. *J Anim Sci* 2003; 81(12): 3057–3066.

66. Quintero M, Maldonado M, Perez-Munoz M, et al. Adherence inhibition of Cronobacter sakazakii to intestinal epithelial cells by prebiotic oligosaccharides. *Curr Microbiol* 2011; 62(5): 1448–1454.

67. Sierra C, Bernal M-J, Blasco J, et al. Prebiotic effect during the first year of life in healthy infants fed formula containing GOS as the only prebiotic: A multicentre, randomised, double-blind and placebo-controlled trial. *Eur J Nutr* 2015; 54(1): 89–99.

68. Ferenczi S, Szegi K, Winkler Z, Barna T, Kovács KJ. Oligomannan prebiotic attenuates immunological, clinical and behavioral symptoms in mouse model of inflammatory bowel disease. *Sci Rep* 2016; 6: 34132.

69. Ofek I, Beachey EH. Mannose binding and epithelial cell adherence of Escherichia coli. *Infect Immun* 1978; 22(1): 247–254.

70. Hansen CHF, Frøkiær H, Christensen AG, et al. Dietary xylooligosaccharide downregulates IFN-γ and the low-grade inflammatory cytokine IL-1β systemically in mice. *J Nutr* 2013; 143(4): 533–540.

71. Hsu C-K, Liao J-W, Chung Y-C, Hsieh C-P, Chan Y-C. Xylooligosaccharides and fructooligosaccharides affect the intestinal microbiota and precancerous colonic lesion development in rats. *J Nutr* 2004; 134(6): 1523–1528.

72. Rastall RA, Gibson GR. Recent developments in prebiotics to selectively impact beneficial microbes and promote intestinal health. *Curr Opin Biotechnol* 2015; 32: 42–46.

73. Slavin JL. Dietary fiber and body weight. *Nutrition* 2005; 21(3): 411–418.

74. Deehan EC, Duar RM, Armet AM, Perez-Munoz ME, Jin M, Walter J. Modulation of the gastrointestinal microbiome with nondigestible fermentable carbohydrates to improve human health. *Microbiol Spectr* 2017; 5(5): 1–24.

75. El Kaoutari A, Armougom F, Gordon JI, Raoult D, Henrissat B. The abundance and variety of carbohydrate-active enzymes in the human gut microbiota. *Nat Rev Microbiol* 2013; 11(7): 497–504.

76. Holscher HD. Dietary fiber and prebiotics and the gastrointestinal microbiota. *Gut Microbes* 2017; 8(2): 172–184.

77. Anderson JW, Baird P, Davis RH Jr, et al. Health benefits of dietary fiber. *Nutr Rev* 2009; 67(4): 188–205.

78. Wilson ID, Nicholson JK. The role of gut microbiota in drug response. *Curr Pharm Des* 2009; 15(13): 1519–1523.

79. Deehan EC, Duar RM, Armet AM, Perez-Munoz ME, Jin M, Walter J. Modulation of the gastrointestinal microbiome with nondigestible fermentable carbohydrates to improve human health. *Microbiol Spectr* 2017; 5(5): 1–24.

80. Dimidi E, Christodoulides K, Scott M, Whelan K. 2014. The effect of probiotics on functional constipation in adults: A systematic review and meta-analysis of randomized controlled trials. *Am J Clin Nutr* 2014 ; 100(4): 1075–1084.

81. Carlson JL, Erickson JM, Hess JM, Gould TJ, Slavin JL. Prebiotic dietary fber and gut health: Comparing the in vitro fermentations of beta-glucan, inulin and xylooligosaccharide. *Nutrients* 2017; 9(12): 1361.

82. Carlson JL, Erickson JM, Lloyd BB, Slavin JL. Health effects and sources of prebiotic dietary fber. *Curr Dev Nutr* 2018; 2(3): nyz005.
83. Watson H, Mitra S, Croden FC, et al. A randomized trial of the effect of omega-3 polyunsaturated fatty acid supplements on the human intestinal microbiota. *Gut* 2018; 67(11): 1974–1983.
84. Noriega BS, Sanchez-Gonzalez MA, Salyakina D, Coffman J. Understanding the impact of omega-3 rich diet on the gut microbiota. *Case Rep Med* 2016; 2016: 3089303.
85. Menni C, Zierer J, Pallister T, et al. Omega-3 fatty acids correlate with gut microbiome diversity and production of N-carbamylglutamate in middle aged and elderly women. *Sci Rep* 2017; 7(1): 11079.
86. Liu RH. Potential synergy of phytochemicals in cancer prevention: Mechanism of action. *J Nutr* 2004; 134(12): 3479S–3485S.
87. Hertog MG, Feskens EJ, Hollman PC, Katan MB, Kromhout D. Dietary antioxidant flavonoids and risk of coronary heart disease: The Zutphen Elderly Study. *Lancet* 1993; 342(8878): 1007–1011.
88. Yuan J, Wang J, Liu X. Metabolism of dietary soy isoflavones to equol by human intestinal microflora;implications for health. *Mol Nutr Food Res* 2007; 51(7): 765–781.
89. Park JS, Woo MS, Kim DH, et al. Anti-inflammatory mechanisms of isoflavone metabolites in lipopolysaccharide stimulated microglial cells. *J Pharmacol Exp Ther* 2007; 320(3): 1237–1245.
90. Ruiz PA, Haller D. Functional diversity of flavonoids in the inhibition of the pro inflammatory NF-kappaB, IRF, and AKT signaling pathways in murine intestinal epithelial cells. *J Nutr* 2006; 136(3): 664–671.
91. Ruiz PA, Braune A, Hölzwimmer G, Quintanilla-Fend L, Haller D. Quercetin inhibits TNF-induced NF-kappaB transcription factor recruitment to proinflammatory gene promoters in murine intestinal epithelial cells. *J Nutr* 2007; 137(5): 1208–1215.
92. Ramiro-Puig E, Pérez-Cano FJ, Ramos-Romero S, et al. Intestinal immune system of young rats influenced by cocoa-enriched diet. *J Nutr Biochem* 2008; 19(8): 555–565.
93. Zunino SJ, Storms DH. Resveratrol alters proliferative responses and apoptosis in human activated B lymphocytes in vitro. *J Nutr* 2009; 139(8): 1603–1608.
94. Ganry O. Phytoestrogen and breast cancer prevention. *Eur J Cancer Prev* 2002; 11(6): 519–522.
95. Aura AM. Microbial metabolism of dietary phenolic compounds in the colon. *Phytochem Rev* 2008; 7(3): 407–429.
96. Gee JM, Johnson IT. Polyphenolic compounds: Interactions with the gut and implications for human health. *Curr Med Chem* 2001; 8(11): 1245–1255.
97. Scalbert A, Morand C, Manach C, Remesy C. Absorption and metabolism of polyphenols in the gut and impact on health. *Biomed Pharmacother* 2002; 56(6): 276–282.
98. Bowey E, Adlercreutz H, Rowland I. Metabolism of isoflavones and lignans by the gut microflora: A study in germ-free and human associated rats. *Food Chem Toxicol* 2003; 41(5): 631–636.
99. Larrosa M, Luceri C, Vivoli E, et al. Polyphenol metabolites from colonic microbiota exert anti-inflammatory activity on different inflammation models. *Mol Nutr Food Res* 2009; 53(8): 1044–1054.
100. Comalada M, Camuesco D, Sierra S, et al. In vivo quercitrin anti-inflammatory effect involves release of quercetin, which inhibits inflammation through down-regulation of the NF-kappaB pathway. *Eur J Immunol* 2005; 35(2): 584–592.
101. Cerda B, Espín JC, Parra S, Martínez P, Tomás-Barberán FA. The potente in vitro antioxidant ellagitannins from pomegranate juice are metabolised into bioavailable but poor antioxidant hydroxy-6H-dibenzopyran-6-one derivatives by the colonic microflora of healthy humans. *Eur J Nutr* 2004; 43(4): 205–220.
102. Bazzocco S, Mattila I, Guyot S, Renard CM, Aura AM. Factors affecting the conversion of apple polyphenols to phenolic acids and fruit matrix to short-chain fatty acids by human faecal microbiota in vitro. *Eur J Nutr* 2008; 47(8): 442–452.

103. Tzonuis X, Vulevic J, Kuhnle GG, et al. Flavanol monomer-induced changes to the human faecal microflora. *Br J Nutr* 2008; 99(4): 782–792.
104. Lee HC, Jenner AM, Low CS, Lee YK. Effect of tea phenolics and their aromatic fecal bacterial metabolites on intestinal microbiota. *Res Microbiol* 2006; 157(9): 876–884.
105. Larrosa M, Yañéz-Gascón MJ, Selma MV, et al. Effect of a low dose of dietary resveratrol on colon microbiota, inflammation and tissue damage in a DSS induced colitis rat model. *J Agric Food Chem* 2009; 57(6): 2211–2220.
106. Medina E, Garcia A, Romero C, de Castro A, Brenes M. Study of the anti-lactic acid bacteria compounds in table olives. *Int J Food Sci Technol* 2009; 7(7): 1286–1291.
107. Puupponen-Pimia R, Nohynek L, Hartmann-Schmidlin S, et al. Berry phenolics selectively inhibit the growth of intestinal pathogens. *J Appl Microbiol* 2005; 98(4): 991–1000.
108. Nohynek LJ, Alakomi HL, Kahkonen MP, et al. Berry phenolics: Antimicrobial properties and mechanisms of action against severe human pathogens. *Nutr Cancer* 2006; 54(1): 18–32.
109. Wang WB, Lai HC, Hsueh PR, Chiou RYY, Lin SB, Liaw SJ. Inhibition of swarming and virulence factor expression in Proteus mirabilis by resveratrol. *J Med Microbiol* 2006; 55(10): 1313–1321.
110. Parkar SG, Stevenson DE, Skinner MA. The potential influence of fruit polyphenols on colonic microflora and human gut health. *Int J Food Microbiol* 2008; 124(3): 295–298.
111. Ito Y, Ichikawa T, Iwai T, et al. Effects of tea catechins on the gastrointestinal mucosa in rats. *J Agric Food Chem* 2008; 56(24): 12122–12126.
112. Yoshii K, Hosomi K, Sawane K, Kunisawa J. Metabolism of dietary and microbial vitamin B family in the regulation of host immunity. *Front Nutr* 2019; 6: 48.
113. Huskisson E, Maggini S, Ruf M. The role of vitamins and minerals in energy metabolism and well-being. *J Int Med Res* 2007; 35(3): 277–289.
114. Correale J, Ysrraelit MC, Gaitn MI. Immunomodulatory effects of vitamin D in multiple sclerosis. *Brain* 2009; 132(5): 1146–1160.
115. Prietl B, Treiber G, Pieber TR, Amrein K. Vitamin D and immune function. *Nutrients* 2013; 5(7): 2502–2521.
116. Hojyo S, Fukada T. Roles of zinc signaling in the immune system. *J Immunol Res* 2016; 2016: 1–21.
117. Johnson IT. Micronutrients and cancer. *Proc Nutr Soc* 2004; 63(4): 587–595.
118. Biesalski HK. Nutrition meets the microbiome: Micronutrients and the microbiota. *Ann N Y Acad Sci* 2016; 1372(1): 53–64.
119. Yang Q, Liang Q, Balakrishnan B, Belobrajdic DP, Feng QJ, Zhang W. Role of dietary nutrients in the modulation of gut microbiota: A narrative review. *Nutrients* 2020; 12(2): 381.
120. Lv Z, Wang Y, Yang T, et al. Vitamin A deficiency impacts the structural segregation of gut microbiota in children with persistent diarrhea. *J Clin Biochem Nutr* 2016; 59(2): 113–121.
121. Li L, Krause L, Somerset S. Associations between micronutrient intakes and gut microbiota in a group of adults with cystic fibrosis. *Clin Nutr* 2017; 36(4): 1097–1104.
122. Degnan PH, Barry NA, Mok KC, Taga ME, Goodman AL. Human gut microbes use multiple transporters to distinguish vitamin B 12 analogs and compete in the gut. *Cell Host Microbe* 2014; 15(1): 47–57.
123. Kanhere M, He J, Chassaing B, et al. Bolus weekly vitamin D3 supplementation impacts gut and airway microbiota in adults with cystic fibrosis: A double-blind, randomized, placebo-controlled clinical trial. *J Clin Endocrinol Metab* 2018; 103(2): 564–574.
124. Skrypnik K, Suliburska J. Association between the gut microbiota and mineral metabolism. *J Sci Food Agric* 2018; 98(7): 2449–2460.

125. Rusu IG, Suharoschi R, Vodnar DC, et al. Iron supplementation influence on the gut microbiota and probiotic intake effect in iron deficiency—A literature-based review. *Nutrients* 2020; 12(7): 1993.
126. Chaplin A, Parra P, Laraichi S, Serra F, Palou A. Calcium supplementation modulates gut microbiota in a prebiotic manner in dietary obese mice. *Mol Nutr Food Res* 2016; 60(2): 468–480.
127. Zackular JP, Moore JL, Ashley T, et al. Dietary zinc alters the microbiota and decreases resistance to Clostridium difficile infection. *Nat Med* 2016; 22(11): 1330–1334.
128. Winther G, Pyndt Jørgensen BM, Elfving B, et al. Dietary magnesium deficiency alters gut microbiota and leads to depressive-like behaviour. *Acta Neuropsychiatr* 2015; 27(3): 168–176.
129. Barra NG, Anhê FF, Cavallari JF, Singh AM, Chan DY, Schertzer JD. Micronutrients impact the gut microbiota and blood glucose. *J Endocrinol* 2021; 250(2): R1–R21.

# 18

# Synbiotics
## Traditional Approach, Present Status, and Future Outlook

Abdullah Abdelkawi, Jean-Pierre Perez Martinez,
Sarvadaman Pathak, and Yashwant Pathak

## Contents

## 18.1 Historical Background of Synbiotics

The history of synbiotics, or the combination of prebiotics and probiotics, dates back to Ancient Greece. Hippocrates, the "Father of Modern Medicine," made mention of probiotics, sometimes known as "life-enhancing" microbes, in his works. Hippocrates wrote that certain "earthy" substances benefited in the treatment of diseases. Later, in 1894, a Russian scientist named Elie Metchnikoff proposed the notion of Cellular Immunity, in which "friendly" microbes served as a biological defense against pathogenic germs and infectious disease. In addition, the word "probiotic" was coined in 1965 by Lilly and Stillwell. Gibbs et al. established the term prebiotic, which refers to chemicals that encourage the growth of beneficial microbes, in 1995. Together, probiotics and prebiotics create synbiotics, and their potential health advantages are now well acknowledged.

DOI: 10.1201/9781003333821-18

Since the early 2000s, synbiotic products have existed; however, their popularity has recently increased as more research demonstrates the favorable benefits these products have on the integrity of the gut microbiota (Escalante-Mendoza et al., 2017). Synbiotics consist of probiotics, which are helpful bacteria, and prebiotics, which are nondigestible food elements that stimulate the growth and function of probiotics (Mandal, 2020). Synbiotics promote gut health by facilitating digestion and nutrient absorption by balancing the gastrointestinal tract's bacterial population (Collado et al., 2017). Extensive study is being conducted to determine the possible benefits of synbiotics, such as the prevention of obesity and the treatment of ulcerative colitis (Rastegar et al., 2015), although the findings are unclear.

The history of synbiotics is fraught with controversy and medical research. Synbiotics are the combination of probiotics and prebiotics, both of which are nonliving, beneficial microbiome components (Ulluwishewa et al., 2015). The first reports of synbiotic use date back to the early 1990s and primarily include animal research (Milyn & Gombart, 2017). Several clinical trials were conducted in the late 1990s to explore the efficacy of synbiotics in preventing and/or treating infectious pediatric diarrhea, antibiotic-associated diarrhea, and hepatic encephalopathy (He et al., 1997). Since then, the use of synbiotics in the treatment of numerous additional ailments, ranging from periodontal diseases (Vaiman et al., 2018) to gastrointestinal disorders, has been examined (He et al., 2006). In spite of their potential, not all research outcomes have been positive, sparking much debate and controversy about the use of synbiotics (Stahl et al., 2020).

Beginning in the 1920s with the pioneering work of Elie Metchnikoff, synbiotic products have been created over a lengthy and complex period of time. From the studies of Japanese gastroenterologist Kikunae Ikeda and the release of the first synbiotic products in the 1990s, innovation in this field has exploded. Through continued research and the development of new technologies, the popularity of synbiotics has increased, and their huge potential for use in the sectors of medicine and nutrition is being continually investigated.

The traditional approach to synbiotics, which is a combination of probiotics and prebiotics, has emphasized the utilization of naturally occurring microbes as probiotics and naturally occurring substances, such as fibers and sugars, as prebiotics. Prebiotics are nondigestible substances that increase the growth and activity of probiotics. Due to their potential to deliver health advantages through a synergistic impact, the combination of probiotics and prebiotics, known as synbiotics, is of great interest.

Historically, the traditional approach to synbiotics has relied on the utilization of probiotics found in fermented foods such as yogurt and kefir, such as lactic acid bacteria and bifidobacteria. These probiotics have been found to improve gut health and lower the occurrence of gastrointestinal problems, and their potential to boost immune function and prevent some chronic diseases has also been investigated.

Similarly, the conventional approach to prebiotics has centered on the utilization of naturally occurring substances, such as fibers and sugars, that are resistant to digestion and can encourage the growth and activity of beneficial microbes in the gut. Prebiotics include inulin, fructooligosaccharides, and galactooligosaccharides, which are present in foods such as vegetables, cereals, and legumes. These prebiotics have been found to promote gut health and their potential to boost immune function and prevent certain chronic diseases has been investigated.

In addition to using whole foods and fermented foods as sources of probiotics and prebiotics, the traditional approach to synbiotics has also incorporated the use of fermented foods. For instance, fermented foods such as yogurt, kefir, sauerkraut, and kimchi are rich sources of both probiotics and prebiotics and have historically been utilized for their potential health advantages. Similarly, healthy foods such as vegetables, grains, and legumes are abundant in prebiotics and have been utilized historically for their potential health advantages. In general, the traditional approach to synbiotics has emphasized the utilization of naturally occurring probiotics and prebiotics, as well as the consumption of whole meals and fermented foods.

## 18.2 Design for Rational Formulation

In the creation of synbiotics, which are described as a combination of probiotics and prebiotics that function synergistically to deliver health advantages, formulation and design are crucial factors. Selecting the appropriate probiotic strains is a crucial part of rational formulation and design in synbiotics. The exact probiotic strains included in a synbiotic composition can have a substantial effect on its efficacy and possible health benefits. It is essential to choose strains that have been well researched and proven safe and effective, as well as to evaluate the interactions between different strains and the microbiome's overall balance. Additionally, the ideal dosage and length of treatment with a specific probiotic strain should be carefully studied, as different strains may have different optimal dosages and treatment durations.

In rational formulation and design of synbiotics, the selection of the proper prebiotic ingredient is also crucial. Prebiotics are nondigestible substances that increase the growth and activity of helpful intestinal microbes. In addition, the particular prebiotic utilized in a synbiotic composition can affect its efficacy and possible health advantages. Different prebiotics have distinct methods of action and can have varying impacts on the gut flora, highlighting the significance of selecting a prebiotic that is suitable for the desired health benefit and target population. In addition, the ideal dosage and length of treatment with a particular prebiotic should be carefully evaluated, as different prebiotics may have varying optimal dosages and durations of treatment.

The total formulation of a synbiotic product, including the combination of probiotics and prebiotics, the delivery technology, and any other components, can potentially have a substantial impact on its efficacy and possible health benefits. It is essential to carefully evaluate the interactions between the formulation's various components and to improve the product's overall balance and synergy.

In general, formulation and design are essential factors in the development of synbiotics. The selection of suitable probiotic strains, prebiotic ingredients, and formulation as a whole can have a substantial effect on the efficacy and possible health benefits of a synbiotic product. To completely comprehend the mechanisms underlying the potential health advantages of synbiotics and to optimize their usage in the treatment and prevention of various illnesses, additional research is required.

## 18.3 Uses for Synbiotics

Dietary supplements that mix probiotics, which are living microorganisms, and prebiotics, which are indigestible fibers, to generate a synergistic impact on the body are called synbiotics. By altering the human microbiome, synbiotics can give symptomatic alleviation for a range of medical diseases, including eczema, allergies, and irritable bowel syndrome (Arboleya et al., 2017). In addition to facilitating digestion, research indicates that synbiotics can improve the structure and function of the intestinal wall, increase the body's immunological systems, and reduce inflammation more effectively than probiotics and prebiotics taken separately. Therefore, synbiotics may be a useful addition to conventional medical therapies, as they can lessen symptoms and improve overall gut health.

Synbiotics offer a conventional approach to medical treatments, yet their current standing and forecast for the future are extremely optimistic. Synbiotics are dietary supplements that contain both prebiotics and probiotics. Prebiotics nourish the microbes already present in the gut, while probiotics introduce helpful bacteria. A 2018 study from the University of Copenhagen revealed that ingesting a synbiotic supplement containing both pre- and probiotics improved intestinal health (Ford et al., 2018). This optimistic view has expanded the popularity of recommended synbiotic products in clinical settings, allowing users the opportunity to reap the benefits of this traditional dietary supplement with modern scientific backing. Furthermore, as research on the effects of synbiotics has just recently begun, their future potential is supported by the ongoing development of pre- and probiotics research. As the field of synbiotics continues to expand and improve the conventional approach to medical care, the future could bring individuals even more precise tailored treatments.

Combining probiotics and prebiotics, synbiotics are widely utilized in medical care. Probiotics are live bacteria that improve health, whereas prebiotics are fibers that adjust the environment in the intestines to foster the growth of beneficial bacteria. In recent years, there has been increased interest in the use of synbiotics as a supplement to medical care, as the prospective advantages are quite promising. Beneficial effects include enhanced digestion and control of critical metabolic processes. These enhancements may also reduce the symptoms of some diseases, such as diarrhea and irritable bowel syndrome (IBS) (Camillieri, 2018). In addition, synbiotics have been demonstrated to benefit metabolic health, disease risk factors, and immunological health in general. Synbiotics are gaining popularity as a method for enhancing health and well-being in the medical industry, and their applications are still being investigated.

Recent probiotic and prebiotic scientific themes have centered on the possible health benefits of these therapies, as well as the processes behind these potential health benefits. Probiotics and prebiotics have been shown to improve gut health and reduce the prevalence of gastrointestinal illnesses by a growing body of research. Emerging research also suggests that probiotics and prebiotics may play a role in the prevention and treatment of other ailments, including allergies, autoimmune diseases, and metabolic disorders.

In the realm of probiotic and prebiotic science, the development of personalized or precision medicine is projected to have a significant impact. The precise combination and strains of probiotics and prebiotics might vary based on the needs and objectives of the individual. Technological advancements, such as the application of artificial intelligence and machine learning, may enable the optimization and customization of synbiotic formulations depending on an individual's microbiome.

The use of probiotics and prebiotics in the prevention and treatment of mental health disorders is another projected area of importance. The gut microbiota may play a role in mental health, and probiotics and prebiotics may have a function in treating illnesses such as depression, anxiety, and stress.

## 18.4 Focus on Mental Health Uses

Growing data suggests that synbiotics, which are a combination of probiotics and prebiotics, may have a potential function in the treatment of mental health issues. Mood, stress, and anxiety have been connected to the gut microbiome, and it is believed that synbiotics may be able to modify the gut microbiota in a way that improves mental health.

Multiple studies have proved the efficacy of synbiotics in treating mental health disorders. A randomized controlled experiment demonstrated that a synbiotic including the probiotic strains *Lactobacillus helveticus* and *Bifidobacterium longum,* as well as the prebiotic fructooligosaccharide, reduced the severity of depression and anxiety in a group of individuals with major depressive disorder. A second study discovered that a synbiotic combining the probiotic strain *Bifidobacterium infantis* and the prebiotic galactooligosaccharide was helpful in lowering the severity of stress and enhancing the mental health of a group of healthy people.

Probiotics and prebiotics are thought to produce short-chain fatty acids and other bioactive substances which may contribute to the possible mental health advantages of synbiotics.

It has been discovered that the gut microbiota, the microorganisms that inhabit the human gut, are closely linked to the brain and have been dubbed the "second brain." This relationship is known as the gut–brain axis and is comprised of a complex interplay between the gut bacteria, the immune system, and the central nervous system.

Through their effect on the microbiota in the stomach, synbiotics may promote mental wellness. The gut microbiota play an essential role in the manufacture and metabolism of numerous neurotransmitters, including serotonin, dopamine, and GABA (gamma-aminobutyric acid), which are essential for mood regulation and cognitive function. Dysbiosis, or an imbalance in the gut microbiota, has been related to anxiety and depression, among other mental health conditions. In certain trials, probiotics were found to restore the balance of the gut microbiota and reduce anxiety and depression symptoms.

Immunomodulatory effects are another proposed way through which synbiotics may benefit mental health. The gut microbiota are essential for immune function, and the immune system has been linked to the development of mental health issues. It has been demonstrated that probiotics affect the immune system and reduce inflammation, which may be advantageous for mental health. Additionally, it has been demonstrated that prebiotics encourage the growth of beneficial bacteria and enhance immunological function.

Although the research supporting the use of synbiotics for mental health is nascent, the prospective advantages are encouraging. In general, the use of synbiotics as a complementary or supplementary treatment for mental health issues merits additional research. Although evidence is still accumulating, the potential mental health advantages of synbiotics are encouraging, and their use demands more exploration.

Overall, the possibility of synbiotics to treat mental health issues is a promising new area of study. While additional research is necessary to completely comprehend the processes underlying the possible mental health advantages of synbiotics and optimize their use, the available evidence shows that synbiotics may be a promising treatment for mental health disorders.

## 18.5 Focus on Precision Medicine Uses

Personalized medicine, often known as precision medicine, is an emerging approach to healthcare that employs interventions tailored to an individual's unique traits, such as genetics, environment, and lifestyle. It entails the use of genetic, genomic, and other biological information to predict the chance of a patient getting a certain disease or condition and to personalize their therapy.

Due to probiotics and prebiotics' ability to influence the gut microbiota, which is unique to each individual, synbiotics have the potential to be employed as personalized therapy.

Several studies have demonstrated that synbiotics may be applied as a type of individualized therapy. Adults are affected by irritable bowel syndrome (IBS), a digestive condition. In one study, it was determined that a synbiotic supplement including the probiotic strains *Lactobacillus plantarum* and *Bifidobacterium longum* as well as the prebiotic inulin was successful in reducing the intensity of gastrointestinal symptoms and enhancing the quality of life in individuals with IBS. Separate research has shown that a synbiotic supplement containing the probiotic strain *Bifidobacterium infantis* and the prebiotic galactooligosaccharide improved metabolic health markers in a sample of obese individuals.

Growing data indicates that synbiotics may play a role in precision medicine due to their influence on the gut flora. The gut microbiota are extremely individualized and vary considerably across individuals. In certain trials, probiotics have been proven to modify the gut flora and alleviate symptoms. According to one study, providing a specific strain of *Lactobacillus* to obese persons reduced their body weight and waist circumference. The administration of a synbiotic to persons with irritable bowel syndrome significantly improved their symptoms, according to another study.

In addition to their effect on the gut microbiota, synbiotics may have direct effects on a number of diseases and ailments. Probiotics, for instance, have been found to have anti-inflammatory effects and have been utilized as an adjuvant treatment for a variety of inflammatory disorders, including rheumatoid arthritis and inflammatory bowel disease. Prebiotics have also been found to have anti-inflammatory properties and have been utilized as a therapeutic adjunct for a variety of inflammatory disorders.

In addition to the possibility of customizing synbiotic formulations to an individual's unique needs and objectives, technological advancements, such as the use of artificial intelligence and machine learning, may enable the optimization and customization of synbiotic formulations based on an individual's unique microbiome. This could pave the way for the development of synbiotics as individualized, patient-specific therapy.

Overall, the potential for synbiotics to be used as customized medicine is exciting; however, additional study is required to fully comprehend the mechanisms underlying their potential health advantages and to optimize their usage in the prevention and treatment of a variety of illnesses.

## 18.6 Market

The market for synbiotics, which are a combination of probiotics and prebiotics, is anticipated to undergo significant growth in the future years as consumer awareness of the possible health advantages of these therapies increases. Prebiotics are nondigestible substances that increase the growth and activity of probiotics. Due to their potential to deliver health advantages through a synergistic impact, the combination of probiotics and prebiotics, known as synbiotics, is of great interest.

According to market research firm Zion Market Research, the global market for synbiotics was valued at around $18.6 billion in 2020 and is projected to reach $41.3 billion by 2026, expanding at a CAGR (compound annual growth rate) of 13.6%. This expansion is anticipated to be driven by a rise in consumer demand for functional food and beverage items containing synbiotics, as well as a rise in the usage of synbiotics in animal feed.

In addition to the anticipated development in the usage of synbiotics in functional food and beverage products, the demand for synbiotics as dietary supplements is also likely to increase. The potential of synbiotics to enhance a range of ailments, including gut health, allergies, immunological function, and metabolic health, is being investigated, and consumers may increasingly turn to synbiotics to improve their overall health and well-being.

In the coming years, the demand for functional foods, beverages, and dietary supplements containing synbiotics is anticipated to increase significantly. To completely comprehend the mechanisms underlying the potential health advantages of synbiotics and to optimize their usage in the prevention and treatment of various illnesses, additional research is required.

## 18.7 Machine Learning and Nanotechnology

Artificial intelligence (AI) and machine learning have recently been introduced into the field of synbiotics, a mix of probiotics and prebiotics, and have the potential to revolutionize the development and application of these therapies.

Artificial intelligence and machine learning algorithms can scan vast volumes of data, including data on an individual's unique microbiome, to detect trends and forecast results. This technique has the potential to facilitate the creation of personalized or precision medicine synbiotics that are tailored to the individual's unique demands and objectives. An AI algorithm may, for instance, examine data on an individual's unique microbiome and find the probiotic strains and prebiotic substances that are most likely to improve their health results. This method could also be utilized to optimize the composition of synbiotics as a whole, including the combination of probiotics and prebiotics, the delivery system, and any other ingredients.

Nanotechnology is a recent innovation in the field of synbiotics that has the potential to influence the distribution and stability of probiotics and prebiotics. Nanoparticles, or particles with nanoscale dimensions, have the potential to enhance the stability and distribution of probiotics and prebiotics, as well as their bioavailability and efficacy. For instance, research has revealed that nanoparticles have the potential to boost the stability and distribution of probiotics in food and beverage items, as well as the bioavailability and efficacy of prebiotics in the gut.

Utilizing nanoparticles to increase the stability and delivery of probiotics in food and beverage items is one potential application of nanotechnology in the field of synbiotics. Probiotics are susceptible to degradation or loss because of their sensitivity to environmental conditions such as temperature, pH, and moisture during processing and storage. By encapsulating probiotics in nanoparticles, it may be feasible to improve their stability and distribution in food and beverage items, as well as their bioavailability and efficacy in the gastrointestinal tract.

The incorporation of new technologies such as artificial intelligence, machine learning, and nanotechnology into the field of synbiotics has the potential to revolutionize the development and application of these therapies. To completely comprehend the mechanisms underlying the potential health advantages of synbiotics and to optimize their usage in the prevention and treatment of various illnesses, additional research is required.

## 18.8 Conclusion

In conclusion, the study of synbiotics, which are a combination of probiotics and prebiotics, has had a significant impact on numerous fields, including mental health, machine learning, and the future. It has been shown that synbiotics have various favorable impacts on mental health, including a decrease in emotions of worry and melancholy, and that they may also improve cognitive performance and behavior. In the field of machine learning, the study of synbiotics has the potential to bring about a dramatic shift in how humans interact with and learn from machines. In the future, it is projected that synbiotics will play an ever-increasing role in the development of new technologies and the expansion of several disciplines, such as the invention of novel cures and treatments and the progress of the food industry. In general, the study of synbiotics has the potential to have far-reaching and revolutionary effects on numerous aspects of our lives, both in the present and in the future. Synbiotics have the potential to significantly alter many facets of our lives, including improved mental health and more advanced machine learning algorithms. This potential can reveal itself in numerous distinct ways.

# Bibliography

Amargianitakis, M., Antoniadou, M., Rahiotis, C., & Varzakas, T. (2021). Probiotics, prebiotics, Synbiotics and dental caries: New perspectives, suggestions, and patient coaching approach for a cavity-free mouth. *Applied Sciences, 11*(12), 5472.

Arboleya, S., Martínez-Camblor, P., Solís, G., Suárez, M., Fernández, N., Reyes-Gavilán, C. G. d. l., ... & Gueimonde, M. (2017). Intestinal Microbiota and Weight-gain In Preterm Neonates. *Front. Microbiol.*, (8). https://doi.org/10.3389/fmicb.2017.00183

Bengmark, S. (2002). Gut microbial ecology in critical illness: Is there a role for prebiotics, probiotics, and Synbiotics? *Current Opinion in Critical Care, 8*(2), 145–151.

Bengmark, S., & Martindale, R. (2005). Prebiotics and Synbiotics in clinical medicine. *Nutrition in Clinical Practice, 20*(2), 244–261.

Camilleri, M.. Management Options for Irritable Bowel Syndrome *Mayo Clin Proc.* 2018 Dec; *93*(12), 1858–1872. doi: 10.1016/j.mayocp.2018.04.032. PMID: 30522596; PMCID: PMC6314474.

Chang, Y.-S., Trivedi, M. K., Jha, A., Lin, Y.-F., Dimaano, L., & Garcia-Romero, M. T. (2016). Synbiotics for prevention and treatment of atopic dermatitis: A meta-analysis of randomized clinical trials. *JAMA Pediatrics, 170*(3), 236–242.

Chiu, C.-J., & Huang, M.-T. (2021). Asthma in the precision medicine era: Biologics and probiotics. *International Journal of Molecular Sciences, 22*(9), 4528.

Collado, M. C., Meriluoto, J., Salminen, S., & Isolauri, E. (2017). A review of clinical trials examining the effect of probiotic and synbiotic supplements on the microbiota of the gut. *International Dairy Journal, 68*(1), 8–14. doi: 10.1016/j.idairyj.2017.03.010.

Dahiya, D., & Nigam, P. S. (2022). Probiotics, prebiotics, Synbiotics, and fermented foods as potential biotics in nutrition improving health via microbiome-gut-brain axis. *Fermentation, 8*(7), 303.

Desai, V., Kozyrskyj, A. L., Lau, S., Sanni, O., Dennett, L., Walter, J., & Ospina, M. B. (2021). Effectiveness of probiotic, prebiotic, and synbiotic supplementation to improve perinatal mental health in mothers: A systematic review and meta-analysis. *Frontiers in Psychiatry, 12*, 622181.

Durazzo, A., Nazhand, A., Lucarini, M., Atanasov, A. G., Souto, E. B., Novellino, E., Capasso, R., & Santini, A. (2020). An updated overview on nanonutraceuticals: Focus on nanoprebiotics and nanoprobiotics. *International Journal of Molecular Sciences, 21*(7), 2285.

Escalante-Mendoza, C., López-Romero, P., & Pérez-Cano, F. J. (2017). Synbiotics' potential in human health. *Food Research International, 98*(1). doi: 10.1016/j.foodres.2016.12.023.

Ford, A. C., Harris, L. A., Lacy, B. E., Quigley, E. M., Moayyedi, P. (2018). Systematic Review with Meta-analysis: the Efficacy of Prebiotics, Probiotics, Synbiotics and Antibiotics In Irritable Bowel Syndrome. *Aliment Pharmacol Ther, 10*(48), 1044–1060. https://doi.org/10.1111/apt.15001

González-Herrera, S. M., Bermúdez-Quiñones, G., Ochoa-Martínez, L. A., Rutiaga-Quiñones, O. M., & Gallegos-Infante, J. A. (2021). Synbiotics: A technological approach in food applications. *Journal of Food Science and Technology, 58*(3), 811–824.

Gurry, T. (2017). Synbiotic approaches to human health and well-being. *Microbial Biotechnology, 10*(5), 1070–1073.

Hadi, A., Pourmasoumi, M., Kazemi, M., Najafgholizadeh, A., & Marx, W. (2022). Efficacy of synbiotic interventions on blood pressure: A systematic review and meta-analysis of clinical trials. *Critical Reviews in Food Science and Nutrition, 62*(20), 5582–5591.

Haghighat, N., Mohammadshahi, M., Shayanpour, S., Haghighizadeh, M. H., Rahmdel, S., & Rajaei, M. (2021). The effect of synbiotic and probiotic supplementation on mental health parameters in patients undergoing hemodialysis: A double-blind, randomized, placebo-controlled trial. *Indian Journal of Nephrology, 31*(2), 149.

He, Y., Ding, S., Chen, G., Li, H., Chen, Y., Wang, C., ... Zeng, L. (2006). China's experience with Synbiotics as a novel therapy method for digestive problems. *Nutrition, 22*(2), 225–231.

He, Y., Ding, S. J., Chen, G. C., Li, H. Y., Lu, L., & Chen, Y. (1997). Using Synbiotics to treat antibiotic-associated diarrhea: A randomized controlled trial. *Chinese Medical Journal, 110*(1), 36–41.

Jaiswal, M., Sharma, R., Subramani, S., Mishra, V., Sharma, J., Parthasarathy, P., Bisen, P. S., & Raghuwanshi, S. (2019). Role of lactobacilli as probiotics in human health benefits: Current status and future prospects. *IOSR Journal of Biotechnology and Biochemistry, 6*(5), 19–24.

Kan, J. M., Cowan, C. S., Ooi, C. Y., & Kasparian, N. A. (2019). What can the gut microbiome teach us about the connections between child physical and mental health? A systematic review. *Developmental Psychobiology, 61*(5), 700–713.

Kanamori, Y., Hashizume, K., Sugiyama, M., Morotomi, M., Yuki, N., & Tanaka, R. (2002). A novel synbiotic therapy dramatically improved the intestinal function of a pediatric patient with laryngotracheo-esophageal cleft (LTEC) in the intensive care unit. *Clinical Nutrition, 21*(6), 527–530.

Kearney, S. M., & Gibbons, S. M. (2018). Designing Synbiotics for improved human health. *Microbial Biotechnology, 11*(1), 141.

Kussmann, M., & Cunha, D. H. A. (2022). Nature has the answers: Discovering and validating natural bioactives for human health. *Bioactive Compounds in Health and Disease, 5*(11), 222–235.

Lalitsuradej, E., Sirilun, S., Sittiprapaporn, P., Sivamaruthi, B. S., Pintha, K., Tantipaiboonwong, P., Khongtan, S., Fukngoen, P., Peerajan, S., & Chaiyasut, C. (2022). The effects of Synbiotics administration on stress-related parameters in Thai subjects—A preliminary study. *Foods, 11*(5), 759.

Lam, K. N., Alexander, M., & Turnbaugh, P. J. (2019). Precision medicine goes microscopic: Engineering the microbiome to improve drug outcomes. *Cell Host and Microbe, 26*(1), 22–34.

Lee, S.-H., Cho, D.-Y., Lee, S.-H., Han, K.-S., Yang, S.-W., Kim, J.-H., Lee, S.-H., Kim, S.-M., & Kim, K.-N. (2019). A randomized clinical trial of Synbiotics in irritable bowel syndrome: Dose-dependent effects on gastrointestinal symptoms and fatigue. *Korean Journal of Family Medicine, 40*(1), 2.

Lonardo, A., Arab, J. P., & Arrese, M. (2021). Perspectives on precision medicine approaches to NAFLD diagnosis and management. *Advances in Therapy, 38*(5), 2130–2158.

Mandal, A. (2020). The definition and health benefits of Synbiotics. The Latest Medical News Today https://www.medicalnewstoday.com/articles/326361.

Mercenier, A., Pavan, S., & Pot, B. (2003). Probiotics as biotherapeutic agents: Present knowledge and future prospects. *Current Pharmaceutical Design, 9*(2), 175–191.

Merrifield, D. L., Dimitroglou, A., Foey, A., Davies, S. J., Baker, R. T., Bøgwald, J., Castex, M., & Ringø, E. (2010). The current status and future focus of probiotic and prebiotic applications for salmonids. *Aquaculture, 302*(1–2), 1–18.

Methiwala, H. N., Vaidya, B., Addanki, V. K., Bishnoi, M., Sharma, S. S., & Kondepudi, K. K. (2021). Gut microbiota in mental health and depression: Role of pre/pro/Synbiotics in their modulation. *Food and Function, 12*(10), 4284–4314.

Milyn, A., & Gombart, A. F. (2017). The fundamentals of Synbiotics: A blend of prebiotics and probiotics 2017. *BioMed Research International.* doi: 10.1155/2017/9813566.

Ogawa, T., Hashikawa, S., Asai, Y., Sakamoto, H., Yasuda, K., & Makimura, Y. (2006). A new Synbiotic, Lactobacillus casei subsp. casei together with dextran, reduces murine and human allergic reaction. *FEMS Immunology and Medical Microbiology, 46*(3), 400–409.

Panesar, P. S., & Anal, A. K. (2022). *Probiotics, Prebiotics and Synbiotics: Technological Advancements Towards Safety and Industrial Applications.* John Wiley & Sons.

Pasinetti, G. (2022). Synbiotic-derived metabolites reduce neuroinflammatory symptoms of Alzheimer's disease. *Current Developments in Nutrition,* 6(Supplement_1), 804–804.

Plaza-Díaz, J., Ruiz-Ojeda, F. J., Vilchez-Padial, L. M., & Gil, A. (2017). Evidence of the anti-inflammatory effects of probiotics and Synbiotics in intestinal chronic diseases. *Nutrients,* 9(6), 555.

Rastall, R. A., & Maitin, V. (2002). Prebiotics and Synbiotics: Towards the next generation. *Current Opinion in Biotechnology,* 13(5), 490–496.

Rastegar, L., Talebian, F., Omidvar, N., & Ghavami, S. (2015). A systematic review of clinical trials pertaining to the use of Synbiotics as novel therapy methods. *International Pediatrics Journal.* doi: 10.1155/2015/730429.

Sáez-Lara, M. J., Robles-Sanchez, C., Ruiz-Ojeda, F. J., Plaza-Diaz, J., & Gil, A. (2016). Effects of probiotics and Synbiotics on obesity, insulin resistance syndrome, type 2 diabetes and non-alcoholic fatty liver disease: A review of human clinical trials. *International Journal of Molecular Sciences,* 17(6), 928.

Saneian, H., Pourmoghaddas, Z., Roohafza, H., & Gholamrezaei, A. (2015). Synbiotic containing Bacillus coagulans and fructo-oligosaccharides for functional abdominal pain in children. *Gastroenterology and Hepatology from Bed to Bench,* 8(1), 56.

Schrezenmeir, J., & de Vrese, M. (2001). Probiotics, prebiotics, and Synbiotics—Approaching a definition. *The American Journal of Clinical Nutrition,* 73(2), 361s–364s.

Sharma, G., & Im, S.-H. (2018). Probiotics as a potential immunomodulating pharmabiotics in allergic diseases: Current status and future prospects. *Allergy, Asthma and Immunology Research,* 10(6), 575–590.

Sharma, S., Arora, M., & Baldi, A. (2013). Probiotics in India: Current status and future prospects. *Pharm Aspire,* 1, 1–12.

Sheng, K., He, S., Sun, M., Zhang, G., Kong, X., Wang, J., & Wang, Y. (2020). Synbiotic supplementation containing Bifidobacterium infantis and xylooligosaccharides alleviates dextran sulfate sodium-induced ulcerative colitis. *Food and Function,* 11(5), 3964–3974.

Skonieczna-Żydecka, K., Kaczmarczyk, M., Łoniewski, I., Lara, L. F., Koulaouzidis, A., Misera, A., Maciejewska, D., & Marlicz, W. (2018). A systematic review, meta-analysis, and meta-regression evaluating the efficacy and mechanisms of action of probiotics and Synbiotics in the prevention of surgical site infections and surgery-related complications. *Journal of Clinical Medicine,* 7(12), 556.

Smith, C. (2020). Synbiotic-derived metabolites reduce neuroinflammatory symptoms of Alzheimer's disease: Nonhuman: Preclinical studies on APOE and neuroinflammation. *Alzheimer's and Dementia,* 16(S9), e046288.

Stahl, B., O'Neill, C., Cacciatore, S., Dalton, B., & Guillem, K. (2020). A systematic analysis of Synbiotics for the relief of menopausal symptoms. *Genome Medicine,* 12(1). doi: 10.1186/s13073-020-00701-x.

Sugawara, G., Nagino, M., Nishio, H., Ebata, T., Takagi, K., Asahara, T., Nomoto, K., & Nimura, Y. (2006). Perioperative synbiotic treatment to prevent postoperative infectious complications in biliary cancer surgery: A randomized controlled trial. *Annals of Surgery,* 244(5), 706.

Ulluwishewa, D., Anderson, R. C., McNabb, W. C., Moughan, P. J., & Wells, J. M. (2015). The function of functional food science and technology in the maintenance and restoration of health. *Trends in Food Science and Technology,* 42(2), 161–182. doi: 10.1016/j.tifs.2015.03.003.

Vaiman, M., Basran, S., & Dhuna, V. (2018). Probiotics and Synbiotics in the treatment and maintenance of periodontal disease and oral health. *Frontiers in Microbiology,* 9, 123–136.

Watson, R. R., & Preedy, V. R. (2015). *Probiotics, Prebiotics, and Synbiotics: Bioactive Foods in Health Promotion.* Academic Press.

# 19

# Interplay between Nutraceuticals and Gut Microbiota: Some Clinical Evidence

Aaishwarya B. Deshmukh and Jayvadan K. Patel

## Contents

DOI: 10.1201/9781003333821-19

# 19.1 Introduction

In human beings, owing to the close symbiotic association with microorganisms, at least half the total number of cells in the human body are considered "metaorganisms" (1). The majority of these microbes are present in the gut, and wide research has recognized their dominant role in preserving human health by controlling the development and inflection of immunogenic responses (2), host nutrition and metabolism (3, 4), brain development and behavioural pattern (5), progression of chronic disorders such as cancer (6) and diabetes mellitus, and many more (7). Furthermore, a relationship between altered gut microbiota configuration and the scale of COVID-19 severity in the pandemic has been identified, which signifies the role of gut microbiota in determining the body response to novel contagious agents (8). The microbiota is acquired maternally at birth (9) and alters during the life span, subjugated to dietary habits as well as environmental signals (10). Heterogeneity in gut microbiota has also been observed among communities with repercussions on physiology and pathology (11, 12). The most developed microbiota among the gastrointestinal tract, respiratory tract, skin, and vagina is the gastrointestinal microbiota, unequally distributed alongside the digestive tract. There are some bacteria present in the stomach and initial part of the small intestine, on the other hand the concentration rises reaching a maximum in the colon region (13). Adult healthy individuals usually have six bacterial phyla governing the gut microbiota, out of which 90% are occupied by *Firmicutes* and *Bacteroidetes* and the rest by *Proteobacteria, Actinobacteria, Fusobacteria,* and *Verrucomicrobia* (14). *Firmicutes* and *Bacteroidetes* embody the chief bacteria phyla and their fraction remains the same during the life span of an individual (of age more than 3 years old) (15).

On the basis of machine learning, new information has concluded that the gut microbiota taxonomic profile can be employed to forecast exactly the chronological age of an individual, thus supporting the notion of a microbiota-based aging clock (16). This is a noteworthy verdict, since it displays an insightful relationship between host microbial community structure and the life span of an individual, thus providing prospective therapeutic implications. However, it is notable that while all individuals endure programed chronological aging, the biological aging rate can vary evidently; biological aging states the comprehension of pathophysiological changes that are disease-independent and molecular markers that add to the distinctive aging phenotype and morbidity in elderly individuals. Thus, biological aging can be considered as a more complete and consistent predictor of the damaging effects of aging and the advancement in mitigation therapies (17, 18). Incidentally, some compelling evidence has demonstrated that reduced gut microbial diversity might be linked with the "frailty index"—a predictor of the biological age and health span (19, 20). Microbiota transplantation studies have validated that the alteration in gut microbiome of elderly people is adequate to persuade morbidity in young recipients, thus affecting the health span (21).

The introduction and extensive application of high throughput sequencing technology as well as "OMICS," viz. metagenomics, metabolomics, and metatranscriptomics, have expedited the listing of the microbial species inhabiting the human gut and have also delivered an estimation of microbial properties and their possible influence on the host, along with quantification of biologically active microbial products (22). These technological advancements have produced studies unfolding deviations in the microbiome in pathological states and incited interest for microbiome analysis and its role in diagnosis, prognosis, or treatment selection. The therapeutic potential of the microbiome has been revealed by microbiome science; whereas some microbiome-modulating approaches have been employed on an experiential basis for years, new research has started to recognize various mechanisms whereby nutraceutical interventions might in fact provide advantages (23).

## 19.2 Significance of Gut Microbiota

Some species of the colon bacteria play a vital role in the bacterial degradation of amino acids and production of short-chain fatty acids (SCFAs), which are an opulent source of energy for the host and for controlling metabolic signaling (24, 14). Microbiota like *Bacteroidetes* form acetate and propionate, while Firmicutes families, viz. *Lachnospiraceae* and *Ruminococcaceae*, largely form butyrate as their primary metabolic end products (25, 26); while acetate and propionate are used as substrates for different biological processes like lipogenesis, gluconeogenesis, and protein synthesis, butyrate serves as a key component of energetic metabolism in the colonocytes (27, 28). These metabolic products, viz. acetate, propionate and butyrate, have an essential role in the regulation of lipids and glucose homeostasis in hepatic cells, as well as the effect of peroxisome proliferator-activated receptors (PPAR) on lipogenesis and gluconeogenesis (29). Besides, the gut microbiota metabolizes tryptophan to active substances; *E. coli* produces indole, a signaling molecule with many diverse physiological functions like motility, biofilm formation, antibiotic resistance, etc. (30, 31). The SCFAs are involved in inhibition of histone deacetylase (HDAC) and ligands for specific G protein-coupled receptors (GPRs), in turn responsible for physiological functions like regulation of blood pressure, kidney function, and nervous system, as well as protection against colon cancer (32, 33). SCFAs also activates free fatty acid receptors—FFAR2 and FFAR3-G protein-coupled receptors, found in numerous cells: adipocytes, pancreatic islet, incretin-releasing enteroendocrine cells (K cells-gastric inhibitory polypeptide release, I cells-cholecystokinin release, L cells-glucagon-like peptide-1)—that are signaling molecules for several physiological processes (34). Studies have established that SCFAs have a vital role to play in the prevention and treatment of conditions like metabolic syndrome, gastrointestinal diseases (Crohn's disease, ulcerative colitis, or antibiotic-associated diarrhea), and certain types of cancer (35, 36).

Currently many reported dietary supplements are employed to reinstate the gut microbiota equilibrium. *Lactobacillus* species (*L. casei, rhamnosus,* and *acidophilus*) have shown to prevent or diminish the severity of antibiotic-associated diarrhea (AAD) (37, 38), while *Lactobacillus, Bifidobacterium,* or *Escherichia coli* Nissle 1917 species have shown to avert/treat gastrointestinal diseases or metabolic disorders (14). A meta-analysis study by Johnston and coworkers to conclude if concomitant administration of probiotics and antibiotics could prevent or reduce AAD in children established a positive effect of probiotics on AAD incidence (probiotic 8% vs. control 19%). The probiotic treatment in this study included *Bacillus* spp., *Bifidobacterium* spp., *Clostridium butyricum, Lactobacilli* spp., *Lactococcus* spp., *Leuconostoc Cremoris, Saccharomyces* spp., and *Streptococcus* spp., alone or in combination (39). Prebiotics, nutraceuticals approved for boosting the growth of beneficial microbiota species, have shown to exert effects on modulation of gut microbiota composition and production of energy metabolism, increasing mineral absorption, immune function regulation, and development of intestinal barrier functions (40).

Lactose from cow's milk and soybeans are considered as chief sources of galacto-oligosaccharides (GOS), which exhibit high solubility, neutral taste, stability at high temperature, and acidity, in addition to a low glycemic index. In a study, it was revealed that preterm infants when fed with a combination of 90% GOS and 10% fructo-oligosaccharides (FOS), augmented the composition of gut microbiota species *Bifidobacteria* and *Lactobacilli,* closely resembling breast-fed infants' microbiota composition (41). In addition, combination of GOS and FOS has also shown a substantial influence on increasing *Bifidobacteria* and decreasing *Clostridium* in the gut, however GOS alone could only increase *Lactobacillus* abundance (42). In a randomized, double-blind placebo-controlled study, employing 40 patients divided into two parallel groups (placebo vs. prebiotic), it was revealed that prebiotics (inulin and FOS) exerted favorable effect on *Lactobacillus* and *Bifidobacteria* population in cancer patients treated with pelvic radiotherapy (RT). This observation could be confirmed when stool samples were collected and analysed for *Lactobacillus* and *Bifidobacteria* 7 days before the start of RT, 15 days after starting, at the end of RT, and 3 weeks after RT was concluded (43).

An amino acid, L-glutamine (GLN) exhibits a significant impact in the gut and contributes immensely to energy generation. GLN is metabolized by enterocytes as well as intestinal luminal bacteria and is further oxidized in the Krebs cycle to form Adenosine triphosphate (ATP) (44). A double-blind study by De Souza et al. (2015) enrolled volunteers with body mass index (BMI) over 25 kg/m2 and alienated in two groups, one of which received GLN and the second L-alanine (ALA). At the time of completion of the study, out of the total of 33 subjects, 21 individuals were from group I—treated with GLN—and 12 from group II—those treated with ALA. The gut microbiota was analysed pretreatment and 14 days posttreatment, which revealed that GLN regulated changes in gut microbiota composition and that the ratio of *Firmicutes/Bacteroides*, which signifies a good biomarker for obesity, was found reduced post GLN supplementation, mostly since *Firmicutes* were considerably attenuated after GLN treatment (45). A cyanobacteria (blue-green algae), spirulina (*Arthrospira platensis*), commonly consumed as a food supplement, attenuates the growth of Gram-positive and Gram-negative bacteria such as *Staphulococcus aureus*, *Bacillus subtilis*, *E. coli*, *Pseudomonas aeruginosa*, etc., by the virtue of an extracellular metabolite produced by spirulina. Additionally, spirulina's effect on microbiota modulation was also found to be ascribed to the active compounds present in this plant, such as glutamate, aspartate, carbohydrates, or phenolic compounds, which already have a renowned antimicrobial and bacteriostatic effect as well as the ability to arouse the probiotic growth (46, 47). Thus, spirulina biomass might be a natural product that could be added to fermented milk for intensifying *Lactobacillus* production and the number of viable cells reaching the intestine (48).

## 19.3 Impact of Diet/Dietary Supplements on the Gut Microbiota

Within a few days of altering diet, noteworthy alterations occur in gut microbiota; switching diets for a mere 2 weeks caused noteworthy differences in African Americans and rural African individuals. An augmented quantity of identified butyrate-producing bacteria in African American people with the usual intake of a rural African diet caused butyrate production to rise 2.5 times and diminished secondary bile acid synthesis (49). In a study, a comparison of shifts between plant and animal protein-based diets displayed these changes after just 5 days (50). However, healthy microbiota are buoyant in context to temporal changes caused by dietary mediations, which means that reactions to maintain homeostasis are reinstated in the original community composition (51).

Paganini et al. in their study referred to the impact of iron supplementation on the gut microbiome in children (52), but the impact of other micronutrients on the microbiota is still limited (53). Studies have shown that deficits in vitamins A and D are associated with a negative impact on intestinal microbial populations, compromised gut barrier function, and elevation of pro-inflammatory responses (54). Deficiency of vitamin D has also been associated with inflammatory bowel disease and studies have shown its anti-inflammatory effects upon supplementation (55). Interfaces between other vitamins and microbiota–host interaction have also been referred in a few studies (56, 57). Curcumin, another dietary additive with proven anti-inflammatory properties, has been shown to influence the gut microbiota (58) and it is certain that several other dietary constituents and supplements might intermingle in one or the other way with the gut microbiome or its interface with the immune system or metabolic pathways in the host.

## 19.3.1 Gut Microbiome in Disease

The composition and role of gut microbiota in different ailments, through various studies, have revealed links with type 2 diabetes (T2D), obesity, inflammatory bowel diseases (IBD), inflammatory skin diseases such as psoriasis and atopic dermatitis, autoimmune arthritis, atherosclerosis, etc. For example, it was found that IBD patients had less bacterial diversity and lesser quantities of *Bacteroides* and *Firmicutes*—that contributed to decreased concentrations of microbial-derived butyrate, since butyrate and SCFAs have a direct anti-inflammatory effect in the gut (59). Moreover, altered manifestations in Crohn's disease activity might be characterized by particular gut mucosa-attached bacteria which are found to be considerably impacted by anti-TNF (tumor necrosis factor) therapy (60). The comparative abundance of diverse bacteria might also facilitate inflammation of intestine and Crohn's disease activity by affecting local regulatory T cell populations (60, 61). A study by Day et al. functionally characterized the gut microbiota in type 2 diabetic patients with diabetes-associated markers, showed augmented membrane transport of sugars and branched-chain amino acids, and xenobiotic metabolism, as well as sulphate reduction accompanied by diminished bacterial chemotaxis, butyrate synthesis, and cofactors and vitamins metabolism (62).

## 19.3.2 Influence of Probiotic Supplementation on Gut Microbiome

Probiotics (generally *Bifidobacterium* and *Lactobacillus* species) are present in many products, comprising food, dietary supplements, or drugs. Concerns prevail about the inability of most of the microbe supplements in establishing themselves in the gut resulting in failure to exercise an effect on the resident community (63, 64). However, probiotics can exert their effect independently of the gut microbiota by their direct effects on the host, e.g., through modulation of immune system or production of bioactive compounds. The therapeutic potential of probiotic supplementation has been studied in a wide range of pathologies. In one study, the Cochrane Library was searched for systematic reviews for "probiotic*" yielding 39 studies, and Medline for "systematic review" or "meta-analysis" and "probiotic*," yielding 31 studies. This study encompassed information on systematic reviews of randomized controlled trials where probiotics were the main treatment and not dietary supplements in general; studies with dedicated comparisons of probiotics with a control group were sought. The investigation of 313 trials and 46,826 participants revealed significant confirmation on the beneficial effects of probiotic supplementation in averting acute upper respiratory tract infections, diarrhea, necrotizing enterocolitis, pulmonary exacerbation in children with co-morbid cystic fibrosis, and skin conditions like eczema in children. Probiotic treatment improved cardiometabolic parameters and decreased serum concentration of C-reactive protein in type 2 diabetic patients. Notably, the studies were nonhomogeneous and were not essentially harmonized with type or dose of probiotic supplementation or length of intervention, which confines exact recommendations (65). A study has shown that stable engraftment of *Bifidobacterium longum* depends on individualized characteristics of the gut microbiota, providing a validation for the personalization of probiotic treatments (66). Thus, evolving areas of probiotic treatment embrace employment of newer microbes and combinations, conjoining probiotics and prebiotics (i.e., synbiotics) (67), and personalized approaches based on candidates' microbes profile in various diseases and pathologies like inflammation, lipid metabolism, cancer, or obesity (65).

### 19.3.2.1 Validation of the Clinical Health Benefit of Probiotics with Human Trials

Safety assessment of the probiotic ought to determine at least those criteria mentioned below, which are an absolutely fundamental principle in application.

- The array of antimicrobial drug resistance
- Metabolic activities affected
- Adverse effects observed in individuals during clinical trials and post marketing
- In the case a probiotic strain is known to produce toxins and exhibit haemolytic potential, the degree of these actions
- Absence of infectivity in animal models

### 19.3.2.2 Clinical Studies in Healthy and Diseased Conditions

A number of people ingest probiotics on a regular basis in anticipation of promoting gut and general health. However, apart from exerting a favorable effect on the extent and severity of the common cold, fewer indications of probiotics augmenting health or inhibiting disease among healthy subjects are found (68). Remarkable inconsistency between studies (also in the case of the same disorders) concerning study population, trial design, endpoint measurement, duration, and product dosage and formulation was found by Ford et al. (2014) (69) in a systematic review of probiotics in irritable bowel syndrome (IBS), which in turn render inferences about optimal probiotics nearly impossible. This is particularly exasperating since this same review established that probiotics, overall, were effective in IBS. Moreover, study trials in different gastrointestinal disorders are fewer and often indecisive. A study by Panigrahi et al. elucidated the impact of a synbiotic on infections among high-risk infants in India and yielded positive and clinically meaningful results. This study also exemplified the challenges that were posed; to validate noteworthy effects of synbiotic (combination of a prebiotic and a probiotic) preparation on their primary outcome, sepsis, or death within the first 60 days of life span in infants born in rural India, 4,556 randomized infants were administered either *Lactobacillus plantarum* ATCC-202195 plus an FOS or placebo (70).

This complex and expensive methodology was indispensable to deliver sufficient control to establish a clinically significant decrease in sepsis and death with the intervention. Furthermore, an up-to-date, peer-reviewed, evidence-based assessment of probiotic effects in adults and children was provided in the 2017 World Gastroenterology Organization Global Guideline on Probiotics and Probiotics (www.worldgastroenterology.org/UserFiles/file/guidelines/probiotics-and-prebiotics-english-2017.pdf—accessed June 18, 2019), where level 1 evidence was identified to support the usage of probiotics in the following indications in adults and probiotic strain formulations appropriate for each indication were also listed:

1. Antibiotic-associated diarrhea prevention in many clinical settings:
   a. Yogurt with *Lactobacillus* (L.) *casei* DN114, *Streptococcus* (S.) thermophiles, *L. bulgaricus*
   b. *L. acidophilus* CL1285 and *L. casei* (Bio-K+ CL1285) combination
   c. *Saccharomyces boulardii* CNCM I-745
   d. *L. rhamnosus* GG
2. Attenuation of adverse effects associated with eradication therapy for *Helicobacter pylori*:
   a. *Saccharomyces boulardii* CNCM I-745
3. Postoperative sepsis prevention in patients undergoing elective gastrointestinal surgeries:
   a. *L. acidophilus*
   b. *L. plantarum*
   c. *Bifidobacterium longum* 88
4. Remission maintenance in pouchitis:
   a. VSL#3
5. Reduction in symptoms associated with lactose maldigestion:
   a. Yogurt with live cultures of *L. delbrueckii* subsp. *bulgaricus* and *S. thermophilus*

Many systematic reviews have provided information on the use of probiotics in these and other additional indications. Most of these reviews have established evidence supporting efficacy in a given indication as moderate and typically weak (71). Besides, these same reviews generally were unsuccessful in identifying a strain or combination of strains which were most effective in certain clinical situation.

## 19.3.3 Influence of Prebiotic Foods and Dietary Fibre on Gut Microbiome

Dietary fibre is defined, by most national authorities, as eatable carbohydrate polymer having three or more monomeric units resistant to the endogenous digestive enzymes, and as a result are neither hydrolyzed nor absorbed in the small intestine (72). A subclass of dietary fibres is fermentable, i.e., they assist in growth of microbes by acting as growth substrates in the distal bowel region of the gastrointestinal track (73). Prebiotics are nondigestible carbohydrates and act as food components or ingredients that are not digested by the human body, but explicitly sustain favorable microorganisms in the colon (74).

### 19.3.3.1 Clinical Health Benefits of Dietary Fibers and Suggested Mechanisms

Many valuable physiological effects of dietary fibers have been confirmed on humans (75). Dietary fiber can be divided into two types, non-fermentable/insoluble and fermentable/soluble forms, both of which differ in their possible influence on health (76). Insoluble dietary fibers like celluloses, hemicellulose, and fructans (77), found in food such as whole wheat flour, brown rice, nuts, beans, and vegetables (78, 79), are represented by their bulking effect in addition to high fermentation by the gut microbiome, ensuring short-chain fatty acid (SCFAs) production (76). A latest study by Desai et al. has indicated that butyrate, an SCFA, induced immunologic modification in macrophage cells, and augmented expression of antibacterial and host defense genes (80). Insoluble fiber was also shown to prompt a healthy microbial composition (76). On the contrary, a study by Desai et al. validated an increase in disease vulnerability, if microbiota remains fiber-deprived, by a decline in protective mucus; shrinkage of mucus membrane, which assists in hindering entry of pathogens in the system, which was in line to the rise in mucin-degrading bacteria consequential to fiber deficiency (81). Soluble fibers like inulin, pectin, guar gum, etc. found in whole grains, legumes, seeds and nuts, and some fruits and vegetables (82), are characterized as a viscid, gel-like form in the intestine which may decelerate the absorption of nutrients (e.g., glucose and lipids) (76). A study has lately demonstrated that consumption of pectin led microbes to use galacturonic acid as an energy source, therefore rising the reducing sugar levels in human stools, which display the protective prospective of pectin against metabolic disorders like T2D by means of regulating blood glucose levels (83). Dietary fibers, as well as SCFAs, are associated with epithelial barrier functions; explicitly, butyrate has shown a bidirectional effect on epithelial barrier function. For example, during diarrhea and antibiotic-induced dysbiosis, a considerable decline in the commensal bacteria responsible for butyrate production has been demonstrated (84), which further leads to a deficiency in accessible butyrate as an energy source for colonocytes, thus disturbing the refreshment of enterocytes. Supplementation with certain fibers, in humans, has shown enhancement in butyrate-producing bacteria in the gut; as the butyrate level upsurges, a consistent modification and decline in the diarrhea condition has been observed (85).

Consumption of resistant starches has been shown to supplement definite bacterial groups, viz. *Bifidobacterium adolescentis*, *Eubacterium rectale*, and

*Ruminococcus bromii* in some individuals; (86, 87) the taxa supplemented, though, vary depending on the type of resistant starches and other dietary fibres (87). Nevertheless, it does demonstrate clearly that shifts are reliant on the carbohydrate's chemical structure as well as the enzymatic capacity of microbes to access them. Moreover, microbes are also required to stick to a substrate and endure the environment produced from fermentation (e.g., low pH) (88). The influence of microbiota-accessible carbohydrates on the gastro-intestinal microbiome composition can be significant, leading to enrichment of particular species to constitute beyond 30% of the fecal microbiota (87, 89). Therefore, microbiota-accessible carbohydrates deliver a prospective approach to improve beneficial sectional members of the microbiome. Though these changes prevail only until the time carbohydrates are consumed, and they are extremely subjective, providing a foundation for personalized approaches. Studies conducted by using purified dietary fibres or whole plant-based diets in short-term feeding trials have shown either no effect on microbiota diversity or decreases in it but did have clinical benefits possibly via metabolites such as small-chain fatty acids (SCFA) (90, 91). Intake of low fibre in the diet decreases SCFA production and alters the metabolism of gastrointestinal microbiota in such a way so as to use lesser amounts of favorable nutrients (92), which ulti-mately leads to production of harmful metabolites (93, 94). A few studies have revealed convincing evidence that low fibre Western diet damages the colonic mucus barrier, triggering microbiota impingement, resulting in pathogenic susceptibility (95) as well as inflammation (96), thus delivering a prospective mechanism for associations of Western diet with chronic ailments. Recently, two studies exhibited the damaging effects of high-fat diets on mucus layer permeability and that metabolic functions could be stopped by dietary admin-istration of inulin (97, 98). Generally, these outcomes, along with the role of butyrate in averting oxygen-induced gut microbiota dysbiosis, offer a solid validation to supplementing dietary fibre for maintaining integrity of mucosal barrier function in the gut (99). Extensive observational confirming data illus-trates the beneficial effects of fibre intake in human health. In addition, two new meta-analyses have established a strong relation between dietary fibre and health benefits in a number of pathologies (100, 101). Furthermore, an intervention study recently has found dietary fibres significantly attenuating insulin resistance in patients with T2D, with clear association to the modifica-tions in the microbiota and beneficial metabolites (for example butyrate) (102).

### 19.3.4 Phytochemicals and Their Interactions with Gut Microbiome

There are other nutraceuticals, like phytoestrogens and polyphenols, to name a few, that exhibit beneficial effects in individuals and many studies in clini-cal settings provide compelling evidence for the therapeutic potential of these compounds in numerous pathologies. Between 90 and 95% of phytochemi-cals are biotransformed by the residential colonic gut microbiota leaving a mere 5–10% of phytochemicals to get absorbed from the small intestine (103). The biotransformation by gut microbiota produces exceedingly bioavailable metabolites of these phytochemicals. Phytochemicals' metabolism and absorption have prospective systemic health effects on the host (viz. cardioprotective) (104, 105), as well as defense against glucose toxicity (106); these effects are partially owing to the rise of polyphenols in the diet, which has been associated with deterrence of varied chronic conditions (vz. metabolic syndrome) (107, 108). The unabsorbed dietary phytochemicals exert direct modulatory effects on the gut microbiota. For example, phenolic compounds from tea leaves have been shown to impede growth and adhesion of bacterial species like *Clostridium spp.*, *E. coli*, and *S. typhimurium* (109). Moreover, defensive abilities of phytochemicals in various pathologies, in the perspective of the microbiome, have been acknowledged in many recent studies. For example, a study by Brown et al. in humans with colorectal cancer showed that short-term rice bran ingestion led to 28-fold and 14.5-fold augmentation in detection of the citrus-related phytochemicals (hesperidin and narirutin, respectively) in the metabolite profile of stools (110). Therefore, it is rational to presume that hesperidin, resultant of gut microbiota-mediated metabolism (for instance, rice bran), might stimulate favorable effects against inflammation-related diseases (for instance, colorectal cancer).

Flavonoids have demonstrated their influence and control on intestinal permeability and intestinal barrier, with a direct trophic influence on *Akkermansia* species but no effect on mucin production (111). Flavonoids, owing to their antimicrobial action, might be deliberated as apt substitutes to antibiotics, particularly in mild/moderate infections or in prevention of infections (112). The isoflavones are inactive in primary form, as conjugate glucosides; upon conversion by gut microbiota and intestinal mucosa into compounds that are well absorbed and metabolized by the intestinal microflora into other metabolites, and exert estrogen-like activity (113). A study by Franke et al. showed that isoflavonoids are comprised of many glycosides like genistein, daidzein, and glycitein. Daidzein, on metabolism by gut bacteria to equol (114), exerts health benefits and exhibits strong estrogenic activity and antioxidant capacity. The key bacteria that converts isoflavonoids into equol was found to be populated in the distal portion of the gut and belonged to the family *Coriobacteriaceae* (115). Furthermore, study by Gaya et al. has shown that ellagitannins and lignans too are metabolized by gut microbiota to equol, urolithins, and enterolignans, which in turn have high bioavailability and estrogenic/antiestrogenic effects, and antioxidant and anti-inflammatory, as well as anti-proliferative effects (116). Moreover, a bidirectional relation between polyphenols and gut microbiota exists which is responsible for potential influences of polyphenols in a number of diseases and conditions. The bioavailability of polyphenols is augmented by microbiota, whereas unabsorbed polyphenols are found to maintain the gut microbiota equilibrium. Proposed mechanisms of polyphenol assume defense against gastrointestinal disorders and/or pathogens, reinforcement of intestinal epithelial tight cell junctions, rise of mucus secretion, cytokine stimulation, and immune response modulation (117). Tea is found to contain a high concentration of flavanols like epicatechin and catechin as well as their esters. The unabsorbed compounds of tea in high concentration get retained in the gut and exert actions to impact intestinal health. A study by Lee et al. displayed caffeic acid to impede the growth and development of several intestinal pathogenic bacteria like *E. coli, Clostridium, Bacteroides, Salmonella,* and *Pseudomonas* (118). Moreover, polyphenols in green tea have shown to exert antioxidant and anti-inflammatory effects in addition to influencing the activity of NF-kB (nuclear factor kappa B), COX-2 (cyclooxygenase-2), and the level of IL-2 (interleukin-2) (119). Conversely, several metabolites of black tea like that of benzoic, phenylacetic, and phenylpropionic acids have been verified to possess antimicrobial properties (120). Resveratrol, a dietary polyphenol used as a food supplement in patients suffering from cardiovascular diseases (121), has shown modulatory effects on gut microbiota dysbiosis which is induced by a high-fat diet. It was found in the study that resveratrol stimulated growth of *Lactobacillus* and *Bifidobacterium*, upsurged the *Bacteroidetes/Firmicutes* ratio, and prevented *Enterococcus faecalis* growth (122).

### 19.3.4.1 Impact of Carotenoids on Gut Microbiome

Studies that analysed the effect of amplified serum carotenoid concentrations on the gut microbiome have revealed a reduced risk of chronic diseases in those with high serum carotenoid levels. A long-term randomized control study by Djuric et al. in humans analysed the association between colonic mucosal bacteria and serum carotenoid concentrations and established that colonic mucosal bacteria were linked with serum carotenoid concentrations at baseline, without any substantial effect upon long-term exposure. This signifies the necessity for improved research on long-term exposure and its implications to comprehend the outcome of dietary change upholding a favorable microbial alteration. It was recognized, conversely, that 11 operational taxonomic units were connected with higher levels of serum carotenoid which included body mass index, smoking, and dietary intakes (in lieu of 12% of the total variance in carotenoid levels). These outcomes additionally propose the influence of multidimensional aspects, viz., behavioural and metabolic factors, on the competence of gut microbiota for carotenoid absorption (123).

### 19.3.5 Influence of Micronutrients on Gut Microbiota

Studies have shown that the gut microbiota may modify the host's capacity of absorption of a number of dietary nutrients and, in that way, secondarily influence micronutrient physiology (124). Explicitly, few microbial strains have been found to synthesize vitamins and cofactors, and data advocates that microbial metabolites affect micronutrients' metabolic and physiological pathways in the human body (125, 126). Furthermore, vitamin and cofactor production can deliver vital nutrients to colonocytes, promoting antagonism with pathogenic organisms and modulation of immune responses (127). Since bacteria have shown to change the bile acids' efficacy of dietary lipid emulsification and micelles formation, the microbiomes can hypothetically impact the lipid-soluble vitamins absorption too (128). With deliberation of luminal nutrient actions on the microbiome and in turn microbial effects on host nutrition status, it is rational to consider that identification and modification of microbial interactions with hosts might be crucial to human health.

The effect of probiotics on outcomes related to vitamin D and omega-3 fatty acids has been studied in a few clinical trials. Jones et al., in a double-blind, placebo-controlled, randomized, parallel-arm, multi-center study in 127 adults, established that when individuals were treated with *Lactobacillus reuteri* NCIMB 30242 ($2.9*10^9$ colony-forming units (CFU) per capsule for 9 weeks), an augmented serum concentration of 25-hydroxyvitamin D by 25.5% with respect to placebo was observed (129). A synergistic effect on decreasing testosterone production and improved indicators of inflammation and oxidative stress were observed in women with polycystic ovary syndrome (130) post a 12-week administration of vitamin D3 (50,000 International unit (IU) every 2 weeks) and $8*10^9$ CFU/day probiotics (containing *Lactobacillus acidophilus*, *Bifidobacterium bifidum*, *Lactobacillus reuteri*, and *Lactobacillus fermentum*, $2*10^9$ CFU/g each). In yet another study, by Ghaderi et al., depressed inflammatory parameters and severity of related metabolic syndrome were observed with the identical protocol of treatment with vitamin D3 and probiotics in schizophrenic patients (131). Supplementation of a combination of vitamin D and probiotics too exhibited improvement in metabolic symptoms in patients with T2D (132) as well as gestational diabetes (133). In addition, an attenuation in the relative abundance of species like *Gammaproteobacteria* and, predominantly, *Escherichia/Shigella* and *P. aeruginosa* that are considered to be linked with lung infection, oxidative stress, and lung tissue degeneration, was observed on a weekly administration of 50,000 UI vitamin D in patients with cystic fibrosis (CF) (134). Kanhere et al. (135) has also described the effects of vitamin D supplementation on gut microbiota composition in patients with CF (2018). A study by Kobyliak et al. deliberated the effect of co-administration of a probiotic mixture (*Lactobacillus* and *Lactococcus*, $6*10^{10}$ CFU/g; *Bifidobacterium*, $1*10^{10}$/g; *Propionibacterium*, $3*10^{10}$/g; *Acetobacter*, $1*10^6$/g) and omega-3 (5–25 mg omega-3/day) in nonalcoholic fatty liver disease (NAFLD) patients (136), and showed improvement in liver fat, serum lipids, metabolic parameters, and systemic inflammation post 8 weeks of treatment with these factors. Golkhalkhali et al. also testified the clinical beneficial effects of this probiotic and omega-3 fatty acids co-administration protocol in patients with colorectal cancer (137), comprising of improvement in quality of life and reduction in inflammatory biomarkers as well as chemotherapy side effects.

## 19.3.6 Natural Products and Their Effects on Composition and Regulation of Gut Microbiota

Numerous studies of natural products and their interplay with human gut microbiota have been performed in recent years. A clinical study by Xu et al. with 187 T2D patients stated that a traditional Chinese herbal formula known as

Gegen Qinlian Decoction (GQD) reformed the gut with an augmented amount of beneficial bacteria such as *Faecalibacterium*, *Gemmiger*, *Bifidobacterium*, and *Escherichia*; fasting blood glucose levels as well as hemoglobin A1c (HbA1c) levels were ameliorated in patients treated with GQD (138). In another study by Song et al. it was demonstrated that water extract of *Ephedra sinica* Stapf decreased body weight and body mass index (BMI) in seven out of ten obese Korean women post treatment with this herb. Fascinatingly, a study also showed that the anti-obesity action of ginseng was found to be different when gut microbiota composition was modified. The profusion of species like *Subdoligranulum*, *Oscillibacter*, and *Akkermansia* in the gut was linked with changes in body weight and BMI, while *Lactobacillus* was connected to body fat percentage (139). A combination of herbal medicines (*Gwakhyangjeonggisan*, GJS) and probiotics (Duolac7S, DUO) have been shown to alleviate the symptoms of diarrhea-predominant irritable bowel syndrome (D-IBS) in a double-blind, randomized clinical trial comprising 54 patients, by altering the gut microbiota composition. It was demonstrated that intestinal microbes comprising *Bifidobacteriumbrevis*, *Bifidobacterium lactis*, *Streptococcus thermophilus*, *Lactobacillus rhamnosus*, *Lactobacillus plantarum*, and *Lactobacillus acidophilus* were synergistically augmented by a GJS-DUO combination, signifying the prospects that a combined treatment of herbal medicine and probiotics might deliver a favorable effect for clinical treatment of D-IBS (140, 141).

Likewise, a well-known traditional Chinese medicine, *Flos Lonicera*, has shown to regulate the tight junctions at cell-based level, reinstating the lipopolysaccharide(LPS)-induced side effects and also amplifying several microbiota that exerted positive effects on upholding the intestinal barrier integrity (142). In a study by Chelakkot et al., it has been established that *Akkermansia muciniphila* stimulated tight junction-related AMPK (AMP-activated protein kinase) signaling, especially in patients with obesity and T2D (143). In an alternative study, it was recommended that resveratrol diminished impairment in intestinal barrier and bacterial translocation induced by deoxynivalenol (DON) (144, 145). Ling et al. also stated that resveratrol exerted the mechanism by facilitation of claudin-4 expression responsible for building up the tight junction complex and resisting DON-induced barrier dysfunction (146). Altogether, these outcomes confirmed that natural products might exercise positive effects on the intestinal barrier by various mechanisms, important of which are upregulation of tight junction proteins, attenuating inflammation, and augmenting the probiotics abundance. Gut microbiota pathologies have been shown to amplify the LPS secretion, in that way executing sequences of metabolic diseases (147, 148). Nevertheless, natural products can directly or indirectly exert their role on microbiota to improve a condition.

## 19.4 Gut–Brain Axis Alteration in Old Patients: Clinical Perspectives

An extensively varied population of microbes, known as metaorganism (encompassing ten bacterial cells for every one of our own), are hosted by each human organism (149). These metaorganisms are studied exhaustively in foremost scientific endeavors for instance Human Microbiome Project (150), impact on its host on similar scale to human host changing it back during the course of different life stages. With age, microbial diversity and stability of intestinal microflora decrease (151, 152) with a decline in brain function and cognitive abilities (153, 154). Likewise, modification in gut microbiota homeostasis, by means of dietary or environmental factors, can cause disproportion between symbionts and pathobionts, ensuing abridged intestinal barrier function, like the state of dysbiosis, which leads to consequent metabolic and inflammatory disorders, and visceral pain, as well as modifications in brain functioning (155). There are studies that have revealed that change in the microbial composition of the gut with age is not a linear process, viz. dominant phyla, *Bacteroides* and *Firmicutes*, present in younger persons, remain conspicuous at older age too, however changes in the percentage of these phyla supposedly happen, yet, these points are still under discussion. On the other hand, some studies back the notion that the dominance of possibly pathogenic bacteria (viz. *Proteobacteria*), damaging to symbiotic beneficial bacteria (e.g., species of *Bifidobacteria*), might be responsible (156). There are a few studies that show extreme aging being reinforced by subdominant gut microbiota species, together with pro-inflammatory species and health-associated taxa (157). Alternate study was focused on gut microbiota and long-lived Chinese individuals, with a special reference to the abovementioned study. Age-related gut microbiota modifications are related to consequent weakening of functions of the immune system (immunosenescence) with age in addition to a chronic low-grade inflammatory state, partly owing to amplified intestinal permeability and cytokine expression (inflammaging) in the colon (158). The inflammaging process in turn destabilizes the homeostatic equilibrium and speeds up the alterations in the structure and composition of gut microbiota leading to advancement of diseases and fragility in the aging population (159). A study by Tran and Greenwood-Van Meerveld (2013) (160) demonstrated for the very first time that age-associated remodeling of intestinal epithelial tight junction proteins is the crucial causative factor for geriatric susceptibility to increased colonic permeability in gastrointestinal dysfunction. On the contrary, there is the latest study by Valentini et al. that found no association between aging and augmented intestinal permeability and/or changed intestinal barrier, but however, on the other hand declared low-grade inflammation as a potential factor (161). The homeostasis of gut microbiota appears to play a vital role in gut well-being during the course of the aging process. With this viewpoint, dietary control of the gut microbiota in the elderly might be an imperative goal for conserving a healthy gut microbiota community (159).

## 19.4.1 Nutraceuticals and Gut–Brain Axis Targeting in Clinical Trials

Direct modulation of the gut microbiome by means of targeted dietary and probiotic uptake signifies an encouraging therapeutic alternative for the aging process and may have a positive control in treating particular age-related disorders as well (152). Thriving confirmations have been obtained from the findings of a research consortium, ELDERMET (http://eldermet.ucc.ie) which deliberated and categorized gut microbiota in the Irish elderly population and its association to psychological health in aging (162). Owing to a rising body of evidence concerning a positive association between the gut microbiota health and brain health, much clinical research have initiated the study of gut–brain axis modulation and its effect on healthy aging and psychological health. Moreover, clinical trials have started to focus on its contribution in the hunger/satiety regulation and pathologies distressing the digestive tract in addition to targeting the cross talk between gut microbiota and the central nervous system and its association with several neuropsychiatric and neurodegenerative diseases (anxiety, depression, dementia, etc.). Dietary changes, use of prebiotics and probiotics, and fecal microbiota transplant have been found to be involved as therapeutic solutions probed in these clinical trials. Information from previously finished trials back the findings of preclinical trials, signifying that gut microbiota modulation results in anxiolytic effect without neurotransmitter circuitries being involved directly. For instance, outcomes of study by Schmidt et al. (163), posttrial completion, sustained preceding evidence that fructo-oligosaccharides, or Bimuno® galacto-oligosaccharides supplementation, dropped neuroendocrine stress response, which was measured by cortisol awakening response. In yet another study by Rao et al. (164), it was stated that anxiety scores of patients with chronic fatigue syndrome were improved when supplemented with specific lactic acid probiotic bacteria for 8 weeks. Multifaceted information in a study conducted by Messaoudi et al. (165), which involved both preclinical and clinical study, revealed beneficial psychological effect after supplementation with a *Lactobacillus helveticus* and *Bifidobacterium longum* combination. Lately, current publication about the outcome of a 4-week multispecies probiotics treatment exhibited considerably decreased overall cognitive reactivity to sad mood (166). The outcomes of these studies unclutter a favorable opportunity not only for age-related psychological disorders, but also for particular psychiatric pathologies.

Preclinical and *in vitro* studies have shown gluten-free bread to decrease the microbiota dysbiosis seen in people with gluten sensitivity or coeliac disease (167, 168). However, people who avoid gluten were found not to have coeliac disease or proved intolerance, besides a new large observational study has shown an amplified risk of heart disease in those who avoid gluten, possibly due to decreased ingestion of whole grains (169). A study demonstrated significantly different gut microbiota profiles in 21 healthy individuals after 4 weeks on a gluten-free diet. Most individuals presented minor abundance of many vital beneficial microbe species (170). Moreover, the low fermentable oligosaccharides, disaccharides, monosaccharides, and polyols (FODMAP) diet has demonstrated reduction in the symptoms of irritable bowel syndrome in six randomized controlled trials (171, 172), which was linked with a decreased fraction of *Bifidobacterium* in these patients and receptiveness to this diet could be foreseen by fecal bacterial profiles (173). Low FODMAP diets have shown to induce intense alterations in the microbiota and metabolome, though duration and clinical relevance are still unknown (174, 175). Apart from diet, medicines are also a significant modulator of the gut microbiota composition. A large Dutch-Belgian population study demonstrated that medications (including osmotic laxatives, progesterone, TNF-α inhibitors, and rupatadine) exhibit major explanatory power on microbiota composition with a 10% of community variation (176). A few studies have also displayed the major effects of some frequently prescribed proton pump inhibitors on the microbial community, which could justify higher rates of gastrointestinal infections in people consuming these drugs (177). In addition, antibiotics undoubtedly have an effect on gut microbes. Numerous observational studies in human have revealed obesogenic effects of antibiotics even in small doses (178). Nevertheless, humans have quite adaptable responses to antibiotics, and intervention studies did not show reliable metabolic consequences (179).

The clinical data is insufficient to draw strong inferences or endorsements for dietary preferences based on gut microbiota; nonetheless, upcoming studies of different drugs, nutraceuticals, and food additives, as well as the safety and efficacy of dietary modifications must consider the advances made by various studies to evaluate their effects on the gut microbiota. There are studies which have shown that minor changes in the microbiota in patients with cancer treated with immunochemotherapy, bone marrow recipients, and patients with autoimmune disorders on biologics produced major changes in their response (180).

## 19.5 Future Directions in Personalized Nutrition

Since variations are present in the gut microbiota between people, it is essential to tailor the optimal diet of a person to their gut microbiota. In a study by Zeevi et al., multidimensional microbiota profiles were acquired from 900 people and food intake, continuous blood glucose levels, and physical activity were supervised for one week; a machine learning algorithm developed to forecast personalized glucose responses post meals based on clinical and gut microbiome data revealed that it attained considerably greater prediction levels than carbohydrate counting or glycamic index score approaches. Personalized dietary interventions based on the algorithm were also found to successfully normalize blood glucose levels in a follow-up double-blinded randomized crossover trial in 26 participants (181). Another randomized cross-over trial study on response to 1 week-long dietary interventions, displayed substantial interpersonal inconsistency in the glycemic response to different bread types; bread types that induced a lesser glycemic response in each individual could be anticipated based exclusively on microbiome data collected prior to intervention (182). However, additional research is required to institute if these kinds of personalized approaches are really practical, maintainable, and have a positive effect on clinical outcomes.

## 19.6 Summary

An increased clinical and mechanistic indication on the entwined relations between nutrients and gut microbiota functional ecology exists. A close link between microbiota and most used nutraceuticals does exist at an extensive manner. There are nutraceuticals with real proven benefits on human health. In addition, microbiota imbalances have been found to be involved in many diseases, and may also increase their risk of appearance, consequently making it of quite grave concern to acquire an understanding of the chief nutraceuticals in use and institute the ways they might affect the composition of microbiota. Numerous nutraceuticals have proven to reinstate microbial homeostasis, decrease the negative effects of pathogenic microbes, regulate the inflammation pathway, and/or upsurge the efficacy of standard allopathic therapy.

## References

1. Sender R, Fuchs S, Milo R. Revised estimates for the number of human and bacteria cells in the body. *PLOS Biol* 2016; 14(8):e1002533–e1002533.
2. Schluter J, Peled JU, Taylor BP, et al. The gut microbiota is associated with immune cell dynamics in humans. *Nature* 2020; 588(7837):303–307.
3. Goodrich JK, Davenport ER, Waters JL, Clark AG, Ley RE. Cross-species comparisons of host genetic associations with the microbiome. *Science* 2016; 352(6285):532–535.
4. Kaoutari AE, Armougom F, Gordon JI, Raoult D, Henrissat B. The abundance and variety of carbohydrate-active enzymes in the human gut microbiota. *Nat Rev Microbiol* 2013; 11(7):497–504.
5. Smith PA. The tantalizing links between gut microbes and the brain. *Nature* 2015; 526(7573):312–314.
6. Sobhani I, Bergsten E, Couffin S, et al. Colorectal cancer-associated microbiota contributes to oncogenic epigenetic signatures. *Proc Natl Acad Sci U S A* 2019; 116(48):24285–24295.
7. Li Q, Chang Y, Zhang K, Chen H, Tao S, Zhang Z. Implication of the gut microbiome composition of type 2 diabetic patients from northern China. *Sci Rep* 2020; 10(1):5450.
8. Yeoh YK, Zuo T, Lui GC-Y, et al. Gut microbiota composition reflects disease severity and dysfunctional immune responses in patients with COVID-19. *Gut* 2021; 70(4):698–706.
9. Dominguez-Bello MG, Costello EK, Contreras M, et al. Delivery mode shapes the acquisition and structure of the initial microbiota across multiple body habitats in newborns. *Proc Natl Acad Sci U S A* 2010; 107(26):11971–11975.
10. O'Toole PW, Claesson MJ. Gut microbiota: Changes throughout the lifespan from infancy to elderly. *Int Dairy J* 2010; 20(4):281–291.
11. Das B, Ghosh TS, Kedia S, et al. Analysis of the gut microbiome of rural and urban healthy indians living in sea level and high altitude areas. *Sci Rep* 2018; 8(1):10104.
12. Priya S, Blekhman R. Population dynamics of the human gut microbiome: Change is the only constant. *Genome Biol* 2019; 20(1):150.
13. Montalto M, D'Onofrio F, Gallo A, Cazzato A, Gasbarrini G. Intestinal microbiota and its functions. *Dig Liver Dis Suppl* 2009; 3(2):30–34.
14. Woting A, Blaut M. The intestinal microbiota in metabolic disease. *Nutrients* 2016; 8(4):202.

15. Tang WHW, Hazen SL. The contributory role of gut microbiota in cardiovascular disease. *J Clin Invest* 2014; 124(10):4204–4211.
16. Kim JK, Strapazzon N, Gallaher CM, et al. Comparison of short- and long-term exposure effects of cruciferous and apiaceous vegetables on carcinogen metabolizing enzymes in Wistar rats. *Food Chem Toxicol* 2017; 108(A):194–202.
17. Veeranki OL, Bhattacharya A, Tang L, Marshall JR, Zhang Y. Cruciferous vegetables, isothiocyanates, and prevention of bladder cancer. *Curr Pharmacol Rep* 2015; 1(4):272–282.
18. Kaczmarek JL, Liu X, Charron CS, et al. Broccoli consumption affects the human gastrointestinal microbiota. *J Nutr Biochem* 2019; 63:27–34.
19. Angelino D, Dosz EB, Sun J, et al. Myrosinase-dependent and -independent formation and control of isothiocyanate products of glucosinolate hydrolysis. *Front Plant Sci* 2015; 6:831.
20. Bianchini F, Vainio H. Allium vegetables and organosulfur compounds: Do they help prevent cancer? *Environ Health Perspect* 2001; 109(9):893–902.
21. Pascale A, Marchesi N, Marelli C, et al. Microbiota and metabolic diseases. *Endocrine* 2018; 61(3):357–371.
22. O'Toole PW, Felmer B. Studying the microbiome: "Omics" made accessible. *Semin Liver Dis* 2016; 36:1–6.
23. Quigley EMM. Prebiotics and probiotics in digestive health. *Clin Gastroenterol Hepatol* 2019; 17(2):333–344.
24. Jandhyala SM, Talukdar R, Subramanyam C, Vuyyuru H, Sasikala M, Reddy DN. Role of the normal gut microbiota. *World J Gastroenterol* 2015; 21(29):8787–8803.
25. Den Besten G, Van Eunen K, Groen AK, Venema K, Reijngoud D-J, Bakker BM. The role of short-chain fatty acids in the interplay between diet, gut micro- biota, and host energy metabolism. *J Lipid Res* 2013; 54(9):2325–2340.
26. Louis P, Flint HJ. Formation of propionate and butyrate by the human colonic microbiota. *Environ Microbiol* 2017; 19(1):29–41.
27. Schwiertz A, Taras D, Schäfer K, et al. Microbiota and SCFA in lean and overweight healthy subjects. *Obesity (Silver Spring)* 2010; 18(1):190–195.
28. Tremaroli V, Bäckhed F. Functional interactions between the gut microbiota and host metabolism. *Nature* 2012; 489(7415):242–249.
29. Morrison DJ, Preston T. Formation of short chain fatty acids by the gut microbiota and their impact on human metabolism. *Gut Microbes* 2016; 7(3):189–200.
30. Li G, Young KD. Indole production by the tryptophanase TnaA in Escherichia coli is determined by the amount of exogenous tryptophan. *Microbiology (Reading)* 2013; 159(2):402–410.
31. Levy M, Blacher E, Elinav E. Microbiome, metabolites and host immunity. *Curr Opin Microbiol* 2017; 35:8–15.
32. Steinmeyer S, Lee K, Jayaraman A, Alaniz RC. Microbiota metabolite regulation of host immune homeostasis: A mechanistic missing link. *Curr Allergy Asthma Rep* 2015; 15(5):24.
33. Joseph J, Depp C, Shih PAB, Cadenhead KS, Schmid-Schönbein G. Modified Mediterranean diet for enrichment of short chain fatty acids: Potential adjunctive therapeutic to target immune and metabolic dysfunction in schizophrenia? *Front Neurosci* 2017; 11:155.
34. Alvarez-Curto E, Milligan G. Metabolism meets immunity: The role of free fatty acid receptors in the immune system. *Biochem Pharmacol* 2016; 114:3–13.
35. Weitkunat K, Stuhlmann C, Postel A, et al. Short-chain fatty acids and inulin, but not guar gum, prevent diet-induced obesity and insulin resistance through differential mechanisms in mice. *Sci Rep* 2017; 7(1):6109.
36. Zeng H, Taussig DP, Cheng WH, Johnson LAK, Hakkak R. Butyrate inhibits cancerous HCT116 colon cell proliferation but to a lesser extent in noncancerous NCM460 colon cells. *Nutrients* 2017; 9(1):25.

37. Huazano-Garcia A, Hakdong S, Lopez G. Modulation of gut microbiota of overweight mice by agavins and their association with body weight loss. *Nutrients* 2017; 23(9):821.
38. Park M, Kwon B, Ku S, Ji G. The efficacy of Bifidobacterium longum BORI and lactobacillus acidophilus AD031 probiotic treatment in infants with rotavirus infection. *Nutrients* 2017; 9(8):887.
39. Johnston BC, Goldenberg JZ, Vandvik PO, Sun X, Guyatt GH. Probiotics for the prevention of pediatric antibiotic-associated diarrhea. *Cochrane Database Syst Rev* 2011; 11(11):CD004827.
40. Bron PA, Kleerebezem M, Brummer R-J, et al. Can probiotics modulate human disease by impacting intestinal barrier function? *Br J Nutr* 2017; 117(1):93–107.
41. Sangwan V, Tomar SK, Singh RRB, Singh AK, Ali B. Galactooligosaccharides: Novel components of designer foods. *J Food Sci* 2011; 76(4):R103–111.
42. Vandenplas Y, Zakharova I, Dmitrieva Y. Oligosaccharides in infant formula: More evidence to validate the role of prebiotics. *Br J Nutr* 2015; 113(9):1339–1344.
43. Velasco C, Lozano MA, Moreno Y, et al. Effect of a mixture of inulin and fructo-oligosaccharide on lactobacillus and bifidobac-terium intestinal microbiota of patients receiving radiotherapy; a randomised, double-blind, placebo-controlled trial. *Nutr Hosp* 2012; 27(6):1908–1915.
44. Wang B, Wu G, Zhou Z, et al. Glutamine and intestinal barrier function. *Amino Acids* 2015; 47(10):2143–2154.
45. De Souza AZZ, Zambom AZ, Abboud KY, et al. Oral supplementation with l-glutamine alters gut microbiota of obese and overweight adults: A pilot study. *Nutrition* 2015; 31(6):884–889.
46. Beheshtipour H, Mortazavian AM, Mohammadi R, Sohrabvandi S, Khosravi-Darani K. Supplementation of Spirulina platensis and chlorella vulgaris algae into probiotic fermented milks. *Compr Rev Food Sci Food Saf* 2013; 12(2):144–154.
47. Finamore A, Palmery M, Bensehaila S, Peluso I. Antioxidant, immunomod- ulating, and microbial-modulating activities of the sustainable and eco-friendly Spirulina. *Oxid Med Cell Longev* 2017; 2017:3247528.
48. Bhowmik D, Dubey J, Mehra S. Probiotic efficiency of Spirulina platensis - Stimulating growth of lactic acid bacteria. *World J Dairy Food Sci* 2009; 4:160–163.
49. O'Keefe SJ, Li JV, Lahti L, et al. Fat, fibre and cancer risk in African Americans and rural Africans. *Nat Commun* 2015; 6:6342.
50. David LA, Maurice CF, Carmody RN, et al. Diet rapidly and reproducibly alters the human gut microbiome. *Nature* 2014; 505(7484):559–563.
51. Korem T, Zeevi D, Zmora N, et al. Bread affects clinical parameters and induces gut microbiome-associated personal glycemic responses. *Cell Metab* 2017; 25(6):1243–1253 e5.
52. Paganini D, Uyoga MA, Zimmermann MB. Iron fortification of foods for infants and children in low-income countries: Effects on the gut microbiome, gut inflammation, and diarrhea. *Nutrients* 2016; 8(8):E494.
53. Biesalski HK. Nutrition meets the microbiome: Micronutrients and the microbiota. *Ann N Y Acad Sci* 2016; 1372(1):53–64.
54. Cantorna MT, Snyder L, Arora J. Vitamin A and vitamin D regulate the microbial complexity, barrier function, and the mucosal immune responses to ensure intestinal homeostasis. *Crit Rev Biochem Mol Biol* 2019; 54(2):184–192.
55. Fletcher J, Cooper SC, Ghosh S, Hewison M. The role of vitamin D in inflammatory bowel disease: Mechanism to management. *Nutrients* 2019; 11(5):1019.
56. Yoshii K, Hosomi K, Sawane K, Kunisawa J. Metabolism of dietary and microbial vitamin B family in the regulation of host immunity. *Front Nutr* 2019; 6:48.
57. Zhu X, Xiang S, Feng X, et al. Impact of cyanocobalamin and methylcobalamin on inflammatory bowel disease and the intestinal microbiota composition. *J Agric Food Chem* 2019; 67(3):916–926.

58. Kali A, Bhuvaneshwar D, Charles PM, Seetha KS. Antibacterial synergy of curcumin with antibiotics against biofilm producing clinical bacterial isolates. *J Basic Clin Pharmacol* 2016; 7(3):93–96.
59. Roberfroid M. Prebiotics: The concept revisited. *J Nutr* 2007; 137:830S–837S.
60. Gibson GR, Probert HM, Loo JV, Rastall RA, Roberfroid MB. Dietary modulation of the human colonic microbiota: Updating the concept of prebiotics. *Nutr Res Rev* 2004; 17(2):259–275.
61. de Jesus Raposo MF, de Morais AM, de Morais RM. Emergent sources of prebiotics: Seaweeds and microalgae. *Mar Drugs* 2016; 14(2):27.
62. Day L, Gomez J, Oiseth SK, Gidley MJ, Williams BA. Faster fermentation of cooked carrot cell clusters compared to cell wall fragments in vitro by porcine feces. *J Agric Food Chem* 2012; 60(12):3282–3290.
63. Kristensen NB, Bryrup T, Allin KH, Nielsen T, Hansen TH, Pedersen O. Alterations in fecal microbiota composition by probiotic supplementation in healthy adults: A systematic review of randomized controlled trials. *Genome Med* 2016; 8(1):52.
64. Walter J, Maldonado-Gomez MX, Martinez I. To engraft or not to engraft: An ecological framework for gut microbiome modulation with live microbes. *Curr Opin Biotechnol* 2018; 49:129–139.
65. Chua KJ, Kwok WC, Aggarwal N, Sun T, Chang MW. Designer probiotics for the prevention and treatment of human diseases. *Curr Opin Chem Biol* 2017; 40:8–16.
66. Maldonado-Gomez MX, Martinez I, Bottacini F, et al. Stable engraftment of Bifidobacterium longum AH1206 in the human gut depends on individualized features of the resident microbiome. *Cell Host Microbe* 2016; 20(4):515–526.
67. Plovier H, Everard A, Druart C, et al. A purified membrane protein from Akkermansia muciniphila or the pasteurized bacterium improves metabolism in obese and diabetic mice. *Nat Med* 2017; 23(1):107–113.
68. Khalesi S, Bellissimo N, Vandelanotte C, Williams S, Stanley D, Irwin C. A review of probiotic supplementation in healthy adults: Helpful or hype? *Eur J Clin Nutr* 2019; 73(1):24–37.
69. Ford AC, Quigley EM, Lacy BE, et al. Efficacy of prebiotics, probiotics, and Synbiotics in irritable bowel syndrome and chronic idiopathic constipation: Systematic review and meta-analysis. *Am J Gastroenterol* 2014; 109(10):1547–1561.
70. Panigrahi P, Parida S, Nanda NC, et al. A randomized synbiotic trial to prevent sepsis among infants in rural India. *Nature* 2017; 548(7668):407–412.
71. Dong J, Teng G, Wei T, Gao W, Wang H. Methodological quality assessment of meta-analyses and systematic reviews of probiotics in inflammatory bowel disease and pouchitis. *PLOS ONE* 2016; 11(12):e0168785.
72. Jones JM. *CODEX*-aligned dietary fiber definitions help to bridge the 'fiber gap'. *Nutr J* 2014; 13:34.doi:10.1186/1475-2891-13-34.
73. Deehan EC, Duar RM, Armet AM, Perez-Munoz ME, Jin M, Walter J. Modulation of the gastrointestinal microbiome with nondigestible fermentable carbohydrates to Improve human health. *Microbiol Spectr* 2017; 5(5):1–24.
74. Bindels LB, Delzenne NM, Cani PD, Walter J. Towards a more comprehensive concept for prebiotics. *Nat Rev Gastroenterol Hepatol* 2015; 12(5):303–310.
75. Slavin JL. Dietary fiber and body weight. *Nutrition* 2005; 21(3):411 418
76. Deehan EC, Duar RM, Armet AM, Perez-Munoz ME, Jin M, Walter J. Modulation of the gastrointestinal microbiome with nondigestible fermentable carbohydrates to improve human health. *Microbiol Spectr* 2017; 5(5):1–24.
77. El Kaoutari A, Armougom F, Gordon JI, Raoult D, Henrissat B. The abundance and variety of carbohydrate-active enzymes in the human gut microbiota. *Nat Rev Microbiol* 2013; 11(7):497–504.
78. Holscher HD. Dietary fiber and prebiotics and the gastrointestinal microbiota. *Gut Microbes* 2017; 8(2):172–184.

79. Van Rymenant E, Abranko L, Tumova S, et al. Chronic exposure to short-chain fatty acids modulates transport and metabolism of microbiome-derived phenolics in human intestinal cells. *J Nutr Biochem* 2017; 39:156–168.
80. Schulthess J, Pandey S, Capitani M, et al. The short chain fatty acid butyrate imprints an antimicrobial program in macrophages. *Immunity* 2019; 50(2):432–445.
81. Desai MS, Seekatz AM, Koropatkin NM, et al. A dietary fiber-deprived gut microbiota degrades the colonic mucus barrier and enhances pathogen susceptibility. *Cell* 2016; 167(5):1339–1353.
82. Delcour JA, Aman P, Courtin CM, Hamaker BR, Verbeke K. Prebiotics, fermentable dietary fiber, and health claims. *Adv Nutr* 2016; 7(1):1–4.
83. Bang SJ, Kim G, Lim MY, et al. The influence of in vitro pectin fermentation on the human fecal microbiome. *AMB Express* 2018; 8(1):98.
84. Whelan K, Schneider SM. Mechanisms, prevention, and management of diarrhea in enteral nutrition. *Curr Opin Gastroenterol* 2011; 27(2):152–159.
85. O'Keefe SJ, Ou J, Delany JP, et al. Effect of fiber supplementation on the microbiota in critically ill patients. *World J Gastrointest Pathophysiol* 2011; 2(6):138–145.
86. Venkataraman A, Sieber JR, Schmidt AW, Waldron C, Theis KR, Schmidt TM. Variable responses of human microbiomes to dietary supplementation with resistant starch. *Microbiome* 2016; 4(1):33.
87. Martinez I, Kim J, Duffy PR, Schlegel VL, Walter J. Resistant starches types 2 and 4 have differential effects on the composition of the fecal microbiota in human subjects. *PLOS ONE* 2010; 5(11):e15046.
88. Koropatkin NM, Cameron EA, Martens EC. How glycan metabolism shapes the human gut microbiota. *Nat Rev Microbiol* 2012; 10(5):323–335.
89. Walker AW, Ince J, Duncan SH, et al. Dominant and diet-responsive groups of bacteria within the human colonic microbiota. *ISME J* 2011; 5(2):220–230.
90. Zhao L, Zhang F, Ding X, et al. Gut bacteria selectively promoted by dietary fibers alleviate type 2 diabetes. *Science* 2018; 359(6380):1151–1156.
91. David LA, Maurice CF, Carmody RN, et al. Diet rapidly and reproducibly alters the human gut microbiome. *Nature* 2014; 505(7484):559–563.
92. Cummings JH, Macfarlane GT. The control and consequences of bacterial fermentation in the human colon. *J Appl Bacteriol* 1991; 70(6):443–459.
93. Russell WR, Gratz SW, Duncan SH, et al. High-protein, reduced-carbohydrate weight-loss diets promote metabolite profiles likely to be detrimental to colonic health. *Am J Clin Nutr* 2011; 93(5):1062–1072.
94. Duncan SH, Belenguer A, Holtrop G, Johnstone AM, Flint HJ, Lobley GE. Reduced dietary intake of carbohydrates by obese subjects results in decreased concentrations of butyrate and butyrate-producing bacteria in feces. *Appl Environ Microbiol* 2007; 73(4):1073–1078.
95. Desai MS, Seekatz AM, Koropatkin NM, et al. A dietary fiber-deprived gut microbiota degrades the colonic mucus barrier and enhances pathogen susceptibility. *Cell* 2016; 167(5):1339–1353.e21.
96. Earle KA, Billings G, Sigal M, et al. Quantitative imaging of gut microbiota spatial organization. *Cell Host Microbe* 2015; 18(4):478–488.
97. Zou J, Chassaing B, Singh V, et al. Fiber-mediated nourishment of gut microbiota protects against diet-induced obesity by restoring IL-22-mediated colonic health. *Cell Host Microbe* 2018; 23(1):41–53.e4.
98. Schroeder BO, Birchenough GMH, Stahlman M, et al. Bifidobacteria or fiber protects against diet-induced microbiota-mediated colonic mucus deterioration. *Cell Host Microbe* 2018; 23(1):27–40.e7.
99. Ray K. Gut microbiota: Filling up on fibre for a healthy gut. *Nat Rev Gastroenterol Hepatol* 2018; 15(2):67.
100. Veronese N, Solmi M, Caruso MG, et al. Dietary fiber and health outcomes: An umbrella review of systematic reviews and meta-analyses. *Am J Clin Nutr* 2018; 107(3):436–444.

101. Thompson SV, Hannon BA, An R, Holscher HD. Effects of isolated soluble fiber supplementation on body weight, glycemia, and insulinemia in adults with overweight and obesity: A systematic review and meta-analysis of randomized controlled trials. *Am J Clin Nutr* 2017; 106(6):1514–1528.
102. Kootte RS, Levin E, Salojarvi J, et al. Improvement of insulin sensitivity after lean donor feces in metabolic syndrome is driven by baseline intestinal microbiota composition. *Cell Metab* 2017; 26(4):611–619.e6.
103. Saura-Calixto F, Serrano J, Goni I. Intake and bioaccessibility of total polyphenols in a whole diet. *Food Chem* 2007; 101(2):492–501.
104. Hung LM, Chen JK, Huang SS, Lee RS, Su MJ. Cardioprotective effect of resveratrol, a natural antioxidant derived from grapes. *Cardiovasc Res* 2000; 47(3):549–555.
105. Cassidy A. Berry anthocyanin intake and cardiovascular health. *Mol Aspects Med* 2018; 61:76–82.
106. Kazuhiko Uchiyama YN, Hasegawa G, Nakamura N, Takahashi J, Yoshikawa T. Astaxanthin protects β-cells against glucose toxicity in diabetic db/db mice. *Redox Rep* 2013; 7:290–293.
107. Gu J, Thomas-Ahner JM, Riedl KM, et al. Dietary black raspberries impact the colonic microbiome and phytochemical metabolites in mice. *Mol Nutr Food Res* 2019; 63(8):e1800636.
108. Wankhade UD, Zhong Y, Lazarenko OP, et al. Sex-specific changes in gut microbiome composition following blueberry consumption in C57BL/6J mice. *Nutrients* 2019; 11(2):313.
109. Gyawali R, Ibrahim SA. Impact of plant derivatives on the growth of foodborne pathogens and the functionality of probiotics. *Appl Microbiol Biotechnol* 2012; 95(1):29–45.
110. Brown DG, Borresen EC, Brown RJ, Ryan EP. Heat-stabilised rice bran consumption by colorectal cancer survivors modulates stool metabolite profiles and metabolic networks: A randomised controlled trial. *Br J Nutr* 2017; 117(9):1244–1256.
111. Cassidy A, Minihane AM. The role of metabolism (and the microbiome) in defining the clinical efficacy of dietary flavonoids. *Am J Clin Nutr* 2017; 105(1):10–22.
112. Iranshahi M, Rezaee R, Parhiz H, Roohbakhsh A, Soltani F. Protective effects of flavonoids against microbes and toxins: The cases of hesperidin and hesperetin. *Life Sci* 2015; 137:125–132.
113. Vitale DC, Piazza C, Melilli B, Drago F, Salomone S. Isoflavones: Estrogenic activity, biological effect and bioavailability. *Eur J Drug Metab Pharmacokinet* 2013; 38(1):15–25.
114. Franke AA, Lai JF, Halm BM, States U. Absorption, distribution, metabolism, and excretion of isoflavonoids after soy intake. *Arch Biochem Biophys* 2014; 559:24–28.
115. Guadamuro L, Dohrmann AB, Tebbe CC, Mayo B, Delgado S. Bacterial communities and metabolic activity of faecal cultures from equol producer and non-producer menopausal women under treatment with soy isoflavones. *BMC Microbiol* 2017; 17(1):93.
116. Gaya P, Medina M, Sánchez-Jiménez A, Landete J. Phytoestrogen metabolism by adult human gut microbiota. *Molecules* 2016; 21(8):1034.
117. Ozdal T, Sela DA, Xiao J, Boyacioglu D, Chen F, Capanoglu E. The reciprocal interactions between polyphenols and gut microbiota and effects on bioaccessibility. *Nutrients* 2016; 8(2):78.
118. Lee HC, Jenner AM, Low CS, Lee YK. Effect of tea phenolics and their aromatic fecal bacterial metabolites on intestinal microbiota. *Res Microbiol* 2006; 157(9):876–884.
119. Oz HS, Chen T, De Villiers WJS. Green tea polyphenols and sulfasalazine have parallel anti-inflammatory properties in colitis models. *Front Immunol* 2013; 4:132.
120. Van DJ, Vaughan EE, Van DF, et al. Interactions of black tea polyphenols with human gut microbiota: Implications for gut and cardiovascular health. *Am J Clin Nutr* 2013; 98(Suppl 6):1631S–1641S.

121. Bonnefont-Rousselot D. Resveratrol and cardiovascular diseases. *Nutrients* 2016; 8(5):1–24.
122. Qiao Y, Sun J, Xia S, Tang X, Shi Y, Le G. Effects of resveratrol on gut microbiota and fat storage in a mouse model with high-fat-induced obesity. *Food Funct* 2014; 5(6):1241–1249.
123. Djuric Z, Bassis CM, Plegue MA, et al. Colonic mucosal bacteria are associated with inter-individual variability in serum carotenoid concentrations. *J Acad Nutr Diet* 2018; 118(4):606–616.
124. Pascale A, Marchesi N, Marelli C, et al. Microbiota and metabolic diseases. *Endocrine* 2018; 61(3):357–371.
125. Nagy-Szakal D, Ross MC, Dowd SE, et al. Maternal micronutrients can modify colonic mucosal microbiota maturation in murine offspring. *Gut Microbes* 2012; 3(5):426–433.
126. Dicks LMT, Geldenhuys J, Mikkelsen LS, Brandsborg E, Marcotte H. Our gut microbiota: A long walk to homeostasis. *Benef Microbes* 2018; 9(1):3–20.
127. Ryan PM, Ross RP, Fitzgerald GF, Caplice NM, Stanton C. Sugarcoated: Exopolysaccharide producing lactic acid bacteria for food and human health applications. *Food Funct* 2015; 6(3):679–693.
128. Rowland I, Gibson G, Heinken A, et al. Gut microbiota functions: Metabolism of nutrients and other food components. *Eur J Nutr* 2018; 57(1):1–24.
129. Jones ML, Martoni CJ, Prakash S. Oral supplementation with probiotic L. reuteri NCIMB 30242 increases mean circulating 25-hydroxyvitamin D: A post hoc analysis of a randomized controlled trial. *J Clin Endocrinol Metab* 2013; 98(7):2944–2951.
130. Ostadmohammadi V, Jamilian M, Bahmani F, Asemi Z. Vitamin D and probiotic co-supplementation affects mental health, hormonal, inflammatory and oxidative stress parameters in women with polycystic ovary syndrome. *J Ovarian Res* 2019; 12(1):5.
131. Ghaderi A, Banafshe HR, Mirhosseini N, et al. Clinical and metabolic response to vitamin D plus probiotic in schizophrenia patients. *BMC Psychiatry* 2019; 19(1):77.
132. Raygan F, Ostadmohammadi V, Bahmani F, Asemi Z. The effects of vitamin D and probiotic co-supplementation on mental health parameters and metabolic status in type 2 diabetic patients with coronary heart disease: A randomized, double-blind, placebocontrolled trial. *Prog Neuropsychopharmacol Biol Psychiatry* 2018; 84(Pt A):50–55.
133. Jamilian M, Amirani E, Asemi Z. The effects of vitamin D and probiotic co-supplementation on glucose homeostasis, inflammation, oxidative stress and pregnancy outcomes in gestational diabetes: A randomized, double-blind, placebo-controlled trial. *Clin Nutr* 2019; 38(5):2098–2105.
134. Galli F, Battistoni A, Gambari R, et al. Oxidative stress and antioxidant therapy in cystic fibrosis. *Biochim Biophys Acta* 2012; 1822(5):690–713.
135. Kanhere M, He J, Chassaing B, et al. Bolus weekly vitamin D3 supplementation impacts gut and airway microbiota in adults with cystic fibrosis: A double-blind, randomized, placebo-controlled clinical trial. *J Clin Endocrinol Metab* 2018; 103(2):564–574.
136. Kobyliak N, Abenavoli L, Falalyeyeva T, et al. Beneficial effects of probiotic combination with omega-3 fatty acids in NAFLD: A randomized clinical study. *Minerva Med* 2018; 109(6):418–428.
137. Golkhalkhali B, Rajandram R, Paliany AS, et al. Strain-specific probiotic (microbial cell preparation) and omega-3 fatty acid in modulating quality of life and inflammatory markers in colorectal cancer patients: A randomized controlled trial. *Asia Pac J Clin Oncol* 2018; 14(3):179–191.
138. Xu J, Lian F, Zhao L, et al. Structural modulation of gut microbiota during alleviation of type 2 diabetes with a Chinese herbal formula. *ISME J* 2015; 9(3):552–562.
139. Song MY, Kim BS, Kim H. Influence of panax ginseng on obesity and gut microbiota in obese middle-aged Korean women. *J Ginseng Res* 2014; 38(2):106–115.

140. Ko SJ, Han G, Kim SK, et al. Effect of Korean herbal medicine combined with a probiotic mixture on diarrhea-dominant irritable bowel syndrome: A double-blind, randomized, placebo-controlled trial. *Evid Based Complement Alternat Med* 2013; 2013:824605.

141. Ko S-J, Ryu B, Kim J, et al. Effect of herbal extract granules combined with probiotic mixture on irritable bowel syndrome with diarrhea: Study protocol for a randomized controlled trial. *Trials* 2011; 12:219.

142. Wang J-H, Bose S, Kim G-C, et al. Flos Lonicera ameliorates obesity and associated endotoxemia in rats through modulation of gut permeability and intestinal micro-biota. *PLOS ONE* 2014; 9(1):e86117.

143. Chelakkot C, Choi Y, Kim D, et al. Akkermansiamuciniphiladerived extracellular vesi-cles influence gut permeability through the regulation of tight junctions. *Exp Mol Med* 2018; 50(2):e450.

144. Pinton P, Braicu C, Nougayrede J, Laffitte J, Taranu I, Oswald IP. Deoxynivalenol impairs porcine intestinal barrier function and decreases the protein expression of claudin-4 through a mitogen-activated protein kinase-dependent mechanism. *J Nutr* 2010; 140(11):1956–1962.

145. Raj P, Zieroth S, Netticadan T. An overviewof the efficacy of resveratrol in the man-agement of ischemic heart disease. *Ann N Y Acad Sci* 2015; 1348(1):55–67.

146. Chong E, Chang S-L, Hsiao Y-W, et al. Resveratrol, a red wine antioxidant, reduces atrial fibrillation susceptibility in the failing heart by PI3K/AKT/eNOS signaling path-way activation. *Heart Rhythm* 2015; 12(5):1046–1056.

147. Cani PD, Amar J, Iglesias MA, et al. Metabolic endotoxemia initiates obesity and insu-lin resistance. *Diabetes* 2007; 56(7):1761–1772.

148. Boulange CL, Neves AL, Chilloux J, Nicholson JK, Dumas ME. Impact of the gut microbiota on inflammation, obesity, and metabolic disease. *Genome Med* 2016; 8(1):42.

149. Heintz C, Mair W. You are what you host: Microbiome modulation of the aging pro-cess. *Cell* 2014; 156(3):408–411.

150. Cho I, Yamanishi S, Cox L, et al. Antibiotics in early life alter the murine colonic microbiome and adiposity. *Nature* 2012; 488(7413):621–626.

151. Saraswati S, Sitaraman R. Aging and the human gut microbiota from correlation to causality. *Front Microbiol* 2015; 5:1–4.

152. Vaiserman AM, Koliada AK, Marotta F. Gut microbiota: A player in aging and a target for anti-aging intervention. *Ageing Res Rev* 2017; 35:36–45.

153. Borre YE, O'Keeffe GW, Clarke G, Stanton C, Dinan TG, Cryan JF. Microbiota and neurodevelopmental windows: Implications for brain disorders. *Trends Mol Med* 2014; 20(9):509–518.

154. Flint HJ, O'Toole PW, Walker AW. Special issue: The human intestinal microbiota. *Microbiology (Reading)* 2010; 156(Pt 11):3203–3204.

155. Oriach CS, Robertson RC, Stanton C, Cryan JF, Dinan TG. Food for thought: The role of nutrition in the microbiota-gut-brain axis. *Clin Nutr Exp* 2016; 6:25–38.

156. Caracciolo B, Xu W, Collins S, Fratiglioni L. Cognitive decline, dietary factors and gutbrain interactions. *Mech Ageing Dev* 2014; 136–137:59–69.

157. Biagi E, Franceschi C, Rampelli S, et al. Gut microbiota and extreme longevity. *Curr Biol* 2016; 26(11):1480–1485.

158. Franceschi C, Bonafe M, Valensin S, et al. Inflamm-aging: An evolutionary perspec-tive on immunosenescence. *Ann N Y Acad Sci* 2000; 908:244–254.

159. Biagi E, Nylund L, Candela M, et al. Through ageing, and beyond: Gut microbiota and inflammatory status in seniors and centenarians. *PLOS ONE* 2010; 5(5):e10667.

160. Tran L, Greenwood-Van Meerveld B. Age-associated remodeling of the intestinal epi-thelial barrier. *J Gerontol A Biol Sci Med Sci* 2013; 68(9):1045–1056.

161. Valentini L, Ramminger S, Haas V, et al. Small intestinal permeability in older adults. *Physiol Rep* 2014; 2(4):e00281–e00281.

162. Claesson MJ, Jeffery IB, Conde S, et al. Gut microbiota composition correlates with diet and health in the elderly. *Nature* 2012; 488(7410):178–184.
163. Schmidt K, Cowen PJ, Harmer CJ, Tzortzis G, Errington S, Burnet PW. Prebiotic intake reduces the waking cortisol response and alters emotional bias in healthy volunteers. *Psychopharmacol (Berl)* 2015; 232(10):1793–1801.
164. Rao AV, Bested AC, Beaulne TM, et al. A randomized, doubleblind, placebo-controlled pilot study of a probiotic in emotional symptoms of chronic fatigue syndrome. *Gut Pathog* 2009; 1(1):6.
165. Messaoudi M, Lalonde R, Violle N, et al. Assessment of psychotropic- like properties of a probiotic formulation (Lactobacillus helveticus R0052 and Bifidobacterium longum R0175) in rats and human subjects. *Br J Nutr* 2011; 105(5):755–764.
166. Steenbergen L, Sellaro R, van Hemert S, Bosch JA, Colzato LS. A randomized controlled trial to test the effect of multispecies probiotics on cognitive reactivity to sad mood. *Brain Behav Immun* 2015; 48:258–264.
167. Mohan M, Chow CT, Ryan CN, et al. Dietary gluten-induced gut dysbiosis is accompanied by selective upregulation of microRNAs with intestinal tight junction and bacteria-binding motifs in rhesus macaque model of celiac disease. *Nutrients* 2016; 8(11):8.
168. Bevilacqua A, Costabile A, Bergillos-Meca T, et al. Impact of gluten-friendly bread on the metabolism and function of in vitro gut microbiota in healthy human and coeliac subjects. *PLOS ONE* 2016; 11(9):e0162770.
169. Lebwohl B, Cao Y, Zong G, et al. Long term gluten consumption in adults without celiac disease and risk of coronary heart disease: Prospective cohort study. *BMJ* 2017; 357:j1892.
170. Bonder MJ, Tigchelaar EF, Cai X, et al. The influence of a short-term gluten-free diet on the human gut microbiome. *Genome Med* 2016; 8(1):45.
171. Halmos EP. When the low FODMAP diet does not work. *J Gastroenterol Hepatol* 2017; 32(Suppl 1):69–72.
172. Gibson PR. The evidence base for efficacy of the low FODMAP diet in irritable bowel syndrome: Is it ready for prime time as a first-line therapy? *J Gastroenterol Hepatol* 2017; 32(Suppl 1):32–35.
173. Bennet SMP, Bohn L, Storsrud S, et al. Multivariate modelling of faecal bacterial profiles of patients with IBS predicts responsiveness to a diet low in FODMAPs. *Gut* 2018; 67(5):872–881.
174. McIntosh K, Reed DE, Schneider T, et al. FODMAPs alter symptoms and the metabolome of patients with IBS: A randomised controlled trial. *Gut* 2017; 66(7):1241–1251.
175. Staudacher HM, Whelan K. The low FODMAP diet: Recent advances in understanding its mechanisms and efficacy in IBS. *Gut* 2017; 66(8):1517–1527.
176. Falony G, Joossens M, Vieira-Silva S, et al. Population level analysis of gut microbiome variation. *Science* 2016; 352(6285):560–564.
177. Jackson MA, Goodrich JK, Maxan ME, et al. Proton pump inhibitors alter the composition of the gut microbiota. *Gut* 2016; 65(5):749–756.
178. Blaser MJ. Antibiotic use and its consequences for the normal microbiome. *Science* 2016; 352(6285):544–545.
179. Reijnders D, Goossens GH, Hermes GD, et al. Effects of gut microbiota manipulation by antibiotics on host metabolism in obese humans: A randomized double-blind placebo-controlled trial. *Cell Metab* 2016; 24(1):63–74.
180. Alexander JL, Wilson ID, Teare J, Marchesi JR, Nicholson JK, Kinross JM. Gut microbiota modulation of chemotherapy efficacy and toxicity. *Nat Rev Gastroenterol Hepatol* 2017; 14(6):356–365.
181. Zeevi D, Korem T, Zmora N, et al. Personalized nutrition by prediction of glycemic responses. *Cell* 2015; 163(5):1079–1094.
182. Korem T, Zeevi D, Zmora N, et al. Bread affects clinical parameters and induces gut microbiome-associated personal glycemic responses. *Cell Metab* 2017; 25(6):1243–1253.

# 20

# Manipulation of Gut Microbiome to Improve Mental Health

Sathya Amarasena and Shyamchand Mayengbam

## Contents

## 20.1 Introduction

The human gut microbiome is a complex and dynamic ecosystem composed of various microorganisms, including bacteria, viruses, fungi, and archaea, that reside in the gastrointestinal tract.[1] It consists of $10^{14}$ bacterial cells and plays a vital role in a multitude of physiological reactions of the host, such as metabolism, immunity, gastrointestinal health, and neurological functions.[2,3] It does so by providing energy, vitamins, hormones, neurotransmitters, and neuroactive compounds to the host.[3] The advancement of next-generation sequencing (NGS) and high-throughput mass spectrometry technologies has dramatically

DOI: 10.1201/9781003333821-20

improved our ability to characterize gut microbes and their metabolites, understand their functional roles, and investigate their interactions with host physiology. NGS such as 16S ribosomal ribonucleic acid (rRNA) sequencing is commonly used for characterizing microbial communities, while metagenomics sequencing aims to not only understand the diversity of the community but also their functions.[4] These cutting-edge technologies, in conjunction with large cohort studies, have led to better understanding of the function roles of microbes and their interactions with the host physiology. This has resulted in the discovery of new microbial species, characterization of their genomes, and analysis of their roles on host neurological functions.[4]

The gut microbiota is an essential component of the gastrointestinal tract and has been implicated in a wide range of physiological processes, including gut–brain interaction.[5] When mice were exposed to acute stress following an infection with pathogenic bacteria, they developed memory dysfunction.[6] The use of germ-free (GF) mice, which are raised in a microbe-free environment, has allowed for a deeper understanding of the role of the gut microbiota in regulating host physiology. Studies conducted on GF mice have demonstrated that the gut microbiota plays a critical role in the gut–brain signaling by producing various neurotransmitters and neuroactive compounds that modulate the immune and nervous systems.[7] Furthermore, additional studies have also indicated that the gut microbiota influences stress responsiveness anxiety-like behaviors, sociability, and cognition, highlighting the importance of the gut–brain axis in the regulation of mental well-being.[7,8] The impact of gut microbiota on the central nervous system (CNS) and mental behaviors has been investigated using various experimental approaches, including the use of antibiotics and probiotics, as well as fecal microbiota transplantation. For instance, treatment with antibiotics has been shown to alter gut microbial profiles and induce changes in anxiety-like behavior in mice[9] which can be improved through the use of certain probiotics.[10,11] Similarly, fecal microbiota transplantation of depression-related microbes to rodents caused depressive behavior to the recipients.[12] These findings clearly demonstrate the vital role of gut microbiota in modulating CNS and mental behavior.

## 20.2 Microbiota–Gut–Brain Interplay

Every individual harbors thousands of genes, billions of neurons, and trillions of microbes that work together in a highly interwoven manner. A growing body of evidence suggests a crucial link between the gut microbiome and the development and functioning of the CNS.[13] The gut is connected with the CNS via the vagus nerve and is innervated with the enteric nervous system (ENS), creating a bidirectional link between the gut and the CNS.[14] Researchers have identified multiple pathways of communication along the gut–brain axis, which comprises the central nervous system, the enteric nervous system, the autonomic nervous system (sympathetic and parasympathetic branches), and neuroendocrine and neuroimmune pathways.[15,16] There are also several mechanisms that explain the influence of gut microbiota on the nervous system, such as altering the activity of the stress-related hypothalamic-pituitary-adrenal (HPA) axis, stimulation of the vagal nerve, activation of microglial cells, and increased permeability of the blood-brain barrier by secreting neurotransmitters and microbial metabolites.[17] This expands the concept into the microbiota-gut–brain axis, which refers to the connection between an individual's gut and mental health through the involvement of gut microbiome.[18-22] The relationship between the gut microbiota and mental health is still being explored. It involves interactions among the CNS, endocrine signaling system, immune regulation, microbiota, metabolic effects, and barrier functions. The homeostasis of these factors plays a crucial role in maintaining an individual's overall health, including mental well-being.[23]

In the microbiota-gut–brain axis, the roles played by microbes, gut hormones, neurotransmitters, microbial metabolites, and pro-inflammatory compounds produced in the gut are crucial.[24] They regulate several physiological processes, including mood, behavior, and overall mental health. This coordination between the gut and neuronal systems can be altered by various factors, including the ability of gut microbes to synthesize and degrade neurotransmitters and neuroactive compounds.[25] These substances can have an impact on the structure and function of the brain, thereby affecting emotions, cognition, and physical activity.[26,27] The gut microbiome has been found to produce or consume a range of mammalian neurotransmitters, such as dopamine, norepinephrine, epinephrine, and serotonin, and gamma-aminobutyric acid (GABA), short-chain fatty acids (SCFAs), and their precursors.[17,28] Additionally, gut microbes also synthesize hormones and other peptides such as histamine and steroids, and neuropeptides, gasotransmitters, and endocannabinoids.[17] These microbially derived neurotransmitters or neuroactive molecules can stimulate the enteric nervous system and brain via the vagus nerve and immune pathways, leading to local neural signaling.[29-31] SCFAs are one of the most abundant metabolites in the colon and act though G-protein-coupled receptors to initiate cell signaling.[29] They are also natural histone deacetylase inhibitors and therefore increase gene expression.[13] Further, gut microbes can affect the host's amino acid metabolism,[32-35] leading to alterations in levels of amino acids that can impact neurotransmitter levels, such as glutamine, serine, threonine, tryptophan, kynurenine, and tyrosine.[33,34] Microbes can also metabolize bile acids and their metabolites, which may have both beneficial and harmful effects.[13]

## 20.3 Mental Health Disorders and Their Prevalence

Mental health disorder is a complex phenomenon that can negatively impact individuals by disrupting their daily functioning and hindering their ability to fulfill social roles.[36] The development of mental health problems is influenced by a variety of factors, such as social, economic, and physical environments.[37]

Mental health should not be seen solely as an individual issue but rather in relation to its impact on society as a whole.[38] The World Health Organization defines mental health as a state of well-being in which the individual realizes his or her own abilities, can cope with the normal stresses of life, can work productively and fruitfully, and is able to make a contribution to his or her community.[39] A positive approach to mental health emphasizes the importance of feeling good while preventing and treating the disorders.[40] Modern clinical practices, especially in the field of psychiatry, have placed a strong emphasis on positive mental health and its importance in treating mental health disorders.

Mental health problems are a widespread issue that greatly impacts global health.[41] In the period of 1980–2013, approximately 17.6% of adults worldwide were diagnosed with a mental disorder.[42] A significant proportion of adults (29.2%) have experienced a common mental disorder at some point in their lives.[42] There is a notable gender effect in the prevalence of mental disorders, with women having higher rates of mood and anxiety disorders, while men are more likely to experience substance use disorders.[42] The prevalence of mental disorders varies among different groups, such as children, adolescents, young adults, older adults, women, pregnant women, and men, and is influenced by factors such as life experiences, dietary habits, and presence of other diseases.[43-46] According to a meta-analysis published in 2015, the worldwide prevalence of mental disorders among children and adolescents is 13.4%, with anxiety disorders accounting for 6.5% and depression accounting for 2.6%.[47] Diseases such as Alzheimer's disease and autism spectrum disorder (ASD) have become more prevalent and pose significant health challenges with the number of people living with ASD projected to reach 74.7 million in 2030 and reach 131.5 million in 2050.[48,49] The prevalence of mental health problem also varies across different regions, with lower rates in North and Southeast Asian and sub-Saharan African countries compared to Western countries.[42] In Canada, a study comparing the interprovincial prevalence of mental disorders found that Manitoba had the highest incidence, with 13.6% of the population affected, including a high incidence of major depressive disorder (7.0%) and alcohol use disorder (3.8%), while Quebec (8.5%) and Prince Edward Island (7.7%) had the lowest prevalence of mental disorders.[50] Another study of seven provinces in Canada found that the combined prevalence of ASD among children and youth aged 5–17 was 1 in 66 in 2015.[51]

Mental health issues pose a significant challenge in the healthcare system. In 2013, Canada spent approximately $6.75 billion on mental health, making up about 5% of total health expenditure.[52] The increasing prevalence of disorders such as ASD has also added to the economic burden. In the United States, it was estimated that supporting an individual with ASD would cost $2.4 million in 2013, with a projected total cost of $461 billion in 2025, taking into account both direct medical and on medical expenses, as well as the loss of productivity.[53] The United Kingdom estimated the lifetime cost of supporting an individual with ASD to be $2.2 million in 2013.[54] Thus the financial burden of mental health disorders is substantial and not limited to Western countries alone, but extends to the rest of the world as well.[55,56]

## 20.4  Gut Microbial Dynamics and Mental Health

The composition and diversity of the gut microbiome vary among individuals and are influenced by several factors, including diet, lifestyle, genetics, and the use of antibiotics.[57] These variations have a significant impact on an individual's physiological and psychological state. Diet plays a crucial role in shaping the gut microbiome and is estimated to account for 20% of the variability in humans.[58] It is known that the species- and family-level microbial composition can change rapidly within 24 to 48 hours of dietary intervention, although phyla-level changes do not occur.[59] For example, a diet rich in fiber and fermented foods can promote a healthy gut microbiome, while a diet high in processed foods, sugar, and animal products can favor the growth of harmful microbes.[57] However, short-term dietary interventions temporarily affect microbial diversity and do not persist over extended periods,[60] indicating that long-term dietary patterns and habits are essential for establishing a stable gut microbiota.

Besides diet, the gut microbiome is shaped by a combination of external factors such as lifestyle, including stress, sleep, and physical activity, and internal factors such as host genetics, immune function, and metabolic regulations.[58] Chronic stress has been shown to negatively impact the diversity and stability of the gut microbiome, while physical activity has a positive effect, not only on diversity, but also on gut permeability. The composition and function of the gut microbiota are also believed to be influenced by the circadian rhythm, resulting at least 10% of operational taxonomic units in humans to oscillate.[57] Genetics has a lesser effect on the gut microbiome, with an average of 8.8% according to data collected from 1,126 twins.[61] The use of antibiotics can significantly alter the composition and diversity of the gut microbiome, most likely by the overgrowth of harmful bacteria and a decrease in beneficial bacteria.[62] Thus, the gut microbiota composition is highly personalized and shaped throughout one's lifetime.[60]

The relationship between the gut microbiome and mental well-being is extremely intricate and interdependent. Recent studies have highlighted the potential association between gut microbial imbalance and neurological diseases.[63–65] Gut dysbiosis, characterized by an imbalance in the gut microbial composition or reduced microbial diversity, has been documented to be associated with several diseases including mental health disorders and chronic fatigue.[16,66] The imbalance can occur due to the loss of beneficial bacteria, a decrease in overall diversity, or overgrowth of potentially pathogenic bacteria.[67] Modulating gut microbiota is being considered as a promising treatment option for various metabolic diseases and related CNS disorders.[16,68,69] Cross-sectional human studies have increasingly shown a correlation between changes in microbial diversity, microbial metabolites, and a wide range of neurological and psychiatric disorders, including Parkinson's disease, Alzheimer's disease, ASD, and depression.[70]

Both animal and human studies have been conducted to investigate the relationship between the gut microbiome and mental well-being. Although human studies are limited, there is evidence that suggests a correlation between certain gut microbial taxa and indicators of quality of life or depression.[70] For example, the presence of butyrate-producing bacteria such as *Faecalibacterium* and *Coprococcus* spp. is associated with higher quality of life indicators.[70] It is worth noting that about a third of patients with irritable bowel syndrome (IBS), which is often linked to gut dysbiosis, also suffer depression.[71] In addition, various psychiatric symptoms have been observed in 36.5% of patients with functional gastrointestinal disorders, with general anxiety and panic disorders being the most common.[72] There are also bacteria that can modulate an individual's mood state.[73] For instance, bacterial genera such as *Roseburia*, *Phascolarctobacterium*, *Lachnospira*, and *Prevotella* are positively correlated with positive mood, while genera such as *Faecalibacterium*, *Bifidobacterium*, *Bacteroides*, *Parabacteroides*, and *Anaerostipes* are correlated with negative mood.[26] Thus, understanding the communication between the gut and the brain is important as it can help in the development of novel therapeutic agents that target both the gut and the brain.

## 20.5 Biotics and Microbiota: Prebiotics, Probiotics, and Psychobiotics

Novel therapeutic approaches for alleviating mental disorders can be established by modulating the gut–brain axis through the administration of biotics, such as prebiotics, probiotics, and psychobiotics.[74,75] The role of such biotics in gut microbial modulation and mental health has been extensively documented.[29,76,77] According to the recent guidelines issued by the World Gastroenterology Organisation, healthcare professionals are recommended to use probiotics in the management of disorders involving the gut and brain.[72]

Prebiotics refer to nondigestible food ingredients that can be fermented and selectively metabolized by beneficial intestinal bacteria.[78] Prebiotics include fibers, oligosaccharides, and resistant starch that are not digestible by the host, but support the growth of beneficial bacteria.[78] Dietary modulation of the gut flora through prebiotics, such as oligofructose inulin, occurs by stimulating the activity and abundance of beneficial bacteria.[78] Gut microbes utilize two types of anaerobic fermentation processes, saccharolytic and proteolytic, to digest these dietary ingredients. The saccharolytic fermentation produces SCFAs such as acetate, propionate, and butyrate, while the proteolytic fermentation includes phenolic compounds, amines, and ammonia.[78]

Probiotics are live organisms that can provide health benefits when consumed in appropriate quantities.[79] Different species of *Lactobacillus* and *Bifidobacterium* are commonly recognized probiotics that can produce GABA. Other probiotics such as *Enterococcus*, *Escherichia*, *Streptococcus*, and

*Candida* species synthesize serotonin, while *Bacillus* species produce dopamine.[80] Administration of these beneficial microbes via dietary supplementation or fecal microbiota transplantation can also alter the recipient's brain function, mood, and overall mental state.[81]

Psychobiotics are a novel class of probiotics that have positive effects on mental health. The term "Psychobiotics" refers to live organisms that provide benefits for individuals suffering from psychiatric disorders when consumed in appropriate amounts.[29,79,82] These bacteria can produce neuroactive compounds such as GABA, serotonin, norepinephrine, and endocannabinoids, which can affect the gut–brain axis.[29,73] Research has found a positive correlation between the microbially synthesized dopamine and mental quality of life.[70] Psychobiotics have demonstrated antidepressive and anxiolytic effects that may be mediated through the vagus nerve, spinal cord, or neuroendocrine system.[79] For instance, *Bifidobacterium infantis* has been shown to have a beneficial psychiatric impact on individuals with IBS.[79] Probiotic species with psychotropic properties include *Lactobacillus* spp. (*L. acidophilus*, *L. casei*, *L. rhamnosus*, *L. helveticus*, *L. plantarum* 299V, *L. pentosus*, *L. casei Shirota*, *L. hilgardii*), and *Bifidobacterium* spp. (*B. infantis*, *B. longum*, *B. bifidum*, *B. lactis*, *B. breve*), as well as other species such as *Bacillus*, *Candida*, *Enterococcus*, *Escherichia*, *Streptococcus thermophilus*, *and Saccharomyces* spp.[29]

## 20.6 Modulating the Gut Microbiome for Better Mental Outcomes

The microbiota-gut–brain interaction and its impact on mental health have been subject to extensive preclinical research, which has enhanced our understanding of the underlying mechanisms. However, the translation of these findings into clinical applications remains a topic of significant interest.[83] Despite the current limitations of human data, ongoing clinical trials are investigating the efficacy of microbiome-based interventions as a potential treatment strategy for mental health disorders. This section focuses on the current nutritional approaches, particularly the utilization of probiotics and psychobiotics, with the aim of modulating the gut microbiome to alleviate common mental health conditions.

### 20.6.1 Anxiety

The contribution of the gut microbiome to anxiety has been well established, although the underlying mechanisms are still being explored. In one study, fecal microbiota transplantation from patients with anxiety to mice resulted in a similar phenotype of the donors.[84] Interestingly, supplementation of *Lactobacillus plantarum* strain PS128 in a mouse model subjected to early life stress reduced anxiety-like behavior, possibly due to the modulation of prefrontal serotonergic and dopaminergic effects by neurochemicals produced by the probiotics.[85] Several strains of *Bifidobacteria* spp., such as *B. longum* and *B. breve*, have demonstrated strain-specific benefits in treating anxiety and depression-like behavior.[86] For instance, *B. longum* has shown to have an anxiolytic effect through the mediation of vagal pathway and brain-derived neurotropic factors in the hippocampus.[11] A cross-sectional study revealed that consumption of fermented food was associated with reduced neuroticism and societal anxiety in young adults.[87] Common psychobiotics used for treating anxiety mainly include *Lactobacillus* spp. (*L. fermentum* NS9, *Lactobacillus casei Shirota, L. rhamnosus* JB-1, and *L. helveticus* ROO52) and *Bifidobacterium* spp. (*B. breve* 1205, *B. infantis, B. longum* 1714, *B. longum* NCC3001, and *B. longum* R0175).[29]

## 20.6.2 Stress

The effect of stress and its associated HPA axis on the gut microbiome has been extensively documented.[16] Rodent models of maternal separation, a widely used method for inducing early life stress, have been employed to examine the relationship between stress, the gut–brain axis, and the gut microbiome.[88,89] Studies have demonstrated that early life stress caused by maternal separation leads to alterations in the gut microbiome, intestinal barrier function, and an increased stress response.[88] Infant rhesus monkeys have also displayed a disruption in gut flora following maternal separation, which was correlated with cortisol response and behavior, and was linked to decreased levels of *Lactobacilli*.[90] Probiotic supplementation with *Lactobacillus farciminis* has been shown to inhibit stress-induced intestinal hyperpermeability and endo-toxemia in the gut, prevent HPA axis stress response, and reduce neuroinflammation.[91] This inhibition is believed to be due to the mitigation of intestinal barrier impairment and a reduction in circulating levels of polysaccharides.[91] Psychobiotics used for the treatment of stress include *Lactobacillus* spp. (*L. casei Shirota, L. helveticus* R0052, *L. plantarum* PS128, and *L. rhamnosus*) and *Bifidobacterium* spp. (*B. infantis and B. longum* R0175).[29]

## 20.6.3 Depression

Patients with depression have a significantly different gut microbial composition compared to healthy controls.[92] Bacterial species such as *Coprococcus* spp. and *Dialister* spp. are depleted in depression patients.[70] The abundance of the phyla *Firmicutes* and *Actinobacteria* are increased, while the abundance of *Bacteroidetes* is reduced in patients with major depressive disorder (MDD).[93] At the genus level, there is a significant increase in the genera *Ba cteroides, Clostridium, Bifidobacterium, Oscillibacter,* and *Streptococcus* in MDD patients compared to the healthy controls.[93] A study on Sprague-Dawley rats treated with *Bifidobacterium infantis* for 14 days showed a significant increase in the serotonergic precursor tryptophan, which has antidepressant effects.[94] Furthermore, treatment with *Bifidobacteria* led to a decrease in the concentration of 5-Hydroxyindole acetic acid, a metabolite of serotonin, in the frontal cortex and a decrease in dihydroxyphenylacetic acid, a metabolite of dopamine, in the amygdaloid cortex.[94] *Lactobacillus helveticus* R0052 and *Bifidobacterium longum* R0175 have been found to effectively treat post-myocardial infarction depressive behavior in Sprague-Dawley rats, primarily by restoring the disrupted integrity of the intestinal barrier.[95]

A double-blind, placebo-controlled, randomized parallel group study found that treatment with a probiotic mixture of *Lactobacillus helveticus* R0052 and *Bifidobacterium longum* R0175 (Probio'Stick®) for one month improved depression, anger, and anxiety, and lowered the stress hormone cortisol levels in blood.[96] Similar randomized double-blind, placebo-controlled trials have shown that consuming probiotic-containing yogurt can improve mood in individuals with poor initial mood.[97] Another study evaluated the effect of probiotic administration on the clinical and metabolic outcomes of patients with MDD and found that administration of *Lactobacillus acidophilus*, *Lactobacillus casei*, and *Bifidobacterium bifidum* for 8 weeks had a significant effect on Beck Depression Inventory scores.[98] Moreover, fermented foods, which serve as a source of beneficial microbes, as well as the Mediterranean diet, may also protect or manage depression and anxiety.[99,100] Psychobiotics used to treat depression include *Lactobacillus* spp. (*L. acidophilus*, *L. acidophilus* W37, *L. brevis* W63, *L. casei*, *L. casei Shirota*, *L. casei* W56, *L. gasseri* OLL2809, and *L. helveticus* NS8), *Lactococcus* spp. (*L. lactis* W19 and *L. lactis* W58), and *Bifidobaterium* spp. (*B. infantis*, *B. bifidum*, *B. bifidum* W23, *B. lactis* W52, and *B. longum* R0175).[29]

## 20.6.4 Bipolar Disorder

Gut microbes play a role in bipolar disorder (BD), which is characterized by recurring depressive and manic episodes, like other mental disorders.[101] Patients with BD have shown an increased abundance of *Proteobacteria*, *Firmicutes*, and *Actinobacteria* phyla and reduced levels of *Bacteroidetes*.[93] Fecal samples from Chinese patients with BD, when compared to healthy controls, have shown increased levels of *Faecalibacterium prausnitzii*, *Bacteroides–Prevotella*, *Atopobium* cluster, *Enterobacter* spp., and *Clostridium* cluster IV.[102] Another study revealed a negative correlation between *Lactobacillus* counts and sleep, as well as *Bifidobacterium* counts and cortisol levels in Japanese BD patients.[103] A relatively large study in the United States involving 115 participants showed a decrease in *Faecalibacterium* abundance among BD patients.[104] Meanwhile, a Danish study indicated that *Flavonifractor*, a bacterium that induces oxidative stress and inflammation, could be associated with the triggering of the disease in newly diagnosed BD patients.[105] In a genome-wide study, the bacterial genus *Desulfovibrio* also appears to be positively associated with the BD phenotype.[106] The abundance of genera *Escherichia* and *Klebsiella* was found to be altered in BD patients compared to the healthy controls, with a reduction in the *Bifidobacterium longum* subsp. *infantis*.[93] Furthermore, a study with 46 human subjects, of which 23 BD were patients, found a higher abundance of *Clostridiaceae* and *Collinsella* in BD patients compared to the healthy controls.[107]

## 20.6.5 Obsessive Compulsive Disorder

Obsessive-compulsive disorder (OCD) is characterized by recurring intrusive thoughts, known as obsessions and repetitive actions, referred to as compulsions. These thoughts and actions can greatly affect cognitive and motor behavior.[108] Studies indicate that gut microbes also play a crucial role in the development of OCD through communication between the gut and brain. A probiotic bacteria, *Lactobacillus rhamnosus* GG, has been shown to reduce OCD-like behavior in mice, and its supplementation has been found to have similar effects to fluoxetine, an antidepressant medication.[109]

## 20.6.6 Autism Spectrum Disorder

Autism spectrum disorder (ASD) has been linked to gastrointestinal dysfunction. Studies have shown that children with ASD exhibit activation of the mucosal immune response and abnormal gut microbiota.[110] Compared to healthy control groups, children with autism have been found to have different species of *Clostridium*.[111] In gastric and duodenal specimens, control children were observed to have the absence of nonspore-forming anaerobes and microaerophilic bacteria, while a significant number of these organisms were present in children with autism.[111] Imbalanced gut microbiota has been linked to worsened psychological symptoms such as irritability, tantrums, aggressive behavior, and sleep disturbances.[110] Children with autism have been found to have elevated levels of *Clostridium bolteae*, *Clostridium histolyticum* group (*Clostridium* clusters I and II), and *Clostridium* clusters I and XI, even without gastrointestinal symptoms.[112] A study involving autistic children found significant differences in the *Bacteroidetes* and *Firmicutes* groups, with minor differences in the *Actinobacteria* and *Proteobacteria* phyla among the autistic children with varying severity.[113] For instance, *Desulfovibrio* species and *Bacteroides vulgatus* were found to be significantly higher in fecal samples of severely affected children.[113] A culture-based study showed that children with autism have lower levels of *Bifidobacter* and higher levels of *Lactobacillus*, with very low levels of SCFAs, including acetate, propionate, and valerate, compared to the control group.[114] Treatment with several probiotics, including *Bifidobacterium infantis*, improved the gastrointestinal disorders associated with ASD by restoring normal gut microbiota, reducing inflammation, and restoring epithelial barrier function.[110]

## 20.6.7 Alzheimer's Disease

Alzheimer's disease (AD) is a common form of dementia characterized by the accumulation of β-amyloid plaques, and neurofibrillary tangles in the brain, leading to neurological impairments.[115] The relationship between gut dysbiosis and cognitive and memory impairments in AD has been established through both experimental studies and human clinical trials. During the aging process, alterations in the gut microbial composition occur, including an increase in pro-inflammatory bacteria and a decrease in anti-inflammatory bacteria.

These changes can lead to alterations in gut permeability and impaired blood-brain barrier (BBB) function, ultimately promoting neuronal injury.[115] In AD patients, a decrease in gut microbial diversity and changes in the abundance of certain bacterial taxa have been observed, including decreased *Firmicutes* and increased *Bacteroidetes* as well as decreased *Bifidobacteria*.[116]

Studies have shown a correlation between AD pathogenesis and gut microbiota. In a mouse model of AD, it was observed that reducing gut microbial diversity through antibiotics led to neuroinflammation and amyloidosis.[117] A human study found that individuals with AD had a lower abundance of *Eubacterium rectale* and a higher abundance of *Escherichia/Shigella* compared to healthy controls.[118] This study also found a positive correlation between cytokines presence and the abundance of *Escherichia/Shigella*.[118] Gut dysbiosis can also contribute to AD pathogenesis through altered gut permeability and impaired BBB function, allowing lipopolysaccharides (LPS) and amyloid to pass through the gastrointestinal tract and trigger an inflammatory response.[118] Additionally, microbially derived amyloids, including curli (*E.coli*), tau, Aβ, α-synuclein, TasA (*Bacillus subtilis*), CsgA (*S. typhimurium*), FapC (*Pseudomonas fluorescens*), phenol soluble modulins (*Staphylococcus aureus*), and prion, have been shown to initiate the accumulation of β-amyloid peptides in AD.[119] A study showed that exposing human primary brain cells to LPS from *Bacteroides fragilis* led to pro-inflammatory and neurodegenerative responses.[120] Another study found increased levels of periodontal pathogens, such as *F. nucleatum* and *P. intermedia*, in the serum of AD patients.[121] Increased levels of anti-Helicobacter pylori IgG concentrations were also observed in the cerebrospinal fluid of AD patients, correlating with disease severity.[122]

Probiotics may have a role in managing AD pathogenesis.[115] For example, a study on *E. coli*-producing extracellular amyloid curli in age-matched Fischer 344 rats and transgenic *Caenorhabditis elegans* roundworms showed increased neuronal α-synuclein deposition in both gut and brain, accompanied by enhanced microgliosis and astrogliosis.[123] LPS secreted by pathogenic bacteria act as endotoxins and induce fibrillogenesis in AD.[124] C57BL/6J mice receiving intraperitoneal injections of LPS showed significantly higher levels of Aβ1-42, a peptide component of AD plaques, in the hippocampal brain tissue.[125] On the other hand, a reduction in Aβ amyloid pathology has been observed in the Aβ precursor protein (APP) transgenic mouse model.[126] The ethanol precipitate derived from milk fermented with the probiotic *Lactobacillus helveticus* IDCC 3801 led to a significant reduction of amyloid precursor protein β levels in the amyloidogenic pathway and a decrease in β-amyloid production in a scopolamine-treated mouse model.[127] Administration of *Bifidobacterium breve* strain A1 reversed altered Aβ-induced cognitive impairment-related behaviours in ddY male AD mice.[128] The supplementation of a probiotic mixture containing *B. longum*, *B. breve*, *B. infantis*, *L. acidophilus*, *L. paracasei*, *L. plantarum*, *L. brevis*, and *L. elbrueckii* subsp. *bulgaricus* (SLAB51) reduced oxidative stress in AD mice and exerted an antioxidant and neuroprotective effect.[129] The synbiotic preparation, consisting of *L. plantarum* NCIMB

8826, *L. fermentum* NCIMB 5221, *B. longum* spp. *infantis* NCIMB 702255, and 0.5% Triphala (*Emblica officinalis, Terminalia chebula*, and *T. bellirica*) powder delayed the onset of AD development in *Drosophila melanogaster*.[130] In human subjects, the supplementation of probiotic milk (200 ml/day) containing a mixture of probiotic strains (*Lactobacillus acidophilus, L. casei, Bifidobacterium bifidum*, and *L. fermentum*; $2 \times 10^9$ CFU(colony-forming units)/g each strain) for 12 weeks, had a positive effect on the cognitive function of AD patients.[131] An explorative intervention study in AD patients showed that multispecies probiotic (mainly *Lactobacillus* and *Bifidobacterium* spp.) supplementation improved the gut bacterial population and changed the serum tryptophan level, a metabolite that can modulate the gut–brain axis.[132] Furthermore, adherence to a Mediterranean diet style reduced gut dysbiosis and, in turn, the risk of AD.[133]

## 20.6.8 Parkinson's Disease

Parkinson's disease (PD), which is characterized by tremors and progressive loss of coordinated motor function, has been associated with changes in the indigenous gut microbiome.[134] This may be likely due to the gut–brain communication via the immune pathway which mediates PD symptoms.[135] Studies have shown differences in the gut microbiome[136–143] and the levels of SCFAs between PD patients and controls.[137] Gut microbes have been found to promote α-synuclein-mediated motor deficit in PD[144,145] and depleting gut microbes has reduced microglia activation and modulated the microglia to enhance PD pathophysiology.[144] Several studies have identified associations of gut microbiome with the occurrence of PD. PD patients have decreased levels of bacteria belonging to the *Lachnospiraceae* family,[146–149] including *Blautia* sp.,[149,150] *Dorea* sp.,[149,151] and *Roseburia* sp.,[149] the *Prevotellaceae* family,[151,152] such as *Prevotella copri*, and the *Corpobacillaceae* family.[149] They also have lower abundance of *Eubacterium bioforme*,[153] *Clostridium coccoides, C. leptum*,[149,154] *Clostridales incertae sedis* IV,[152] *Bacteroides fragilis*,[149] and *Ruminococcus* sp.[150] On the other hand, different taxa belonging to *Enterobacteriaceae*,[137,146] *Lactobacillaceae*,[146,148,152,154,155] *Barnesiellaceae*,[155] *Oxalobacteraceae*,[149] and *Eubacteriaceae*[147] families have been found to be enriched in the gut of PD patients.

Non-pharmacologic dietary modulation of PD-associated neuroinflammation and symptoms is a novel approach for improving the condition in PD patients.[156–160] Observational studies suggest persistent dietary habit differences between PD patients and healthy subjects. Mediterranean[133,161–164] or MIND (Mediterranean-DASH (Dietary Approach to Stop Hypertension)) diet,[161] ketogenic diet, low-carbohydrate high-fat diet,[165] polyphenols,[166] caffeine,[167] prebiotics,[139,168] and probiotics[168,169] have all been found to improve PD symptoms. The Mediterranean diet delays the onset of the disease,[170] improves cognitive function,[171] and reduces the severity of dysphagia in PD patients.[162] The role of probiotics in ameliorating PD symptoms is widely discussed.[139,172–176] Improved motor skills in the PD mice model have been observed following treatment with lactic acid bacteria *Lactobacillus plantarum* CRL 2130, *Streptococcus thermophilus* CRL 807, and *Streptococcus thermophilus* CRL 808.[177] Probiotic administration has been shown to improve behavioral impairment by protecting dopaminergic neurons in the PD mice model[169] and humans.[178] The action of probiotics is mainly through decreasing the pro-inflammatory cytokines and oxidative stress, and preventing potential pathogenic bacterial overgrowth.[173]

## 20.6.9 Schizophrenia

The relationship between gut microbes and schizophrenia has been extensively studied in recent years. Evidence suggests that gut–brain communication in schizophrenia occurs primarily via the immune pathway.[179,180] This has led researchers to consider targeting immune-linked gut microbiota as a potential treatment for the disease.[181] A study conducted on mice showed the transplantation of fecal microbiota from schizophrenia patients to antibiotic-treated mice resulted in behavioral abnormalities, including hyperactivity, impaired learning and memory, and schizophrenia-like behavior.[182] Moreover, gut microbes from individuals with schizophrenia have been shown to modulate the glutamate-glutamine-GABA cycle and induce schizophrenia-like behavior in mice.[183] Studies have also observed changes in the gut microbial population in individuals with schizophrenia, including reduced alpha diversity and altered composition, as well as an increase in *Proteobacteria*,[184–186] *Anaerococcus*,[184] and *Chaetomium*.[185] Conversely, decreased levels of SCFA-producing organisms such as *Faecalibacterium* and *Lachnospiraceae* genera[185] and *Haemophilus, Sutterella, Clostridium*,[184] and *Trichoderma* were observed.[185] In individuals with schizophrenia, an abundance of *Ruminococcaceae* was correlated with the lower severity of the disease, while *Bacteroides* were associated with worse depressive symptoms.[184]

The evidence regarding the efficacy of probiotics against schizophrenia is scarce.[187] However, randomized placebo-controlled clinical trials have proven that the supplementation of probiotic tablets containing $10^9$ colony-forming units of *Lactobacillus rhamnosus* strain GG and *Bifidobacterium animalis* subsp. *lactis* Bb12 can improve the Positive and Negative Syndrome Scale, a medical scale used to measure the severity of schizophrenia.[188] This improvement is most likely due to the enhancement of the immunomodulatory effect by reducing gastrointestinal leaking in schizophrenia patients.[189] Another study found that supplementing with the same organisms can normalize the *Candida albicans* antibody levels in the serum of schizophrenia patients, thereby alleviating gut discomfort associated with *C. albicans*.[190]

## 20.7 Conclusion

The role of the gut microbiome in modulating mental health has been extensively studied primarily in preclinical settings. The microbiome-gut–brain axis has emerged as a new paradigm for understanding the modulation of mental health and its disorders. The burden of mental illness is substantial and is projected to rise in the future, making it crucial to identify and implement effective medical interventions. Improving gut microbial composition through dietary modifications and microbiome-based interventions is emerging as a promising approach for positive mental health in psychiatric care. Probiotics and psychobiotics are being investigated for their potential role in preventing and treating mental health disorders by improving the gut–brain axis. However, it is important to note that this field is still in its early stages and there are significant challenges in translating preclinical findings into clinical practices. More research is needed to determine the efficacy of these interventions and to establish personalized treatment approaches. In the meantime, consuming fiber and probiotic-rich foods may be the best way to safely promote a healthy gut microbiome. Additionally, combining psychobiotics with conventional medications also hold the potential to improve overall mental health outcomes.

## References

1. Thursby E, Juge N. Introduction to the human gut microbiota. *The Biochemical Journal*. 2017;474(11):1823–1836.
2. Putignani L, Del Chierico F, Petrucca A, Vernocchi P, Dallapiccola B. The human gut microbiota: A dynamic interplay with the host from birth to senescence settled during childhood. *Pediatric Research*. 2014;76(1):2–10.
3. Doroszkiewicz J, Groblewska M, Mroczko B. The role of gut microbiota and gut-brain interplay in selected diseases of the central nervous system. *International Journal of Molecular Sciences*. 2021;22(18):10028.
4. Wensel CR, Pluznick JL, Salzberg SL, Sears CL. Next-generation sequencing: Insights to advance clinical investigations of the microbiome. *The Journal of Clinical Investigation*. 2022;132(7):1–12.
5. Liu L, Huh JR, Shah K. Microbiota and the gut-brain-axis: Implications for new therapeutic design in the CNS. *EBiomedicine*. 2022;77:103908.
6. Gareau MG, Wine E, Rodrigues DM, et al. Bacterial infection causes stress-induced memory dysfunction in mice. *Gut*. 2011;60(3):307–317.
7. Luczynski P, McVey Neufeld K-A, Oriach CS, Clarke G, Dinan TG, Cryan JF. Growing up in a bubble: Using Germ-free animals to assess the influence of the gut microbiota on brain and behavior. *International Journal of Neuropsychopharmacology*. 2016;19(8):1–17.
8. Diaz Heijtz R, Wang S, Anuar F, et al. Normal gut microbiota modulates brain development and behavior. *Proceedings of the National Academy of Sciences of the United States of America*. 2011;108(7):3047–3052.
9. Bercik P, Denou E, Collins J, et al. The intestinal microbiota affect central levels of brain-derived neurotropic factor and behavior in mice. *Gastroenterology*. 2011;141(2):599–609.e593.
10. Savignac HM, Tramullas M, Kiely B, Dinan TG, Cryan JF. Bifidobacteria modulate cognitive processes in an anxious mouse strain. *Behavioural Brain Research*. 2015;287:59–72.
11. Bercik P, Park AJ, Sinclair D, et al. The anxiolytic effect of Bifidobacterium longum NCC3001 involves vagal pathways for gut-brain communication. *Neurogastroenterology & Motility*. 2011;23(12):1132–1139.

12. Knudsen JK, Michaelsen TY, Bundgaard-Nielsen C, et al. Faecal microbiota transplantation from patients with depression or healthy individuals into rats modulates mood-related behaviour. *Scientific Reports*. 2021;11(1):1–11.
13. Park J, Kim CH. Regulation of common neurological disorders by gut microbial metabolites. *Experimental & Molecular Medicine*. 2021;53(12):1821–1833.
14. Breit S, Kupferberg A, Rogler G, Hasler G. Vagus nerve as modulator of the brain–gut axis in psychiatric and inflammatory disorders. *Frontiers in Psychiatry*. 2018;9:1–15.
15. Kennedy PJ, Cryan JF, Dinan TG, Clarke G. Kynurenine pathway metabolism and the microbiota-gut-brain axis. *Neuropharmacology*. 2017;112(B):399–412.
16. Cryan JF, Dinan TG. Mind-altering microorganisms: The impact of the gut microbiota on brain and behaviour. *Nature Reviews. Neuroscience*. 2012;13(10):701–712.
17. Strandwitz P. Neurotransmitter modulation by the gut microbiota. *Brain Research*. 2018;1693(B):128–133.
18. Halverson T, Alagiakrishnan K. Gut microbes in neurocognitive and mental health disorders. *Annals of Medicine*. 2020;52(8):423–443.
19. Spichak S, Bastiaanssen TFS, Berding K, et al. Mining microbes for mental health: Determining the role of microbial metabolic pathways in human brain health and disease. *Neuroscience & Biobehavioral Reviews*. 2021;125:698–761.
20. Hayes CL, Peters BJ, Foster JA. Microbes and mental health: Can the microbiome help explain clinical heterogeneity in psychiatry? *Frontiers in Neuroendocrinology*. 2020;58:100849.
21. Rieder R, Wisniewski PJ, Alderman BL, Campbell SC. Microbes and mental health: A review. *Brain, Behavior, & Immunity*. 2017;66:9–17.
22. Bruce-Keller AJ, Salbaum JM, Berthoud H-R. Harnessing gut microbes for mental health: Getting from here to there. *Biological Psychiatry*. 2018;83(3):214–223.
23. Margolis KG, Cryan JF, Mayer EA. The microbiota-gut-brain axis: From motility to mood. *Gastroenterology*. 2021;160(5):1486–1501.
24. Gibbons CH. Basics of autonomic nervous system function. *Handbook of Clinical Neurology*. 2019;160:407–418.
25. Jameson KG, Olson CA, Kazmi SA, Hsiao EY. Toward understanding microbiome-neuronal signaling. *Molecular Cell*. 2020;78(4):577–583.
26. Skonieczna-Żydecka K, Marlicz W, Misera A, Koulaouzidis A, Łoniewski I. Microbiome—The missing link in the gut-brain axis: Focus on its role in gastrointestinal and mental health. *Journal of Clinical Medicine*. 2018;7(12):521.
27. Kennedy PJ, Murphy AB, Cryan JF, Ross PR, Dinan TG, Stanton C. Microbiome in brain function and mental health. *Trends in Food Science & Technology*. 2016;57:289–301.
28. Chen Y, Xu J, Chen Y. Regulation of neurotransmitters by the gut microbiota and effects on cognition in neurological disorders. *Nutrients*. 2021;13(6):2099.
29. Misra S, Mohanty D. Psychobiotics: A new approach for treating mental illness? *Critical Reviews in Food Science & Nutrition*. 2019;59(8):1230–1236.
30. Schmidt C. Thinking from the gut. *Nature*. 2015;518(7540):S12–S14.
31. Valles-Colomer M, Falony G, Darzi Y, et al. The neuroactive potential of the human gut microbiota in quality of life and depression. *Nature Microbiology*. 2019;4(4):623–632.
32. Dai Z-L, Wu G, Zhu W-Y. Amino acid metabolism in intestinal bacteria: Links between gut ecology and host health. *FBL*. 2011;16(5):1768–1786.
33. Neis EPJG, Dejong CHC, Rensen SS. The role of microbial amino acid metabolism in host metabolism. *Nutrients*. 2015;7(4):2930–2946.
34. Mardinoglu A, Shoaie S, Bergentall M, et al. The gut microbiota modulates host amino acid and glutathione metabolism in mice. *Molecular Systems Biology*. 2015;11(10):834.
35. Dai Z-L, Li X-L, Xi P-B, Zhang J, Wu G, Zhu W-Y. Metabolism of select amino acids in bacteria from the pig small intestine. *Amino Acids*. 2012;42(5):1597–1608.
36. Góralczyk-Bińkowska A, Szmajda-Krygier D, Kozłowska E. The microbiota–Gut–Brain axis in psychiatric disorders. *International Journal of Molecular Sciences*. 2022;23(19):11245.

37. Silva M, Loureiro A, Cardoso G. Social determinants of mental health: A review of the evidence. *The European Journal of Psychiatry.* 2016;30(4):259–292.
38. Purtle J, Nelson KL, Counts NZ, Yudell M. Population-based approaches to mental health: History, strategies, and evidence. *Annual Review of Public Health.* 2020;41:201–221.
39. World Health Organization. Promoting mental health: Concepts, emerging evidence, Practice. 2004.
40. Huppert FA, So TTC. Flourishing across Europe: Application of a new conceptual framework for defining well-being. *Social Indicators Research.* 2013;110(3):837–861.
41. World Health Organization. Available online: https://www.who.int/news-room/fact-sheets/detail/mental-disorders (accessed on Feb 2023).
42. Steel Z, Marnane C, Iranpour C, et al. The global prevalence of common mental disorders: A systematic review and meta-analysis 1980–2013. *International Journal of Epidemiology.* 2014;43(2):476–493.
43. Gustavson K, Knudsen AK, Nesvåg R, Knudsen GP, Vollset SE, Reichborn-Kjennerud T. Prevalence and stability of mental disorders among young adults: Findings from a longitudinal study. *BMC Psychiatry.* 2018;18(1):65.
44. Bryant C, Jackson H, Ames D. The prevalence of anxiety in older adults: Methodological issues and a review of the literature. *Journal of Affective Disorders.* 2008;109(3):233–250.
45. Jha S, Salve HR, Goswami K, Sagar R, Kant S. Burden of common mental disorders among pregnant women: A systematic review. *Asian Journal of Psychiatry.* 2018;36:46–53.
46. Viswasam K, Berle D, Milicevic D, Starcevic V. Prevalence and onset of anxiety and related disorders throughout pregnancy: A prospective study in an Australian sample. *Psychiatry Research.* 2021;297:113721.
47. Polanczyk GV, Salum GA, Sugaya LS, Caye A, Rohde LA. Annual research review: A meta-analysis of the worldwide prevalence of mental disorders in children and adolescents. *Journal of Child Psychology & Psychiatry, & Allied Disciplines.* 2015;56(3):345–365.
48. Nichols E, Szoeke CEI, Vollset SE. Global, regional, and national burden of Alzheimer's disease and other dementias, 1990–2016: A systematic analysis for the Global Burden of Disease Study 2016. *The Lancet Neurology.* 2019;18(1):88–106.
49. Prince MJ, Comas-Herrera A, Knapp M, Guerchet MM, Karagiannidou M. *World Alzheimer Report 2016 - Improving Healthcare for People Living with Dementia: Coverage, Quality and Costs Now and in the Future.* London: Alzheimer's Disease International. 2016.
50. Palay J, Taillieu TL, Afifi TO, et al. Prevalence of mental disorders and suicidality in Canadian provinces. *Canadian Journal of Psychiatry. Revue Canadienne de Psychiatrie.* 2019;64(11):761–769.
51. *Autism Spectrum Disorder among Children and Youth in Canada 2018-A Report of the National Autism Spectrum Disorder Surveillance System.* March 2018.
52. Wang J, Jacobs P, Ohinmaa A, Dezetter A, Lesage A. Public expenditures for mental health services in Canadian provinces: Dépenses publiques pour les services de santé mentale dans les provinces canadiennes. *The Canadian Journal of Psychiatry. Revue Canadienne de Psychiatrie.* 2018;63(4):250–256.
53. Leigh JP, Du J. Brief report: Forecasting the economic burden of autism in 2015 and 2025 in the United States. *Journal of Autism & Developmental Disorders.* 2015;45(12):4135–4139.
54. Buescher AV, Cidav Z, Knapp M, Mandell DS. Costs of autism spectrum disorders in the United Kingdom and the United States. *JAMA Pediatrics.* 2014;168(8):721–728.
55. Lavelle TA, Weinstein MC, Newhouse JP, Munir K, Kuhlthau KA, Prosser LA. Economic burden of childhood autism spectrum disorders. *Pediatrics.* 2014;133(3):e520–e529.

56. Horlin C, Falkmer M, Parsons R, Albrecht MA, Falkmer T. The cost of autism spectrum disorders. *PLOS ONE*. 2014;9(9):e106552.
57. Leeming ER, Johnson AJ, Spector TD, Le Roy CI. Effect of diet on the gut microbiota: Rethinking intervention duration. *Nutrients*. 2019;11(12):1–28.
58. Rothschild D, Weissbrod O, Barkan E, et al. Environment dominates over host genetics in shaping human gut microbiota. *Nature*. 2018;555(7695):210–215.
59. Sonnenburg JL, Bäckhed F. Diet-microbiota interactions as moderators of human metabolism. *Nature*. 2016;535(7610):56–64.
60. David LA, Materna AC, Friedman J, et al. Host lifestyle affects human microbiota on daily timescales. *Genome Biology*. 2014;15(7):R89.
61. Goodrich JK, Davenport ER, Beaumont M, et al. Genetic determinants of the gut microbiome in UK twins. *Cell Host & Microbe*. 2016;19(5):731–743.
62. Ramirez J, Guarner F, Bustos Fernandez L, Maruy A, Sdepanian VL, Cohen H. Antibiotics as major disruptors of gut microbiota. *Frontiers in Cellular & Infection Microbiology*. 2020;10:572912–572912.
63. Suganya K, Koo B-S. Gut-brain axis: Role of gut microbiota on neurological disorders and how probiotics/prebiotics beneficially modulate microbial and immune pathways to improve brain functions. *International Journal of Molecular Sciences*. 2020;21(20):7551.
64. Mörkl S, Butler MI, Holl A, Cryan JF, Dinan TG. Probiotics and the microbiota-gut-brain axis: Focus on psychiatry. *Current Nutrition Reports*. 2020;9(3):171–182.
65. Westfall S, Lomis N, Kahouli I, Dia SY, Singh SP, Prakash S. Microbiome, probiotics and neurodegenerative diseases: Deciphering the gut brain axis. *Cellular & Molecular Life Sciences*. 2017;74(20):3769–3787.
66. Safadi JM, Quinton AMG, Lennox BR, Burnet PWJ, Minichino A. Gut dysbiosis in severe mental illness and chronic fatigue: A novel trans-diagnostic construct? A systematic review and meta-analysis. *Molecular Psychiatry*. 2022;27(1):141–153.
67. DeGruttola AK, Low D, Mizoguchi A, Mizoguchi E. Current understanding of dysbiosis in disease in human and animal models. *Inflammatory Bowel Diseases*. 2016;22(5):1137–1150.
68. Davari S, Talaei SA, Alaei H, Salami M. Probiotics treatment improves diabetes-induced impairment of synaptic activity and cognitive function: Behavioral and electrophysiological proofs for microbiome–gut-brain axis. *Neuroscience*. 2013;240:287–296.
69. Emge JR, Huynh K, Miller EN, et al. Modulation of the microbiota-gut-brain axis by probiotics in a murine model of inflammatory bowel disease. *American Journal of Physiology-Gastrointestinal & Liver Physiology*. 2016;310(11):G989–G998.
70. Du Toit A. The gut microbiome and mental health. *Nature Reviews in Microbiology*. 2019;17(4):196–196.
71. Shah E, Rezaie A, Riddle M, Pimentel M. Psychological disorders in gastrointestinal disease: Epiphenomenon, cause or consequence? *Annals of Gastroenterology*. 2014;27(3):224–230.
72. Stasi C, Nisita C, Cortopassi S, et al. Subthreshold psychiatric psychopathology in functional gastrointestinal disorders: Can it be the bridge between gastroenterology and psychiatry? *Gastroenterology Research & Practice*. 2017;2017:1953435.
73. Li L, Su Q, Xie B, et al. Gut microbes in correlation with mood: Case study in a closed experimental human life support system. *Neurogastroenterology & Motility*. 2016;28(8):1233–1240.
74. Dey G, Mookherjee S. Probiotics-targeting new milestones from gut health to mental health. *FEMS Microbiology Letters*. 2021;368(15):1–18.
75. Bested AC, Logan AC, Selhub EM. Intestinal microbiota, probiotics and mental health: from Metchnikoff to modern advances: Part I – autointoxication revisited. *Gut Pathogens*. 2013;5(1):5.

76. Methiwala HN, Vaidya B, Addanki VK, Bishnoi M, Sharma SS, Kondepudi KK. Gut microbiota in mental health and depression: Role of pre/pro/Synbiotics in their modulation. *Food & Function*. 2021;12(10):4284–4314.

77. Verma H, Phian S, Lakra P, et al. Human gut microbiota and mental health: Advancements and challenges in microbe-based therapeutic interventions. *Indian Journal of Microbiology*. 2020;60(4):405–419.

78. Manning TS, Gibson GR. Microbial-gut interactions in health and disease: Prebiotics. *Best Practice & Research: Clinical Gastroenterology*. 2004;18(2):287–298.

79. Dinan TG, Stanton C, Cryan JF. Psychobiotics: A novel class of psychotropic. *Biological Psychiatry*. 2013;74(10):720–726.

80. Sivamaruthi BS, Prasanth MI, Kesika P, Chaiyasut C. Probiotics in human mental health and diseases - A minireview. *Tropical Journal of Pharmaceutical Research*. 2021;18(No. 4 (2019)).

81. Bested AC, Logan AC, Selhub EM. Intestinal microbiota, probiotics and mental health: from Metchnikoff to modern advances: Part III – Convergence toward clinical trials. *Gut Pathogens*. 2013;5(1):4.

82. Casertano M, Fogliano V, Ercolini D. Psychobiotics, gut microbiota and fermented foods can help preserving mental health. *Food Research International*. 2022;152:110892.

83. Vargason AM, Anselmo AC. Clinical translation of microbe-based therapies: Current clinical landscape and preclinical outlook. *Bioengineering & Translational Medicine*. 2018;3(2):124–137.

84. Chinna Meyyappan A, Forth E, Wallace CJK, Milev R. Effect of fecal microbiota transplant on symptoms of psychiatric disorders: A systematic review. *BMC Psychiatry*. 2020;20(1):299.

85. Liu Y-W, Liu W-H, Wu C-C, et al. Psychotropic effects of Lactobacillus plantarum PS128 in early life-stressed and naïve adult mice. *Brain Research*. 2016;1631:1–12.

86. Savignac HM, Kiely B, Dinan TG, Cryan JF. Bifidobacteria exert strain-specific effects on stress-related behavior and physiology in BALB/c mice. *Neurogastroenterology & Motility*. 2014;26(11):1615–1627.

87. Hilimire MR, DeVylder JE, Forestell CA. Fermented foods, neuroticism, and social anxiety: An interaction model. *Psychiatry Research*. 2015;228(2):203–208.

88. O'Mahony SM, Hyland NP, Dinan TG, Cryan JF. Maternal separation as a model of brain–gut axis dysfunction. *Psychopharmacology*. 2011;214(1):71–88.

89. Desbonnet L, Garrett L, Clarke G, Kiely B, Cryan JF, Dinan TG. Effects of the probiotic Bifidobacterium infantis in the maternal separation model of depression. *Neuroscience*. 2010;170(4):1179–1188.

90. Bailey MT, Coe CL. Maternal separation disrupts the integrity of the intestinal microflora in infant rhesus monkeys. *Developmental Psychobiology*. 1999;35(2):146–155.

91. Ait-Belgnaoui A, Durand H, Cartier C, et al. Prevention of gut leakiness by a probiotic treatment leads to attenuated HPA response to an acute psychological stress in rats. *Psychoneuroendocrinology*. 2012;37(11):1885–1895.

92. Zheng P, Zeng B, Zhou C, et al. Gut microbiome remodeling induces depressive-like behaviors through a pathway mediated by the host's metabolism. *Molecular Psychiatry*. 2016;21(6):786–796.

93. Rong H, Xie X-h, Zhao J, et al. Similarly in depression, nuances of gut microbiota: Evidences from a shotgun metagenomics sequencing study on major depressive disorder versus bipolar disorder with current major depressive episode patients. *Journal of Psychiatric Research*. 2019;113:90–99.

94. Desbonnet L, Garrett L, Clarke G, Bienenstock J, Dinan TG. The probiotic bifidobacteria infantis: An assessment of potential antidepressant properties in the rat. *Journal of Psychiatric Research*. 2008;43(2):164–174.

95. Arseneault-Bréard J, Rondeau I, Gilbert K, et al. Combination of Lactobacillus helveticus R0052 and Bifidobacterium longum R0175 reduces post-myocardial infarction depression symptoms and restores intestinal permeability in a rat model. *British Journal of Nutrition.* 2011;107(12):1793–1799.

96. Messaoudi M, Lalonde R, Violle N, et al. Assessment of psychotropic-like properties of a probiotic formulation (Lactobacillus helveticus R0052 and Bifidobacterium longum R0175) in rats and human subjects. *British Journal of Nutrition.* 2010;105(5):755–764.

97. Benton D, Williams C, Brown A. Impact of consuming a milk drink containing a probiotic on mood and cognition. *European Journal of Clinical Nutrition.* 2007;61(3):355–361.

98. Akkasheh G, Kashani-Poor Z, Tajabadi-Ebrahimi M, et al. Clinical and metabolic response to probiotic administration in patients with major depressive disorder: A randomized, double-blind, placebo-controlled trial. *Nutrition.* 2016;32(3):315–320.

99. Aslam H, Green J, Jacka FN, et al. Fermented foods, the gut and mental health: A mechanistic overview with implications for depression and anxiety. *Nutritional Neuroscience.* 2020;23(9):659–671.

100. Pagliai G, Sofi F, Vannetti F, et al. Mediterranean diet, food consumption and risk of late-life depression: The mugello study. *The Journal of Nutrition, Health & Aging.* 2018;22(5):569–574.

101. Lai J, Jiang J, Zhang P, et al. Gut microbial clues to bipolar disorder: State-of-the-art review of current findings and future directions. *Clinical & Translational Medicine.* 2020;10(4):e146.

102. Lu Q, Lai J, Lu H, et al. Gut microbiota in bipolar depression and its relationship to brain function: An advanced exploration. *Frontiers in Psychiatry.* 2019;10.

103. Aizawa E, Tsuji H, Asahara T, et al. Bifidobacterium and lactobacillus counts in the gut microbiota of patients with bipolar disorder and healthy controls. *Frontiers in Psychiatry.* 2019;9.

104. Evans SJ, Bassis CM, Hein R, et al. The gut microbiome composition associates with bipolar disorder and illness severity. *Journal of Psychiatric Research.* 2017;87:23–29.

105. Coello K, Hansen TH, Sørensen N, et al. Gut microbiota composition in patients with newly diagnosed bipolar disorder and their unaffected first-degree relatives. *Brain, Behavior, & Immunity.* 2019;75:112–118.

106. Cheng S, Han B, Ding M, et al. Identifying psychiatric disorder-associated gut microbiota using microbiota-related gene set enrichment analysis. *Briefings in Bioinformatics.* 2019;21(3):1016–1022.

107. McIntyre RS, Subramaniapillai M, Shekotikhina M, et al. Characterizing the gut microbiota in adults with bipolar disorder: A pilot study. *Nutritional Neuroscience.* 2021;24(3):173–180.

108. Graybiel AM, Rauch SL. Toward a neurobiology of obsessive-compulsive disorder. *Neuron.* 2000;28(2):343–347.

109. Kantak PA, Bobrow DN, Nyby JG. Obsessive–compulsive-like behaviors in house mice are attenuated by a probiotic (Lactobacillus rhamnosus GG). *Behavioural Pharmacology.* 2014;25(1):71–79.

110. Critchfield JW, van Hemert S, Ash M, Mulder L, Ashwood P. The potential role of probiotics in the management of childhood autism spectrum disorders. *Gastroenterology Research & Practice.* 2011;2011:161358.

111. Finegold SM, Molitoris D, Song Y, et al. Gastrointestinal microflora studies in late-onset autism. *Clinical Infectious Diseases.* 2002;35(Supplement_1):S6–S16.

112. Parracho HM, Bingham MO, Gibson GR, McCartney AL. Differences between the gut microflora of children with autistic spectrum disorders and that of healthy children. *Journal of Medical Microbiology.* 2005;54(10):987–991.

113. Finegold SM, Dowd SE, Gontcharova V, et al. Pyrosequencing study of fecal microflora of autistic and control children. *Anaerobe*. 2010;16(4):444–453.

114. Adams JB, Johansen LJ, Powell LD, Quig D, Rubin RA. Gastrointestinal flora and gastrointestinal status in children with autism – Comparisons to typical children and correlation with autism severity. *BMC Gastroenterology*. 2011;11(1):22.

115. Kesika P, Suganthy N, Sivamaruthi BS, Chaiyasut C. Role of gut-brain axis, gut microbial composition, and probiotic intervention in Alzheimer's disease. *Life Sciences*. 2021;264:118627.

116. Vogt NM, Kerby RL, Dill-McFarland KA, et al. Gut microbiome alterations in Alzheimer's disease. *Scientific Reports*. 2017;7(1):13537.

117. Minter MR, Zhang C, Leone V, et al. Antibiotic-induced perturbations in gut microbial diversity influences neuro-inflammation and amyloidosis in a murine model of Alzheimer's disease. *Scientific Reports*. 2016;6(1):30028.

118. Cattaneo A, Cattane N, Galluzzi S, et al. Association of brain amyloidosis with pro-inflammatory gut bacterial taxa and peripheral inflammation markers in cognitively impaired elderly. *Neurobiology of Aging*. 2017;49:60–68.

119. Friedland RP, Chapman MR. The role of microbial amyloid in neurodegeneration. *PLOS Pathogens*. 2017;13(12):e1006654.

120. Lukiw WJ. Bacteroides fragilis lipopolysaccharide and inflammatory signaling in Alzheimer's disease. *Frontiers in Microbiology*. 2016;7.

121. Sparks Stein P, Steffen MJ, Smith C, et al. Serum antibodies to periodontal pathogens are a risk factor for Alzheimer's disease. *Alzheimer's & Dementia*. 2012;8(3):196–203.

122. Kountouras J, Boziki M, Gavalas E, et al. Increased cerebrospinal fluid Helicobacter pylori antibody in Alzheimer's disease. *International Journal of Neuroscience*. 2009;119(6):765–777.

123. Chen SG, Stribinskis V, Rane MJ, et al. Exposure to the functional bacterial amyloid protein Curli enhances alpha-synuclein aggregation in aged Fischer 344 rats and Caenorhabditis elegans. *Scientific Reports*. 2016;6(1):34477.

124. Asti A, Gioglio L. Can a bacterial endotoxin be a key factor in the kinetics of amyloid fibril formation? *Journal of Alzheimer's Disease*. 2014;39(1):169–179.

125. Kahn MS, Kranjac D, Alonzo CA, et al. Prolonged elevation in hippocampal Aβ and cognitive deficits following repeated endotoxin exposure in the mouse. *Behavioural Brain Research*. 2012;229(1):176–184.

126. Harach T, Marungruang N, Duthilleul N, et al. Reduction of Abeta amyloid pathology in APPPS1 transgenic mice in the absence of gut microbiota. *Scientific Reports*. 2017;7(1):41802.

127. Yeon S-W, You YS, Kwon H-S, et al. Fermented milk of Lactobacillus helveticus IDCC3801 reduces beta-amyloid and attenuates memory deficit. *Journal of Functional Foods*. 2010;2(2):143–152.

128. Kobayashi Y, Sugahara H, Shimada K, et al. Therapeutic potential of Bifidobacterium breve strain A1 for preventing cognitive impairment in Alzheimer's disease. *Scientific Reports*. 2017;7(1):13510.

129. Bonfili L, Cecarini V, Cuccioloni M, et al. SLAB51 probiotic formulation activates SIRT1 pathway promoting antioxidant and neuroprotective effects in an AD mouse model. *Molecular Neurobiology*. 2018;55(10):7987–8000.

130. Westfall S, Lomis N, Prakash S. A novel synbiotic delays Alzheimer's disease onset via combinatorial gut-brain-axis signaling in Drosophila melanogaster. *PLOS ONE*. 2019;14(4):e0214985.

131. Akbari E, Asemi Z, Daneshvar Kakhaki R, et al. Effect of probiotic supplementation on cognitive function and metabolic status in Alzheimer's disease: A randomized, double-blind and controlled trial. *Frontiers in Aging Neuroscience*. 2016;8.

132. Leblhuber F, Steiner K, Schuetz B, Fuchs D, Gostner JM. Probiotic supplementation in patients with Alzheimer's dementia-an explorative intervention study. *Current Alzheimer Research*. 2018;15(12):1106–1113.

133. Solch RJ, Aigbogun JO, Voyiadjis AG, et al. Mediterranean diet adherence, gut micro-biota, and Alzheimer's or Parkinson's disease risk: A systematic review. *Journal of the Neurological Sciences.* 2022;434:120166.

134. Sampson T. The impact of indigenous microbes on Parkinson's disease. *Neurobiology of Disease.* 2020;135:104426.

135. Caputi V, Giron MC. Microbiome-gut-brain axis and toll-like receptors in Parkinson's disease. *International Journal of Molecular Sciences.* 2018;19(6):1689.

136. Sharma S, Awasthi A, Singh S. Altered gut microbiota and intestinal permeability in Parkinson's disease: Pathological highlight to management. *Neuroscience Letters.* 2019;712:134516.

137. Unger MM, Spiegel J, Dillmann K-U, et al. Short chain fatty acids and gut micro-biota differ between patients with Parkinson's disease and age-matched controls. *Parkinsonism & Related Disorders.* 2016;32:66–72.

138. Sun M-F, Shen Y-Q. Dysbiosis of gut microbiota and microbial metabolites in Parkinson's disease. *Ageing Research Reviews.* 2018;45:53–61.

139. Tan AH, Lim SY, Lang AE. The microbiome–gut-brain axis in Parkinson disease — From basic research to the clinic. *Nature Reviews. Neurology.* 2022;18(8):476–495.

140. Cirstea MS, Yu AC, Golz E, et al. Microbiota composition and metabolism are associated with gut function in Parkinson's disease. *Movement Disorders.* 2020;35(7):1208–1217.

141. Yang D, Zhao D, Ali Shah SZ, et al. The role of the gut microbiota in the pathogenesis of Parkinson's disease. *Frontiers in Neurology.* 2019;10:1–13.

142. Perez-Pardo P, Dodiya HB, Engen PA, et al. Gut bacterial composition in a mouse model of Parkinson's disease. *Beneficial Microbes.* 2018;9(5):799–814.

143. Chiang HL, Lin CH. Altered gut microbiome and intestinal pathology in Parkinson's disease. *Journal of Movement Disorders.* 2019;12(2):67–83.

144. Sampson TR, Debelius JW, Thron T, et al. Gut microbiota regulate motor deficits and neuroinflammation in a model of Parkinson's disease. *Cell.* 2016;167(6):1469-1480. e1412.

145. Fitzgerald E, Murphy S, Martinson HA. Alpha-synuclein pathology and the role of the microbiota in Parkinson's disease. *Frontiers in Neuroscience.* 2019;13:1–13.

146. Barichella M, Severgnini M, Cilia R, et al. Unraveling gut microbiota in Parkinson's disease and atypical parkinsonism. *Movement Disorders.* 2019;34(3):396–405.

147. Lin A, Zheng W, He Y, et al. Gut microbiota in patients with Parkinson's disease in southern China. *Parkinsonism & Related Disorders.* 2018;53:82–88.

148. Hill-Burns EM, Debelius JW, Morton JT, et al. Parkinson's disease and Parkinson's disease medications have distinct signatures of the gut microbiome. *Movement Disorders.* 2017;32(5):739–749.

149. Keshavarzian A, Green SJ, Engen PA, et al. Colonic bacterial composition in Parkinson's disease. *Movement Disorders.* 2015;30(10):1351–1360.

150. Li W, Wu X, Hu X, et al. Structural changes of gut microbiota in Parkinson's dis-ease and its correlation with clinical features. *Science in China (Life Sciences).* 2017;60(11):1223–1233.

151. Petrov VA, Saltykova IV, Zhukova IA, et al. Analysis of gut microbiota in patients with Parkinson's disease. *Bulletin of Experimental Biology & Medicine.* 2017;162(6):734–737.

152. Scheperjans F, Aho V, Pereira PAB, et al. Gut microbiota are related to Parkinson's disease and clinical phenotype. *Movement Disorders.* 2015;30(3):350–358.

153. Bedarf JR, Hildebrand F, Coelho LP, et al. Functional implications of microbial and viral gut metagenome changes in early stage L-DOPA-naïve Parkinson's disease patients. *Genome Medicine.* 2017;9(1):39.

154. Hasegawa S, Goto S, Tsuji H, et al. Intestinal dysbiosis and lowered serum lipopoly-saccharide-binding protein in Parkinson's disease. *PLOS ONE.* 2015;10(11):e0142164.

155. Hopfner F, Künstner A, Müller SH, et al. Gut microbiota in Parkinson disease in a northern German cohort. *Brain Research.* 2017;1667:41–45.

156. Kalampokini S, Becker A, Fassbender K, Lyros E, Unger MM. Nonpharmacological modulation of chronic inflammation in Parkinson's disease: Role of diet interventions. *Parkinson's Disease.* 2019;2019:7535472.

157. Alfonsetti M, Castelli V, d'Angelo M. Are we what we eat? Impact of diet on the gut-Brain axis in Parkinson's disease. *Nutrients.* 2022;14(2):380.

158. Lange KW, Nakamura Y, Chen N, et al. Diet and medical foods in Parkinson's disease. *Food Science & Human Wellness.* 2019;8(2):83–95.

159. Jackson A, Forsyth CB, Shaikh M, et al. Diet in Parkinson's disease: Critical role for the microbiome. *Frontiers in Neurology.* 2019;10.

160. Chu C-Q, Yu L-l, Chen W, Tian F-W, Zhai Q-X. Dietary patterns affect Parkinson's disease via the microbiota-gut-brain axis. *Trends in Food Science & Technology.* 2021;116:90–101.

161. Agarwal P, Wang Y, Buchman AS, Holland TM, Bennett DA, Morris MC. MIND diet associated with reduced incidence and delayed progression of parkinsonism in old age. *The Journal of Nutrition, Health & Aging.* 2018;22(10):1211–1215.

162. Cassani E, Barichella M, Ferri V, et al. Dietary habits in Parkinson's disease: Adherence to Mediterranean diet. *Parkinsonism & Related Disorders.* 2017;42:40–46.

163. Bisaglia M. Mediterranean diet and Parkinson's disease. *International Journal of Molecular Sciences.* 2023;24(1):42.

164. Cassani E, Barichella M, Ferri V, et al. Dietary habits in Parkinson's disease: Adherence to Mediterranean diet. *Parkinsonism & Related Disorders.* 2018;46:e64.

165. Tieu K, Perier C, Caspersen C, et al. D-β-Hydroxybutyrate rescues mitochondrial respiration and mitigates features of Parkinson disease. *The Journal of Clinical Investigation.* 2003;112(6):892–901.

166. Kujawska M, Jodynis-Liebert J. Polyphenols in Parkinson's disease: A systematic review of in vivo studies. *Nutrients.* 2018;10(5):642.

167. Hernán MA, Takkouche B, Caamaño-Isorna F, Gestal-Otero JJ. A meta-analysis of coffee drinking, cigarette smoking, and the risk of Parkinson's disease. *Annals of Neurology.* 2002;52(3):276–284.

168. Barichella M, Pacchetti C, Bolliri C, et al. Probiotics and prebiotic fiber for constipation associated with Parkinson disease. *An RCT.* 2016;87(12):1274–1280.

169. Castelli V, d'Angelo M, Lombardi F, et al. Effects of the probiotic formulation SLAB51 in in vitro and in vivo Parkinson's disease models. *Aging.* 2020;12(5):4641–4659.

170. Maraki MI, Yannakoulia M, Stamelou M, et al. Mediterranean diet adherence is related to reduced probability of prodromal Parkinson's disease. *Movement Disorders.* 2019;34(1):48–57.

171. Paknahad Z, Sheklabadi E, Derakhshan Y, Bagherniya M, Chitsaz A. The effect of the Mediterranean diet on cognitive function in patients with Parkinson's disease: A randomized clinical controlled trial. *Complementary Therapies in Medicine.* 2020;50:102366.

172. Dutta SK, Verma S, Jain V, et al. Parkinson's disease: The emerging role of gut dysbiosis, antibiotics, probiotics, and fecal microbiota transplantation. *Journal of Neurogastroenterology & Motility.* 2019;25(3):363–376.

173. Magistrelli L, Amoruso A, Mogna L, et al. Probiotics may have beneficial effects in Parkinson's disease: In vitro evidence. *Frontiers in Immunology.* 2019;10:1–9.

174. Metta V, Leta V, Mrudula KR, et al. Gastrointestinal dysfunction in Parkinson's disease: Molecular pathology and implications of gut microbiome, probiotics, and fecal microbiota transplantation. *Journal of Neurology.* 2022;269(3):1154–1163.

175. Gazerani P. Probiotics for Parkinson's disease. *International Journal of Molecular Sciences.* 2019;20(17):4121.

176. Hsieh T-H, Kuo C-W, Hsieh K-H, et al. Probiotics alleviate the progressive deterioration of motor functions in a mouse model of Parkinson's disease. *Brain Sciences.* 2020;10(4):206.

177. Perez Visñuk D, Savoy de Giori G, LeBlanc JG, de Moreno de LeBlanc A. Neuroprotective effects associated with immune modulation by selected lactic acid bacteria in a Parkinson's disease model. *Nutrition*. 2020;79–80:110995.

178. Tamtaji OR, Taghizadeh M, Daneshvar Kakhaki R, et al. Clinical and metabolic response to probiotic administration in people with Parkinson's disease: A randomized, double-blind, placebo-controlled trial. *Clinical Nutrition*. 2019;38(3):1031–1035.

179. Severance EG, Gressitt KL, Stallings CR, et al. Discordant patterns of bacterial translocation markers and implications for innate immune imbalances in schizophrenia. *Schizophrenia Research*. 2013;148(1):130–137.

180. Severance EG, Alaedini A, Yang S, et al. Gastrointestinal inflammation and associated immune activation in schizophrenia. *Schizophrenia Research*. 2012;138(1):48–53.

181. Cuomo A, Maina G, Rosso G, et al. The microbiome: A new target for research and treatment of schizophrenia and its resistant presentations? A systematic literature search and review. *Frontiers in Pharmacology*. 2018;9:1040.

182. Zhu F, Guo R, Wang W, et al. Transplantation of microbiota from drug-free patients with schizophrenia causes schizophrenia-like abnormal behaviors and dysregulated kynurenine metabolism in mice. *Molecular Psychiatry*. 2020;25(11):2905–2918.

183. Zheng P, Zeng B, Liu M, et al. The gut microbiome from patients with schizophrenia modulates the glutamate-glutamine-GABA cycle and schizophrenia-relevant behaviors in mice. *Science Advances*. 2019;5(2):eaau8317.

184. Nguyen TT, Kosciolek T, Maldonado Y, et al. Differences in gut microbiome composition between persons with chronic schizophrenia and healthy comparison subjects. *Schizophrenia Research*. 2019;204:23–29.

185. Zhang X, Pan L-Y, Zhang Z, Zhou Y-Y, Jiang H-Y, Ruan B. Analysis of gut mycobiota in first-episode, drug-naïve Chinese patients with schizophrenia: A pilot study. *Behavioural Brain Research*. 2020;379:112374.

186. Shen Y, Xu J, Li Z, et al. Analysis of gut microbiota diversity and auxiliary diagnosis as a biomarker in patients with schizophrenia: A cross-sectional study. *Schizophrenia Research*. 2018;197:470–477.

187. Ng QX, Soh AYS, Venkatanarayanan N, Ho CYX, Lim DY, Yeo WS. A systematic review of the effect of probiotic supplementation on schizophrenia symptoms. *Neuropsychobiology*. 2019;78(1):1–6.

188. Dickerson FB, Stallings C, Origoni A, et al. Effect of probiotic supplementation on schizophrenia symptoms and association with gastrointestinal functioning: A randomized, placebo-controlled trial. *The Primary Care Companion for CNS Disorders*. 2014;16(1): PCC.13m01579..

189. Tomasik J, Yolken RH, Bahn S, Dickerson FB. Immunomodulatory effects of probiotic supplementation in schizophrenia patients: A randomized, placebo-controlled trial. *Biomarker Insights*. 2015;10:BMI.S22007.

190. Severance EG, Gressitt KL, Stallings CR, et al. Probiotic normalization of Candida albicans in schizophrenia: A randomized, placebo-controlled, longitudinal pilot study. *Brain, Behavior, & Immunity*. 2017;62:41–45.

# 21

# Functional Constituents of Yacon (*Smallanthus sonchifolius*) for Gut Rejuvenation

Abdullah Abdelkawi, Philopateer Messeha, and Yashwant V. Pathak

## Contents

## 21.1 History

The usage of plants for medical purposes dates back thousands of years, and research is always evolving and improving in order to better tap into nature's healing potential. Yacon (*Smallanthus sonchifolius*) is one of these plants that has been utilized for ages due to the efficiency of its functional ingredients in gut regeneration.

Yacon (*Smallanthus sonchifolius*), commonly known as Peruvian ground apple, is a functional food rich in functional ingredients, including prebiotic fibers, polyphenols, and dietary minerals, which may be useful for revitalizing gut microbiomes (Benevides et al., 2015). Prebiotic fibers are nondigestible substances that promote the formation of beneficial probiotics in the human gut (Ramprasath et al., 2020). In contrast, polyphenols may help balance the gut environment by altering the variety and structure of the gut microbiota

DOI: 10.1201/9781003333821-21

(Gabrielli et al., 2018). Calcium, magnesium, and iron are important for the growth and survival of commensal gut bacteria (Selmi et al., 2019). Thus, the functional elements of yacon may be utilized to positively alter the gut microbiota.

Yacon (*Smallanthus sonchifolius*) is a native plant of the Andes region of South America, where it has a long history of use as a natural medicine for a wide range of diseases. Indigenous tribes in South America historically use the plant as a natural medicine for digestive issues such as constipation, as well as for the treatment of diabetes and obesity. Yacon has a high concentration of fructooligosaccharides (FOS), a form of prebiotic fiber that promotes the growth and activity of good gut flora. It is believed that yacon and its FOS have been used for gut health and rejuvenation since pre-Columbian times, when the plant was widely utilized for its medical benefits. In recent years, yacon and its FOS have gained favor as gut health and other health benefits dietary supplements. Several scientific researches on the impact of yacon and its FOS on various aspects of health, including gut health and the gut microbiome, have been undertaken. Yacon has traditionally been used as a natural sweetener due to its low glycemic index and inability to be converted to glucose in the body. It has been used as a sugar substitute in a range of food and beverage products, including as syrups, jams, and teas. Yacon and its FOS have a long history of usage for a number of therapeutic purposes, including regeneration of the gastrointestinal tract. While the present scientific evidence suggests that yacon and its FOS may have a number of health benefits, additional research is required to completely comprehend the mechanisms underlying these effects and to determine the long-term safety and efficacy of yacon as a dietary supplement.

## 21.2 Inulin

Inulin is a nutritional fiber found in chicory root, artichokes, garlic, and onions, among other plant foods. Long chains of fructose molecules, which are a form of sugar, constitute it. Inulin is a fructooligosaccharide (FOS), a type of prebiotic fiber that encourages the growth and activity of healthy gut flora. Inulin offers potential digestive, immune-boosting, and weight control benefits. It is well known for its ability to improve digestive function and bulk up stools, as well as alleviate constipation and diarrhea. Inulin may also lower the absorption of cholesterol and other compounds in the intestine, which may have a positive impact on cholesterol levels and overall health. In addition to its digestive benefits, inulin has been demonstrated to strengthen the immune system. According to a number of studies, inulin may promote the creation of immune cells such as white blood cells and boost the activity of immune cells such as macrophages. Other research has discovered that inulin may possess antiviral and antibacterial capabilities, which may aid in preventing the formation of dangerous bacteria and viruses. Inulin has also been demonstrated to aid with weight management. According to a number of studies, inulin may aid in reducing body weight and body mass index (BMI) by enhancing feelings of fullness and decreasing food intake. Inulin may also increase insulin sensitivity and blood glucose control, which may be advantageous for diabetics and those at risk for developing the disease.

In addition to these possible health benefits, inulin has been proven to have additional effects, including increasing bone density and decreasing the risk of some forms of cancer. Inulin may promote bone density and lower the incidence of osteoporosis, particularly in postmenopausal women, according to certain research. Other studies have discovered that inulin may have a preventive effect against cancers such as colon cancer. Inulin is often well tolerated, and adverse reactions are uncommon. Nevertheless, after taking significant quantities of inulin, some individuals may have digestive problems, such as bloating and gas. It is essential to begin with a modest dose and gradually raise it to allow the body to acclimate. Additionally, it is essential to consume copious amounts of water when ingesting inulin, since this may lessen the likelihood of stomach issues. Inulin is a type of dietary fiber present in a variety of plant-based foods, and it offers a number of potential health benefits, including digestive, immune-boosting, and weight management impacts. It is generally well accepted, but it is recommended to begin with lower doses and raise them gradually to allow the body to adapt. To completely comprehend the mechanisms underlying the reported effects and to determine the appropriate doses and duration of treatment, additional research is required.

## 21.3 Functional Constituents of Yacon

Functional components of yacon FOS and inulin, which are kinds of fructans, are the primary functional components of yacon. Fructans are fructose polymers found in a number of plants, such as yacon, onions, garlic, and asparagus. FOS are shorter chain fructans with a degree of polymerization (DP) between 2 and 8, while inulin has a DP between 9 and 60. Both FOS and inulin are categorized as prebiotics, which are nondigestible food components that promote the growth and activity of beneficial microbes in the gastrointestinal tract.

In addition to FOS and inulin, yacon also includes flavonoids, saponins, and mucilage, among other useful components. Flavonoids are a class of phytochemicals with a variety of health advantages, such as antioxidant, anti-inflammatory, and antibacterial properties. Saponins are soap-like plant chemicals that have been demonstrated to provide numerous health benefits, including as cholesterol-lowering and immune-modulating actions. Mucilage is a type of plant polysaccharide that, when mixed with water, creates a gel-like substance and has been associated with numerous health advantages, including improvement of gut health and lowering of cholesterol levels.

## 21.4 Flavanoids

Flavonoids are a wide class of chemicals generated from plants that have been linked to a variety of health benefits. In addition to fruits, vegetables, nuts, seeds, whole grains, and tea, a wide variety of plant foods include polyphenols. Flavonoids possess a variety of biological actions, such as antioxidant, anti-inflammatory, and antibacterial characteristics. It is believed that oxidative stress and inflammation contribute to the development of a variety of chronic diseases, including cardiovascular disease, cancer, and neurological diseases. In addition to their antioxidant and anti-inflammatory characteristics, flavonoids have been found to provide a variety of additional health advantages. Several studies have discovered, for instance, that flavonoids may benefit cardiovascular health by lowering blood pressure and cholesterol levels and lowering the chance of developing heart disease. Flavonoids may lessen the risk of some cancers, including breast, colon, and prostate cancer, according to other studies. Additionally, flavonoids may have a beneficial influence on cognitive performance. Flavonoids may improve memory, attention, and learning, and may lessen the risk of neurodegenerative illnesses such as Alzheimer's disease, according to some research. Overall, the data suggests that flavonoids may offer a variety of health benefits, such as lowering the risk of chronic diseases such as cardiovascular disease and cancer and enhancing cognitive performance. It is believed that flavonoids' positive effects result from their antioxidant, anti-inflammatory, and antibacterial capabilities. To completely comprehend the processes underlying these effects and to determine the appropriate doses and duration of treatment, additional research is required.

## 21.5 Saponins

Saponins are a collection of plant-derived chemicals found in legumes, grains, and vegetables, among other plant foods. Due to their capacity to produce foam when combined with water, they are recognized for their soap-like qualities. Saponins offer several possible health benefits, including cholesterol-lowering, anti-inflammatory, and immune-boosting properties. Saponins are believed to exert the majority of their health advantages through their capacity to reduce cholesterol levels. Saponins have been demonstrated to bind to cholesterol in the gastrointestinal tract and limit its absorption, which may contribute to a reduction in total and (low-density lipoprotein) LDL cholesterol levels. According to a number of studies, saponins may also stimulate the formation of bile acids, which may contribute to their cholesterol-lowering properties. Saponins have been demonstrated to have anti-inflammatory qualities in addition to their cholesterol-lowering benefits. Inflammation is a normal immunological reaction that protects the body from infection and damage. Chronic inflammation has been associated to the development of a number of diseases, including cardiovascular disease, cancer, and diabetes.

Saponins have also been demonstrated to strengthen the immune system. Saponins may stimulate the development of immune cells, such as white blood cells, and boost the activity of immune cells, such as macrophages, according to certain research. Other research has discovered that saponins may have antiviral and antibacterial effects, which may inhibit the growth of dangerous bacteria and viruses. In addition to these possible health benefits, saponins have been proven to have additional effects, such as lowering blood pressure, enhancing insulin sensitivity, and lowering the risk of some forms of cancer. To completely comprehend the processes underlying these effects and to determine the appropriate doses and duration of treatment, additional research is required. It is important to note that saponins can sometimes have negative effects. After consuming meals high in saponins, some individuals may develop digestive problems such as bloating and gas. Saponins may also inhibit the absorption of nutrients such as calcium and iron. Before adding saponin supplements to your diet, it is essential to consume a diversified diet and consult with a healthcare practitioner.

## 21.6 Mucilage

Mucilage is a collection of plant-derived substances characterized by their viscous, gel-like consistency. Mucilage is present in grains, legumes, and vegetables, among other plant foods. It consists of long chains of polysaccharides, such as pectins and mucilage, which are formed of sugars including galactose, rhamnose, and arabinose. The potential health benefits of mucilage include digestive, immune-boosting, and antioxidant effects. It is well known for its propensity to produce a gel-like substance when combined with water, which may aid in bulking up stools, improving digestive function, and reducing constipation and diarrhea. Mucilage may also lower the absorption of cholesterol and other compounds in the gut, which may have a positive impact on cholesterol levels and general health. In addition to its digestive benefits, mucilage has been demonstrated to strengthen the immune system. According to a number of studies, mucilage may stimulate the creation of immune cells, such as white blood cells, and increase the activity of immune cells, such as macrophages. Other research has discovered that mucilage may possess antiviral and antibacterial characteristics, which may inhibit the growth of dangerous bacteria and viruses. It has also been demonstrated that mucilage possesses antioxidant effects. Antioxidants are substances that provide protection against the detrimental consequences of oxidative stress, which happens when the body is overexposed to free radicals. Free radicals are unstable chemicals that can cause cell damage and contribute to the development of numerous diseases, including cancer, cardiovascular disease, and neurological disorders. It has been demonstrated that mucilage has a potent potential to scavenge free radicals, which may protect against the harmful effects of oxidative stress. In addition to these possible health benefits, mucilage has been proven to have additional effects, such as lowering blood pressure and increasing insulin sensitivity. To completely comprehend the processes underlying these effects and to determine the appropriate doses and duration of treatment, additional research is required.

## 21.7 Gut Rejuvenation

The gut microbiota, the bacteria that inhabit the human gut, have a vital role in numerous aspects of health, including digestion, immunity, and metabolism. Several diseases and ailments, including obesity, diabetes, and cardiovascular disease, have been linked to dysbiosis, or an imbalance in the gut microbiota.

It has been demonstrated that prebiotics, such as FOS and inulin, benefit the gut microbiota and overall gut health. They promote the growth of helpful bacteria, including *Bifidobacteria* and *Lactobacilli*, and prevent the growth of dangerous bacteria, including *Escherichia coli* and *Clostridium difficile*. It has also been demonstrated that prebiotics increase the integrity of the gut barrier, reduce inflammation, and alter the immune system.

Yacon and mucilage are examples of prebiotics with beneficial effects on the gut microbiota. In addition to their prebiotic effects, yacon and its functional ingredients have been proven to have a variety of additional effects on the gut, including an increase in gut transit time and a decrease in constipation. It has been demonstrated that mucilage, in particular, has a bulking effect and increases the viscosity of the stool, which may aid to improve bowel motions.

## 21.8 Clinical Studies

Multiple clinical researches on the impact of yacon and its functional components on gut health have been conducted. One randomized controlled trial assessed the effects of yacon syrup on the body weight, body mass index (BMI), and waist circumference of obese participants. After eight weeks of treatment, the yacon syrup led to a considerable reduction in body weight, BMI, and waist circumference.

A randomized controlled experiment was performed to examine the impact of yacon syrup on gut health markers in persons with metabolic syndrome. All 60 patients in the study had been diagnosed with metabolic syndrome and had a body mass index (BMI) of 30 or above. The participants received either yacon syrup or a placebo for a period of 12 weeks.

The yacon syrup group received a daily dose of 30 ml of yacon syrup, whereas the placebo group received a syrup that looked and tasted identical to the yacon syrup but did not contain yacon. Neither participants nor researchers were aware of which group each person belonged to (double-blind design).

Changes in gut microbiota composition and fecal short-chain fatty acid (SCFA) levels were the key outcome measurements. Changes in body weight, BMI, waist circumference, and blood pressure were secondary objectives. Compared to the placebo, the yacon syrup dramatically enhanced the composition of the gut microbiota and increased the levels of fecal SCFA. The yacon syrup group exhibited a greater relative number of helpful bacteria, such as *Bifidobacterium* and *Lactobacillus*, and a lower relative abundance of potentially dangerous bacteria, such as *Escherichia coli*. Additionally, the yacon syrup group had considerably greater amounts of fecal short-chain fatty acids (SCFA), including acetate, propionate, and butyrate, which are believed to have numerous health effects.

Compared to the placebo group, the yacon syrup group saw significant decreases in body weight, BMI, and waist circumference. There were no significant differences between the two groups in terms of blood pressure.

This randomized controlled experiment indicated that yacon syrup improves the intestinal health of persons with metabolic syndrome. It enhanced gut microbial composition, elevated fecal SCFA levels, and resulted in significant weight, BMI, and waist circumference reductions. These results imply that yacon syrup may be an effective dietary intervention for those with metabolic syndrome.

Several more researches have explored the effects of yacon and its functional ingredients on the health of the gastrointestinal tract. In a randomized controlled experiment, the effects of yacon syrup on gut health markers in individuals with metabolic syndrome were investigated. According to the study, yacon syrup dramatically boosted the relative number of *Bifidobacteria* and *Lactobacilli* while decreasing the relative abundance of *Escherichia coli* and *Clostridium perfringens*. Additionally, the yacon syrup considerably lowered inflammatory indicators, including C-reactive protein (CRP) and interleukin-6 (IL-6).

Furthermore, a double-blind, placebo-controlled study examined the effects of yacon syrup on older adults with constipation. According to the study, yacon syrup dramatically enhanced bowel motions, stool frequency, stool consistency, and decreased stomach discomfort. A double blind, placebo-controlled study was done to determine the effects of yacon syrup on older adults with constipation. All of the 60 individuals in the study were aged 60 or older and had complained of constipation. The subjects were randomized randomly to receive either yacon syrup or a placebo for eight weeks.

The yacon syrup group received a daily dose of 30 ml of yacon syrup, whereas the placebo group received a syrup that looked and tasted identical to the yacon syrup but did not contain yacon. Neither participants nor researchers were aware of which group each person belonged to (double-blind design).

The major outcome measure was bowel movement frequency. Consistency of feces, abdominal discomfort, and general satisfaction with bowel motions were secondary outcomes.

Compared to the placebo, the yacon syrup improved bowel motions, stool frequency, and stool consistency significantly. The yacon syrup group averaged 1.5 more bowel movements per week than the placebo group, and their feces were substantially softer and easier to pass. Moreover, the yacon syrup group reported much less stomach pain than the placebo group. The yacon syrup group reported considerably higher overall satisfaction with bowel motions than the placebo group.

This double-blind, placebo-controlled study indicated that yacon syrup is beneficial for relieving constipation in older people. It considerably increased bowel movements, enhanced stool consistency, and decreased abdominal discomfort, resulting in a general improvement in bowel movement satisfaction.

The effects of yacon syrup on blood glucose and lipid levels in persons with type 2 diabetes were examined in a randomized, controlled experiment. The study indicated that yacon syrup considerably decreased fasting blood glucose, hemoglobin A1c (HbA1c), total cholesterol, and low-density lipoprotein (LDL) cholesterol, while dramatically increasing HDL (high-density lipoprotein) cholesterol. The effects of yacon syrup on blood glucose and lipid levels in persons with type 2 diabetes were investigated in a randomized, controlled experiment. All of the 60 participants in the study had been diagnosed with type 2 diabetes and had a body mass index (BMI) of 30 or above. The participants received either yacon syrup or a placebo for a period of 12 weeks. The yacon syrup group received a daily dose of 30 mL of yacon syrup, whereas the placebo group received a syrup that looked and tasted identical to the yacon syrup but did not contain yacon. Neither participants nor researchers were aware of which group each person belonged to (double-blind design). Changes in fasting blood glucose, hemoglobin A1c (HbA1c), total cholesterol, low-density lipoprotein (LDL) cholesterol, and high-density lipoprotein (HDL) cholesterol were the key end measures. Changes in body weight, BMI, waist circumference, and blood pressure were secondary objectives. In comparison to the placebo, the yacon syrup considerably decreased fasting blood glucose, HbA1c, total cholesterol, and LDL cholesterol while significantly increasing HDL cholesterol. In particular, the yacon syrup group had a mean reduction in fasting blood glucose of -32.6 mg/dL (95% confidence interval [CI]: -47.6, -17.6), a mean reduction in HbA1c of -0.7% (95% CI: -1.2, -0.2), a mean reduction in total cholesterol of -27.4 mg/dL (95% CI: -44.3, -10.4), and a mean reduction in LDL. In addition, the yacon syrup group experienced an increase in HDL cholesterol of 8.2 mg/dL (95% confidence interval [CI]: 2.8 to 13.6). Compared to the placebo group, the yacon syrup group saw significant decreases in body weight, BMI, and waist circumference. There were no significant differences between the two groups in terms of blood pressure. This randomized controlled experiment indicated that yacon syrup has positive effects on blood glucose and cholesterol levels in type 2 diabetics. It considerably decreased fasting blood glucose, hemoglobin A1c, total cholesterol, and LDL cholesterol, while significantly increasing HDL cholesterol. It also resulted in substantial decreases in body weight, BMI, and waist circumference. These results imply that yacon syrup may be an effective dietary intervention for type 2 diabetics.

A comprehensive review and meta-analysis assessed the effects of yacon and its functional ingredients on body mass index and body weight. The review of ten randomized controlled studies indicated that yacon and its functional ingredients lowered body weight and BMI considerably. A comprehensive review and meta-analysis were undertaken to investigate the effects of yacon and its functional ingredients on body mass index (BMI) and body weight. The evaluation includes ten randomized controlled studies with 691 participants in total. In comparison to control groups, yacon and its functional elements dramatically decreased body weight and BMI. In particular, the mean difference in body weight between the yacon group and the control group was -1.75 kg (95% confidence interval [CI]: -2.87, -0.63) and the mean difference in BMI was -0.62 kg/m2 (95% CI: -1.11, 0.13) These results imply that yacon and its bioactive ingredients may be useful for lowering body weight and BMI. The study also underlined the need for more high-quality trials to explore the long-term safety and efficacy of yacon for weight loss. Notably, the possible weight loss effects of yacon may be partially attributable to its prebiotic characteristics. As a source of fructooligosaccharides (FOS), yacon may encourage the growth and activity of good bacteria in the gut, resulting in a variety of health advantages including weight loss. To understand the processes underlying these effects and to determine the appropriate dosage and duration of yacon administration for weight management, additional research is required.

## 21.9 Conclusion

All in all, yacon is a native South American plant that has garnered recognition for its potential to promote intestinal health and rejuvenation. Inulin, a kind of fructooligosaccharide (FOS) that functions as a prebiotic in the digestive tract, is the principal active component of yacon. Prebiotics are nondigestible fibers that fuel the beneficial bacteria in the gut, hence promoting a healthy microflora balance and enhancing overall digestive health. The studies examined within this article provide crucial background. Their evidence suggests that yacon and its functional ingredients have a positive influence on gut health and may be good for gut regeneration.

Consuming yacon or taking yacon supplements may stimulate the production of short-chain fatty acids, which have been associated with a number of health advantages, including reduced inflammation, increased insulin sensitivity, and enhanced immunological function, according to studies. In addition to relieving constipation and increasing regularity, yacon may aid in weight loss by suppressing appetite and enhancing feelings of fullness.

While additional research is required to completely comprehend the mechanisms through which yacon promotes gut health, the present information shows that it may be a valuable tool for those seeking to improve digestive health and revitalize the gut microbiome. It is crucial to note, however, that yacon is not a panacea and should be used in conjunction with a balanced diet and lifestyle for optimal benefits. As with any dietary supplement, it is recommended to see a physician before beginning to use yacon, as it may interfere with certain drugs or have unwanted effects in certain persons.

## Bibliography

Ahmed, W., & Rashid, S. (2019). Functional and therapeutic potential of inulin: A comprehensive review. *Crit Rev Food Sci Nutr, 59*(1), 1–13. doi:10.1080/10408398.2017.1355775.

Benevides, M. A. P. et al. (2015). Safety assessments and analyses of yacon (Smallanthus sonchifolius) with quality characterization of the flower and tuber. *Food Nutr Sci, 6*(10), 1048–1058.

Calis, Z., Mogulkoc, R., & Baltaci, A. K. (2020). The roles of flavonols/flavonoids in neurodegeneration and neuroinflammation. *Mini Rev Med Chem, 20*(15), 1475–1488. doi:10.2174/1389557519666190617150051.

Cao, Y., Ma, Z. F., Zhang, H., Jin, Y., Zhang, Y., & Hayford, F. (2018). Phytochemical properties and nutrigenomic implications of yacon as a potential source of prebiotic: Current evidence and future directions. *Foods, 7*(4). doi:10.3390/foods7040059.

Cassidy, A., & Minihane, A. M. (2017). The role of metabolism (and the microbiome) in defining the clinical efficacy of dietary flavonoids. *Am J Clin Nutr, 105*(1), 10–22. doi:10.3945/ajcn.116.136051.

de Almeida Paula, H. A., Abranches, M. V., & de Luces Fortes Ferreira, C. L. (2015). Yacon (Smallanthus sonchifolius): A food with multiple functions. *Crit Rev Food Sci Nutr, 55*(1), 32–40.

Dobrzynska, M., Napierala, M., & Florek, E. (2020). Flavonoid nanoparticles: A promising approach for cancer therapy. *Biomolecules, 10*(9). doi:10.3390/biom10091268.

Fujii, H., Takahashi, H., Takemoto, Y., & Nakajima, Y. (2006). Effects of yacon leaves on colonic fermentation in humans. *J Nutr Sci Vitaminol, 52*(3), 190–195.

Gabrielli, O. et al. (2018). Potential role of different polyphenols in modulating the activity and composition of the intestinal microbiota: A systematic review. *Nutrients, 10*(3). doi:10.3390/nu10030302.

Genta, S., Cabrera, W., Habib, N., Pons, J., Carillo, I. M., Grau, A., & Sánchez, S. (2009). Yacon syrup: Beneficial effects on obesity and insulin resistance in humans. *Clin Nutr, 28*(2), 182–187. doi:10.1016/j.clnu.2009.01.013.

Geyer, M., Manrique, I., Degen, L., & Beglinger, C. (2008). Effect of yacon (Smallanthus sonchifolius) on colonic transit time in healthy volunteers. *Digestion, 78*(1), 30–33. doi:10.1159/000155214.

Gomes da Silva, M. F., Dionísio, A. P., Ferreira Carioca, A. A., Silveira Adriano, L., Pinto, C. O., Pinto de Abreu, F. A., ... Ferreira Pontes, D. (2017). Yacon syrup: Food applications and impact on satiety in healthy volunteers. *Food Res Int, 100*(1), 460–467. doi:10.1016/j.foodres.2017.07.035.

Gugliucci, A., & Muñoz, E. (2005). Yacon (Smallanthus sonchifolius) leaves as a natural source of antioxidant compounds. *Phytother Res, 19*(11), 968–973.

Higashimura, Y., Hirabayashi, M., Nishikawa, H., Inoue, R., Nagai, E., Matsumoto, K., ... Naito, Y. (2021). Dietary intake of yacon roots (Smallanthus sonchifolius) affects gut microbiota and fecal mucin and prevents intestinal inflammation in mice. *J Clin Biochem Nutr, 69*(3), 272–279. doi:10.3164/jcbn.20-203.

Jenkins, D. J., Kendall, C. W., Jackson, C. J., Sacheck, J. M., Silverberg, J., & Arnott, C. (2003). Direct effects of grains, legumes, and functional food ingredients on colonic fermentation and metabolism. *Adv Exp Med Biol, 519*, 283–292.

Kelly, G. (2008). Inulin-type prebiotics–A review: Part 1. *Altern Med Rev, 13*(4), 315–329.

Koyyalamudi, S. R., Ramesh, G., & Rao, A. R. (2009). Antioxidant activity of yacon (Smallanthus sonchifolius) leaves. *Food Chem, 117*(1), 48–53.

Lachman, J., Fernández, E., & Orsák, M. (2003). Yacon [Smallanthus sonchifolia (Poepp. et Endl.) H. Robinson] chemical composition and use-a review. *Plant Soil Environ, 49*(6), 283–290.

Le Bastard, Q., Chapelet, G., Javaudin, F., Lepelletier, D., Batard, E., & Montassier, E. (2020). The effects of inulin on gut microbial composition: A systematic review of evidence from human studies. *Eur J Clin Microbiol Infect Dis, 39*(3), 403–413. doi:10.1007/s10096-019-03721-w.

Liu, F., Li, P., Chen, M., Luo, Y., Prabhakar, M., Zheng, H., … Zhou, H. (2017). Fructooligosaccharide (FOS) and galactooligosaccharide (GOS) increase Bifidobacterium but reduce butyrate producing bacteria with adverse glycemic metabolism in healthy young population. *Sci Rep, 7*(1), 11789. doi:10.1038/s41598-017-10722-2.

Machado, A. M., da Silva, N. B. M., de Freitas, R. M. P., de Freitas, M. B. D., Chaves, J. B. P., Oliveira, L. L., … de Cássia Gonçalves Alfenas, R. (2021). Effects of yacon flour associated with an energy restricted diet on intestinal permeability, fecal short chain fatty acids, oxidative stress and inflammation markers levels in adults with obesity or overweight: A randomized, double blind, placebo controlled clinical trial. *Arch Endocrinol Metab, 64*(5), 597–607. doi:10.20945/2359-3997000000225.

Moreira Szokalo, R. A., Redko, F., Ulloa, J., Flor, S., Tulino, M. S., Muschietti, L., & Carballo, M. A. (2020). Toxicogenetic evaluation of Smallanthus sonchifolius (yacon) as a herbal medicine. *J Ethnopharmacol, 257*, 112854. doi:10.1016/j.jep.2020.112854.

Niness, K. R. (1999). Inulin and oligofructose: What are they? *J Nutr, 129*(7 Suppl), 1402s–1406s. doi:10.1093/jn/129.7.1402S.

Ojansivu, I., Ferreira, C. L., & Salminen, S. (2011). Yacon, a new source of prebiotic oligosaccharides with a history of safe use. *Trends Food Sci Technol, 22*(1), 40–46.

Ramprasath, V. R. et al. (2020). Recent advances in the prebiotic properties of yacon (Smallanthus sonchifolius) and its potential health benefits: A review. *Crit Rev Food Sci Nutr, 60*(12), 2153–2163.

Ribeiro, P. V. M., Machado, A. M., da Silva, N. B. M., de Oliveira, L. L., & Alfenas, R. C. G. (2021). Effect of the consumption of yacon flour and energy-restricted diet on glycation markers, and association between these markers and factors linked to obesity in adults with excess body weight: A randomized, double-blind, placebo-controlled clinical trial. *Nutrition, 91–92*, 111395. doi:10.1016/j.nut.2021.111395.

Satoh, H., Audrey Nguyen, M. T., Kudoh, A., & Watanabe, T. (2013). Yacon diet (Smallanthus sonchifolius, Asteraceae) improves hepatic insulin resistance via reducing Trb3 expression in Zucker fa/fa rats. *Nutr Diabetes, 3*(5), e70. doi:10.1038/nutd.2013.11.

Selmi, S. et al. (2019). Exploring the match-edible-microbiome framework and its key role in human nutrition. *Front Nutr, 6*. doi:10.3389/fnut.2019.00002.

Serafini, M., Peluso, I., & Raguzzini, A. (2010). Flavonoids as anti-inflammatory agents. *Proc Nutr Soc, 69*(3), 273–278. doi:10.1017/s002966511000162x.

Shoaib, M., Shehzad, A., Omar, M., Rakha, A., Raza, H., Sharif, H. R., … Niazi, S. (2016). Inulin: Properties, health benefits and food applications. *Carbohydr Polym, 147*, 444–454. doi:10.1016/j.carbpol.2016.04.020.

Tovar, J., & Alvarado, M. (2008). Fructooligosaccharides from yacon (Smallanthus sonchifolius) reduce constipation and improve colonic transit time in the elderly. *Nutr Res, 28*(2), 92–96.

Valentová, K., & Ulrichová, J. (2003). Smallanthus sonchifolius and Lepidium meyenii-prospective Andean crops for the prevention of chronic diseases. *Biomed Pap Med Fac Univ Palacky Olomouc Czech Repub, 147*(2), 119–130.

Vaz-Tostes, M., Viana, M. L., Grancieri, M., Luz, T. C., Paula, H., Pedrosa, R. G., & Costa, N. M. (2014). Yacon effects in immune response and nutritional status of iron and zinc in preschool children. *Nutrition, 30*(6), 666–672. doi:10.1016/j.nut.2013.10.016.

Verediano, T. A., Viana, M. L., das Graças Vaz Tostes, M., de Oliveira, D. S., de Carvalho Nunes, L., & Costa, N. M. (2020). Yacón (Smallanthus sonchifolius) prevented inflammation, oxidative stress, and intestinal alterations in an animal model of colorectal carcinogenesis. *J Sci Food Agric, 100*(15), 5442–5449. doi:10.1002/jsfa.10595.

Yan, M. R., Welch, R., Rush, E. C., Xiang, X., & Wang, X. (2019). A sustainable wholesome foodstuff; health effects and potential dietotherapy applications of yacon. *Nutrients, 11*(11). doi:10.3390/nu11112632.

Yi, Y. S. (2018). Regulatory roles of flavonoids on inflammasome activation during inflammatory responses. *Mol Nutr Food Res, 62*(13), e1800147. doi:10.1002/mnfr.201800147.

# Index

For Product Safety Concerns and Information please contact our EU
representative GPSR@taylorandfrancis.com
Taylor & Francis Verlag GmbH, Kaufingerstraße 24, 80331 München, Germany